Biomechanics
of Human
Movement

SECOND EDITION

Biomechanics of Human Movement

Marlene J. Adrian, D.P.E

Professor Emerita of Kinesiology, Rehabilitation, Bioengineering
Director of Biomechanics Research Laboratory
University of Illinois at Urbana-Champaign

John M. Cooper, Ed.D.

Professor Emeritus of Physical Education
Indiana University

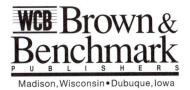

WCB Brown & Benchmark
PUBLISHERS

Madison, Wisconsin • Dubuque, Iowa

Book Team

Editor *Scott Spoolman*
Production Editor *Jayne Klein*
Art Editor *Tina Flanagan*
Photo Editor *Rose Deluhery*
Visuals/Design Freelance Specialist *Mary L. Christianson*
Marketing Manager *Pamela S. Cooper*
Production Manager *Beth Kundert*

WCB Brown & Benchmark

A Division of Wm. C. Brown Communications, Inc.

Executive Vice President/General Manager *Thomas E. Doran*
Vice President/Editor in Chief *Edgar J. Laube*
Vice President/Marketing and Sales Systems *Eric Ziegler*
Director of Production *Vickie Putman Caughron*
Director of Custom and Electronic Publishing *Chris Rogers*
National Sales Manager *Bob McLaughlin*

Wm. C. Brown Communications, Inc.

President and Chief Executive Officer *G. Franklin Lewis*
Senior Vice President, Operations *James H. Higby*
Corporate Senior Vice President and Chief Financial Officer *Robert Chesterman*
Corporate Senior Vice President and President of Manufacturing *Roger Meyer*

Cover and interior designs by Lesiak/Crampton Design Inc.

Cover image by © William R. Sallaz/Duomo Photography Inc.

Copyedited by Jeffrey Putnam

Library of Congress Catalog Card Number: 93–74411

ISBN 0–697–16242–7

Printed in the United States of America by Wm. C. Brown Communications, Inc.,
2460 Kerper Boulevard, Dubuque, IA 52001

10 9 8 7 6 5 4 3 2 1

To Charlianna Cooper, from both of us

CONTENTS IN BRIEF

CONTENTS

Contents   **xi**

FOREWORD

Little did Aristotle, the acknowledged father of kinesiology, realize where his practical observations on animal locomotion and human performance would lead. The study of biomechanics, as we know it today, is based on his work and those whose curiosity led them to follow in his footsteps. Those footsteps have led to what the present biomechanists consider to be the major purpose of biomechanics. That purpose is to scientifically analyze the techniques involved in the performance of human movement skills. It allows one to look at movement in terms of space, time, and direction (kinematics), or in terms of the forces responsible for causing motion (kinetics). Further, it allows one to examine the environment in which the movement is performed. No matter whether the movement is a daily movement task or whether the movement is a sport-related skill, the joy and satisfaction of performance occurs when it is done correctly, effortlessly, and safely.

When the first edition of this text was written, the 1988 Olympic Games had just been completed. Nowhere was the importance of biomechanics more evident. For the athletes and coaches, the very motto of the Olympics, *Citius, Altius, Fortius*—Swifter, Higher, Stronger—, implied a reliance on the knowledge inherent in the field of biomechanics. Their goal was to compete in an event in the most effective and efficient

manner possible. While this book was in revision, another Olympic Games passed. Performances were even better than the previous Olympic Games, with World and Olympic records being broken. The goal of all athletes in the Olympics was to be the best that they could be. Achieving these goals could not have been possible without the advances in the field of the sport sciences, among them biomechanics.

In a sense, Adrian and Cooper have used the motto of the Olympics as their guiding theme in writing this revised text. The first edition of the text provided a comprehensive exploration of every aspect of human movement and biomechanics. They provided the background material for understanding movement effectiveness and efficiency. However, just as the athletes from one Olympics to another strived to improve the quality of their performances, the authors also strived to improve the quality of their text. They reorganized sections of the text for better clarity, strengthened some of the material on basic biomechanical concepts, and added new information to the application section.

This text represents one of the most comprehensive undertakings in the writing of texts for biomechanics. It covers almost every aspect involved in the living human body. For the teacher or student in biomechanics, the text provides a blend of theory and practice. Learning is enhanced with motivational tools, such as mini-laboratory learning experiences, and excellent illustrations, tables, and graphs.

Adrian and Cooper long have been recognized as pioneers and leaders in the field of biomechanics. Their experience and wealth of knowledge have added to the value of this text. There is no doubt that they will take their place in history along with the others who have so ably promoted the study of human movement. Their enthusiasm for the field is contagious and their dedication to the field second to none.

Carole J. Zebas, P.E.D.
Past Chair, Kinesiology Academy
Past President, CSC-ACSM

PREFACE

This edition has been revised to provide the ideas, concepts, and facts for today's students of biomechanics that will enable them to adapt to changing technology, changing social demographics, and the unknown requirements of the future. This book is based on the premise that facts of today may not be facts of tomorrow. But we hope that our presentation of ideas and diversity of perspectives will provide the foundation for adapting to and optimizing our tomorrows.

New Knowledge

As we have repeatedly seen in the past, the introduction of new techniques of analysis result in new knowledge. For example, the electron microscope "saw" new information about bone morphology and the telescope "saw" errors in our thinking about the planets Pluto and Saturn. As we explored the world of kinanthropometry, we came to realize why tall golfers use the predominance of arm actions when they hit a golf ball and shorter golfers emphasize the actions of the trunk. We also see shot putters, especially shorter athletes, using a discus-style turn when putting the shot. New perspectives and greater interrelationships of a multiplicity of factors must be woven into existing knowledge. This we have tried to do in this volume.

Diversity

The amount of material is certainly more than might be discussed in one semester of class meetings. But students and teachers should not be hampered because of the size of this book. Books such as this one are resources to stimulate discussion among students and between students and teachers. The large amount of material is vital to enable students to learn the broad scope of biomechanics and all its applications. Our educational objective is to teach to the diversity of our students. Each student has unique prior experiences. Each has unique objectives and will select a vocational career that will require different aspects of biomechanics. Each student is also endowed with uniquely different cultural and familial backgrounds. With this book, we have tried to provide for the diversity and individuality of our readers. We hope it includes areas of study that will be exciting and motivating to every reader.

Suggestions on Using the Book

This book is designed to be nontraditional, although it can be used in a traditional manner. Since no two classes of students are alike, the order of presentation of material may differ from class to class. We envisage that graduate or second-course level students might wish to start with Chapters 7 and 8 to study movement analysis. Some teachers may wish to begin with Chapter 24 as a motivating beginning; others will use it as the final session of a class to stimulate thinking for postcollege applications. An idea mentioned in one chapter may be further explored in one or more sections of the book. As the need arises, the student can explore the same concept from several perspectives, or choose to acquire only the basics. The teacher, therefore, can assign a portion of a chapter together with an application from another chapter, and recommend optional sections to read on the same general topic. It is not necessary to read the same number of pages or the same number of chapters for each successive class session. Some material is more difficult or less familiar than other material. Moreover, what is familiar to one student may not be familiar to another student.

Instructor's Manual

We would also mention that the instructor's manual is designed to provide hints for teachers in selecting appropriate key concepts, discussion topics, objectives, evaluation materials, and mini-laboratory experiences. The latter include mathematical problem-solving tasks. Some of the material is photocopy-ready for transparency displays on overhead projectors. The instructor's manual is a resource for the teachers to further enhance learning and provide additional experiences of biomechanical topics, emphasizing the problem-solving analysis approach.

Varied Presentations

The general format of the book is consistent throughout, but we believe that some variation in the presentation of material is refreshing to the student. Therefore, we have not followed a standardized style of writing. The freedom of presentation of ideas from new perspectives seems to be somewhat inconsistent, but we view it as providing the reader with one unique "feel" of each topic. This decision is congruous with the belief that change is inherently valuable for education and that the students of today are a diverse group.

Changes in This Edition

Adrian and Cooper acknowledge the pioneers' work, specifically that of Lawrence Morehouse and Ruth Glassow who wrote with us on previous editions of *Biomechanics of Human Movement*. Morehouse should be cited for his insight into the value of biomechanics as it related to sports. Glassow's pioneer work involved the synthesis of theory and application to the study of human movement. We are grateful for their outstanding foresights. We also are grateful for the contributions of those who contributed to the previous edition. We also acknowledge the many experts in biomechanics, teaching, coaching, therapy, anatomy, and related fields who have contributed to this edition.

Contributors are a Unique Source of Strength

One of the unique features of our book is the valuable insights and knowledge presented by our contributors. They have enabled us to continue to provide our readers with application concepts, knowledge, and issues in a wide spectrum of movement environments. We include a multitude of sports, activities of daily living, music and other arts, occupational tasks, rehabilitation, exercise, and developmental movement patterns. Thus, with this new edition, we have again presented a comprehensive textbook of biomechanics of human movement. This book continues to have the most complete description of analysis techniques, instrumentation systems, and methods of displaying and interpreting data in the field.

New Topics

New sports topics include soccer, team handball, and wrestling. Sections of many of the chapters have been expanded, and new research findings have replaced outdated material. We have particularly expanded the information on dance movements, dysfunctional patterns of disabled people, aging patterns, cycling, and exercise. Some sections have been rearranged and/or merged with others. All sections have been revised extensively.

Organization

The format has been redefined to include the highlighting of key concepts in each section and topics for discussion and movement pattern analysis. The material in the book's sections is consistent with Kinesiology Academy Guidelines, but goes far beyond these requirements.

The book consists of six parts:

Part I.   Basic Biomechanical Concepts

Part II.   Tools for Human Movement Analysis

Part III.   Movements Across the Entire Spectrum of Life

Part IV.   Sports Movements on Land

Part V.   Sports Movements in Air, Ice, Snow, and Water Environments

Part VI.   The Future

Main Authors

Marlene J. Adrian, DPE, FSM
Professor Emerita of Kinesiology, Rehabilitation, Bioengineering
University of Illinois at Urbana–Champaign
Urbana, Illinois

John M. Cooper, Ed.D., FSM
Professor Emeritus
Former Director, Biomechanics Laboratory
Indiana University
Bloomington, Indiana

Contributors

Hobie Billingsley, M.S.
Former US Olympic Diving Coach
Indiana University
Bloomington, Indiana
Consultant for Chapter 23

Connie Bothwell-Meyers, Ph.D.
University of New Brunswick
Fredericton, New Brunswick, Canada
Curling in Chapter 17

Douglas Briggs, Ph.D.
Eastern Michigan University
Ypsilanti, Michigan
Cycling in Chapter 22

Carol Brink, Ph.D.
St. Cloud State University
St. Cloud, Minnesota
Chapter 13 jointly with Lela June Stoner

Eugene W. Brown, Ph.D.
Michigan State University
East Lansing, Michigan
Soccer in Chapters 18 and 19

Dayna Daniels, Ph.D.
University of Lethbridge
Lethbridge, Canada
Chapter 23

Terence M. Freeman, Col.
US Army, West Point, New York
Team Handball in Chapter 19

Paula Richley Giegle, M.S., PT
Outpatient Therapy, Services Manager
Carle Foundation Hospital
Urbana, Illinois
Consultant for Chapters 10 and 11

Joy Hendrick, Ph.D.
State University College at Cortland
Cortland, New York
Chapter 5

Phillip Henson, Ph.D.
Assistant Track Coach, Indiana University and Olympic Facilities Manager for the 1996 Olympics
Bloomington, Indiana
Consultant for Chapters 15, 16, and 17

Lois Klatt, PED
Concordia University
River Forest, Illinois
Rating sheets in several chapters
Field Hockey in Chapter 19

Anne Klinger, Ph.D.
Clatsop Community College
Astoria, Oregon
Consultant for Chapter 20

Sharol Laczkowski, M.S.
Fitness Expert, Student Health Center
Indiana University
Bloomington, Indiana
Power Skating and In-line Skating in Chapter 22

Cheryl Maglischo, Ed.D.
California State University
Chico, California
Jointly with Ernie Maglischo, Chapter 21

Ernie Maglischo, Ph.D.
California State University
Arizona State
Tempe, Arizona
Jointly with Cheryl Maglischo, Chapter 21

Dawn L. Orman Patel, M.S.
Indianapolis University
Indianapolis, Indiana
Badminton in Chapter 18

Michael Purcell, M.S., Kodan
Member of Kodokan Scientific Study Group, Japan
Richland, Washington
Judo in Chapter 20

Lynda Randall, PED
California State University
Fullerton, California
Clinical Diagnosis in Chapter 9

James Richards, Ph.D.
University of Delaware
Newark, Delaware
Bobsled and Luge in Chapter 22

Mary Ridgway, Ph.D.
University of Texas, Arlington
Arlington, Texas
Volleyball in Chapter 19

Paul Smith, Ph.D.
West Chester University
West Chester, Pennsylvania
Karate in Chapter 20

Lela June Stoner, Ph.D.
University of Minnesota
Minneapolis, Minnesota
Chapter 13 jointly with Carol Brink

Tonya Toole, Ph.D.
Florida State University
Tallahassee, Florida
Aging in Chapter 9

Reviewers

David A. Barlow
University of Delaware

Cheryl Maglischo
California State University–Chico

Helen Miles
Fort Hays State University

Mary E. Ridgeway
University of Texas–Arlington

Carole J. Zebas
University of Kansas

Basic Biomechanical Concepts

1

Fundamental Biomechanical Concepts

Biomechanics is a synthesis of biology and mechanics that seeks to understand and explain human movement. This chapter is an introduction to the fundamental concepts of all types of human movements.

Welcome to the exciting and diversified world of biomechanics! When you explore this world, you will be embarking on an immense journey that has intrigued people since time's beginning. The human body contains more mysteries than the cosmos or the deep. Studying how it thinks, dreams, imagines, feels, and moves is more fascinating than the best novel or greatest movie.

Through biomechanical studies, physical educators, physical therapists, occupational therapists, engineers, mathematicians, zoologists, biologists, computer scientists, and others strive to measure, model, explain, equate, categorize, and catalog not only the movement patterns of all sorts of living creatures, but also the movements of the internal components of the body. Some specialists concentrate on such areas of study as snake biomechanics, amoeba biomechanics, equine biomechanics, and human biomechanics.

Human biomechanics is divided into areas such as sports, occupational, activities of daily living (ADL), rehabilitative, and exercise biomechanics. In addition, these subject areas often focus on special populations. The athlete is most frequently studied in sports biomechanics. The disabled and the elderly are frequently studied in ADL biomechanics. Moreover, some human biomechanists are interested in specific areas, such as bone biomechanics, muscle biomechanics, lung biomechanics, or blood biomechanics.

■ Biomechanics can be broad or narrow in application. We can look within the body or we can look outside the body. We can also look at the interaction between the internal and the external.

A study of specific parts of the body usually has clinical objectives. Two prominent areas of study with clinical applications are orthopedic and podiatric biomechanics. If you were interested in orthopedic biomechanics, you would investigate movement patterns and forces acting at the joints and on the bones of individuals before—and after—surgery or treatment. Podiatric biomechanics—how and why the feet and legs function or malfunction—is probably less than twenty years old. Interest in this area has been sparked by improved technology and the popularity of fitness running and high-impact aerobics, as well as the concomitant high numbers of injuries that have resulted from these activities.

What Is Human Biomechanics?

Biomechanics is the physics of human (or another living organism's) motion. It is an integrated study of forces produced by the human body and forces acting on the human body and the consequences of motion and tissue deformation. An expanded definition is: *Biomechanics is that branch of science concerned with understanding the interrelationships of structure and function of living beings with respect to the kinematics and kinetics of motion.* Anatomy, physics, and mathematics are used to determine and measure the quantities of motion (time, space, and force) and to fully understand movements of living things.

The biomechanical approach to the study of movement also involves the integration of concepts from biology and mechanics. It is important to remember that human movement occurs in an environment that is constantly changing, even as the person changes biologically. Nothing is static. The body is always adjusting to an ever-present force in its environment—the force of gravity. The task you choose to perform, as well as how you perceive the task, influences the movement. For example, if you want to throw a ball, you can select from one of many goals. One goal might be to throw the ball as far as possible. Another goal might be to throw the ball as accurately as possible. The movement patterns will be different depending on which goal you choose. It is the interaction of the person, the task, and the environment that determines the movement. (See Figure 1.1.)

The Person

What Is This Thing Called Human?

The human organism is comprised not only of physical matter, but also of the chemical and electrical changes that take place in this matter to create responses that produce movement. How the person moves and reacts to the task and environment to produce a movement depends on such factors as perception, physical ability, and goals. Perception is the receiving and processing of stimuli through the visual, auditory, tactile, olfactory, and kinesthetic senses.

Perception

What the person senses

What the person chooses to process

What the congruence between sensing and reality is

What cultural constraints exist

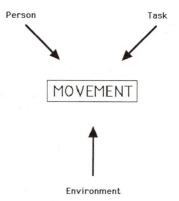

FIGURE 1.1 Movement Schema. The person, task, and environment interact to produce, modify, and otherwise influence the characteristics of the movement.

Although the study of goals is not actually a part of biomechanics, it is important to consider in order to correctly interpret the data from an analysis of the movement.

Goals

Why the person performs the task

What the movement represents to the person

What the cultural, gender, lifestyle, and age constraints are

Physical ability is also a major biomechanical concern.

Physical ability

What can be performed

What the anatomical characteristics are

What the anthropometric characteristics are

What the neurological abilities are

What the muscular abilities are

What Are the Physical Characteristics of Humans?

The adult human organism consists of

more than 200 major muscles that supply energy (out of a total of over 400 muscles).

more than 206 bones that provide the framework for movement, with over half found in the hands and feet.

43 major joints of the appendages (126 bones involved), about which body parts rotate.

approximately 14 billion nerve cells and over 100 trillion other cells.

over 60,000 miles of blood/lymph vessels.

Levers and the insertion points of muscles affect performance. The angle of the bony lever that is assumed in action likewise influences the action. Usually, the arms are placed at approximately 90° and the legs at 112° in order to sustain great weight or exert great force. It takes thirty to forty times more energy to carry messages along the nervous system than to move muscles. The fastest-moving muscles are fast-twitch (type II), or white, muscles. The slow-twitch (type I), or red, are slow-sustaining muscles. Usually, 60–70% of the muscles in the legs of sprinters are the fast-twitch type. The opposite is true for distance runners, whose leg muscles may be 70–80% slow-twitch muscles.

The human body has often been compared to a machine. The human motor is probably best described as an "electro-capillary" engine in which nervous excitation modifies the tension of the muscles and produces contractions (Amar 1910). Compared with the steam engine, the efficiency of the human machine is high. Steam engines require about double the relative fuel consumption of the human body. Walking is one of the most efficient forms of human locomotion, varying from 25 to 30% efficiency, based on caloric intake and work output. The human body is able to develop sustained power of less than one horsepower. (Contrast this output with the horsepower developed in an automobile engine.) The human organism can, however, develop 6–12 HP for a fraction of a second during activities such as shot putting.

The human body is not a machine, but a living and changing entity. Many different factors can affect human performance. Muscle coordination, health and general condition of the person, level and type of techniques, readiness for action, previous experience, temperature, fatigue, anxiety, motivation, cultural setting, social expectations, gender, and age of participant all help determine movement performance achievements. Another major factor is heredity.

Men and women perform skills in much the same manner. Anatomical and physiological differences are evident, but only to a degree. Since strength depends in part on the cross-sectional area of muscle, and because men possess greater muscle mass, the strength factor favors the male. This difference in strength, however, is evident only on an absolute basis. When strength is equated with lean body weight pound for pound, there is little difference in strength between males and females. The ability, however, to move quickly in a small space favors the female. Top women athletes now perform certain skills, especially in swimming and track and field events, as well as Olympic male athletes did only a few years ago.

MINI-LABORATORY LEARNING EXPERIENCE

1. Search sports magazines, record books, sports organization newsletters, and newspapers for performance records in your favorite sport.
2. Construct graphs of the best performances of men and women, juniors, and masters competitors.
3. Determine improvements over a period of years.

■ Human beings possess unique modifications of their common anatomical structure and, therefore, do not have the same potential to perform all movements to the same level of success.

What Are the Performance Feats of Humans?

You do not have to read Ripley's Believe It or Not books to know that humans are astonishing and mysterious creatures capable of almost unbelievable motor tasks. One of the most commonly cited examples is the lifting of an automobile by a 90-pound (400 N) woman when she saw her child pinned under the tire. We have also noted that, under hypnosis, weightlifters have lifted greater loads than at any other time in their weightlifting careers, prior or future. Consider some achievements of elite athletes.

Many people have swum the rough and stormy English Channel. It can take 20 or more hours of continuous swimming to perform this feat. One of the oldest persons to perform this task was James Counsilman (former U.S. Olympic swimming coach), at age 58.

Some quadruple amputees have been able to participate in many physical activities, including sports.

A few people have fallen from great heights without permanent injury.

One man walked around the world's land masses in four years.

Human beings have the ability to pace themselves over a long-distance run. Native Americans, often in relay fashion, were able to run down a deer.

A blind person can play golf. With the aid of an assistant for posture placement, one blind man shot an 85 on a typical 18-hole course.

Human beings have reached running speeds of 35–45 kmph (22–27 mph). This is remarkable when you realize a human being has only two legs with which to propel a cylindrical body moving upright and offering maximum wind resistance.

Other feats include marathon dancing, running, sailing, and cardiopulmonary resuscitation performed for hours, and even days.

The fastest and strongest movements tend to be seen in the sports arena. Baseballs can be thrown overarm at 167 kmph (103 mph), and softballs are pitched underarm at a slightly faster speed. The volleyball overarm serve attains speeds of 117 kmph (72 mph), which must be dissipated by the receiver. Tennis balls are projected at 257 kmph (160 mph), badminton smashes travel at 400 kmph (249 mph), and the slap shot in ice hockey has been timed at 197 kmph. Although locomotor speeds are not as fast, human beings ride skateboards at 100 kmph (62 mph) and take off at 110 kmph (68 mph) from a ski jump. Contrast these speeds with such ADL movements as walking at 5–8 kmph (3–5 mph) and mopping a floor at 6–9 kmph (3½–6 mph).

These are feats of today. Future performances will exceed these as people train harder, use more scientific knowledge to plan optimum training protocols, and improve nutrition and mental health. The biomechanist can help people reach the limits of their potential by recognizing their unique human characteristics and the requirements of the task to be performed in its specific environment.

MINI-LABORATORY LEARNING EXPERIENCE

1. Scan some recent sports magazines.
2. Note the limits of the performances in different sports. For example, look for ice skating and soccer kick speeds, pole vault heights, long jumping distances, surfboarding rotational speeds, etc.
3. Note whether specific ranges in height, weight, or other physical characteristics seem to be common to athletes in a particular sport, for example divers, sumo wrestlers, basketball players, gymnasts, and horse racing jockeys.

Why can some people produce higher speeds of movement than others? Is it only because of differences in technique and training? One important determinant of level of performance is related to anthropometry, the study of the measurement of the human body.

Anthropometry. Basic information concerning the structure of the human body can be used to estimate forces acting on the joints and other body tissues and the forces produced by or on them. **Anthropometry** is the measurement of the human body. Scientists can measure the body and its segments with respect to lengths, widths, diameters, circumferences (girths), and areas. They calculate ratios and proportions based on two or more of these measurements and identify shapes, sizes, and topography. One of the earliest studies in anthropometry related to human movement, gait in particular. In 1889 two German scientists, Braune and Fischer, published a comprehensive paper on an experimental method that they had developed to determine the center of gravity of the human body. Adolf Eugen Fick (1829–1901) drew on their work and eventually became one of the outstanding authorities in the field of joint mechanics.

Today's concepts on **posture** have had their origin in the experiments of Braune and Fischer. Earlier methods of locating the center of gravity of the human body had proved to be ineffective, and Braune and Fischer modified some earlier procedures. First, they conceived of a way of freezing a dead body so that it remained unchanged while they made mathematic calculations. They compared the frozen posture of a cadaver with the posture of a living person and found the two postures to be markedly similar. They located the center of gravity not only of the body as a whole but also of each segmental component. They were the first to estimate the percentage of total body weight of body segments. After they located the center of gravity of the total body of the frozen cadavers, they cut two of them into body segments and located the center of gravity of each.

Segmental body weights and centers of mass of each segment are indispensable to modeling and simulating **static postures.** Other inertial characteristics of the human body and its parts, moments of inertia and radii of gyration, are required for modeling dynamic movement. Selected values and detailed descriptions of anthropometric techniques appear in Chapter 12, Appendix E, and in the resources at the end of this chapter, especially the anthropometric databases and review articles. Common anthropometric tools are shown in Figure 1.2.

Kinanthropometry. The field of **kinanthropometry** is a relatively new scientific discipline that focuses solely on the measurement of size, shape, proportion, composition, maturation, and gross function as related to such concerns as growth, exercise, performance, and nutrition.

Widths, lengths, girths, and other single anthropometric measurements do not correlate highly with any known skill. Ratios, indexes, and comparisons of one measurement with another have shown higher correlations with performance than do single measurements, but even these parameters do not provide more than a group predictability. A more complete approach is the use of a unisex phantom, or representation of a bilaterally symmetric average human body. Ross et al. (1978) applied the unisex phantom model to data collected by Eiben on 125 women athletes participating in the European Track and Field Championships, 1966. They found the following significant differences among long jumpers, shot putters, discus throwers, and the phantom.

1. Long jumpers had smaller arm breadth and girth measurements than did the phantom.
2. Long jumpers had greater tibial heights than shot putters.

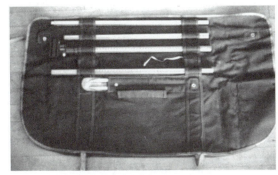

a

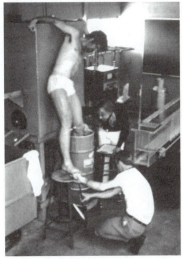

b

FIGURE 1.2 (a) Anthropometric kit for measuring body lengths, widths, and circumferences. Identification of anatomical landmarks is crucial if accurate measurements are to be obtained. (b) Water-immersion method for determining center of gravity and weight of body segment. In this procedure the scale is used to measure the weight of the tank, water, and immersed body segment. **How can the center of mass of the body segment be determined using this method?**

3. The shot putters and discus throwers had much greater chest depth and bitrochanteric width than did the phantom.
4. Long jumpers' thigh circumference and body weight were equal to the phantom's. The discus throwers' were greater than the phantom's, and the shot putters' measurements were greater than the discus throwers'.

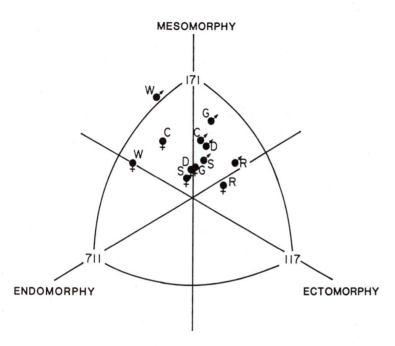

MESOMORPHY

171

W

G

C   C

D

W   D S R

S G

R

711   117

ENDOMORPHY   ECTOMORPHY

FIGURE 1.3 Mean somatotypes of sports groups participating in the Mexico City Olympic Games, ♂, male; ♀, female; W, weight throwers; C, canoeists; G, gymnasts; S, swimmers; D, divers; R, middle-distance runners.

(Based on data presented by de Garay, A. L., Levine, L., and Carter, J. E. L. 1974. *Genetic and anthropological studies of Olympic athletes.* New York: Academic Press.)

More than 100 measurements are taken on a person to construct an anthropometric profile. Anthropometricists then compare the profile with profiles at various times with respect to age, sports participation, nutrition, and other factors, as well as with profiles of other persons, including elite performers.

Somatotyping. One of the methods more commonly used to study proportionality characteristics is the body-typing method called **somatotyping** (Sheldon et al. 1954). Since people tend to observe the total body in general terms such as skinny, fat, or muscular, the somatotype has been very popular. The **ectomorph** is the linear or lean person, the **endomorph** is the person with excess adipose tissue, and the **mesomorph** is the person with a high proportion of muscle. Few exhibit only one of these attributes; most people have a combination of all three. On a 7-point scale, the average person would be rated 4, 4, 4 (endo-, meso-, ecto-). Athletes tend to be more mesomorphic, except for the ectomorphs found in events such as long-distance running. Athletes also are usually taller than the average population. In addition, numerous researchers, more recently those using the Carter anthropometric somatotyping method, have shown that athletes in certain sports cluster in unique places on

the somatotype chart (Figure 1.3). One consequence of these findings is the preselection and training of young children for national and international sports competition on the basis of the child's anatomic characteristics. Unfortunately, we do not know whether athletes develop their body characteristics because of the sport or choose the sport because of their body characteristics.

■ **The gymnast is short; the high hurdler is tall; the basketball player is tallest.**

From a biomechanical perspective, the athlete who projects his or her body into space must be proportionally different from the one who projects objects. Just as Morpurgo (1889) found that exercise changed the body, we cannot be sure how much the body is changed through participation in an activity and how much of its size and shape is inherited, and which proportion of each is vital to success in a motor skill. High correlations merely show relationships; that is, one item is likely to occur with another item related positively to it. One must be cautious, however, not to confuse relationships with cause and effect. It has been shown that both bone and muscle hypertrophy with use. Tennis players, bowlers, baseball pitchers, and other unilateral sports performers have heavier and larger limbs on one side of the body than on the other.

The Task

Any number of classification systems describe the specific task to be performed. One classification consists of work, activities of daily living (ADL), and leisure. The kinesiologist, biomechanics specialist, or human engineer interested in greater work productivity might well be concerned only with movement patterns related to the work situation. The physical therapist might be concerned with ADL and the restoration of independent living for the physically disabled. The physical educator and coach might be concerned only with leisure activities of sports and dance. This broad classification system is not always effective, however, since many movement patterns do not exist exclusively in one of each of these categories. For example, walking is an activity of daily living, but is also used in the work situation in folk and disco dancing, and in several sports, including golf.

Higgins (1977) has grouped movement patterns into three categories: locomotion (ambulation), manipulation, and a combination of the two. Although these categories are useful, many biomechanists have preferred to further subdivide movement patterns into more specific, yet rather broad categories, such as locomotion on land, locomotion in water, locomotion in the air, projecting oneself into the air, returning to earth, swinging and suspending one's body, projecting external objects, receiving external objects, and manipulating objects. Manipulation has been divided into gross motor skills such as using long-handled instruments, and into fine motor skills such as piano playing, using a fork and spoon, and typing.

Each action of the task must be identified and described with respect to space, time, and force and the relationship of the person to objects used or constraints on the human-movement system. Table 1.1 lists the factors to be considered in describing and analyzing the task.

The Environment

More definitive analysis of the task requires an investigation of environment. Within the earth's environment, bodies are attracted to the earth at an acceleration rate of approximately 9.8 m/sec^2. This rate varies with the distance of the body from the center of the earth, but any attempt to move the body upward requires muscular force in opposition to this attraction, known as gravity.

TABLE 1.1 Four major factors to consider when describing and analyzing a motor task.

Posture:	stand, sit, stoop, supine, prone, lean, twist, flex, hyperextend
Ambulate:	step, walk, run, jump, climb, sidestep
Manipulate:	push, pull, reach, grasp, press, rotate, lift, carry
Actions:	swing, forceful, circular, linear, percussive, quick, slow

The required force is directly proportional to body mass, which is the quantity of matter the body possesses. The product of mass and acceleration of gravity is equal to body weight. The effectiveness and efficiency of upward movement is therefore determined to a major degree by the relationship of body weight to the force that the muscles of the body can produce, as well as to the speed of this force production.

According to physicists, although gravity is one of the often unnoticed forces in nature, it is a real influence with respect to movement. For example, a shot putter will put the shot a few inches further at the equator than at the Tropic of Capricorn. Also, at a higher altitude such as Denver, the shot put will travel a longer distance than at sea level. Every movement of a body part upward or downward is influenced by gravitational force; it facilitates downward movement and inhibits or indirectly causes an upward movement.

Since every volitional movement of body parts is rotary, there will always exist a vertical component for every movement. Furthermore, since the force of gravity is a vertical vector (an arrow having a vector quantity, or magnitude of force, acting toward the center of the earth), it influences the efficiency of every posture or stance, as well as every movement. When muscle force is required to maintain a posture, the amount of force required is directly proportional to the efficiency of that posture. To determine whether muscles will need to contract, thereby exerting a counterforce to the gravitational force, one must resolve the gravitational force vectors acting on every particle of the body either into one force vector or into one force vector per body segment. The supporting surface for the feet (floor), the masses of the objects being manipulated and their balance points, and the relative placements of tools, sports equipment, furniture, and other objects to the person are potential positive or negative influences on the execution of the task. If the task is performed outdoors, the forces of air flow and climate will affect performance. In water, snow, ice, and free-fall environments, movement patterns must be adjusted to resultant forces of these environments.

MINI-LABORATORY LEARNING EXPERIENCE

1. Simulate on four different surfaces the skating action used in cross-country skiing, ice skating, or in-line skating. Select such environments as a carpet, a glossy, slippery tile, a rubber traction-treaded shoe, etc.
2. Note the ease and difficulty in executing an identical skating action during each of the environments.
3. Draw conclusions from this experiment.

Newton's laws of motion are the basis for understanding the environment. They are:

1. The law of **inertia:** A body will remain at rest or in uniform motion unless a force causes it to move or change motion.
2. The law of **acceleration:** Movement is proportional to the force causing it and inversely proportional to the mass that is moved.
3. The law of **interaction:** For each action there is an equal and opposite reaction.

The Movement

When a person performs a task in a given environment, the resultant movement pattern (performance) cannot be analyzed independently of either the task or the environment. The basis for the movement analysis is our spatial field within our time frame and relative to forces existing and produced during the movement. A schematic of movement components is given in Table 1.2.

The description of movement with respect to time and space is known as the kinematics of movement. There is no consideration of force characteristics. When

TABLE 1.2 A schematic of movement characteristic components.

TIME	SPACE	FORCE	ABSTRACTION
duration	self	internal-external	quality
sequencing	world	biological-physical	
		INTERRELATIONSHIPS	

force is analyzed, this analysis is called a kinetic analysis. Although biomechanical analyses of movements always consist of the analysis of time, space, and force, rarely is any thought given to the fourth factor listed in Table 1.2, abstraction. This factor exists, but is difficult to observe and probably cannot be measured. But it is listed because observers and feelers of movement, especially dancers who perform for the movement rather than for an external goal, can sense the difference between two performances that spatially and temporally look alike, but create a totally different essence of movement. Since the movements look alike, the forces also would be measured as being identical.

Dancers may refer to this abstraction as the quality of the movement, but it is something more. It is similar to what is being realized in the study of non-linear dynamical system and chaos theory. Movement is complex and greater than the sum of its parts. There may be some factor we cannot measure because we cannot find it. For our purposes with movement analysis, we will be content with studying the time, space, and force factors and their interrelationships.

Temporal Aspects of Movement

The duration of human movement and the separate actions or phases of a movement pattern are usually measured in milliseconds, seconds, and minutes. Sports movements are generally faster than movements in the workplace or daily activity movements. Some hand movements during the playing of musical instruments, in particular the classical guitar, are faster than sports movements. Thus, the initial analysis of a movement pattern is to determine the duration of each body segment movement and changes of direction of movements. When compared with the total time of the movement, the relationship of movements with respect

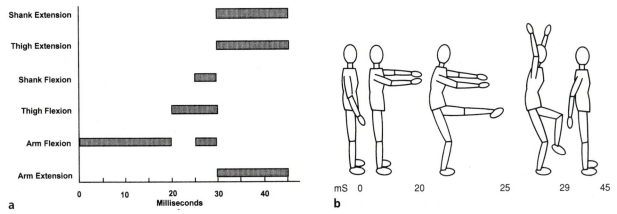

FIGURE 1.4 Kinematic sequencing contourograms with histogram display of temporal sequencing of movements of body parts.

to different body parts can be determined. This is known as the sequencing of actions. When different performances are normalized (one common standard scale), scientists can compare the temporal aspects of movements of different persons or of the same person. Movements have definite rhythms, or temporal sequencing patterns, that we can use to define or describe each type of movement. When time is related to space, we can determine the positions, displacements, velocities, and accelerations of body parts.

Spatial Aspects of Movement

Spatial analysis uses several different spatial frames of reference: the self (anatomical framework); the world (polar coordinate framework); orthogonal framework (Cartesian coordinate framework); personal space (Laban framework); or combinations of these.

The anatomical framework is based on the spatial orientation and relationship of one body segment to another. The anatomical terms of flexion, supination, etc. are used to describe movement. Refer to Figures 3.5 and 3.6 for a complete description of these movements. Figure 1.4 shows the use of the anatomical framework to create a kinematic sequencing graph. Study it and the exercise sequence shown in Figure 1.5. Create a kinematic sequencing graph for the exercise sequence.

Because we move in external space, the orthogonal Cartesian coordinate system has become the common method for describing and analyzing movement. Using this system we relate movement to three orthogonal (at 90°-angles to each other) planes and to a multitude of tilts or diagonals from these planes. You can visualize the basic orthogonal planes of motion as a cube, representing a piece of cheese being sliced (Figure 1.6). The top and bottom are horizontal planes. If the cheese is sliced parallel to the top surface, the cutter moves in a transverse (horizontal) plane. The front and back of the cube are vertical slices in the frontal plane. The two sides are parallel to each other and vertical. The slices are made by movements in the sagittal plane. The planes as slices through the center of gravity of a human being are depicted in Figure 1.7.

Although locomotion tends to be in a vertical plane known as the sagittal, or anteroposterior (AP), plane, the anatomy of the body is such that some horizontal motion occurs as the body alternates between right-leg support and left-leg support. Only during imposed conditions and during limited single-limb movements used in exercising is pure planar motion likely to occur. Human movement usually occurs in two or more planes and is referred to as nonplanar or three-dimensional.

If movement is primarily in one plane and movement in a second plane is negligible, the movement may be

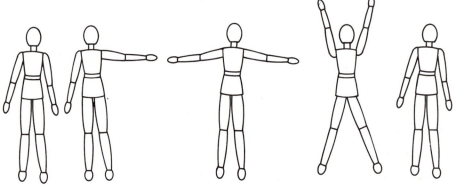

FIGURE 1.5 Kinematic sequencing contourograms. **Create the histogram of temporal initiation and duration of movements.**

Assume a .5 second interval between contourograms.

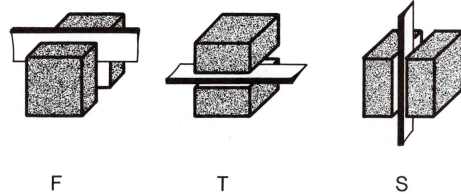

F   T   S

FIGURE 1.6 Three-dimensional space can be visualized as a cube, rectangle, or a room in a house. The surfaces of the structure represent the planes of the body: *F,* the front and back surfaces of the cube lie in the vertical (frontal) plane; *T,* the top and bottom surfaces lie in the horizontal (transverse) plane; *S,* the side surfaces lie in the vertical (sagittal) plane. The movement involved in slicing the cube occurs in the plane of the surface being sliced: *S,* the movement of the knife occurs in the sagittal plane since the slices are separated front-to-back. **Describe the movements of the knife to cut in the frontal, transverse, and oblique planes.**

analyzed as a planar movement for ease of analysis. For example, many movements of human beings and quadrupeds are sagittal-plane movements primarily, since, anatomically, the flexor and extensor muscle groups are the principal locomotor muscles. Birds use their wings in the frontal plane, a vertical plane with movements right and left of body center. Fish move their tails in a horizontal plane. Thus, these three planes (sagittal, frontal, and horizontal) are considered the basic planes of motion in our three-dimensional world. Logan and McKinney (1977) have defined several diagonal planes of motion because many human arm motions occur in diagonal planes. Two of these diagonal planes are right high to left low and right low to left high. Additional planes of motion have been identified in human-factors engineering and aerospace research. The complexity of describing spatial motion increases as the need for more precise location of the path of movement increases. By understanding the planes of movement, the movement analyst can determine the probable muscles involved in producing the movement (Figure 1.8).

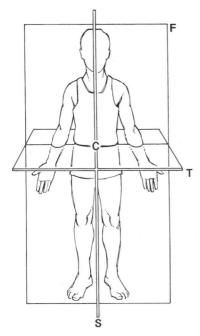

FIGURE 1.7 The center of gravity (center of mass) of the human body is at the intersect (C) of the three cardinal planes: transverse (T), sagittal (S), and frontal (F) (coronal). In this case the body is divided into top and bottom halves (cephalic-caudal halves), right and left halves, and front and back halves (anterior-posterior halves). The human body is depicted in a position known as "the anatomical position."

Translatory and Rotary Movements

The three types of motion that occur within a plane or through several planes may be described as follows.

Translatory motion is motion of a body from one plane to another, with each part of the body moving an equal distance. The movement may be linear, that is, occur in a straight line, as in the movement of a child being carried. Another example of translatory movement is gliding on ice skates. Because we live in a gravitational field, many of the observed translations of objects are curvilinear, or parabolic, such as the flight of a ball.

Contrast translation with the second type of motion, rotary motion. This type of motion differs from translation in that the body or body segment rotates about an axis, causing each part of the body to move a distance proportional to its position from the axis. For example, a

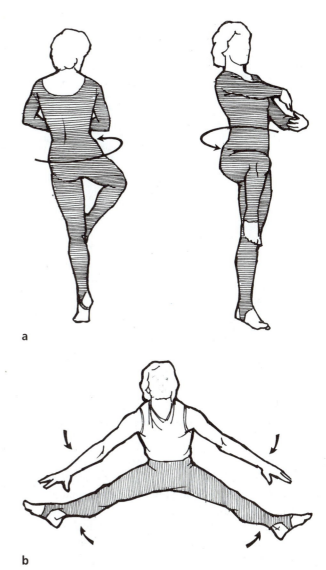

FIGURE 1.8 Movement in the transverse plane about the longitudinal (vertical) axis of the body is depicted in *a*. Oblique or diagonal movements are depicted in the actions of the arms and legs in *b*. The trunk flexes in the sagittal plane. Movements in the sagittal plane also are depicted in Figures 1.4*b* and 1.11. Movements in the frontal plane are depicted in Figure 1.5.

Fundamental Biomechanical Concepts　　**13**

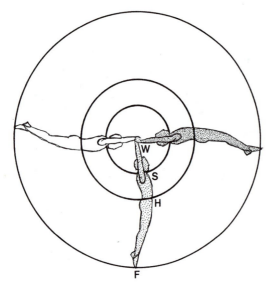

FIGURE 1.9 This giant swing on the gymnastics high bar is an example of rotary motion. The bar is a fixed axis of rotation. The wrist (W) travels a circumferential distance of 2r, where 4 represents the radius of rotation. Note the circumferential distances increase as the body part (S, shoulder; H, hip; and F, foot) is farther from the axis of rotation. The shoulder travels approximately one-fourth the distance the foot travels. The actual distances can be calculated by measuring the figure and multiplying the values by 60 (the figure is 60 times smaller than the actual human being). **What is the approximate distance the hip will travel?**

person performing a giant swing on the high bar (Figure 1.9) will experience only a slight movement of the wrists, while the hips will move a distance equal to 2π, with r equal to the length of the body from hands to hips. Logically the feet travel the greatest distance of all the body parts, a total of 2π, with r now being the length of the body from hands to feet ($\pi = 3.1416$).

Many limb-segment exercises use pure rotation. However, human and animal movements tend to be complex, and a third type of motion, a combination of translation and rotation (general motion) is the more common type of motion produced voluntarily. The human anatomy consists of a number of body parts attached by means of joints, which act as axes of rotation. Locomotion occurs, and the body translates as a result of rotations of two or more body segments. Therefore, one or more of the axes of rotation translate, and only one axis is stationary, or fixed. The complexity of locomotion is illustrated again because the same axis does not remain fixed during

locomotion. At one point, the fixed axis is the intersection of the heel of one foot with the ground. Next, the fixed axis occurs at the intersection of the metatarsal-phalangeal joint and the ground. Later, the fixed axis transfers to the opposite limb. Thus, the human body has been called a kinematic link system. Movement of one segment of the body creates movement and a repositioning of another body segment (Figure 1.10).

Axes and Planes

Several terms are important when discussing the **axes of rotation** and the plane of motion when rotary movement takes place. There are no axes of motion during pure translatory movement. Each anatomic axis and each axis

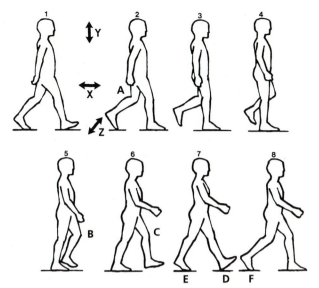

FIGURE 1.10 Using nomenclature of the Cartesian Coordinate Reference System, the common rotary movements are depicted with each major axis of rotation: vertical axis (Y), lateral-horizontal axis (X) and frontal-horizontal axis (Z). Prior to reading the following sentences identify the axis or axes of rotation in each figure and determine the plane of movement of the body parts rotating about the identified axes. During this walking sequence there are six axes present with respect to the movements of the leg (a). The leg rotates in the sagittal plane (flexes) about the frontal-horizontal hip axis; (b) the shank rotates in the sagittal plane (extends) about the frontal-horizontal axis at the knee; and (c) next, both hip and knee axes are present as the thigh flexes and the shank extends. (d) As heel contact is made, the axis of rotation becomes the intersect of the heel with the floor (again a frontal-horizontal axis) as the total body rotates about the axis; (e) next, the body rotates about the metatarsal joints; and (f) lastly, during the toeoff position the axis of rotation becomes the toe-floor intersect. **Select the figures in Chapter 22 to identify axes and planes of movement for airborne activities.**

external to the living body (external axis) may be described with respect to space. The **axis** may be represented as a line passing through the plane of motion and at a right angle to that plane. Therefore, any rotary motion in a horizontal plane will occur about a vertical axis (Y). When rotary motion occurs within one of the two vertical planes of motion, the axis of rotation will be a horizontal axis. The sagittal plane of motion occurs about the horizontal-frontal axis (Z), and the frontal plane of motion occurs about the horizontal-sagittal axis (X). Rotary motion occurring in diagonal planes has diagonal axes.

This way of describing motion provides the basis for analyzing it. From this basis, we can determine linear and angular displacements, velocities, and accelerations. We can estimate forces from the kinematic data and the anthropometry of the person, as well as from the masses of objects being manipulated.

The Force Aspects of Movement. By definition, a **force** is that which causes, or has the potential to cause, divert, or retard, movement of an object upon which it acts. We can divide the forces into external and internal forces for convenience in analysis. Muscle contraction is the major internal force creating movements of body

segments. Ligaments and tendons also apply forces to create and restrict movements. Inspiration and expiration of air produces air flows and, consequently, force, pressure, and stress to the tissues. Likewise, the kinetics of blood flow results in similar effects. We have chosen not to discuss these internal flows. The forces of muscles, tendons, and ligaments, will be discussed with respect to the levels of stress that can be tolerated during movement.

The major external force, gravity, may facilitate or interfere with our volitional execution of movements. It also acts to create internal stresses to the body tissues. Friction is also a prominent force, necessary for all land and water activities. Friction of air may or may not be an important force, depending on the velocities of the person or/and the air. Water exerts a buoyancy force that creates a very different environment for the production of movements and the posturing of the body.

Forces can be identified by magnitude and direction using the linear equations of motion, such as:

$$F = ma$$ the product of the moving mass and its acceleration equals the force

$$F_t = mv$$ the force is equal to the momentum of an object relative to the time during which the momentum acts

$F_d = \frac{1}{2} mv^2$ the force is equal to the energy of an object relative to the distance during which the energy acts

Moments of force, or forces producing rotary movements, can be identified similarly to the linear ones by substituting moment of inertia for mass and angular velocity for linear velocity.

■ The force of gravity is always vertical (downward). The forces of air and water are multidirectional. Frictional forces are always parallel to the acting surfaces. Collision forces have normal and tangential components. Parallel, tangential, and shearing forces are frictional forces. Normal forces are perpendicular to the acting surfaces. All forces act at a point, in a direction, and with a magnitude. All forces can be identified as vectors and measured.

The Why of Biomechanics

Why should we study biomechanics? The reasons are numerous. Athletic competition is one of the most prestigious and favored activities of society. Multitudes of spectators cheer the athlete to victory. Champions earn huge sums of money. It is no wonder that people strive to perfect their technique and train safely to reach their potential. Biomechanical analyses of movements have begun to serve as a database to provide information to improve technique.

There is an epidemic of injuries in the sports world, as well as in the industrial world. Kinetic analysis of the forces acting on the human body can result in valuable information to create safe training programs and other methods to prevent needless injury.

We have a large population of people who are physically disabled because of wars, diseases, accidents, and human assaults. Biomechanical assessment of dysfunction and suggestions for modified movement patterns can enhance their movement functioning and improve their quality of life.

The ever-increasing number of aging individuals has resulted in a segment of the population with loss in ability to independently perform activities of daily living. The most mechanically efficient movement patterns must be developed to assist these individuals in recapturing their independence.

See the Difference with Biomechanical Analyses

S	for safety
E	for effectiveness
E	for enhancement

This biomechanical analysis results in optimization of movement performance, mechanical efficiency, and/or maximum achievement in performance.

Movement Analysis Models

Now that you've read about why to analyze movement we will present three theoretical models for analysis: POSSUM, factors-results, and holistic principles. Use these approaches to analysis, modify them, or develop your own model.

POSSUM

This model was proposed by Jackie Hudson of the University of North Carolina–Greensboro and is an acronym for *Purpose/Observation System of Studying and Understanding Movement.* Three questions are used as guidelines for analysis: What matters? How is it measured? How is it manipulated?

The first step is to classify the movement's purpose. Examples of such purposes are generation of maximum force, maintenance of balance, and intentional loss of balance. Within a purpose category, there should be observable dimensions of movement that correspond with the correct execution of the task. That is to say, the observations that matter are those that can be used to distinguish between levels of skill from the novice to the elite. If an observed item is not useful in evaluating movement, then it does not matter. Once an observation is deemed to matter, we must evaluate its measurability. Since most appliers of biomechanical information do not have access to advanced laboratories, the observations should be measurable qualitatively with the naked eye. Once a measurement is made, the question becomes, Can this observation be manipulated? If it is crucial to performance, performers must be able to

Direction of Force

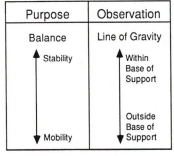

Purpose	Observation
Balance	Line of Gravity
▲ Stability ↕ ▼ Mobility	▲ Within Base of Support ↕ ▼ Outside Base of Support

Purpose	Observation
Projection	Initial Path
▲ Height ↕ Range ↕ ▼ Speed	▲ Vertical ↕ 45° ↕ ▼ Horizontal or Below

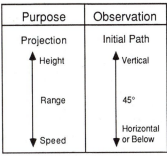

Magnitude of Force

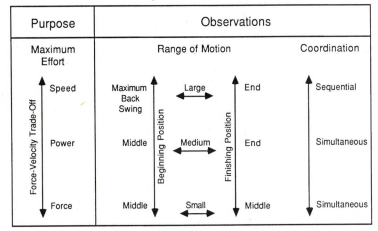

Purpose	Observations		
	Range of Motion		Coordination
Maximum Effort			
▲ Speed (Force-Velocity Trade-Off) ↕ Power ↕ ▼ Force	Maximum Back Swing / Middle / Middle (Beginning Position) — Large / Medium / Small — End / End / Middle (Finishing Position)		▲ Sequential ↕ Simultaneous ↕ ▼ Simultaneous

a   b

FIGURE 1.11 Examples of components of POSSUM model developed by Jackie Hudson. Analysis of balance, projection, and maximum effort purposes are evaluated with respect to direction and magnitude of force. Observations are made and estimates of line of gravity, path, and range of motion are placed on the respective continua. These estimates are then matched to each purpose continuum.

change it. Otherwise it does not matter. Observations that matter (variables) and are observable can be evaluated in relative terms based on a continuum.

Two continuum POSSUM examples addressing direction of force and magnitude of force are analyzed using vertical jumping as the application example. (See Figure 1.11.) The purposes are to remain stable over the base of support and to project the body vertically. We obtain the desired pattern of movement by extending from the purpose continuum horizontally to connect with the observation continuum. Therefore, if stability is desired, the line of gravity should fall within the base of support. If height of projection is desired, the initial path of the projectile should be vertical. Concerning magnitude of force, the purpose of maximum vertical jumping is to display maximum effort with respect to the force-velocity trade-off. Moving horizontally from the power region on the purpose continuum, the beginning position of the range of motion should be in the middle (slightly greater than 90°). Also, a medium excursion is needed to finish with complete extension. The pattern of coordination that connects with powerful efforts is the simultaneous force-production pattern.

Factors-Results Model

This is the name we use to describe the qualitative model developed by Hay. Hay and Reid (1988) describe the model as one in which the analyst identifies the result of the performance and then lists the factors that produce this result. Examples of results of common sports include distance, time, height, points scored, weight lifted, and advantage attained. The result of throwing and jumping competition is *distance,* while running, swimming, and cycling have *time* as their result.

Hay uses hierarchial structure to depict the factors that determine the result. Figure 1.12 applies this model to the standing long jump. Note that the

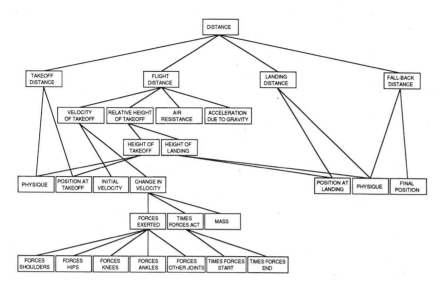

FIGURE 1.12 Factors-results model proposed by Hay for the standing long jump. Note the hierarchial structure. Each lower factor influences the linked factor above. Distance is the goal and four subcomponents of distance are influenced by twenty-three factors as diagrammed. (Reprinted by permission from Hay, James G. and Reid, J. Gavin. 1988. *Anatomy, mechanics and human motion.* Englewood Cliffs, NJ: Prentice Hall: p. 255.)

distance of the jump is determined by four subcomponents: the takeoff distance (how far the center of gravity is in front of the feet); the flight distance (the distance during which the center of gravity does not fall below its elevation at takeoff); the landing distance (that distance reached by the feet beyond the flight distance); and the fall-back distance (distance to be subtracted from total distance). Except for the *physique* factor, the factors evaluated in this model are motion factors (mechanics, velocity, speed, distance, force, mass, acceleration, and resistance of air). This model is a deterministic model in that each factor is determined by those linked to it from the next-lower row of the hierarchy.

Holistic Principle Model

This model (see Figure 1.13) is a holistic approach based on one by Higgins and consists of the following steps:

1. Describing the movement.
2. Setting the performance goal.
3. Identifying the anatomical, mechanical, and environmental considerations.
4. Determining the biomechanical principles for successful and skilled performance of the movement.
5. Assessing the performance based on these principles.

Step 1. Describing the movement: This step consists of a qualitative and general description of the temporal and spatial characteristics of the movement as performed, and an identification of the forces involved in the movement.

Step 2. Setting the performance goal: There may be different goals for different individuals performing the same movement. For example, the competitive breaststroke swimmer will not glide appreciably during the stroke cycle, while the swimmer desiring maximum stroke efficiency of energy output will perform long, optimum glides. Likewise, race walking, walking on ice, and walking wearing snowshoes involve different goals that must be determined.

Step 3. Identifying the anatomical, mechanical, and environmental considerations: The next step is to identify such factors as the size, shape, weight, strength, and speed of the performer and his or her body parts to consider their influence on performance, including limitations. For example, a person with paralysis of one arm will swim differently than an able-bodied person. On earth the laws of mechanics can be used to identify the roles of different body parts in performance execution. The force of gravity and muscle force are the primary considerations for analysis. The environment, however, can restrain, restrict, or facilitate performance. The

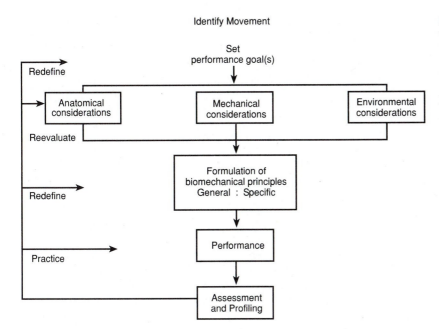

Identify Movement

FIGURE 1.13 Holistic Principle model developed by the authors. The goal of the movement is determined and the anatomical, mechanical, and environmental factors important to the movement success are listed. Basic biomechanical principles are formulated and movement is evaluated according to these principles. Profiles are constructed to aid in evaluation.

terrain, climate, work space, tools, rules of a sport, and anxiety level are common environmental factors to be identified.

■ There is no one ideal biomechanical performance. The uniqueness of each person and the environment determine the ideal biomechanical performance at that instant in time.

Step 4. Biomechanical principles of movement: A principle denotes a statement of fact about a phenomenon, person, object, or event. We formulate principles to reduce the complex movement of living bodies to simpler elements and evaluate or describe them. Principles are usually stated as a relationship about two or more factors or as a cause-and-effect statement. Examples of biomechanical principles are:

Moderate ball speed is required to achieve best pin action in bowling.

Greater kinetic energy is developed by increasing the height of the backswing in bowling.

A body will be in equilibrium if the center of mass remains above the base of support.

Selecting the best combination of principles, or compromising or adapting general principles, is sometimes

necessary because of the goal, individual impairment, or other unique anatomical, mechanical, or environmental considerations. For example, in golf one might sacrifice maximum distance to gain accuracy.

Step 5. Performance and assessment: This step consists of isolating the components of the movement that cause success or failure and then relating those problems to the biomechanical principles.

The Search for the Answers

With today's sophisticated technology, we have been able to learn more about human movement in the past ten years than in any previous decade. Many beginning biomechanics students will soon be able to investigate problems once studied only by the most advanced graduate students. The president of California Polytechnic State University said in the early 1960s that, every ten years, the advancement of knowledge has been so rapid that the level of study has moved downward as much as four years. It is more true today than ever.

Although we are anatomically limited in how we can move, remember the phrase "structure determines function—function determines structure." The human body will change, the devices the human body uses will change, and the environment in which the human body lives will change. Thus, the questions of the next decade are unasked and unknown. How then, can we have the answers? We must use basic concepts about what is known to pose the questions of the future and create more effective, safer, and more rewarding human movement.

Remember also that facts are merely items we know. Facts change and new facts are derived. Human movement is dynamic. We also must be dynamic and receptive to new concepts. The succeeding chapters in this book are designed to present the existing knowledge and help you pose questions for the search for new knowledge. This book also presents guidelines for the study of such topics as how to better understand movement dysfunction and trauma-induced movements and how to optimize performance.

References

Amar, J. 1910. *The human motor*. New York: Dutton.

Braune, G. L. 1941. Kinesiology: From Aristotle to the twentieth century. *Research Quarterly* 12:163.

Carter, J. E. L. 1970. The somatotypes of athletes—a review. *Human Biology* 42: (4)535–69.

Cooper, J. 1979. Biomechanical research in sport: Past, present and future. In *Science in athletics*, eds. J. Terauds and G. Dales, pp. 3–15. Del Mar, CA: Academic Publishers.

deGaray, A. L., Levine, L., and Carter, J. E. L. (1974). *Genetic and anthropological studies of olympic athletes*. New York: Academic Press.

Easterby, R., Kroemer, K. H. E., and Chaffin, D. B. eds. 1982: *Anthropometry and biomechanics: Theory and applications*. Proceedings of the NATO Symposium, Cambridge, England. July 1980. New York: Plenum.

Hay, J. G., and Reid, G. 1988. *Anatomy, mechanics, and human motion*. Englewood Cliffs, NJ: Prentice-Hall.

Logan, G., and McKinney, W. C. 1977. *Anatomic kinesiology*, 2nd ed. Dubuque, IA: Wm. C. Brown.

Morpurgo, Benedetto. 1889. Sur la nature des atrophies par inanition aigue chez/es animaux à sang chaud. *Arch. Ital. Biol.*, 12, xxxii–xxxiii.

NASA. 1978. *Anthropometric source book,* 3 vols. NASA reference publication 1024.

Ross, W., Eiben, O., Ward, R., Martin, A., Drinkwater, D., and Clarys, J. 1984. Alternatives for the conventional methods of human body composition and physique assessment. In *Perspectives in kinanthropometry,* ed. J. Day, pp. 203–20. Champaign, IL: Human Kinetics.

Sheldon, W. H., Dupertuis, C. W., and McDermott, E. 1954. *Atlas of men.* New York: Harper.

Steindler, A. 1955. *Kinesiology of the human body under normal and pathological conditions.* Springfield, IL: Charles C. Thomas.

Tricker, R. A., and Tricker, B. J. K. 1967. *The science of movement.* New York: American Elsevier.

2 Static and Dynamic Posture

This chapter presents the gravitational field, as well as other conditions and their effects on the posture of the human body. Gravity largely determines static and dynamic postures, and subsequent movements in time and space reflect our gravitational environment.

Posture is a static position or a series of sequential positions culminating in a movement pattern. Most of these positions reflect adjustments to the gravitational field. Not only our postures, but also our anatomical structures are, in part, consequences of human beings living on earth.

We would see differences if we lived on Mars, Pluto, or other places in the galaxy. On the sun, for example, body weight would be more than 30 times that on earth. Without some major change in muscle morphology, human beings would weigh two and one-half times their earth body weight if they lived on Jupiter. Contrast this with a weight of approximately 40% on Mars and 17% on the earth's moon. The astronauts had a great deal of difficulty walking on the surface of the moon. Since their bodies kept rising upward, they had to use a short-step pattern with very low accelerations of the body parts. Muscles, particularly those identified as antigravity muscles, would atrophy from living on the moon.

■ Plants, animals, and human beings respond according to their unique structure, and each structure is modified by the environment in which it exists.

Human beings are bipeds whose upright posture makes them distinct from all other animals. Using *man* and *his* as neutral gender, Morton and Fuller (1952) say that "in his body form, in his completely erect bipedism and mental development, Man possesses characteristics that separate him undeniably from all other living creatures." They believe that the physical differences that distinguish the human being from other, closely related animal forms developed as a result of reaction to the force of gravity. (See Figure 2.1.)

To maintain an erect position, human beings had to undergo certain skeletal and muscular changes as compared to animals. The human foot was the sole weight-bearing organ. Concerning the human foot arrangement, Morton and Fuller (1952) state:

1. It permits the body center to occupy its central position over the area of ground contact so that the margin of postural security is equal forward and backward.
2. It places the direction of structural unbalance toward the front so that the muscular tension needed to maintain our erect posture is imposed entirely upon the large and powerful calf muscles.
3. The weaker anterior group of muscles is released from any active counter-balancing tension.

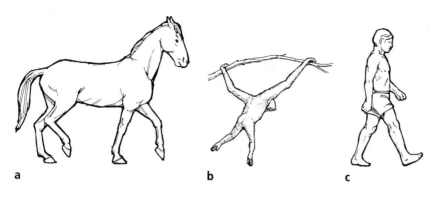

FIGURE 2.1 Anatomical structure is the foundation for functional movement. Quadrupeds, brachiating animals, and human beings have unique structures that favor walking on four legs (*a*); locomotion by swinging from the arms (*b*); and walking on two legs (*c*). **Study the skeletal structure of the horse and human being and postulate what the structure of this brachiating animal would be.**

a   b   c

In addition, this anteriorly unbalanced position of the body center aids in the initiation of forward movement.

The functional locomotor posture of the human, the monkey, and the horse are shown in Figure 2.1. There are other anatomical changes in the human being. For example, compared to quadrupeds, the human has shorter and broader pelvic bones.

Here are some important terms to understand.

Equilibrium is a condition of balance among forces acting within or upon a body. The body is in a state of rest or motion without a change. It might be said that if the sum of the forces and the sum of the moments acting on a body are equal, there is either static equilibrium, as in standing, or action (dynamic) equilibrium, with constant linear and angular velocity. The latter would be rare in a sports setting.

■ Static equilibrium is positively related to mass of the object.

Balance is a constant adaption to forces in order to momentarily attain dynamic equilibrium before adapting and establishing a new equilibrium.

Principles of Equilibrium

The following principles concern the various postures of static positions:

1. To maintain balance, human beings, as with all living beings and inanimate objects, must keep the center of gravity in an area within and directly above the supporting base.

2. The larger the base and the greater the range of support, the greater will be the angle of tilt necessary to move the center of gravity outside the base area. Thus, the stability of the body is often said to increase as the center of gravity is lowered.

3. The closer the center of gravity is to the base of support, the greater will be the angle of tilt necessary to move the center of gravity outside the base area. Thus, the stability of the body is often said to be increased as the center of gravity is lowered.

4. The human body can use many body segments as a base: the feet, one foot, the hands, one finger (in the case of acrobats), the buttocks, the head, the thighs, or the entire body.

5. The segments above the base can be adjusted to bring them into various positions. No general balance pattern exists, but whatever the base and the positions of the segments above it, the center of gravity must be kept over the base area if balance is to be maintained.

Center of gravity is that imaginary point in the body where all forces acting upon it are balanced. Methods of locating this point are discussed later in the chapter. The various postures of the body influence the location, so this location changes as the body moves. It may be located inside or outside the body.

Gravitational line is represented by a single vector passing through the center of gravity. The force of gravity is represented by a force vector passing through the center of gravity vertically.

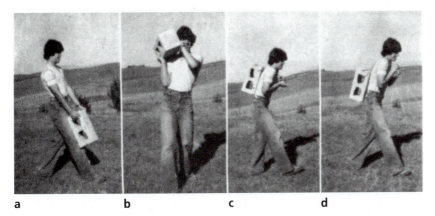

FIGURE 2.2 Variations in body segment alignment as a result of carrying the same load in four positions. (*a*) Functional lordosis; (*b*) functional scoliosis; (*c, d*) trunk flexion with possible functional kyphosis.

a   b   c   d

Normal and Abnormal Postures

Normal Standing and Sitting Positions

Keep in mind that cultural influences have a bearing on posture in moving, sitting, and lying down. Also, there is no one posture, but many. "Normal" is just a name, meaning average or common to a given situation. Individuals, as well as family groups, various cultures, and age groups within cultures, show differences in standing and sitting postures. Although individual differences may be linked to many causes, including attitudes and emotional states, cultures and subcultures appear to develop postures distinct to their groups. The reasons probably are many but certainly include nutrition, climate, and training. Hewes (1957) identified over 1000 different postures ranging from standing, squatting, kneeling, and sitting. Although not common to the United States, at least a fourth of the population of the world habitually crouch in a low squat, both to rest and to work. In certain parts of Africa, India, Australia, and South America, the "nilotic stance" is a common resting position. This stance is a stork-like posture in which the sole of the one foot is planted against the support leg near the knee. Warm climate, bare feet, and unknown cultural reasons are likely reasons for adoption of this stance, as well as occupation or habit of carrying a long staff.

Other influences on posture include clothing, which affects styles of sitting for both men and women. While clothing alone does not explain all posture differences, heavy, bulky, long, light, and skimpy clothing can have an influence on posture. Some sitting postures are predominantly a concern in occupational activities, especially computer work. The biomechanics of sitting posture is discussed in Chapter 12. Equilibrium concerns are quite different for sitting posture than for standing posture. The chair supports the body and eliminates active regulation of balance by the person.

Effects of Carrying a Load

Carrying an object increases the weight the feet must support and affects the position of the gravity planes with reference to the body. If the carrier is to remain upright, these planes must be kept within the area of the supporting foot. The carrier must make segmental adjustments, usually by altering the trunk position. If the object is held in front of the body, the trunk will be inclined backward. If it is held to the side, the trunk will be inclined to the opposite side. The amount of inclination depends on the weight, size, and distribution of weight of the object and on the height at which the object is carried. Figure 2.2 shows the differences in body position when carrying an identical weight, well distributed and poorly distributed, with respect to body symmetry.

Loads carried on the head do not cause inclination of the trunk. Visitors to regions in which carrying objects on the head, especially among women, is common frequently comment on the excellent carriage of these people. Undoubtedly, the additional weight high above the feet requires careful alignment of body segments.

Walking with a heavy load also alters the stepping pattern. The center of gravity is not allowed to move as far forward of the supporting foot as it does in normal walking. With the load the step will be shortened, and the

Static and Dynamic Posture   **23**

center of gravity will be held over the supporting foot for a longer time. It is interesting to note that when bulky packs of produce are loaded onto the backs of Mexican Indian men by fellow workers, the carrier cannot sit down during the 16-km (10-mile) trip from the fields to market. Once the load is lowered, he cannot lift it again without assistance. When carrying a load the center of gravity and gravitational line of the system must be considered, not just the human body or the load independently.

Among the various body types, obese persons are likely to have the most erect posture as a result of the effort required to support excessive fatty tissues. Fat persons twist as they walk, and to reduce the amount of this turning they stiffen and take short steps. Persons with large abdomens often lean slightly backward to balance the weight in front. Some short, stocky people stand erect to make themselves appear taller and slimmer. Extremely thin individuals often lack the muscular strength needed to hold themselves erect. During the teenage years, many tall girls voluntarily slouch to appear more nearly the size of their shorter boy companions.

Specialization in certain forms of hard work or strenuous athletic activity also results in adaptations of posture. A coal miner carries the head and shoulders forward and the arms slightly bent in the position of work. The side-horse specialist in gymnastics tends to become overly round-shouldered and kyphotic if this activity is not balanced by others that exercise contralateral musculature. Posture adaptations to specialized events may also be counteracted by a conscious effort to improve the carriage at all times when the person is not bent to the task.

Effects of Anatomical Abnormality

Abnormalities of the spine (Figure 2.3) and other structural portions of the body often cause adjustments in gait and normal posture. Arthritis of the knees, hands, and even the neck often interfere with normal activities. Osteoporosis, diabetes, and Parkinson's disease are detrimental to performing even daily living activities. A biomechanical evaluation may help in compensating for these abnormalities, so that adherence to normal patterns is possible.

Structural deformities cause postural compensations. A short leg produces scoliosis, which may be corrected by elevating the heel to lengthen the short leg. Pronated feet result in an anteriorly tilted pelvis and lordosis, which are corrected when the pronation is remedied.

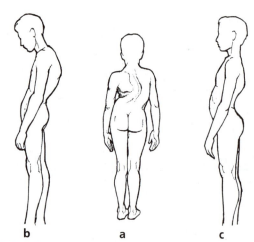

b   a   c

FIGURE 2.3 Standing postures with various spinal column deformities. **Match the following to the appropriate posture:** scoliosis (lateral curvature of the spine); kyphosis (exaggerated posterior thoracic convexity); and lordosis (exaggerated posterior lumbar concavity). The matching is *b, a, c.*

Effects of Pregnancy

The later weeks of pregnancy are marked by a large forward displacement of the center of gravity because of the combined weight of the fetus, its surrounding amniotic fluid, and the massive uterus. The resulting postural compensation is a light backward lean and backward shift of weight in the lumbar region. More weight is borne by the heels. The backward lean (although the center of gravity stays over the base) becomes more exaggerated as the pregnancy progresses. This adaptation occasionally corrects a customary slouch but usually causes increased lumbar stress. (See Figure 2.4.)

Effects of Shoe Heel Height

Julius Caesar is thought to have been the first to discover the advantage of elevating the heels. He observed that when heels were added to the sandals of his legions, the soldiers were able to march farther with less fatigue. When the calcaneus is elevated about 1.27 cm (0.5 inches) above the level of the base of the ball of the foot, its shaft is brought to a tangent with the Achilles tendon, and thus the gastrocnemius and soleus muscles are able to exert a greater force in plantar flexion. If shoes without heels or with higher heels are worn after an individual has become accustomed to wearing heels of a certain height, the legs and feet become fatigued more quickly.

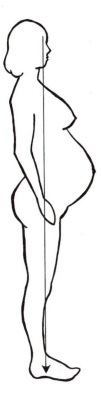

FIGURE 2.4 Changes in anatomy during pregnancy. **Estimate the position of the center of gravity and line of gravity after you have read this chapter.**

The ability of the human body to adjust to heel heights of 7.5 cm or greater is attested to by the skilled movements of women jitterbug dancers of the 1940s and disco dancers of the 1970s. Both men and women wear cowboy boots without mishap. High-heeled pumps, however, appear to be the cause of numerous falling accidents. The high heel, combined with the high sole, may reduce perceptual awareness of the position of the foot and delay the kinesthetic and tactile responses to loss of balance, in addition to elevating the center of gravity of the body about 9 cm. The changes in line of gravity and position of the center of gravity with different heel heights appear in Figure 2.5. Note that similar alignment of body parts, as well as knee angle and trunk position, can be achieved with any of these heel heights.

Effects of Standing for Long Durations of Time

Continued standing may result in a pooling of blood and other fluids in the feet, as well as lowering of the arches to such an extent that the foot may increase in size as much as one or two shoe sizes. Clerks, dentists, ticket takers, and barbers commonly wear shoes at work that are lacerated at the toe, ball, and top to allow for the expansion to take place. Workers in these occupations

MINI-LABORATORY LEARNING EXPERIENCE

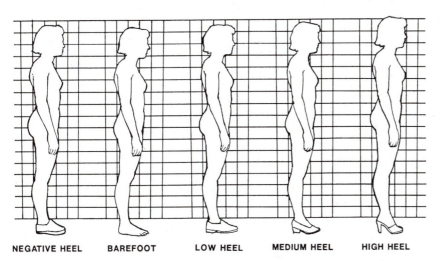

NEGATIVE HEEL   BAREFOOT   LOW HEEL   MEDIUM HEEL   HIGH HEEL

FIGURE 2.5 Effects of changes in elevation of heels on standing posture and forefoot weightbearing. Hip joint and background grid may be used to estimate gravitational line and center of gravity of the body. Note the decrease in forefoot surface area (reproductions of pedographs) and change in weighting of toes and fifth metatarsals as the height of heel increases. **What implications do these changes have for body position and balance?**

should probably wear two pairs of shoes, one in the morning and a larger pair in the afternoon. Some people choose loose-fitting shoes. However, this solution is poor because when no support is given, pronation occurs. A well-designed shoe for standing is constructed so that most of the weight is borne on the outside of the foot. This part of the foot is supported by strong ligaments, while the inside of the foot is supported by long, thin muscles that are easily fatigued.

Posture of Readiness

The standing posture is affected by a person's anticipation of forthcoming action. If no action is anticipated and the conditions of the external environment are unexciting, the response will be a relaxed posture. This is so well known that athletes can simulate a relaxed posture to deceive their opponents. A basketball player about to receive a pass can often deceive a defender by assuming a relaxed posture and passive countenance.

The posture of readiness before performing a rapid or strong movement is an alert one. The peak of attention is reached between one and two seconds after concentration is directed to the situation. The posture adapts to the condition. After the peak of attention is past, the posture either is relaxed or becomes unstable because of extreme tremor, possibly resulting from accommodation of the coordinating centers of the nervous system.

The position assumed during a state of readiness is in accord with the immediate tasks to be accomplished (Figure 2.6). If the direction of movement is not known, the weight should be distributed over the surface of both feet. When the direction is known, the center of gravity should be shifted in the anticipated direction. A slight flexion may occur at the ankle, causing the equilibrium of the body to be unstable, facilitating movement. The head, arm, and leg positions are also adjusted to the action to follow. The infielder in baseball leans forward and rises on the toes as the ball is pitched. The baserunner taking a one-stride lead off the base will lean toward the next base and rise on the toes as the ball is pitched. In each instance, the mechanical equilibrium of the body is disturbed and movement is commenced. The football quarterback crouches with the arms forward and heels of the hands close together in a position of readiness to catch the ball from the center.

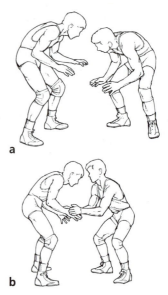

FIGURE 2.6 Postures of readiness. (a) Wrestlers are using staggered stances, which are best for moving rapidly forward or backward. (b) Wrestlers are using parallel stances, which are best for moving right or left. Modifications of these two stances are also used in preparation for certain actions and against certain opponents. (From Boring, W. J. 1975. *Science and skills of wrestling.* St. Louis: Mosby.)

Such postures of readiness should not be held motionless for an extended length of time, since proprioceptor sensations, which govern the senses of position and relationship of the body parts to objects in view, will be diminished and have to be reestablished before accurate movement can be accomplished. For this reason, the golfer waggles the club near the ball while adjusting the stance position in readiness for the swing. While poised for the pitch, the batter in baseball does the same thing to heighten the sensation of the position of the bat in relation to the body and to the path of the ball.

Dynamic Posture

The previous principles apply to situations in which movement does not exist. These principles may or may not be valid for the dynamic situation, since movement itself introduces another force: ma, or I. The mass (m) of the body represents its resistance (inertia) to translation, which is multiplied by acceleration (a) to depict the force of a translating body. I is the moment of inertia, or

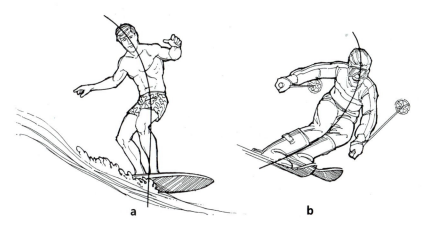

FIGURE 2.7 Typical body leans and curvatures during surfboarding and snow skiing. **Can you list other activities that produce similar curvatures? Note:** Center of gravity is outside the base of support.

the resistance to rotation of a body. This resistance is multiplied by rotary, or angular, acceleration (*a*) to depict the moment of force of a rotating body. Therefore, the moving human body may be in "dynamic balance." In other words, a person may not fall when the line of gravity falls outside the base of support. Note the lean of the bodies depicted in Figure 2.7 during surfboarding and snow skiing. A further explanation of this phenomenon and of situations in which other forces are present will be considered in Chapters 22 and 23.

Determining Center of Gravity

The techniques presented in this section are appropriate for determining the center of gravity of a human body. Some modifications may be made in the size of equipment, but the concepts are valid for all living and inanimate objects. In activities such as horseback riding, finding the center of gravity of the horse, the rider, and the horse-rider system may prove useful in determining the positions of the rider that either interfere with the progress of the horse or enhance it. A review of the concepts involved in the center of gravity is presented first, followed by a discussion of how to find its location.

All masses within the gravitational field of the earth are constantly subjected to a pull toward the earth's center, and the greater the mass, the stronger will be the force of that pull. The force of gravitational attraction that the earth exerts on a body is called its **weight.** Gravitational force pulls downward on each point of a given body. The distribution of these points determines the

position of the center of gravity of the body. If a board is suspended on a support, as in playground teeterboards, a downward pull is exerted on each side of the support. If the board mass on each side is equal in size and in distance from the support, the board will balance. If a child sits on one side of the balanced board, that side will be pushed downward, and the opposite side will move upward. In such unbalanced situations, gravitational force, interestingly, is responsible for the upward as well as the downward movement. We will see later how this upward movement caused by gravitational force is used by the body in many forms of locomotion. On the teeterboard, a second child can take a position on the opposite side of the board; if the distance from the board is adjusted, the board and the two children can be balanced. Within every mass is a point about which the gravitational forces on one side will equal those on the other. This balance point, determined in three planes of the mass, is the center of gravity.

Center of Gravity in the Transverse Body Plane

The point of balance in the human body has long interested investigators. The earliest of these, the Italian physicist, Borelli (1608–1679), employed the teeterboard to locate the transverse plane of that point. He placed a nude subject on a board in the prone position and then moved the board back and forth as it rested on a knife-edged support until the total mass balanced. He reported the balance plane to be one that cut the body "between the genitals and pubis." Somewhere within this plane would lie the subject's center of gravity. In

1836, two German brothers, the Webers, improved Borelli's method by first balancing the board and then sliding the subject back and forth until balance was obtained. They found the transverse plane of the center of gravity to be 56.8% of the height above the heel.

Half a century later (1889), the two Germans Braune and Fischer reported that the center-of-gravity plane was 54.8% of the height measured from the soles. Their conclusion was based on finding the point of balance in four frozen male cadavers. The cadavers were first balanced on a knife-edge, and then a steel rod was driven into the cadaver at the determined plane. Each cadaver was suspended by the steel rod, and gravitational force moved the mass into a balanced position. When the body attained equilibrium, a plumb line was dropped from the point of suspension to locate the transverse plane of the center of gravity. Since fluid volume and tissue weight varies between live and dead bodies, other methods for determination of centers of gravity of bodies and body segments were sought. Hay (1973) has summarized common methods and data on segmental and body weights, centers of gravity, and moments of inertia.

The most convenient early method of locating the plane of the center of gravity was proposed by two Americans, Reynolds and Lovett (1909). (See Figure 2.8.) A board of a known length is supported at either end of a knife-edge. The knife-edges are placed on scales that can be adjusted to eliminate the weight of the board. The subject lies on the board, and the plane of the center of gravity is determined mathematically. It will be at a point on the board determined by multiplying the weight on one scale by the distance from that knife-edge to the plane of the center of gravity. This product will equal that obtained by multiplying the weight on the second scale by the distance between the second knife-edge and the plane of the center of gravity: $w_1 d_1 + w_2 d_2$, where w_1 equals the weight on scale 1, d_1 equals the distance from the line of gravity to w_1, w_2 equals the weight on scale 2, and d_2 equals the distance from the line of gravity to w_2. This equation can be reduced to one unknown by redefining d_2 as the distance between the knife-edge minus d_1. The use of this equation is shown in the solution of the following laboratory experience problem.

Since the head was even with the knife-edge, the distance from the top of the head to the transverse plane of the center of gravity is 77.3 cm. If the subject is 171 cm

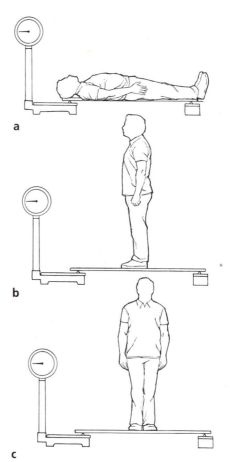

FIGURE 2.8 One method used for determining position of the line of gravity and the center of gravity of the body. The known weight of the human body and the recorded weight acting on the scale are used to mathematically calculate the position of the vertical force vector acting through the center of gravity of the body (line of gravity): (a) line of gravity (balance point) top and bottom halves of body; (b) balance point of front and rear halves of body; (c) balance point of right and left halves of body. The intersect of the position of three calculated force vectors is the site of the center of gravity of the body. **Using the values shown in the text, determine the location of the center of gravity in each of the three planes.**

in height, the plane line of gravity is 45% of the height measured from the top of the head, and 55% of the height measured from the soles of the feet.

This procedure can be used when only one scale is available, since the reading on the second scale will always be the total weight minus the reading on the single scale (Figure 2.8).

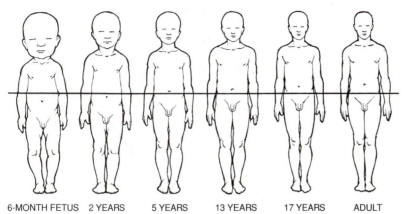

FIGURE 2.9 Contourograms of ventral aspects of body at pre-birth and various ages after birth. Body lengths are scaled to reduce all figures to the same height. The transverse plane at the level of the center of gravity of each body is represented by the transverse line.
(From Palmer, C. E. 1944. *Child Dev.* 15:99. The Society for Research in Child Development, Inc.) **Is it any wonder that infants have locomotor and head control problems?**

6-MONTH FETUS   2 YEARS   5 YEARS   13 YEARS   17 YEARS   ADULT

MINI-LABORATORY LEARNING EXPERIENCE

Problem: A subject weighing 660 N lies on a board, with the top of the head in line with the knife-edge on scale 1. The distance between the knife-edges is 1.50 m. The scale reading on the head scale 1 is 320 N; the other scale 2 reads 340 N. These values are placed appropriately into the previously presented equation, which in essence is the determination of the moments of force about the line of gravity.

Solution:

$$320\,\text{N} \times d_1 = 340\,\text{N}\,(1.50\text{m} - d_1)$$
$$320\,\text{N} \times d_1 = 510\,\text{NM} - 340\,\text{N} \times d_1$$
$$660\,\text{N} \times d_1 = 510\,\text{NM}$$
$$d_1 = 0.773\,\text{m}$$
$$\text{N} = \text{newton}$$
$$\text{NM} = \text{newton-meter}$$

One newton (unit of force) is that force that gives a mass of 1 kg an acceleration of 1 m/sec^2.

Using the scale method, other investigators have reported findings on the location of the transverse plane of the human center of gravity. Croskey and associates reported in 1922 that this plane is slightly higher in men than in women. The average height of the plane in men was 56.18% of the height above the soles; the range of percentages was 55% to 58%. For women, the average was 55.44%; the range was 54% to 58%. Additional observations were made by Hellebrandt and coworkers (1938, 1942, 1943), who found that in 357 college women the transverse plane averaged 55.17% of the height; the lowest observed was 53%, and the highest was 59%.

The most extensive early study is that reported by Palmer (1944), who located the transverse plane of the center of gravity in 1172 subjects—596 boys and 576 girls from birth to 20 years of age—and in 18 fetal cadavers. Palmer concluded that regardless of age or sex, the plane can be estimated as follows:

0.557 × height plus 1.4 cm (0.551 in.) from soles of feet

Since body segments differ in proportion to total height from birth to maturity, the plane of the center of gravity will lie in a different section of the body as age increases. The proportion of height will be constant (Figures 2.9 and 2.10).

Obviously, a change in position of the limbs with reference to the prone torso will change the position of the center of gravity. If the arms are raised overhead or the hips flexed, the plane will move toward the head. Loss of body parts will also alter the position. Amputation of any part of a lower limb will raise the plane,

Static and Dynamic Posture **29**

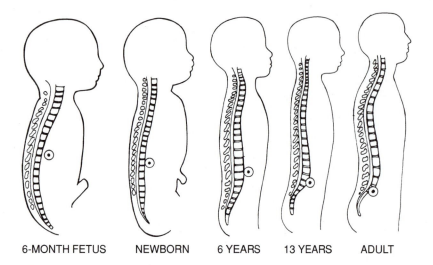

FIGURE 2.10 The positions of center of gravity in the sagittal plane with reference to the spine are depicted as ⊙. Note how the C-curve changes to a 4-curve as the center of gravity drops and the head weight is reduced.
(Modified from Palmer, C. E. 1944. *Child Dev.* 15:99.)

6-MONTH FETUS   NEWBORN   6 YEARS   13 YEARS   ADULT

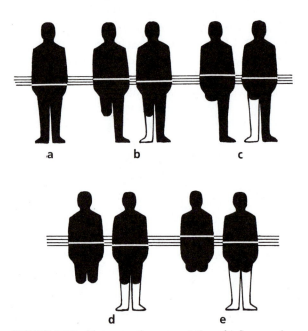

FIGURE 2.11 Diagrammatic representation of influence of amputation of lower extremities on height of center of gravity and compensatory effect of prosthetic limb. The white transverse line represents the plane at the level of the center of gravity. (*a*) able-bodied person; (*b*) below-knee single-leg amputee without and with below-knee prothesis; (*c*) above-knee single-leg amputee without and with above-knee prosthesis; (*d*) below-knee double-leg amputee without and with prosthesis; (*e*) above-knee double-leg amputee without and with prosthesis.
(From Hellebrandt, F. A. 1950. *JAMA*, 142:1353–1356.)

and the height of the center of gravity will increase with the amount of body mass lost. The addition of a prosthetic appliance to replace the amputated limb will lower the center of gravity toward the normal position (Figure 2.11).

Center of Gravity in Frontal and Sagittal Body Planes

In the preceding discussion, the transverse plane of the center of gravity was located at a distance from the top of the head or from the soles of the feet. In balance and locomotor activities, it is important to locate the gravity plane in the frontal and sagittal planes. (See Figure 1.7 for visualization of all three planes.) If the Reynolds-Lovett method is used, the body must be stationary on the board, and some body point must be located with reference to the knife-edges. If the frontal gravity plane is located while the subject is standing, some part of the foot will be taken as the reference point, and the distance of this part from one of the knife-edges must be known. Since it is more convenient to stand near the middle of the board rather than near one end of it, a line on the board halfway between the knife-edges is convenient for measuring distance.

The same mathematical procedure described in the preceding section for finding the center of gravity in the transverse body plane can be used to determine both the frontal gravity plane and the sagittal gravity plane (Figure 1.7). Often it is desirable to locate the frontal plane with reference to the ankle joint. In this case, if the ankle joint is 15 cm from the tip of the toes, the frontal plane is 4.5 cm in front of that joint. A perpendicular line passing through the foot at this point is often called the gravity line. In postural measures, certain body landmarks are described in terms of deviation from this line.

When a person stands erect, the frontal gravity plane lies in front of the ankle joint and in back of the metatarsophalangeal joints. The location between these points differs with individuals and may differ from time to time in the same individual. This location between the ankles and the proximal end of the toes has been so frequently observed that it can be accepted as a human characteristic. Many investigators have studied human postural positions. Over the years, hundreds of students in our biomechanics classes have observed this phenomenon in themselves and in their classmates. Not only have they observed the location, but they have also seen that this plane is rarely stationary. It usually fluctuates, and the degree of fluctuation varies with the individual and the movement.

As the subject stands on the board for gravity-plane determination, the observer finds it difficult to make an exact scale reading because the dial needle fluctuates rapidly. The range of the needle varies with individuals, but rarely exceeds 20 N. If one reading is desired, the best one to take is that about which the needle hovers; however, the extremes will also provide interesting information. The reason for the changes in scale readings is understood when one remembers that the body must balance on the small base provided by the upper surface of the talus at the ankle joint. Since the center of gravity of the body is ahead of the ankle joint, the body is unbalanced on this small surface. Gravitational force would tilt the body forward if no counterforce were present. The ankle extensors provide this force; the tension in these muscles must be sufficient to withstand gravitational pull if the erect position is to be maintained. Any slight change in any body part (solid, liquid, or gas) will change the distribution of weight. Such a change will alter the force of gravitational pull and consequently change the demand on the ankle extensors. The tension

in the muscles may change also. Whatever the cause, the frontal plane is constantly shifting, although it remains within the limits described. Class observations in which students are asked to lean forward as far as possible without raising the heels and then backward as far as possible without lifting the toes (and without falling) rarely find that the gravity plane has moved back of the ankle or ahead of the proximal end of the toes. It does not move beyond the normal limits for the individual.

■ Segmental alignment above the ankle is not a universal characteristic. Individuals differ in degree of pelvic tilt, in depth of lumbar, dorsal, and cervical curves, and in shoulder girdle and head position. All these factors affect the distribution of weight. Yet when an individual stands in a habitual position, the frontal plane of the center of gravity will fall between the ankle and the metatarsophalangeal joints.

For location of the sagittal gravity plane, the subject stands on the board, with the right side toward one knife-edge and the left side toward the other. Locating this plane is useful in determining whether the subject is likely to carry more of the weight on one foot than on the other.

Measurement of Postural Sway

Hellebrandt has said that standing is really movement on a stationary base and that swaying is inseparable from the upright stance. Hellebrandt and others have shown that considerable **postural sway** occurs in forward, backward, and sideward directions. Co-author Cooper has had his students measure the amount of sway that occurs during five- and ten-minute periods of standing erect without moving (other than swaying) and with the feet placed close together. It was found that the longer the individual stands, the greater the amplitude of sway. Usually after 15 minutes, the individual will tend to faint and fall to the floor. One individual in a special experiment was able to stand erect for 25 minutes with his feet in a bucket of ice water. At the end of 25 minutes, he fell to the floor and had to be revived. Hellebrandt and Franseen (1943, p. 220) state, "Sway is reduced when the eyes are open and focused on a fixed point and increased when the eyes are closed."

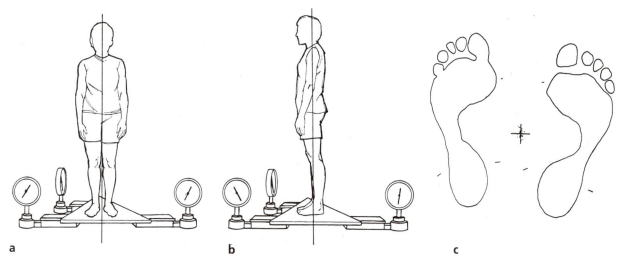

a   b   c

FIGURE 2.12 Non-computerized method for obtaining line of gravity during standing. Equipment used to determine mean gravity line in sagittal (*a*) and frontal (*b*) planes. Front and side view photographs are taken simultaneously; each view presents two of three dial scales. Gravity lines added to photographs after calculations represent mean of 30 determinations; each dot between feet represents one determination; center point of crossed lines represents mean of 30 determinations (*c*).
(From Waterland, J. C., and Shambes, G. M. 1970. Biplane center of gravity procedures, *Percept. Mot. Skills* 30:511.)

Joseph (1960) also investigated sway. He showed that activity in the muscles of the calves of the legs was greater when subjects wore high-heeled shoes (2½ inches) than when they were barefoot. The increased muscular activity was necessary to counteract the otherwise unstable position created by the high-heeled shoes. Activity in the gastrocnemius muscle was increased the most. Recent researchers (Hines-Woollacott 1990) have shown effects of aging, Parkinson's disease, and other factors on postural sway.

An inexpensive arrangement for simultaneously determining the frontal and sagittal planes of the center of gravity has been presented by Waterland and Shambes (1970). The subject takes a position on a base supported by three dial scales. Two photographs, a side and a front view, are taken by a synchronized shutter arrangement. The three scale readings shown in the photographs will equal the total weight of the subject. With these readings the positions of gravity lines in the frontal and sagittal planes can be calculated. These investigators have shown fluctuations of the gravity line in a "static" standing position. By placing on the supported board a paper on which the footprints of the subject were traced, they located the gravity line with reference to the feet (Figure 2.12).

The triangular platform shown in Figure 2.12 was used by Hasselkus (1974) to compare the postural sway of ten women, 21 to 30 years of age, with ten others 73 to 80 years of age. Greater sway was thought to be a possible indication of aging of the neuromuscular system. Each subject stood on the platform for three 18-second periods, during which cameras recorded the scale readings every second. The area enclosed in the outer borders of the 54 calculated positions of gravity lines was expressed as a percentage of the functional base of support, a quadrilateral area enclosed in lines drawn along the lateral borders of the feet and across the back of the heels and connecting the heads of the first metatarsals. The older women's sway area covered an average of 43%, and the younger women's, an average 23%. For all subjects, the position of the gravity line tended to be to left and posterior of the geometric center of the functional base. Today, computerized force platform systems automatically display the magnitude, direction, and pattern of sway.

Xo = -0.35 in, Yo = -2.35 in

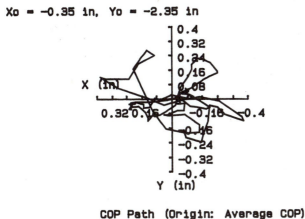

COP Path (Origin: Average COP)

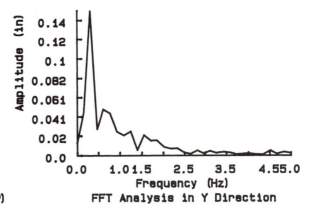

FFT Analysis in Y Direction

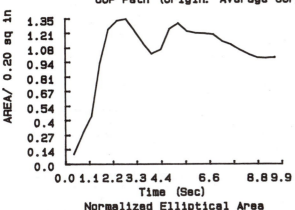

Normalized Elliptical Area

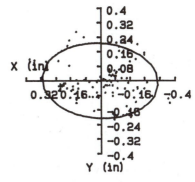

COP Points (Origin: Average COP)

FIGURE 2.13 Graphic outputs of a person standing on an AMTI force platform. The COP Path is a stabilogram depicting the X, Y coordinates of the center-of-pressure. The FFT is a frequency analysis in the X (anteroposterior) direction. The ellipse is an approximation of the data and the area of the ellipse is used to correlate sway data with other factors.

(Courtesy of Advanced Medical Technology, Inc.)

A graphical example of a postural sway pattern generated by a computer from an AMTI force platform is depicted in Figure 2.13. Other platforms have been built that move forward, backward, and tilt up and down. The postural adjustments are automatically recorded and stored in a computer. These platforms have been used in studying clinical patients, different types of shoes, and aging phenomena.

Determining Center of Gravity in a Moving Body

Two methods, the scale (or whole-body) and the segmental (or indirect or parts), have been used to determine the center of gravity in the moving body. Both methods require that the investigator "freeze" the moving body into static positions. This is done by selecting

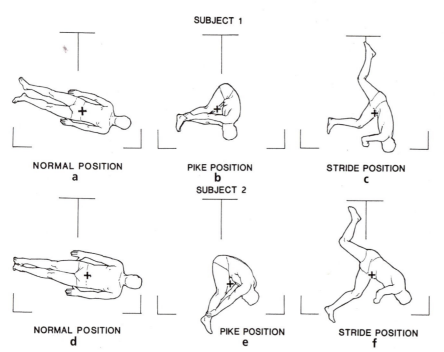

SUBJECT 1

NORMAL POSITION
a

PIKE POSITION
b

STRIDE POSITION
c

SUBJECT 2

NORMAL POSITION
d

PIKE POSITION
e

STRIDE POSITION
f

FIGURE 2.14 Performer-position combinations assumed by two performers on center-of-gravity board. Position of center of gravity in each of the six positions is at the cross (+). Note the differences between subject 1 and subject 2. The center of gravity lies outside the body in the pike positions, and in all conditions, is in the vicinity of the pelvis. (From Davis, M. 1973. Quality of data collected by the segmental analysis technique, Ph.D. dissertation, Indiana University.)

still photographs, frames of movie film, or posed positions determined by the observer and used to represent the sequencing of the movement. It is important to attempt to duplicate exactly the position of all body parts at each of the imposed stationary images of the movement. The position of the center of gravity in two planes can be found from each image.

Scale Method

Triangular and rectangular boards using two-four scales have been used in much the same way as the one-two **scale method** for determining the line of gravity in one plane. Davis (1973) devised a center-of-gravity board with three accompanying scales (Figure 2.14). After the subjects had assumed various performer-position combinations, he determined (1) the center of gravity in the transverse and sagittal planes for the pike and stride positions; and (2) the center of gravity in the transverse and frontal planes for the normal position. Davis also photographed these performer-position combinations and used the segmental method.

TABLE 2.1 Weights of body segments expressed in percentages relative to total body weight for women as cited by various authors.

Segment	Bernstein	Plagenhoef	Kjeldsen
Trunk		55.00	60.20
Upper arm	2.63	2.90	2.74
Forearm	1.82	1.55	1.61
Hand	0.64	0.50	0.51
Thigh	12.48	11.50	8.26
Calf (lower leg)	4.73	5.25	5.49
Foot	1.31	1.20	1.24

Segmental Method

Another method of determining the location of the center of gravity in the moving body is the **segmental method** suggested by Dawson (1935). This method is used when the performer is not present and only a photograph or film of the performance is available. It uses estimations of the weight of each body segment and the

TABLE 2.2 Weights of body segments expressed in percentages relative to total body weight for men as cited by various authors.

Segment	Braune and Fischer	Cleaveland	Williams and Lissner	Dempster
Head and neck	7.06	7.03	7.9	
Trunk	42.70	48.30	51.1	49.4
Upper arm (2)	6.72	6.25	5.4	7.0
Forearm (2)	6.24	4.33	4.4	3.2
Hand (2)	(With forearm)	(With forearm)	(With forearm)	1.0
Thigh (2)	23.16	22.52	19.4	27.4
Calf (lower leg) (2)	14.12	11.52	12.0	9.4
Foot (2)	(With calf)	(With calf)	(With calf)	2.6

Values for upper arm, forearm, hand, thigh, calf, and foot are for both segments in each case.

TABLE 2.3 Locations of centers of gravity of body segments expressed as percentage of total segment length as measured from proximal end for women as cited by two authors.

Segment	Matsui	Bernstein
Head and neck	63	
Trunk	52	
Upper arm	46	48.40
Forearm	42	41.74
Hand	50	
Thigh	42	38.88
Calf	42	42.26
Foot	50	

TABLE 2.4 Locations of centers of gravity of body segments expressed as percentage of total segment length as measured from proximal end for men as cited by various authors.

Segment	Cleaveland	Dempster	Matsui
Head and neck		(With trunk)	65
Trunk	53	60.4	52
Upper arm	42	43.6	46
Forearm	28	43.0	41
Hand	(With forearm)	50.6	50
Thigh	36	43.3	42
Calf	42	43.3	41
Foot	(With calf)	42.9	50

estimation of its center of gravity. Since the position of the center of gravity of the body is changed each time a body segment moves to assume a new position, the effect of this new position must be ascertained. In 1955, Cleaveland using eleven college men, determined these data on live subjects by means of water-submersion technique.

Marks on the body indicated the limits of each segment, and the body was lowered into a tank of water to each mark in succession. The weight of each segment was calculated by the weight lost and the amount of water displaced at each stage of submersion. The center of gravity of each segment was located at the point at which half the amount of weight was lost.

Kjeldsen and Morse (1977) have described significant differences in anthropometric measurements, including percentages of body segment weights, among women gymnasts, women non-gymnasts, and men. To further clarify differences, Hay (1973) presents an excellent compilation and discussion of the extensive data on **segmental body weights** and segmental centers of gravity. Partial listings of these differences are given in Tables 2.1 to 2.4. Note the similarities as well as the differences.

Limitations. Care must be taken when using the segmental method. The precision of the estimation of the center of gravity is significantly affected by the type of segmental data applied. Segmental data collected on men should not be used when analyzing the movements of women and children.

Furthermore, data from older persons, and physically disabled persons need to be acquired for a better understanding of the anatomic differences among people.

Therefore, it might be misleading to analyze the position of the center of gravity of a person based on the data from a small sample of cadavers or live subjects.

Davis (1973) found the reliability and validity of the segmental method acceptable for use in his kinematic analyses. Pike and Adrian (unpublished) used three sets of data to determine forces acting at the knee joint during kicking. Although two sets of data varied less than the third, the third set was significantly different from the other two. Thus, kinetic data, based on cadavers or other values in databases, may not be representative of the true values.

The segmental method is best used with data from the actual performer, at least submersing the limbs and estimating the trunk weight to determine center of gravity location. The segmental method, by means of the computer and without the errors of the scale method, allows the calculation of centers of gravity for many positions. Remember that the scale method requires that the person exactly duplicate the position of the movement.

Simplified Version. We will use a simplified version of the segmental method to illustrate the basic theory underlying the method. Think of three children seated on a teeterboard, with each child representing a part of one human body. For example, child 1 would be the legs, child 2 would be the head and trunk, and child 3 would be the arms of a single human body. One child weighs 240 N and is seated on the board 1 m from the fulcrum. Another child seated on the same side weighs 200 N and is 0.6 m from the fulcrum. The third child is seated on the opposite side, weighs 360 N, and is 0.8 m from the fulcrum. Since these body weights act as rotating forces, the effect of each force, multiplied by the distance from the fulcrum, is known as a moment of force. On the side where the heaviest child is seated, the moment will equal 360 N × 0.8 m, which is 288 NM. On the side where the two lighter children are seated, it will be 240 N × 1.0 m plus 200 N × 0.6 m, which equals 360 NM.

The board will not be balanced with this arrangement. The board can be balanced by using one of two possible methods. First, the positions of the children may be changed. The child weighing 360 N might be moved to a position 1.0 m from the fulcrum, and the

moment on that side of the board would equal the 360 NM moment of the opposite side. The second possibility is to move the fulcrum. To determine the distance that the fulcrum should be moved, use the percentage weight of each child in relationship to total weight of the three children to determine the force of each side:

$$240 \text{ N: } 0.30 \times 1.0 \text{ m} = 0.30 \text{ m}$$
$$200 \text{ N: } 0.25 \times 0.6 \text{ m} = 0.15 \text{ m}$$
$$\text{Total } 0.45 \text{ m}$$
$$360 \text{ N: } 0.45 \times 0.8 \text{ m} = 0.36 \text{ m}$$
$$\text{Total } 100\%$$

The difference between 0.45 and 0.36 (0.09), is the distance (in meters) that the fulcrum should be moved. The board is balanced by increasing the distance between the heaviest child and the fulcrum by 0.09 m. The distance between the fulcrum and each of the lighter children should be decreased 0.09 m. With these distances and the percentage weights, the moment values are:

$$0.30 \times 0.91 \text{ m} = 0.273 \text{ m}$$
$$0.25 \times 0.51 \text{ m} = 0.128 \text{ m}$$
$$\text{Total } 0.401 \text{ m}$$
$$0.45 \times 0.89 \text{ m} = 0.401 \text{ m}$$
$$\text{Total } 100\%$$

This proves that the center of gravity of the body (actually, the line of gravity in one plane) is 0.09 m toward the head, which is represented by the lighter children. We considered one line of gravity, as represented by the fulcrum of the teeterboard, and rejected it as not being the true balance point, or line of gravity, of the system. To find the position of the center of gravity of the total body, one may arbitrarily choose any line (which may or may not pass through some part of the body) as the line from which the position of the segmental centers of gravity will be measured. Moment-of-force values for each segment can be calculated (using percentage weights). The difference between the sums of the values on each side of the line will show the distance that the line should be moved to pass through the total-body center of gravity.

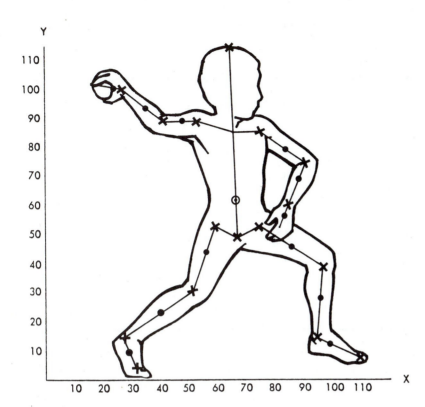

FIGURE 2.15 Tracing from film of young child throwing a ball. The center of gravity (⊙) has been determined using the segmental method. Tabulations are listed in Table 2.5. **X**, end points of segments; •, segmental centers of gravity.

To use the segmental method for determining the location of the center of gravity of the body traced from a film of a boy throwing a ball (Figure 2.15), the investigator must have the following information:

1. The percentage of total body weight of each segment (Tables 2.1 and 2.2).
2. The location of the center of gravity in each segment, usually reported as a percentage of the total segment length as measured from the proximal end of the segment (Tables 2.3 and 2.4).
3. The horizontal and vertical distance of each body segment center of gravity from a vertical and horizontal axis in the form of an x- and y-coordinate system (Figure 2.15).

The steps to follow in calculating the total-body center of gravity from a projected film image are:

1. Project the image onto a piece of graph paper and trace the performer.
2. Establish a coordinate system on the graph paper in such a way that the origin is in the lower left-hand corner (Figure 2.15). This confines all the data to the upper right quadrant, where all x- and y-coordinate values will be positive.
3. From the picture, select two reference points (stationary objects) that can be viewed in all the frames to be analyzed for a given performance, for example, the center of a wall clock or an electric wall socket.
4. Record the x- and y-coordinate values of the two reference points from the graph paper. In analyzing future frames of this same performance, these reference coordinate values must be exactly the same.
5. Record the x- and y-coordinate values of each of the following segmental end points:
   a. Tragus of the ear (cartilage anterior of ear opening)
   b. Sternal notch
   c. Crotch
   d. Right shoulder
   e. Right elbow
   f. Right fingertips (distal point of right fingertips)

Static and Dynamic Posture   **37**

TABLE 2.5 Segmental center of gravity locations determined for position of body and coordinate reference frame in Figure 2.15. Weighted values used in this determination were averages from data listed in previous tables. These weighted values were multiplied by the appropriate coordinate values of each segmental center of gravity to obtain the X value weighted and Y value weighted.

Segment	% of body weight	X-coordinate	X value weighted	Y-coordinate	Y value weighted
Head and neck		(With trunk)		(With trunk)	
Trunk	51.4	65.0	33.41	76.0	39.01
Upper arm (left)	3.0	81.5	2.45	81.0	2.43
Forearm (left)	1.6	88.0	1.41	69.5	1.11
Hand (left)	0.17	83.5	0.50	57.0	0.34
Thigh (left)	12.8	83.5	10.77	48.0	6.19
Calf (left)	4.7	95.5	4.58	30.0	1.44
Foot (left)	1.5	99.0	1.49	13.0	0.20
Upper arm (right)	3.0	48.0	1.44	89.0	2.67
Forearm (right)	1.6	35.0	0.56	93.0	1.49
Hand (right)	.50	23.5	0.14	101.0	0.61
Thigh (right)	12.9	55.5	7.16	44.5	5.74
Calf (right)	4.8	41.0	1.97	24.0	1.15
Foot (right)	1.5	29.0	0.44	10.0	0.15
Total body			66.32		62.53

g. Left shoulder
h. Left elbow
i. Left wrist
j. Left fingertips (distal point of left fingertips)
k. Right hip
l. Right knee
m. Right ankle
n. Right toe
o. Left hip
p. Left knee
q. Left ankle
r. Left toe (distal point of left toes)

These points are marked on Figure 2.15.

6. Connect the segmental end points to form a stick figure.
7. Locate the center of gravity for each segment by the following procedure:

a. Measure the segment lengths.
b. Multiply this value by the appropriate percentage from Table 2.3 or 2.4.

c. Measure this amount from the proximal end of the segment. Mark this spot as the center of gravity for the segment; that is, if the trunk and head measure 10 cm, then the center of gravity for this segment would be $0.604 \times 10 = 6.04$, or 6.04 cm from the crotch (using Dempster data on men, Table 2.2).
d. Repeat the procedure for all segments.

8. Record all the x- and y-coordinate values for each segment's center of gravity.
9. Multiply the x values for each segment's center of gravity by the percentage of the total body weight contributed by that segment (Table 2.3). Sum these values. This sum represents the location of the center of gravity of the total body in the x, or horizontal, plane.
10. Repeat step 9, using the y values for each segment's center of gravity.
11. The x- and y-coordinate total-body center of gravity can be located on the graph paper. Table 2.5 contains sample coordinate values on the image in Figure 2.15.

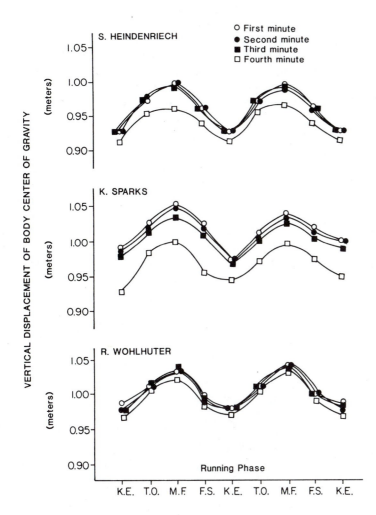

FIGURE 2.16 Vertical displacement (measured from the ground) of body center of gravity of runners was calculated by the segmental method for four positions during each of two cycles each minute in a four-minute-mile run. Only during the fourth minute did the runners show effect of fatigue. The reduced vertical displacement differed among the runners and was due to greater flexion at the knees and general alteration of running style. K.E., knees even; T.O., toe off; M.F., midflight; F.S., foot strike.

(From Sparks, K. E. 1975. Physiological and mechanical alterations due to fatigue while running a four-minute mile on treadmill, Ph.D. dissertation, Indiana University.)

Graphing the Center of Gravity

These measures and calculations illustrate a method to depict the path of the body's center of gravity in any skill. Sparks (1975) used this procedure, as seen in Figure 2.16. To use the method there must be a vertical and a horizontal reference line, neither of which has to pass through some part of the body, as did the lines in the illustration. The number of film frames necessary to determine the path depends on whether the body is in flight or whether segments are changing position while the body is supported on a stationary base.

Once contact with the supporting surface has been broken and the body is in flight, the path of the center of gravity is determined by the velocity and direction imparted to it at takeoff and by gravitational pull. It is now a projectile and can be treated as such. The line of flight can be found by the method described in Appendix C. Once the body is in flight, no segmental movement will affect the path of the center of gravity. Therefore, it is necessary to locate the center of gravity at only two points (and the corresponding times). One point must always be the first frame in which contact has been broken—in which the body has just begun its flight. The second can be any frame before landing, but it is better to select a frame as far as possible from the first. The frame selected depends on the number of frames in the film. The second frame should be as far as possible from the first because there are always likely to be measurement errors; the longer the time and the distance measured, the smaller the percentage of error. Since the in-flight path of the center of gravity will be a parabolic curve, the equation for that curve can be calculated from any two points on the curve. In this text, when we report direction and velocity of body projections, we have determined them by this method.

When the path of the center of gravity is depicted while the base is stationary and segments are moving, its position should be found in every film frame. In such situations, the center of gravity is not a projectile, and movement of a segment will affect its path. To determine the path of the center of gravity in the takeoff phase of a standing long jump, Johnson (1958) drew the vertical reference line through the metatarsophalangeal joints and the horizontal line along the bottom of the toes. At the time the heels left the floor, she found the center of gravity to be 72.6 cm (28.6 in.) above the floor and 7.6 cm (3 in.) ahead of the metatarsal joints. As the flexion occurred at knees and hips and the arms moved downward from the height of the backswing, the center of gravity moved downward and forward to a position 55.6 cm (21.9 in.) above the floor and 26.4 cm (10.4 in.) ahead of the metatarsophalangeal joints.

At takeoff, the center of gravity was 74.4 cm (29.3 in.) above the floor and 57.9 cm (22.8 in.) ahead of the metatarsophalangeal joints. Note that, interestingly, the center of gravity was ahead of the toes at the time the heels were raised—a further indication that gravitational pull, not muscle action, tilts the body (raising the heels). As the muscles act and move body segments, the position of the center of gravity is changed so that it is outside the base of support, and the body falls forward, a fall that is controlled by the ankle extensors.

Calculations to determine the center of gravity by this method involve a relatively long and involved process. Yet actually working a few calculations will further your understanding of the effect of segmental positions. If films are not available, various positions can be taken on the gravity board. For example, the subject either may stand on the board in a stride position with feet separated at a measured distance and trunk flexed at a measured angle or may lie on the board with upper and lower limbs held at measured angles to the trunk. Researchers can then compare segmental calculations with scale determinations.

For more extensive studies, recently developed techniques reduce the amount of work necessary. Motion analyzers and digitizers used in conjunction with computers (on-line or separate) can greatly increase the number of frames a researcher can analyze in a given time.

Human beings possess a diversity of physical (anatomic) characteristics. It is no wonder that researchers, teachers, coaches, physical therapists, and others concerned with education in and improvement of human movement have attempted to relate anatomic characteristics to movement-performance achievements. A new scientific discipline, focusing on the measurement of size, shape, proportion, composition, maturation, and gross function in relation to growth, exercise, performance, and nutrition, has emerged. Termed kinanthropometry, this new discipline is closely aligned with ergometry, the measurement of work of muscles.

In summary, some key comments about the center of gravity in the movement environment relative to **stability** and **mobility** are listed as follows:

1. If center of gravity is lower, the position is more stable; if higher, the position is more mobile.
2. If the size of the base of support is wider, then the body is more stabile. Stability is increased by flexing at the knees and moving the feet farther apart.
3. Size of feet affects mobility and stability; if they are large, there is more stability and less mobility.
4. Positioning the body so that its center is near the edge of the base, but still within the gravitational line, gives some stability and some instability for fast action.
5. The center of gravity is at times outside the body. A sprinter explosively pushes against the starting blocks. A high jumper drapes the body around the bar to clear it.
6. Movement of the limbs changes the position of the center of gravity, affecting the stability and mobility.

MINI-LABORATORY LEARNING EXPERIENCE

1. On graph paper, trace the outline (contourogram) of a performer from one frame of a film, mark the joints, and draw line segments between the joints. Using the segmental method described in this chapter, determine the center of gravity in two planes of the performer, as traced.
2. Using the scale method described in this chapter, determine the center of gravity in three planes of two human beings:
   a. in the anatomic position
   b. in a track starting position
   c. in a posture of your choice

References

Braune, W., and Fischer, O. 1889. Ueber den schwerpunkt des menchilichen korpers mit ruchsicht auf die austtustrung des deutschen infanteristerm. *Abb. D. K. Sachs Ges, Wiss.* 15–2.

Cleaveland, H. G. 1955. The determination of the center of gravity in segments of the body. Ph.D. dissertation, University of California, Los Angeles.

Croskey, M. I., et. al. 1922. The height of the center of gravity in man. *Am. J. Physiol.* 61(171).

Davis, M. 1973. Quality of data collected by the segmental analysis technique. Ph.D. dissertation, Indiana University.

Dawson, P. M. 1935. *The physiology of physical education.* Baltimore: Williams & Wilkins.

Hasselkus, B. R. 1974. Variations in the postural sway related to aging in women. Ph.D. dissertation, University of Wisconsin.

Hay, J. G. 1973. The center of gravity of the human body. *Kinesiology,* vol. III, AAHPER.

Hellebrandt, F. A., and Franseen, E. B. 1943. Physiological study of the vertical stance of man. *Physiol. Rev.* 23(220).

Hellebrandt, F. A., Riddle, K. S., and Fries, E. C. 1942. Influence of postural sway on stance photography. *Physiotherapy Rev.* 22(88).

Hellebrandt, F. A., Tepper, R. H., Braun, G. I., and Elliott, M. C. 1938. The location of the cardinal anatomical orientation planes passing through the center of weight in young adult women. *Am. J. Physiol.* 121(465).

Hewes, G. W. 1957. The anthropology of posture. *Sci. Am.* 196:122–28.

Hines-Woollacott, M. 1990. Changes in posture control across the life span: A systems approach. *Physical Therapy* 70(12):799–807.

Howell, A. B. 1944. Speed in animals. Chicago: University of Chicago Press.

Hudson, J. 1987. POSSUM. Paper presented at AAHPER convention, Las Vegas, NV.

Johnson, B. P. 1958. An analysis of the mechanics of the takeoff in the standing broad jump. Ph.D. dissertation, University of Wisconsin.

Joseph, J. 1960. Man's posture—electromyographic studies. Springfield, IL: Charles C. Thomas.

Kjeldsen, K., and Morse, C. 1977. In *Research reports,* vol. 3, eds. M. Adrian and J. Brame. Washington, DC: American Association for Health, Physical Education and Recreation.

Metheny, J. E. 1952. *Body dynamics.* New York: McGraw-Hill.

Miller, D., et al. 1990. Kinetic and kinematic characteristics of 10-M platform performances of elite divers. *Inter J. Sports Biomechanics* 6(3):283–308.

Morton, D. J., and Fuller, D. D. 1952. *Human locomotion and body form.* Baltimore: Williams & Wilkins.

Palmer, C. E. 1944. Studies of the center of gravity in the human body. *Child Dev.* 15(99).

Pike, N., and Adrian, M. 1985. Effect of body segment parameter data upon generated kinetic parameters. In *Abstracts of research papers,* ed. E. Haymes, p. 46. Reston, VA:AAHPERD.

Plagenhoef, S. 1971. Patterns of human motion. Englewood Cliffs, NJ: Prentice-Hall.

Reynolds, E., and Lovett, R. W. 1909. Method of determining the position of the center of gravity in relation to certain bony landmarks in the erect position. *Amer. J. Physiol.* 24.

Sparks, K. E. 1974. Physiological and mechanical alterations due to fatigue while performing a four-minute mile. Ph.D. dissertation, Indiana University.

Waterland, J. C., and Shambes, G. M. 1970. Biplane center of gravity procedures. *Percept. Mot. Skills* 30:511.

Yeadon, M. 1989. Twisting techniques used in freestyle aerial skiing. *Inter. J. Sports Biomechanics* 5(2).

3 The Human Structural System

The *skeleton* is the framework of the body and is composed of the bones and cartilages. In biomechanical terms, certain parts of the body move by means of muscle contraction. The skeletal parts, such as the hands, actually propel objects such as a ball. The biomechanist analyzes these movements of the skeleton to gain information about the action.

Human beings and other animals do not choose their structure; each structure is inherited. Within limits, structure can be modified by environment, exercise, and nutrition through a process of adaptation. Movements have inherent limitations imposed by the structure of bone, muscle, joints, and nerve innervations. We say that structure influences function, and function influences structure. For example, the tall, thin high jumper and the small monkey in a zoo have inherited different structures. But they have also modified these structures to be able to perform what they best like to do. The high jumper will most likely have a somewhat longer and stronger takeoff leg (if the jumper is right-footed) than left leg. The monkey will have a bilaterally developed strong shoulder girdle and arm muscles. It is important to understand this interrelationship because movements are produced by forces, and forces, in turn, act on body structures.

■ An understanding of the structure of bones and joints is part of the foundation of movement. It is called the muscle-bone lever system.

Framework of the Skeleton

Skeletons of modern terrestrial forms have many similarities. Differences exist in the number of bones and in the types of articulations between the bones that limit the types of locomotion and manipulation possible by any given species. The human skeleton has more than 200 bones, with 126 forming the appendicular skeleton comprising the bones of the upper and lower extremities (Figure 3.1). The appendicular skeletons of hoofed quadrupeds, however, have fewer bones. Because of this, these animals lack versatility in manipulation skills. On the other hand, the lack of a clavicle in the cat allows it to leap farther than would be possible with a clavicle limiting the flexion of its forelimbs.

Joints

Bones articulate with other bones to produce joints. They are important to the biomechanist since they are the locations of movement. Arthrology, the study of

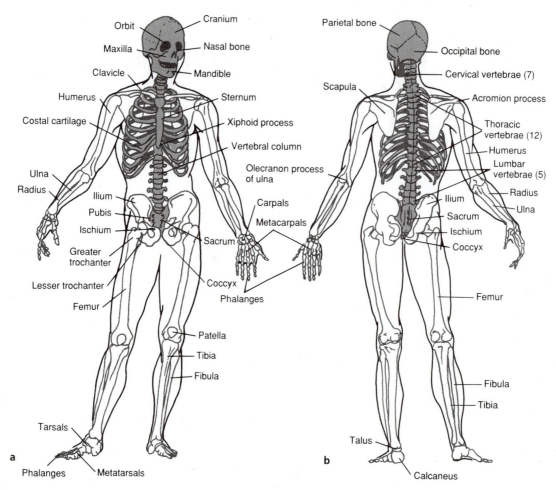

FIGURE 3.1 Anterior view (*a*) and posterior view (*b*) of human skeleton.
(Adapted from Anthony, C. P., and Thibodeau, G. A. *Textbook of anatomy and physiology,* 13th ed. St. Louis: Mosby.)

joints, often begins with the classification of the six major types of diarthrodial joints (Figure 3.2) that are important to movement analysis:

1. The gliding joint (arthrodia), in which either the bones glide over one another or one or more bones glide over another bone, is best illustrated by the articulating surfaces of the vertebrae and the tarsal and carpal bones. Most of the movement between any two surfaces is extremely small, but may be large in the entire segment, such as the whole foot. Each small movement is added to the movement from adjacent joints to achieve a wide range of movement.

2. The hinge joint (ginglymus), in which one surface is round, with a knob-like end that fits into another concave surface, usually moves in only one plane about a single axis. This hinge-like movement is exemplified by the elbow joint as it moves in flexion and extension in the sagittal plane.

3. The ball-and-socket joint (enarthrosis) can move in many planes and many axes. The spherical head of one bone fits into the hollowed concave surface of the other bone, such as the head of the femur fitting into the acetabulum of the hip. This triaxial joint has many actions, such as extension, flexion, abduction, adduction, circumduction (the combined movement

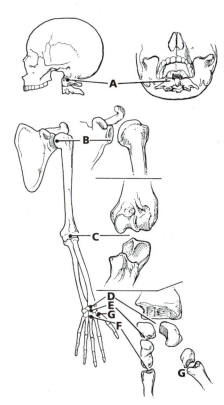

FIGURE 3.2 Major types of diarthrodial joints with respect to articulating surfaces are depicted for the upper extremity and head-neck joint. (a) pivot (atlantoaxial), (b) ball-and-socket (shoulder, also termed humero-scapular), (c) hinge (elbow, also termed humero-ulnar), (d) condyloid (radiocarpal), (e) gliding (intercarpal), (f) condyloid (metacarpophalangeal), (g) saddle (thumb). **Identify the types of diarthrodial joints in the lower extremities.**

of the preceding four movements), horizontal flexion and extension (also termed horizontal adduction and abduction), and rotation.

4. The condyloid joint (ovoid or ellipsoid joint) has movement similar to the ball-and-socket joint, but occurring in only two planes, sagittal and frontal (no rotation is allowed). In this joint, a more oval-shaped head (condyloid) fits into a concave surface. The articulations between the carpal bones of the wrist and the metacarpals of the fingers are examples of this joint.

5. The saddle joint (sellar joint), which may be thought of as a modified condyloid joint with greater freedom of movement, is shaped much like a western saddle, with the ends of a concave surface tipped up to form a convex surface in the other direction. This surface fits over an opposite concave-convex surface that allows for flexion, extension, abduction, adduction, and circumduction. This joint is found only in the carpal-metacarpal joint of the thumb.

6. The pivot joint (trochoid joint) permits only rotary movement about the longitudinal axis of the bone. An example of such uniaxial movement is the radius, rotating about its superior (proximal) articulation with the ulna.

These joints are classified as **diarthrodial joints.** They possess an articular cavity and have a ligamentous capsule that encases the joint and the synovial fluid, which lubricates the joint and regulates the pressure within the capsule. The articular surfaces of these joints are smooth and covered with cartilage. Two other major classifications of joints, synarthrodial and amphiarthrodial, are not discussed here because they allow negligible or no movement, although they may facilitate movement in the diarthrodial joints and cumulatively, as in the spine, have importance.

Stability of Joints

The stability of a joint is important from a safety perspective. Some joints are inherently more stable than others, particularly as one compares the high number of dislocated shoulders with the low number of dislocated hips. The type of joint and the bony articulations of the joint, including the area of bone contact, will affect stability, usually in one plane more than the others. The arrangement of the surrounding ligaments and muscles can also add stability, particularly in the knee, ankle, and shoulder joints. Atmospheric pressure, which caused a vacuum to be formed in the acetabulum of the hip, for example, also adds stability. It is important to understand that flexibility and stability are not inversely related. For example, gymnasts need great flexibility to perform the various routines, but stability is also important. For example, it helps to absorb the forces of landing and rebounding off the floor.

The flexibility and elasticity of the spine diminishes under certain conditions, including age, medication, prolonged work conditions, etc. The mini-laboratory problems deal with these conditions.

1. Do we become shorter during the day? Measure the height of the arch of the foot with a ruler while standing immediately after rising in the morning. Repeat the measurement in the evening. What is the difference? Why?
2. Does a driver adjust the rearview mirror of a car during a day's drive? Measure the sitting height in the morning and in the evening. Are there any differences? Explain.

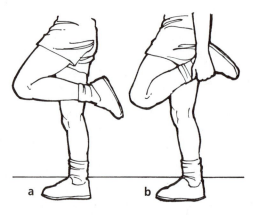

FIGURE 3.3 Range of motion is specific to body parts, orientation to gravity, and other factors. In this figure, active movement (*a*) is less than passive movement (*b*). **Under which circumstances would active movement at this joint be equal to, or greater than, passive movement?**

It is important, however, to note that gravity and other factors influence the measurement of ROM (Figure 3.3).

Range of Motion (ROM) (Flexibility)

The major movements at the primary joints are shown in Figures 3.4, 3.5 and 3.6. The types of anatomic movement are identified.

FIGURE 3.4 Basic movements and normal ranges of motion of skeleton: of the neck; and at the shoulders. The depicted body segment movements are those of the head, arm, and scapula.

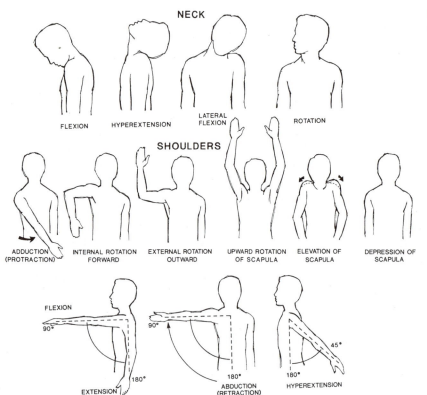

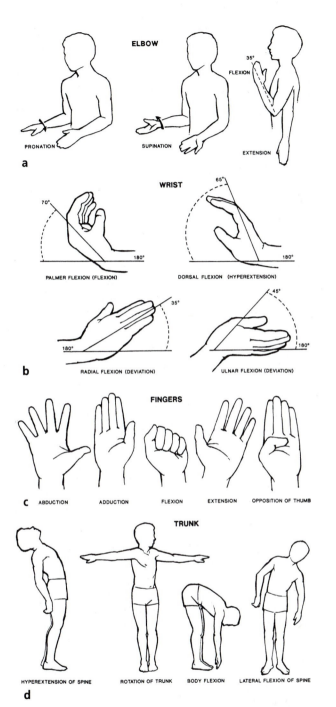

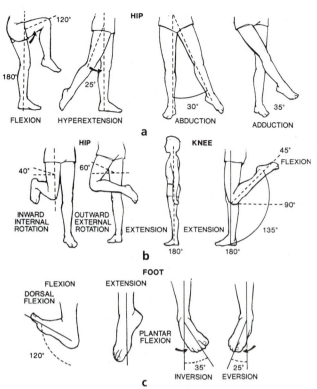

FIGURE 3.6 Basic movements and normal ranges of motion of skeleton: at the hip (a), knee (b), and ankle (c). The depicted body segment movements are those of the thigh, shank, and foot.

■ To better understand ROM, a person should move each joint both to the right and left for evaluation.

Determining Range of Motion. Many types of movements are predetermined by the structure of the joint. The **range of motion (ROM)** is determined not only by the structure of the joint, but by such factors as use, disease, injury, extensibility of muscles, tendons, and ligaments, and by the size of more distal body parts involved in the change of angle at the joint.

The arrangement and number of muscles, ligaments, and tendons surrounding a joint influence ROM at that joint. These tissues are lengthened through use, and ROM increases in the direction of lengthening. If, for example, movement is practiced in the flexion mode but never in the extension mode, ROM of flexion will increase, while ROM of extension will show a decrease.

FIGURE 3.5 Basic movements and normal ranges of motion of skeleton: at the elbow (a), wrist (b), metacarpal and interphalangeal joints (c), and spine (d). The depicted body segment movements are those of the hands and fingers, including the thumb and trunk.

The Human Structural System **47**

Likewise, an injury that separates (tears) the medial collateral ligament at the knee will cause an increased abduction capability, but no change in adduction.

Flexibility of Joints. Very young persons appear to be more **flexible** (have a greater ROM) than any other age group, and females appear to be more flexible than males. This flexibility is often measured by the use of goniometry. (See Chapter 7.) Specific flexibilities, however, may be due to specific adaptations to such factors as exercise routines. Thus, differences that appear as a result of comparisons of age or sex groups can be attributed to primary causes, such as physical activity patterns, participation in specific sports, and habitual postures of work. For example, gymnasts have greater hyperextension at the elbow, baseball pitchers have greater ROM at the wrist, and hurdlers have greater flexion at the hip than do members of an average population. Conversely, persons whose occupations involve constant sitting usually show a decrease in horizontal extension at the shoulder. The ROM at the elbow also may be reduced after a weight-training program designed to cause hypertrophy of the biceps brachii. In the case of extreme development of the biceps brachii, the ROM may be limited to 90° of flexion at the elbow, while the norm shows 120° of flexion before the tissues of the upper arm and forearm contact each other and prevent further change in the angle at the joint. Often it is lack of stretching of the other muscles crossing the joint that limits the range of motion rather than the hypertrophy of the biceps brachii.

Tendonitis, bursitis, calcium deposits in the muscle, osteoarthritis, and other disorders produce pain and resistance to movement at a joint. The ROM can be decreased, or it may be normal, but executed at a slower-than-normal speed. The contralateral (opposite) limb can be used to compare ROM lost as a result of one of these disorders. This comparison, however, may not be totally valid since asymmetry exists in most people.

Types of ROM. Two types of ROM are often determined. Active ROM is that ROM possible by voluntary muscle contraction. Passive ROM is ROM resulting from an application of some external force. Another person is

MINI-LABORATORY LEARNING EXPERIENCE

Study Figures 3.4, 3.5, and 3.6. Move (and measure) the ROM of your body parts as shown to better understand normal ranges of motion of the joints.

often the applicator of this force, pushing the joint beyond its normal active limits. As one would expect, passive ROM should always be greater than active ROM.

Active ROM can be thought of as the range through which one can apply muscular force. The greater time a person can apply a force, the greater will be the resulting impulse. Therefore, as active ROM increases, for example, shoulder flexibility of the baseball pitcher, the resulting impulse will also increase.

Bones

To paraphrase writer Gertrude Stein, a bone is not a bone is not a bone. All are different. Bones constitute the rigid structure of the body that must withstand the forces of all the muscles, tendons, and ligaments, as well as the force of gravity and external forces resulting from blows, falls, or other types of collisions. Bones are classified by their sizes and shapes into four groups. The *long bones,* those most directly involved with movement, have a long shaft with broad knobby ends. Those classified as long bones include the humerus, radius, ulna, metacarpals, phalanges, clavicle, femur, tibia, fibula, and metatarsals. *Short bones,* characterized by their short, chunky shape, include the carpals and tarsals. The *flat bones* have a large flat area for the attachment of muscles and for protection of vital structures and organs. Most flat bones (with the exception of the scapulae) enclose various bony cavities. Flat bones include the ribs, sternum, and several cranial bones. The remaining bones are called the *irregular bones,* due to their irregular shape. These include the vertebrae, sacrum, coccyx, and several facial bones.

Each bone has an outer, compact layer and an inner, cancellous (spongy) layer. The compact layer (cortex)

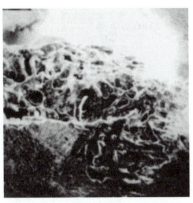

a

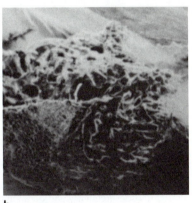

b

FIGURE 3.7 Example of trabecular structure of bone. Note the various orientations within the network as a result of stresses being applied from different directions.

usually is thicker in the cylindrical or long bones forming the appendages than in flat bones, which tend to have large muscle masses attached to them. The cancellous layer consists of a network of trabeculae (see Figure 3.7) enclosing spaces filled with blood vessels and marrow. Bones in general, and the long bones in particular (since long bones have a central cavity), acquire maximal rigidity with minimal weight of material. It is interesting to note that the skeleton accounts for approximately 16% of the total adult body weight; the skeletal muscle proportion is 40–45%! Bones, however, are approximately thirty-two times stronger than muscles!

■ Muscles, ligaments, and tendons exert tensile forces, bending moments, and tension forces on bones.

Forces Acting on Bones

Two major forces act on bones: gravity and muscles. Gravity is always present and acting on bones. It is a major compressing force on the skeleton. In addition, when muscles contract, they exert forces on bones. The forces produce stress, which is the force per unit area. The bone reacts with an equal internal resistance to the force. There are two stresses that act axially (along the longitudinal axis), tending to elongate or to compress a bone. Elongation can be produced by a force that acts to pull the bone apart; this type of stress is termed tension. The bone also becomes narrower as it elongates. The tensile deformation of bone is minuscule. The opposite deformation occurs with a force that tends to shorten and widen the bone. Pure compression and pure tension occur only if the force, also called a load, acts directly along the long axis. Otherwise a bending moment occurs, causing tension in some portions of the bone and compression in other portions. In addition, some portions may have no stress placed on them. When a material is stressed in a way that causes one part to slide over another because of a blow, this stress is termed shear. Shearing stresses also occur when a bone is twisted, due to torsional loading. Examples of various kinds of stress on bones are given in Figure 3.8.

A person in the upright position experiences compression on the skeletal system because of gravity. For example, the weight of the upper body rests on the knee, producing compression at the joint. The alignment of the bones, however, is such that true compression does not exist. Note in Figure 3.8*d* how the weight of the upper body on the hip does not act through the long axis of the femur, but produces a bending moment. The placement of the feet also determines how the line of gravity acts through the bones. Muscle forces act to produce stresses in bone, in addition to causing them to rotate. The usual result of muscle action is a bending moment that produces both compression on the concave side of the bone and tension on the convex side of the bone.

The Human Structural System **49**

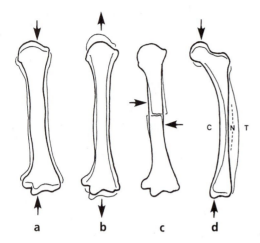

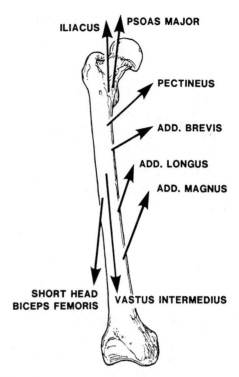

FIGURE 3.8 Forces acting on bone to produce stress are depicted by the arrows (vectors). (a) Compressive stress with potential to shorten and widen the bone; (b) tensile stress with potential to lengthen and narrow the bone; (c) shearing stress with potential to sever the bone; (d) bending moment with both tension (T) and compression (C), the mid-portion experiencing no stress (N).

MINI-LABORATORY LEARNING EXPERIENCE

1. Using a goniometer, measure the range of motion of right and left joints of selected individuals. Identify possible reasons for differences by asking about such factors as sports training, job, and previous injury.
2. Measure both passive and active ranges of motion at various joints. Which joints tend to have the greatest margins between the two measurements? What factor(s) could be limiting the ranges of motion at each joint?

The effect of muscle force and the interplay of muscles on a single bone is complex and interesting. It is valuable to compare the shape of the humerus and that of the femur, for example, by drawing the muscle force vectors and gravitational line vector representing the bone weight. The reason for a normally curved femur, compared with a straight humerus, can clearly be identified in Figure 3.9.

FIGURE 3.9 Muscle forces depicted as vectors capable of deforming and bending the femur. The deformation is influenced by such factors as amount of collagen in bone, amount of potential tensile force in each muscle, frequency and duration of muscular force production, and angle of pull of muscle.

Many materials of the body have a linearly elastic characteristic; that is, they deform at a measurable rate for each increment of stress up to or approaching the breaking point of the material. The result of forces acting on materials is deformation. If the deformation tolerances of the material are exceeded, the material will break. The deformation per unit length is termed strain. Fractures of bone, even the large femur, have occurred simply due to excessive strain caused by muscular force applied at such an angle to overcome the tolerances of the bone (Figure 3.9).

Bone Strength

Bone tissue is anisotropic in nature. Its ability to withstand stress varies according to the direction and site of application of force.

Bones are strongest in compression, next strongest in tension, and least strongest in shear. When a bending moment occurs, the fracture occurs on the tensile side. Take a piece of wood (pencil, ruler, or stick), hold it at each end, and bend it. Notice where the stress fracture appears initially. The same phenomenon is true for ligaments, tendons, and muscles. Although figures are not available on human tolerances in life, the limits of bone strength (ability to withstand stress) have been estimated from cadavers (Nordin and Frankel 1989). For example, in a femur, the limits are: compression, 1406 to 2109 N/cm^2 (20,000 to 30,000 psi); tension, 703 to 1406 N/cm^2 (10,000 to 20,000 psi); and shear 281 N/cm^2 (4000 psi). Naturally, these values differ for each bone and each person. They also differ when rate of loading varies; the higher the rate, the more energy is stored and the less likelihood of bone failure. Physical exercise can increase the strength of bones; disease often decreases it. Fatigue also increases the potential for bone failure, as noted by the skeletal injuries in thoroughbred race horses during the last 25% of a mile race.

The hardness, compressive strength, and rigidity of bone are due to its mineral content. The tensile strength and elasticity of bone—that is, its ability to revert to original form after deformation—are due to the presence of collagen. Young bone is mainly collagenous. With age, the collagen content is reduced, and bone minerals, primarily calcium and phosphate, are increased to constitute 60% to 70% of adult bone. Mineral salts provide strength to withstand compressive loads. Water, primarily in a bound state, constitutes 25% to 30% of adult bone. In old age, the mineral content of bone is reduced, and breaking strength decreases as a result of further loss of collagen, which causes the bone to become brittle and hard, not flexible. The changes in this deformation-strength relationship with age are depicted in Figure 3.10.

Normal Growth of Bones in Children

The bones of infants are mostly cartilaginous and very elastic. Because of this they deform readily, although breakage is rare. As the upright position is achieved, the spinal column, which is C-shaped at birth, begins to acquire the characteristic S-shaped appearance seen in the adult. The weight of the head, the position of the ribs anteriorly to the spinal column, the movement of the arms,

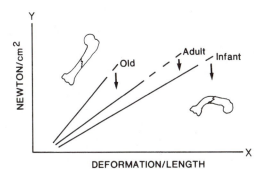

FIGURE 3.10 Changes in stress and strain characteristics of bone with age. Stress is measured on Y-axis, and strain on X-axis. Fracture is depicted with vertical vector, and shape of bone at fracture point is depicted for the old and the young.

and the tilting of the pelvis to a functional sitting position all produce forces that remodel the shape of the spinal column. No two spinal columns are alike. Heredity, nutrition, and specific postures that cause forces to act along certain lines with respect to the spinal column result in differing degrees of curvature in the cervical, thoracic, lumbar, and sacral regions.

Once the child begins to walk, a bowlegged appearance is noted. Since the bones of the legs also tend to deform with body weight, the amount and permanency of bowleggedness depends on the calcium content in the bones, the laying down of new bone in response to the bending moment caused by the upright posture, and other factors. Permanent bowleggedness and other bone deformities affect movement patterns and the ability to perform certain types of movements.

An extreme remodeling of the fibula has been reported in a boy born without a tibia. The fibula (which is not a weight-bearing bone) was made to bear the body weight. After the boy learned to walk, a second x-ray film revealed that the fibula had taken on the normal shape of a tibia.

Ridges, tuberosities, and other protuberances existing at the site of muscle or tendon attachments on the bone are a direct response to the tensile stress at the site. The size of these bony landmarks might well be an indication of early muscle use and strength. The strength of the bone can be exceeded, and sports injuries to young children have included bone pieces being separated from the rest of the bone. Such an injury, called avulsion, occurs at the site of a muscle (or tendon) attachment when the muscles have become too strong too early in relation to the bone strength.

A common site of injury to the long bones is the epiphyseal plate. This plate is a cartilaginous ring separating the long shaft of the bone from the bulbous end (epiphysis). Until this cartilage ossifies (is replaced by bone), it represents a weakness in the otherwise ossified bone and is a probable site for dislocation during instances of trauma to the bone. This cartilage, representing an amphiarthrodial articulation, normally ossifies after puberty, usually before the age of 21 years, but may vary in specific bones.

Ossification of Bones

The primary center for ossification in long bones is the center of the shaft, the diaphysis. As the bone ossifies the center enlarges, spreading towards the ends of the bone where it will eventually meet with the secondary centers, the epiphyses, which are also expanding. The epiphyseal plate separates these centers until ossification is complete, leaving an epiphyseal line on the surface of the bone.

The bones are weakest at the growth plate before ossification. This is why contact sports pose one of the greatest risks of bone fractures to children. Large children are often placed in positions of high injury risk due to their size. A sizable body does not mean that the young bones are mature (ossified). Having large children assume the position of the base of a pyramid in gymnastics, for example, may be very dangerous to their bones, notably the epiphyseal plates.

Bones of Elderly Persons

The later decades of life are high-risk decades with respect to bone fractures. If osteoporosis, or loss of bone minerals, occurs, fractures may occur as a result of forces no greater than those experienced during normal activities of daily living. Since bones protect body organs, act as part of the movement system, and support body weight of terrestrial species, damage to the bones because of their inability to cope with the forces acting on them is a vital concern.

Bone Responses to Treatment, Immobilization, and Changes in Environment

When slight tensile stress is placed on a fractured bone, the bone heals faster and becomes stronger than it does without this stress. Conversely, a bone that is immobilized begins to atrophy, bone cells are resorbed, and the bone loses strength. The influence of gravity as a stressor was recognized when the astronauts returned from space, where the strong gravitational force of the earth was not present. The loss in mineral content—the strength substances of bone—was measurable. This destruction of bone is of major concern to the biomechanist because of increased space travel and the possibility of living in space.

Effects of Sports and Physical Work on Bones

People participating in unilateral sports such as tennis, bowling, baseball (especially a baseball pitcher), and racquetball typically show asymmetric development of bones. The tennis arm shows hypertrophied bones as well as muscles. The bones and muscles of the jumping leg of high jumpers also are hypertrophied. A male high jumper, whose performance was in the 2 m (6½ ft.) range, was able to execute a standing vertical jump twice as high with the left (takeoff) leg as with the right leg. By measuring the girth of the thigh and the diameter of the shank and knee, researchers were able to indirectly measure bone and muscle size. Differences between these anthropometric measurements of the legs corresponded to the differences between the jumping performances.

In summary, bones may be strong or weak, depending on the stresses placed on them. Muscles pulling against weak bones have caused bone fractures, especially in baseball pitching, javelin throwing, and hand grenade throwing. These fractures are due to torsion on the bone. **Torsion** involves a twisting or turning of the bone with one end fixed and is primarily a shearing stress on the bone.

Ethnic and Racial Influence

Although data concerning ethnic or racial influences on bone density are not conclusive, blacks have been found to have denser and, therefore, stronger bones than whites. Men, both whites and blacks, have denser bones than women. The effect of exercise cannot be ruled out as a factor in these differences, since many of the population samples consisted of active, low-income blacks and more affluent, sedentary whites. One study in South Africa indicated that diet was an important influence on bone density. Affluent, presumably better-nourished blacks floated in water as easily as did whites, while the less affluent blacks showed the generally accepted characteristics of low fat, dense bones, and decreased ability to float. Caution is advised when attempting to link a cause and effect to bone strength and ethnic groups.

References

Adrian, M. J. 1981. Flexibility in the aging adult. In *Exercise and aging: The scientific basis,* eds. E. L. Smith and R. C. Serfass. Papers presented at the American College of Sports Medicine annual meeting, Las Vegas, 1980. Hillside, NJ: Enslow Publishers.

Barha, J. N., and Wooten, E. P. 1973. *Structural kinesiology.* New York: Macmillan.

Bosco, C., and Komi, P. V. 1982. Muscular elasticity in athletes. In *Exercise and sport biology,* Champaign, IL: Human Kinetics Publishers.

Butler, D. L., Grood, E. S., Noyes, F. R., and Zernicke, R. F. 1979. Biomechanics of ligaments and tendons. In *Review of exercise and sports sciences,* vol. 6, ed. R. Hutton. Philadelphia: Franklin Institute Press.

Hill, A. V. 1965. *Trails and trials in physiology.* Baltimore: Williams and Wilkins.

Hoeltzel, D. A. 1986. *Orthopedic biomechanics: Keys to the skeleton, mechanical engineering.* New York: Columbia University Press.

Kapandji, I. A. 1974. *The physiology of the joints.* Vol. 3, *The trunk and the vertebral column.* New York: Churchill Livingstone.

Kulig, K., Andrews, J. G., and Hay, J. G. 1984. Human strength curves. *Exercise and Sports Sciences Reviews* 12.

Lindh, M. 1989. Biomechanics of the lumbar spine. In *Basic biomechanics of the musculoskeletal system,* eds. M. B. Nordin and V. H. Frankel. Philadelphia: Lea and Febiger. Also see several other authors in the same book on structural aspects of the human body.

Nordin, M. B., and Frankel, V. H. 1989. *Basic biomechanics of the musculoskeletal system.* Philadelphia: Lea and Febiger.

4 Human Movement Assembly: Muscle-Bone Lever System

This chapter presents the lever system and its component parts. The biomechanical linkage of anatomy to motion and forces acting to produce or prevent movement is described and analyzed. Some mathematics is required to understand the role muscles play in lever action. This chapter's discussion also assumes a basic knowledge of basic human anatomy. The concept of moment arms is essential in analyzing human movement.

Early biomechanists likened the movement apparatus of living bodies to a lever system. Bones were levers rotated by muscles and external forces. Anatomically, each animal and human is born with muscle attachments at particular sites. During body growth and development, the muscles increase in strength, the bones become larger and longer, particularly in the case of the appendages, and the weights of the body segments change. Therefore, the effectiveness of the lever system also changes. During extremely rapid growth periods, such as during puberty in humans, the lever system may seem unwieldy and unfamiliar to the person. The individual must learn again how to use the body. A good example of this is top Olympic-caliber female gymnasts, who were champions at age 14 yet appeared less skilled one or two years later because of changes in distribution of segmental weights and because of longer levers.

This chapter is designed to explain lever systems and their functions, to show effective and efficient use of the muscle-bone lever systems, and to provide a method for analyzing those lever systems.

Definition of a Lever

A **lever** is a machine, a device, for transmitting energy; it is able to do work when energy is transmitted through it. In the human body, energy derived from muscular contraction is applied to the bones, resulting in movement of the body segments. These segments may transmit energy to external objects more efficiently than is possible without a lever system. Figures 4.1 and 4.2 will help you visualize human levers.

■ The lever is commonly defined as a rigid bar that revolves about an axis, or fulcrum.

Identifying Human Levers

There are two basic lever systems. In the first, the forces act at points on both sides of the axis, as in a teeterboard. In the second, the forces act on only one side of the axis, as in a door that rotates about its hinges. The latter is usually subdivided into two types, depending on which of the opposing forces, effort or resistance, is closer to the axis. These three types of lever systems are shown in Figures 4.1 and 4.2.

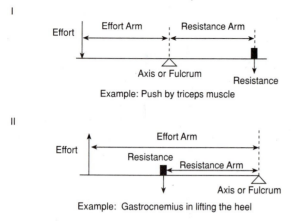

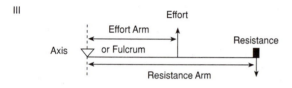

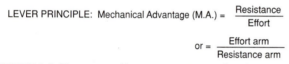

LEVER PRINCIPLE: Mechanical Advantage (M.A.) = $\dfrac{\text{Resistance}}{\text{Effort}}$

or = $\dfrac{\text{Effort arm}}{\text{Resistance arm}}$

FIGURE 4.1 Three types of lever systems. Universal use.

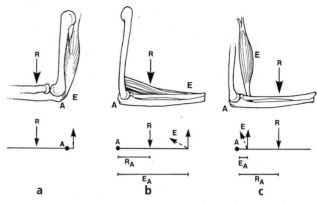

FIGURE 4.2 Types of lever systems relative to the human body. (a) First class—axis lies between effort (E) and resistance (R); (b) second class—resistance lies between axis and effort; (c) third class—effort lies between axis and resistance. EA, effort arm; RA, resistance arm.

In the body, the location of the axis or the fulcrum is readily identified as a line (axis) passing through, or a point (fulcrum) within, the joint in which the movement occurs. Since these joints have widths, and since the bones forming a joint have one or more contact points, such as condyles, the concept of an axis of rotation is more reasonable than that of a fulcrum.

Identification of the rigid bar may be more difficult if the word *bar* suggests a straight mass whose length is considerably greater than its width or thickness. The word *rigid,* too, may present difficulties if it suggests an undivided, continuous mass. It is important to realize that external levers can vary in shape and structure. A hammer can be used as a lever in both driving in and pulling out a nail. Yet the hammer is neither a straight bar nor an undivided mass; the head need only be securely attached to the handle. Even the common crowbar, often cited as an example of an external lever, although usually one continuous mass, could be an effective device for transmitting energy even if it consisted of two or more segments bound together firmly enough to withstand the forces to which it might be subjected.

The student of biomechanics must realize that body levers may vary in shape from the traditional rigid bar. One or more bones may be bound together by muscles firmly enough for them to function as a single mass. For example, the bones of the upper and lower arms can be held together by muscles crossing the elbow joint. The bones of the entire arm, the shoulder girdle, the vertebrae, and the pelvis can be held together by muscles crossing all intervening joints. These variations from the common concept of external levers may suggest that lever identification in human movement is difficult.

Lever Elements

The following is a discussion of the different elements of a lever system.

1. The axis, A, is a real or imaginary line passing through the joint and about which the rigid mass of the limb (lever) rotates. The axis will always be perpendicular to the plane of movement of the lever.

2. The point of application of effort is the point at which the contracting muscle is attached to the moving bone.

3. The effort, *E*, is that force acting at its application site and is represented by a vector. The vector is the muscle that creates the movement volitionally. A vector is a line representing a physical quantity that has magnitude and direction, such as acceleration or force. This is distinguished from a scalar which is definable by a single number or point. A scalar has magnitude but no direction.

4. The effort arm is the moment arm for the effort; that is, the distance from the axis to the site of muscle attachment. All the parts of the rigid mass of the lever between the axis and the point of application of effort compose the effort arm. However, the measurement of the effort arm is the perpendicular distance from the axis to the effort, not the curvature or other conformation distance along the bone.

5. The point of application of resistance is the point at which the external object, or the center of gravity of the mass of the lever, is applied.

6. The resistance, *R*, is that force acting at its application site that is represented as a vector having the opposite direction to that of the effort. In the case of the first-class lever system, the direction is the same, but the effect on the lever is opposite. For example, if the effort direction and site of application cause clockwise rotation, the resistance causes counterclockwise rotation.

7. The resistance arm is the moment arm for the resistance; that is, the distance from the axis to the resistance vector. All the parts of the rigid mass of the lever lying between these two points compose the resistance arm. Again, the measurement of the resistance arm is the perpendicular distance from the axis to the resistance vector. Thus, all three lines —axis, resistance vector, and resistance arm—are mutually perpendicular. Note that in Figure 4.2 all the axes are horizontal, the resistance and effort vectors are vertical, and the moment arms (resistance and effort) are horizontal, but at right angles to the axes. Movement occurs in the plane of the effort and resistance vectors.

In descriptions of the body levers, we will not precisely locate the points E and R. This is because the attachment of a muscle necessarily covers more than one point, or there can be two or more muscles involved in the lever system. We must select an average position arbitrarily. Likewise, R may also cover more than one point. In addition, there are usually at least two resistances; one is the weight of the segment, and the other is an external object, such as a ball. The axis, too, may cause some problems in analysis, since the axis may be a line of intersection of the body and an external object, such as the foot with the floor or the hands with the vaulting horse. Also, some bones may be moving along more than one axis simultaneously. Isolating each movement with the corresponding locations of E and R is very complex. This lack of precision, however, will not prevent you from understanding the lever action in the body or from using the basic concepts of lever systems in analyzing human and animal movements.

Function of Bony Levers

As previously stated, the bony lever, together with the forces acting on this lever, is known as a lever system. If bone and muscle were isolated from the body, the lever system would resemble Figure 4.3.

In Figure 4.3 muscle M attaches to bones V and H. The action of the muscle is one of shortening. The result of this muscle shortening may be movement (rotation) of bone V and bone H, of only bone V, of only bone H, or of neither bone. If bone H is the distal bone, it is the bone more likely to move, since its mass is apt to be less than that of the more proximal bone V. Furthermore, since the distal end of bone H is free to move, the resistance of the lever to movement is minimal. The more proximal attachment of bone V to another body segment adds additional mass to bone V, so bone V will probably remain stationary. Examples of these three movement possibilities are shown in Figure 4.5.

■ One bone or two bones can move, or no bone movement can take place, even though there is muscle contraction.

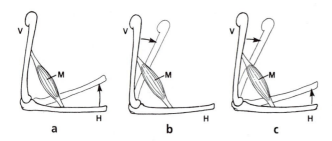

FIGURE 4.3 Effects of muscle (M) contraction on the lever system. (a) Produces movement of distal bone (H); (b) produces movement of proximal bone (V); (c) produces movement of both bones (V and H). **Under what circumstances does each occur?**

MINI-LABORATORY LEARNING EXPERIENCE

Referring again to Figure 4.2A, note that the muscle moment of force is equal in magnitude and opposite in direction of the moment of resistance created by the weight of the forearm, since no rotatory movement is occurring. As shown in Figure 4.4, the attachment of the triceps brachii is about 15 mm from the elbow joint, while the center of gravity of the body segment is approximately 195 mm from the elbow joint. Therefore, the muscle force must be thirteen times that of the weight of the body segment (remember that the moments of force must be equal in magnitude to remain in a static state). The muscle force is calculated by means of the moment-of-force, or levers equation, which states that the product of the force acting perpendicular to a lever and its perpendicular distance (moment arm) from the axis of rotation equals the moment of force about the axis. Note that the line of the muscle vector, the distance from the muscle insertion to the joint, and the axis of rotation are mutually perpendicular to each other. Referring to the coordinate system, y = muscle, x = moment arm, and z = axis. Note that the gravitational vector is also vertical, or in the y direction, its moment arm is x, and the moment of force, again, is about the z axis, but in the counterclockwise direction. What would happen to the amount of E required to hold the arm if a ball were placed in the hand? Hint: what effect does this have on RA? What if the object were moved closer to the axis at the elbow?

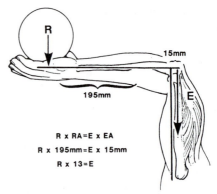

$$R \times RA = E \times EA$$
$$R \times 195mm = E \times 15mm$$
$$R \times 13 = E$$

FIGURE 4.4 Triceps muscle acting as a first class lever (R, resistance; RA, resistance arm; E, effort; EA, effort arm). The muscular effort required to hold the sphere is equal to thirteen times that of the weight of the sphere. **What implications does that have for activities involving the triceps muscle?**

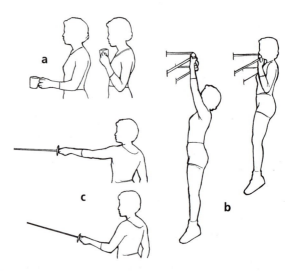

FIGURE 4.5 Examples of three movement possibilities as a result of contraction of biceps brachii. (a) Distal segment moves in lifting cup; (b) proximal segment moves in chin-up because distal end is fixed; (c) both proximal and distal segments move in fencing thrust.

When both bones move, the lever system actually becomes two lever systems, the muscle being the common force for each system. Analyzing the bone-muscle lever system is easiest on a planar level with two opposing forces. In reality, however, a complete analysis necessitates investigating moments of force in a world of three-dimensional forces.

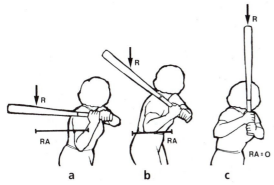

FIGURE 4.6 Three positions of bat during stance phase of batting. Resistance arms (RA) and resistance vectors (R) are depicted for ease of comparison of moments of force acting on wrists. The effort and effort arm must adjust to changes in RA. **Measure the approximate effort arm and compare it to that of the resistance arms in each of the three positions.**

Effect of Positioning of Body Segments on Resistance Arms

Figure 4.6 is an example of the important concept of "mutual perpendicularity." The figure compares the resistance moments produced in each of three options in holding a softball or baseball bat in the ready position for a pitched ball. In all options the wrists represent the axis of rotation, and the resistance arm is measured as the horizontal line (distance) from the extended line of the joint to the line of gravity of the bat. Note how the moment arm (RA) increases as the bat position changes from nearly vertical to nearly horizontal. The longer and heavier the bat (assuming that the center of gravity of the bat is in the same location, proportionally), the more muscle force will be required of the relatively small muscles acting at the wrist. Is it any wonder that the characteristic adjustment that batters make when their muscles are not strong enough for the task is to space the hands 15 to 25 cm apart? With this adjustment, the batter has introduced a first-class lever system into the ready position. The hand closest to the end exerts an opposite force to that of the weight of the bat, while the other hand, which lies between these two forces, acts as the balance point, or fulcrum. The mechanical advantage of the lever system is enhanced. The batter now uses the stronger muscles acting at the shoulder and elbow, as well as the weight of the upper arm, rather than relying on the muscles that cross the wrist.

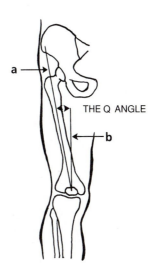

FIGURE 4.7 The Q angle showing the quadriceps muscle pull. (This is a modification of Figure 13.4 found in Atwater, A. Gender differences in distance running. In Cavanagh, P. 1990. *Biomechanics of running.* Champaign, IL: Human Kinetics. Reprinted by permission.)

MINI-LABORATORY LEARNING EXPERIENCE

Determine the resistance, effort, and resistance arms, using several different values for the angles in Figure 4.6.

The Q Angle

The Q (quadriceps) angle, illustrated in Figure 4.7, varies in degrees in many instances between males and females. In males, it generally is 10° and in females 15°. The larger the angle, the more likely it is the patella will be shifted laterally when the quadriceps contracts, for example, in running. The wider the hips, the higher the Q angle, and this explains why females tend to have higher Q angles. However, some males have wide hips and some females have narrow hips. It appears that wider hips are mechanically a disadvantage to long-distance runners. The Q angle results in the inefficient transmission of energy with respect to the lever system.

Muscles

Muscle Composition

Muscles, ligaments, and tendons produce their own forces and, in turn, may be stressed as a result of collisions to the body, shearing forces to the bone, and tensile forces greater than the tolerances of the muscles. The muscles of the body produce stresses on many body parts other than bone, including the skin, organs, and connective tissue. When muscles allow the inhalation and exhalation of air, the airflow produces stresses on the walls of the airways. Similarly, the cardiac muscle initiates blood flow, which causes arterial, capillary, and venous wall stress.

Ligaments passively restrict movement at the joint, and tendons transmit the forces of the muscle to the bone. Since muscles are the prime producers of movement, the remainder of this chapter will describe the muscles, the nature of muscle tension development, and the roles muscles play in movement.

Muscle Anatomy

Approximately 435 voluntary muscles (Figures 4.8 and 4.9) are found in the human body. According to Schottelius and Schottelius (1978), muscles constitute 43 percent of the body weight, contain more than one-third of all the body proteins, and represent approximately one-half of the metabolic activity of the resting body. Simple and complex activities are involved when the muscles are activated against the bones to which they are attached, causing the bony levers to move. Coordination and organization of these muscles in movement often involve not only individual muscles or a group of muscles, but also constituent parts of muscles. To understand muscle function, it is important to learn the basic physics, chemistry, and anatomy of muscles.

Types of Muscle. The three kinds of muscles—cardiac, smooth, and skeletal (striated)—vary by function. Cardiac and smooth muscles have similar functions, and both surround cavities and form walls of our organs. *Cardiac muscle* is the heart muscle. It has some characteristics in common with skeletal muscles and is classified as striated. However, single muscle fibers such as those noted in skeletal and smooth muscle are not obvious in cardiac muscle. *Smooth muscle* is found in blood vessels, the digestive tract, and certain other organs of the viscera. Cardiac and smooth muscles contract slowly, rhythmically, and involuntarily. *Skeletal muscles* are different. They are activated voluntarily, as well as reflexively, and their fibers contract with great rapidity. Huxley (1958) has stated that striated muscles can shorten at speeds of up to ten times their resting length in a second. Skeletal muscles are usually attached to bone and cartilage. Under an ordinary light microscope, these muscles are seen to be crossed by striations, while the smooth muscles have none.

Fiber Arrangements. There are two main types of arrangements of muscle fibers: fusiform and penniform. In the fusiform arrangement, the muscle fibers are distributed in longitudinal fashion in the muscle, allowing for maximal range of contraction. The sartorius is an example of a fusiform muscle. Its long, slender fibers are stretched between two heavy tendons. It is the longest muscle in the body and has the greatest range of contraction. The sartorius in an average-size man will shorten approximately 20 cm (8 in.) during the full action of flexion at the hip and knee joints and when turning the thigh outward. Since the muscle fibers are arranged longitudinally, there are fewer fibers in this type of arrangement than in others. With fewer fibers, muscular force is reduced. The large range of contraction is thus achieved at the sacrifice of strength. In addition, the parallel arrangement of muscle fibers permits such muscles to move body parts with great speed with a small amount of muscle shortening.

The penniform arrangement of muscle fibers is similar to that of the barbs of a feather. A tendon is the position of the quill of a feather. Variations in the penniform arrangement include demipennate, unipennate, bipennate, multipennate, and circumpennate. Some of these arrangements are illustrated in Figure 4.10. In the demipennate muscles, such as the adductor magnus, the fibers are arranged diagonally between two tendons and look like a feather cut in two along the quill. Unipennate muscles, like the semimembranosus and the extensor digitorum longus, have the muscle fibers located to one side of the tendon. Pennate muscles possess a feather-shaped fiber arrangement and include the flexor digitorum longus, peroneus tertius, and flexor pollicus longus. Fibers of bipennate muscles are double-feather shaped,

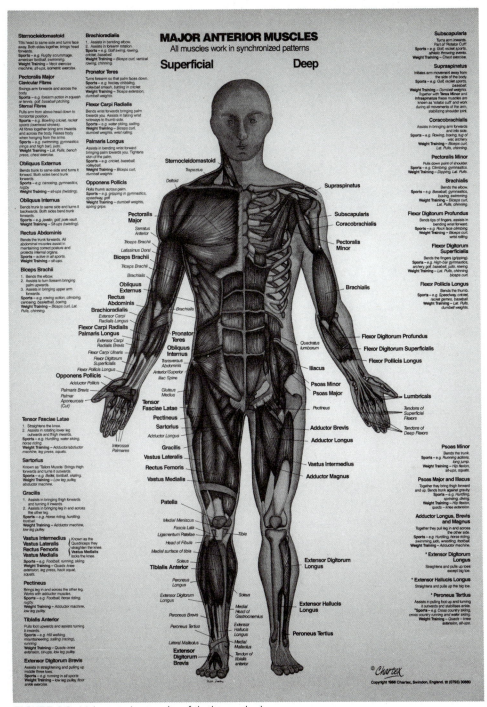

FIGURE 4.8 Major anterior muscles of the human body.
(Courtesy of Chartex.)

Human Movement Assembly: Muscle-Bone Lever System   **61**

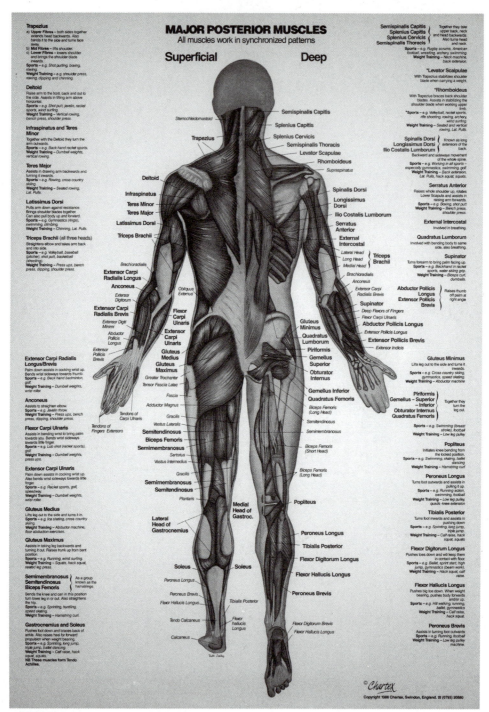

FIGURE 4.9 Major posterior muscles of the human body.
(Courtesy of Chartex.)

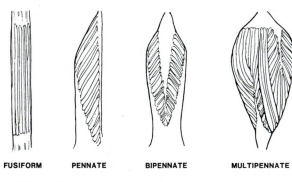

FUSIFORM   PENNATE   BIPENNATE   MULTIPENNATE

FIGURE 4.10 Fiber arrangement in skeletal muscle. **Measure the cross-sectional area orthogonal to the fiber orientation to estimate the amount of force that can be developed in each muscle.**

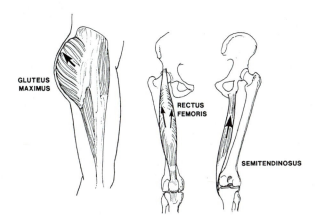

FIGURE 4.11 Force vectors representing lines of contractile forces in three muscles.

as in the vasti medialis and lateralis. Multipennate muscle fibers are found in broad muscles, such as the deltoideus and the pectoralis major.

Diagonal Pull. The diagonal pulling position of the penniform muscles allows a greater number of fibers to act in a given mass, but there is a loss in the range of contraction because these fibers are shorter. As a rule, a long sheath of tendon extends nearly the entire length of penniform muscles. In the peroneus longus, the tendinous sheath is 46 cm (18 in.) long, while the longest muscle fibers measure only 2.5 cm (1 in.). The great number of fibers available for action in the penniform muscles allows only a limited shortening of the muscle, but provides great strength.

Because muscle fibers always contract in a straight line, a three-part muscle may actually have discrete and different actions because of the manner in which its fibers are laid. This is evident in large muscles, such as the deltoideus. However, those muscles with tendinous extensions, such as those to the hand and foot as they cross the wrist and ankle to connect with each finger phalange or toe phalanx, are able to pull at a changed angle to contract in a straight line. Furthermore, in fusiform as compared to multipennate arrangement, the muscle has the advantage of long fibers, but has a narrow origin and insertion. The reverse is true in the multipennate muscle; with broad origin and insertion, muscle fibers run parallel to the contracting ones. Figure 4.11 shows force vectors (direction of muscle tension) for three muscles.

MINI-LABORATORY LEARNING EXPERIENCE

Identify two muscles that have fusiform fiber arrangements and explain how this arrangement can be of value in muscular contraction.

Do the same for pennate fiber arrangement and multipennate.

One might ask the following questions of any muscle:

1. Do muscle fibers always obey the all-or-none law? The variation comes in what all means. If the stimulus is insufficient, it will be nothing, not something.
2. Can a muscle fire a second time without a refractory period? Yes, this is the case.
3. Does myelination really come in degrees of thickness? The measure of thickness of myelin sheath has been given as 180 A. The sheath is described as lamellar, and there may be about 100 layers in a mature sheath.

Muscle Tension

The approximately 150 muscles that are directly involved in moving the levers to maintain posture or in activating movement of all or a part of the body are capable of performing a great amount of mechanical work. The amount of mechanical work done by a muscle is determined by multiplying the newtons of the load lifted by the height to which the load is lifted as measured in millimeters (or meters); the result expresses the work in newton-meters (Schottelius and Schottelius 1978). It is possible for a muscle to contract even if no mechanical work is involved. If a load is too heavy and is not lifted, the muscle has accomplished no mechanical work. The expended energy appears as heat and would be measured by the amount of oxygen consumed. The optimum load for a muscle to lift is one in which maximum work is accomplished each time the muscle contracts. On the other hand, if the muscle can barely lift the load and develops the maximal tension that it can generate in doing so, it lifts the maximal load. It is generally accepted that no muscle can do sustained work when the load that it lifts is greater than one-third to one-half of its total capacity.

It is generally believed that a muscle's strength is directly proportional to its physiological cross-section. This means that the cross-section is measured in such a way that the section is perpendicular to all the fibers of the muscle and not at another angle, as is often the case in an anatomic cross-section measurement. Thus, penniform muscles are considered stronger than quadrilateral muscles. Evans (1971), however, states, "The force which a muscle can exert when it contracts depends upon the number, length, and arrangement of its fibers, the geometric relations of the muscle fibers to the tendon, the angle of insertion of the tendon on the bone, and the distance the tendon inserts from the joint axis about which movements occur." Determining the potential strength of a muscle is a complex task.

Muscle Action. The tension a muscle can exert becomes less as the muscle shortens. It has been postulated by some that this decrease results from internal friction. Since a muscle does not liberate more heat as it rapidly shortens, however, this does not appear to be the case. Huxley (1958) states:

> When the muscle shortens, it exerts less tension: the tension decreases as the speed of shortening increases. One might suspect that the decrease of tension is due to the internal viscosity or friction in the muscle, but it is not. If it were, a muscle shortening rapidly would liberate more heat than one shortening slowly over the same distance, and this effect is not observed.

Hill (1965) has shown that a muscle does liberate more heat while shortening, but only in proportion to the distance that it shortens and not to its speed. When a muscle is stretched between two bones in such a fashion that it is elongated, it gains an advantage, in that the range of contraction is large before tension is significantly reduced (allows for greater momentum to occur).

The techniques of thermography have been used to measure changes in heat within tissues of the body. Researchers in the former USSR found the faster the movement, the more heat and the more ROM existed.

■ Muscle contraction is best understood through a study of a composite of muscle physiology and muscle biomechanics. The terms used in this section can all be found in books on these subjects.

Power is defined as the rate of work, that is, how much work is performed in a given unit of time. Maximum power is the maximum work a muscle can perform in a given unit of time. This is dependent upon the maximum rate of cross-bridge cycling at the level of actin and myosin. This bridging is a function of the total cross-sectional area of a muscle that can be activated. Power can be altered by training although it is not a linear function of total change in cross-sectional area. The angle of pull of muscle fibers may change as muscle hypertrophies (gets larger), and, thus, power and tension potential change.

Striated muscles can shorten to ten times their resting length in a second; relax in a fraction of a second (Huxley 1958). This is because each fiber of a muscle is surrounded by an electrically polarized membrane that has one-tenth of a negative volt. When an impulse travels down a nerve to the motor end plate, which is in contact with the muscle fiber, it depolarizes the membrane. A substance (probably calcium) is released throughout the fiber. Then the process of liberation of energy takes place as mentioned previously, and the fiber contracts.

Changes in Muscle Length. Changes in muscle length are shown in Figure 4.12. The amplitude of a muscle is the range from maximum contraction to maximum stretch. A muscle normally works through a range somewhat less than its total amplitude.

A muscle that shortens (when contracting) to a greater extent than another has the advantage of contracting through a great distance resulting in great speed, but

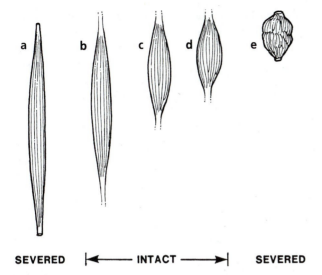

SEVERED |←——— INTACT ———→| SEVERED

FIGURE 4.12 Length of skeletal muscle in five different conditions. (*a*) Maximum resting length after distal end has been severed; (*b*) maximum length of intact muscle when elongated by pull of muscles on opposite side (according to Weber-Fick law, twice the length of condition *d*); (*c*) natural length of noninnervated muscle; (*d*) maximum shortening of intact muscle in extreme flexion (usually half the length of condition *b*); (*e*) length of maximally stimulated muscle after distal end has been severed (one-fourth to one-sixth the length of condition B).

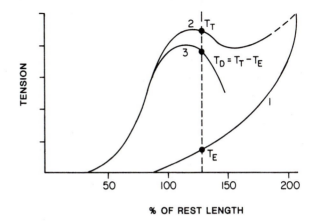

% OF REST LENGTH

FIGURE 4.13 Tension-length curves for isolated muscle. Curve 1, passive elastic tension T_E in a muscle passively stretched to increasing length; curve 2, total tension T_T exerted by muscle contracting actively from increasingly greater initial lengths; curve 3, developed tension calculated by subtracting elastic tension values on curve 1 from total tension values at equivalent lengths on curve 2, i.e., $T_D = T_T - T_E$.
(From Gowitzke, B. A., and Milner, M. 1980. *Understanding the scientific bases of human movement.* Baltimore: Williams and Wilkins.)

lacks strength in lifting a limb. The classic long-fiber muscle is the sartorius, which is reported to be able to contract a maximum of 57% of its resting length. Normally muscles with short fibers contract considerably less than this—some even less than one-third their length.

Force Development in the Muscle. The amount of force development depends on the length of an isolated muscle (Figure 4.13). In the isolated muscle, maximum developed tension occurs with the muscle slightly longer than resting length. As resting length increases, so does the series elastic component, thus reducing the developed tension in the muscle. If the muscle length is shorter than its resting length, the total tension decreases (even though the elastic tension is almost nonexistent). Below 50% of resting length the muscle is unable to develop contractile force. Our movements are often modified to take advantage of this tension-length relationship. The person performing lower-leg extensions on a universal machine leans backward (extending at the hip) as fatigue

sets in, so that the length of the rectus femoris muscle is increased and consequently its force will increase. Two-joint muscles have the advantage of being able to position one joint so that the muscle can be made more productive at the other joint.

Beyond these general applications, however, the isolated muscle experiments on which the length-tension curves are based may not have too much practical value when investigating muscle torque and power in a live human being. Perrine (1986) investigated the biophysics of maximal power output using an isokinetic device (velocity-controlled resistance-producing machine). The torque curves were ascending and descending curves, but not of the same type found by Hill (1965). Perrine's (1986) data were collected from fifteen subjects performing extensions of the lower leg (shank) at different rotational speeds. The subjects achieved peak power at a speed of 240° per second, while peak torques occurred at a much lower speed, i.e., 96° per second.

The tension-velocity curve differs at the two velocities. According to Kulig, Andrews, and Hay (1984), these two curves and a parabolic curve are common in strength curves. The parabolic curve is typical of flexion

Human Movement Assembly: Muscle-Bone Lever System   **65**

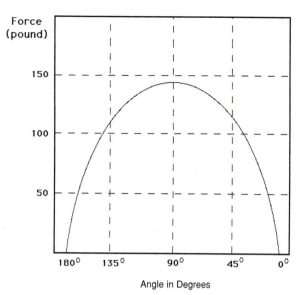

Force (pound)

Angle in Degrees

FIGURE 4.14 A force-angle curve showing graphically the effects of position using the biceps muscle as an example. The muscle-joint was gradually moved from extension to flexion. Note that a 90° angle produced the most force. The mean average of seven female subjects was recorded.
(Data collected by authors.)

at the elbow. A force-angle chart showing joint-angle position in executing movement by the biceps muscle is seen in Figure 4.14. In action, certain positions of the joint enable a muscle to create more force than at other positions.

There is an interaction between the changes in the muscle moment arm and the changes in length as the angle of the joint changes. Therefore, it is difficult to predict the exact angle at which the body will be able to produce the greatest force. This is complicated further by the fact that more than one muscle is usually contracting to produce a movement.

Recently, Herzog et al. (1991) showed that specificity in athletic running and cycling affects strength at different moment arm lengths. Cyclists were stronger during shorter than resting length, while runners tended to be stronger at longer than resting length of the muscle.

■ Strength curves can be altered by activity levels, types of activity, and ranges through which habitual intense movements occur.

Types of Muscle Contraction. Muscle contraction can be classified generally in three types: concentric, eccentric, and static. *Concentric contraction* occurs when a muscle develops sufficient tension to overcome a resistance and shortens. A body lever is moved in opposition to a given resistance. When an individual picks up an object, some of the muscles of the arm, such as the biceps brachii, contract and shorten as the object is lifted. *Eccentric contractions* may occur when muscles are used to oppose a movement, but not to stop it. An example is the action of the biceps brachii in lowering the arm gradually, whether the weight is greater than can be lifted or is a light object being slowly placed on the floor. The main characteristic is that the muscle lengthens during the action and this action is usually in the same direction as the force (for example, in line with gravity). Both concentric and eccentric contractions are called isotonic because the muscle changes length due to its own contraction during a movement with a load (Figure 4.15). Nordin and Frankel (1989) have redefined this as isoinertial, since the inertia (load) is constant.

MINI-LABORATORY LEARNING EXPERIENCE

1. Palpate the muscles of the arm and back while a person performs an isometric contraction against resistance to flexion at the elbow. Describe your findings and explain them with respect to muscle function.
2. Ask this same person to lift a heavy weight, using flexion at the elbow. Palpate the muscles and compare your findings with those in step 1.
3. Have a person perform a half or full squat, first with the trunk in an erect position and then with the trunk in a flexed position. Palpate the thigh muscles during the descending and ascending movements under these two conditions. Discuss your findings with respect to muscle function and stress to joints, including the spine.

A *static contraction* occurs when a muscle that develops tension is unable to move the load and does not change length. The effort exerted by the muscle is

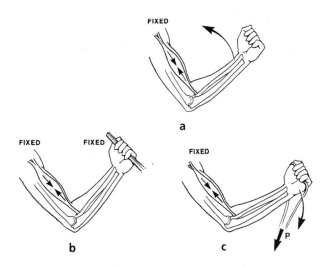

FIGURE 4.15 Concentric, isometric, and eccentric contractions of the biceps brachii muscle. (*a*) Concentric contraction to produce movement of distal segment, muscle shortens; (*b*) isometric contraction with no movement of body segments since they are restrained from responding to muscular contraction, there is no external manifestation of the minute muscle shortening; (*c*) eccentric contraction with movement caused by external force (P) acting in opposition to muscular contraction, muscle lengthens despite its attempt to shorten.

insufficient to move either when the load is too heavy or when opposing muscles contract in opposition to each other, preventing movement. This fixation of a muscle's action into a static contraction is termed **isometric** because the muscle develops tension without changing appreciable length.

Preceding a concentric contraction phase with an eccentric phase is referred to as a stretch-shortening cycle. As noted by Viitasalo, Komi, and Bosco (1984), putting the muscle under stretch in the eccentric phase enables it to store potential (elastic) energy. Bosco and Komi (1982) demonstrated the effect of this stretch-shortening cycle in vertical jumps performed with and without a counter-movement. Jumps using the counter-movement produced higher vertical jump height, average force, and power output than without the counter-movement. Furthermore, factors such as fiber composition (fast-twitch and slow-twitch fibers), length of prestretch, velocity of the stretch, and coupling time between the eccentric and concentric contractions affected the amount of potential energy. It was found that:

> Subjects rich in FT fibers in the vastus lateralis muscle benefit more from the stretching phase performed with high speed and short angular displacement (at the knee). The slow type muscle, on the other hand, may be able to retain the cross-bridge attachment longer and therefore also utilize elastic energy better in a slow type ballistic motion. (Bosco and Komi, p. 215)

The authors also noted that training was another important element in influencing force-time characteristics.

Classification of Muscles According to Function

For action to take place, the muscles of the body develop teamwork through training and practice. However, individually they can do only two things—develop tension to various degrees or relax in various manners.

Since a muscle either develops increased tension within itself or relaxes (in varying degrees), it performs various roles as action of the skeletal levers takes place. The shape, arrangement, size, and location, including whether it is a one- or two-joint muscle, the length and nature of the tendons at the insertions, the type and mechanical advantage(s) of the bone(s) to which it is attached, and the insertion's angle with and distance from the fulcrum of the action bones are all factors in determining how the muscle functions in moving its bony lever. Muscles are normally classified with regard to their direction of pull on the joint and subsequent skeletal movement. Such actions as extension, flexion, adduction, abduction, and lateral and medial rotation are classified according to the direction of the movement produced in the limb. If the proximal and distal insertions of a muscle lie in a single plane, the muscle can carry out only one of the previously defined actions. Muscles that cross one of the cardinal planes usually produce more than one action, a primary one and a secondary one. In the following pages, descriptive terms are used to define and describe these roles and functions.

It has been mentioned previously that muscles seldom operate singly; rather, they act in cooperation with one or more other muscles or as members of a team (sometimes involving most of the major muscles of the body) in a variety of combinations and patterns. Muscles do not always contract for the purpose of causing lever movement. Muscles may contract to help steady or support the lever, to stabilize a body part, to neutralize a body part, or even to neutralize the undesired action of some other muscles. Primarily, then, muscles are movers, stabilizers, and neutralizers.

Roles of Muscles

Mover, or Agonist. A muscle that is known to be the principal mover or one of the principal movers of a lever is called a **mover,** or **agonist.** This muscle, which contracts concentrically, may be directly responsible, along with one or more other muscles, for movement of a lever. The muscle is known as a prime mover when it has or shares primary responsibility for a joint action. When a muscle aids the prime mover in its action, it is known as an assistant mover. For example, the long head of the biceps brachii, although not often involved in shoulder abduction, becomes involved under certain circumstances. Brunnstrom (1946) claims that therapists have taught patients to use this muscle to abduct the shoulder when the deltoideus and supraspinatus have been paralyzed.

Antagonist. A muscle that acts as an **antagonist** is one that in contraction tends to produce movement opposite to that of the mover. In extension, the extensors are the movers and the flexors are the antagonists. After studies of muscle action, Elftman (1938, 1939, 1940) concluded that antagonists play a major role in walking and running. In such actions, when the limbs are about to complete a movement, the pull (eccentrical contraction) of the antagonists in the opposite direction of the agonists helps in the deceleration of the limb. This prevents injury from occurring to the limb. During the maximum effort by the agonists, the antagonists must relax until the very end so that there is no interference in the movement.

Stabilizer, Fixator, or Supporter. A muscle that steadies, fixes, or anchors a bone or body part against contracting muscles is known as a **fixator,** stabilizer, or supporter. The stabilizer may also be used to combat the pull of gravity and the effects of momentum and interaction. For action to take place, one end of a muscle must be free to move and the other end firmly anchored.

A stabilizing muscle is rarely in static contraction, because the part being stabilized is in motion. Actually, the anchoring part may be gradually moved to direct or guide the moving part as it performs its task.

The hip flexors stabilize when the rectus abdominis and other muscles flex the thoracic and lumbar spine (from the supine position). On the other hand, the abdominal muscles and lumbar spine extensors stabilize when the thigh is being extended by the gluteus maximus, hamstrings, and adductor magnus (especially when the knee is extended and the thigh is flexed beyond a 45-degree angle). However, when the foot is fixed and supports the weight, knee action extends the thigh (reversed muscle action). The parallel pull along the long axis of the bone is accomplished by certain muscles that are better suited for stabilizing a joint than others. This arrangement is convenient because the slower, stronger muscles help support the limbs, while the weaker, faster ones produce the limb movement.

Neutralizer, or Synergist. A muscle that acts to prevent an undesired secondary action of another muscle is called a **neutralizer.** Rasch and Burke (1963) use this term to avoid the difficulty with the term **synergist.** Researchers have defined this troublesome term in many different ways. Morris (1955) has stated that writers in this field show little agreement, but the term continues to be used. Some call a muscle that functions as a neutralizer a synergist, and others use this term to mean a muscle that aids and abets the action of other muscles.

If a muscle both extends and adducts, but the performer wishes to extend only, the abductors are activated to prevent adduction. They are neutralizers and prevent the undesired action of the agonist. Wright (1928) classifies synergists as true synergists and helping synergists. The true synergist is a muscle that acts to prevent an undesired action of an agonist, but has no effect on its desired action. A true synergist often contracts statically to prevent undesired action of two-joint muscles. For example, in clenching a fist, the wrist extensors must contract statically to prevent flexion of the wrist. The helping synergist is one that helps another muscle to move a lever in a desired way and at the same time prevents an undesired action. A helping synergist then acts like a neutralizer.

Classification of Movement Type with Respect to Muscle Contraction. Based on studies of the electrical activity and the changes in tension in the various muscles involved in a voluntary movement, we know that a close cooperation exists between anatomically antagonistic muscles. The adjustment of the time relations and the magnitude of the responses to degrees of resistance and velocity of movement are infinitely variable. Nevertheless, rather fixed patterns of responses to different movements have been the basis for another system of classification of movement. Some of these systems have been reviewed and summarized by A. V. Hill. One classification along these lines is: (1) slow tension movements; (2) rapid tension movements; and (3) ballistic movements. In addition, there are oscillating (repetitive) movements.

Slow Tension Movements. Slow movements of body parts and objects that offer great resistance are phasic in character. A phasic movement is indicated by moderate to strong co-contraction of antagonists. The co-contraction fixes the joints involved in the action and aids in accurate positioning of the body part or object being moved.

In the slow, controlled forms of movement, the antagonistic muscle groups are continuously contracted against each other, giving rise to tension. Tremors occur when antagonistic muscles are in contraction and balanced against each other in fixation.

Travis and Hunter (1927) observed voluntary movement to be a continuation of a tremor without interruption of the tremor rhythm. The elementary unit of a slow, controlled movement is the tremor. If a short movement is attempted, its amplitude is determined by that of the tremor. Ability to make movements more and more minute is limited not by sensory methods of control, but by the fundamental tremor element. Stetson and McDill (1923) have determined that the magnification of the visual field does not improve the delicacy of minute movement.

Slow, controlled movements result from a slight increase in the algebraic sum of the number of muscle fibers contracting in the positive muscle as against the number of fibers contracting in the antagonist muscle group. The limb moves in the direction of the group exerting the stronger pull, and tension of the two groups of antagonistic muscles is continually readjusted.

Rapid Tension Movements. A movement in which tension is present in all opposing muscle groups through the motion may be considered a movement of translation superimposed on fixation, with one group of contracting muscles suddenly initiating the movement, followed by contraction of the antagonistic group to stop the movement. Control of these faster movements cannot be attained more often than ten times in a second, since modifying the course of a movement is possible only at the tremor terminations and not at other points in the movement. If the tremor cycles average ten per second, then no modification of the movement could occur in less than one-tenth of a second. This limitation is imposed on the maximal rate of tapping. If the rate of tremor is ten per second, then the rate of tapping cannot exceed that value. Travis (1929) has shown that a majority of movements of the faster type synchronize with the tremor cycle.

Ballistic Movements. A **ballistic movement,** begun by a rapid initial contraction of the prime mover, proceeds relatively unhindered by antagonistic contractions and is followed by a relaxation of the agonist while the movement is still in progress. During a movement such as throwing a baseball, the antagonist progressively decreases in activity during the throw, indicating co-contraction. In comparison with the activity of the prime movers, however, the tension in the antagonists is slight during the ballistic type of movement. Some believe that as one becomes more and more skilled, the amount of co-contraction decreases. Ideally, for a maximal effort, no co-contraction should be present. There is some question whether true ballistic movements occur in sport skills.

One of the greatest differences between skilled and unskilled movements centers around replacing tension movements with ballistic movements. Attempts to perform ballistic movements with muscles that are already fixed are fatiguing. Tension in one group of muscles necessitates an increase in the intensity of contraction of other sets. The spread of intensity results in rigidity, which is wasteful and restrictive.

In a ballistic movement, such as a golf swing, the moving limb swings rapidly about a joint, and the movement is terminated by co-contraction of the opposing muscles and the loss of momentum. It is important that the antagonist contract as late as possible so that force production is not sacrificed. If a movement is arrested by a strong contraction of the antagonistic group of muscles and, as a result, moves in the opposite direction, the movement is said to be oscillatory. Movements of great amplitude are more economical than those of small amplitude because of the intensity and continuity of muscular activity required to stop and start each phase of oscillation. A fast, shallow kick in swimming requires more effort to gain the same propulsive force than a slower, deeper kick requires. Hubbard (1960) has stated that fast action of a limb involves muscular contraction that acts as an impulse (F_t, force applied over a period of time). A limb once set in action by an impulse will continue to move by virtue of its own momentum until acted on by an outside force. The muscle, having developed energy in the limb, then tends to relax.

Components of Muscle Force

Muscles rarely exert forces that are solely perpendicular (90°) to the longitudinal axis of the bone; usually the muscles pull at angles of less than 90°. Furthermore, the angle of pull changes as the angle at the joint changes. The force vector for the muscle, then, is diagonal to the longitudinal axis of the bone and can be resolved into its two components by using the graphic, or trigonometric, method described in Chapter 6.

Muscles, then, provide both a force capable of moving the bone and a force that acts on the joint. In most instances, the force acting on the joint increases the integrity (stability) of that joint. This force is termed a stabilizing component, since it tends to draw the moving bone into the joint, that is, into a closely packed position. This force, which acts along the bone and has no moment of force, is also referred to as a reaction force, or **tangential** force. The movement component of force acts at right angles to both the axis and the bone and is

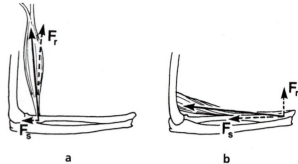

FIGURE 4.16 Examples of spurt (a, biceps brachii) and shunt (b, brachioradialis) muscles. F_r = rotary or movement force (perpendicular to longitudinal axis of forearm), F_s = stabilizing or tangential force (acting along the longitudinal axis of forearm and through the joint). Note that the magnitudes of these forces are represented by the lengths of the vectors. If reverse muscle action would occur (proximal bone moves rather than distal bone), the spurt and shunt roles of these two muscles would also reverse. **Why?**

termed a normal, or rotary force. When the bone to be moved is in a horizontal position, the movement component is a vertical force and the stabilizing component is a horizontal force.

There are instances in which the usual stabilizing force becomes a dislocating force, that is, it acts to pull the bone (lever) away from the second bone forming the joint. This occurs whenever the angle of pull of the muscle exceeds 90°.

The stabilizing component of muscle force is important when the person or animal must exert great isometric forces or move at high speeds. These high speeds create great centrifugal forces, which pull the lever away from the joint. Dislocation would result if this stabilizing component and other assisting muscles did not exist.

Muscles possessing a larger stabilizing component than moving component are called shunt muscles (Figure 4.16). The angle of muscle pull is less than 45°. Muscles having a larger moving component than stabilizing component are called spurt muscles, and their angles of pull are greater than 45°. Although this classification is convenient, some muscles can act as shunt muscles with respect to their action on the distal bone and as spurt muscles with respect to the proximal bone. For example, in most activities of daily living, sports, and work, the brachioradialis functions as a shunt muscle. During the act of chinning, this muscle acts as a spurt muscle as it moves the proximal bone. Therefore, this classification is useful if one remembers to identify the moving bone and the point of attachment of the muscle on that bone. Keep in mind that the angle of the muscle attachment with respect to the bone is a changing angle. Therefore, the amounts of stabilizing and movement force also change as the angle at the joint changes (Figure 4.17).

Figure 4.18 is a mathematic calculation of the forces acting in two static limb positions in which an object is held. Note the use of trigonometry to measure the perpendicular moment arms of the resistance and the perpendicular component of the effort vector.

Producing Movement

If the joint permits movement in a certain plane, the ability of the person to produce movement in that plane will depend on the following:

1. number of muscles capable of moving the body part in that plane
2. force of each muscle and its angle of pull and cross-section as well as its distance from the axis (joint)
3. weight of body part(s) being moved and the distance of its center of gravity from the joint
4. weight of external objects attached to or held by the body part and their distances from the joint
5. number of objects resisting the movement

The ratio of the moment of force produced by the muscles to the moment of force produced by the resistances determines whether movement will occur when muscles contract. The formula is as follows:

$$R \times RA/E \times EA$$

- If the ratio is equal to 1, no movement occurs.
- If the ratio is greater than 1, the resistance produces the movement.
- If the ratio is equal to less than 1, the muscles produce the movement.

These calculations of muscle moments to produce movement presuppose that the body part is stationary and that the body part is accelerated from zero to an undefined acceleration. When a body part is moving, the movement itself is a force ($I\alpha$) because it maintains the object in its path and speed of rotation.

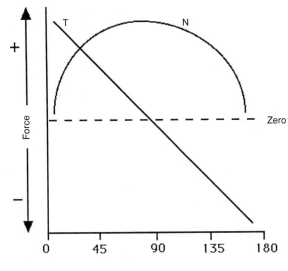

FIGURE 4.17 Relationship of stabilization and movement components of muscular force. (N, movement force that is normal or perpendicular to bone; T, stabilization force that is parallel to bone, either toward or away from joint.) Dislocating force exists at angles greater than 90°, depicted below the zero line.

Muscle force required to stop the motion is equal to the force of the motion plus the resistance moments of force previously described. This relationship is logical because a moment of force greater than the resistance moment was required to cause a certain amount of movement, measured in units of acceleration. Film analysis aids in making these types of calculations. Dillman (1970) was one of the first to estimate moments of force of muscles, which cause both acceleration and deceleration of a body part during running.

Can you do calculations similar to those in Figure 4.18 with another load?

Single-Muscle Levers

We encourage you to measure the moment arms and angles of muscle pull and to estimate the amount of muscle force required to initiate movement as presented in the following analyses of single-muscle lever systems. Any muscle force that produces a moment of force greater than the resistance moment will produce volitional movement.

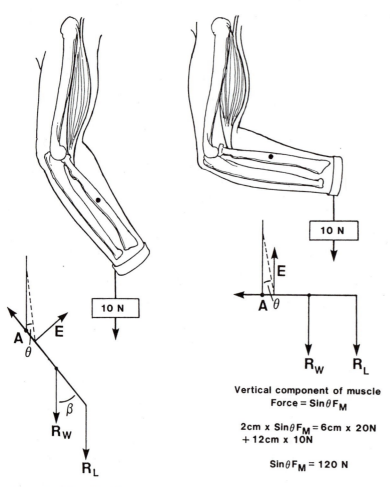

FIGURE 4.18 Free body diagrams for mathematical determination of amount of muscle force required to hold an object in two different positions.

10 N

E

A θ

β

R$_W$

R$_L$

2cm x SinθF$_M$ = Sinβ6cm x 20 N
+ Sinβ12cm x 10 N

10 N

E

A θ

R$_W$ **R$_L$**

**Vertical component of muscle
Force = SinθF$_M$**

2cm x SinθF$_M$ = 6cm x 20N
+ 12cm x 10N

SinθF$_M$ = 120 N

TOTAL MUSCLE FORCE = 120 N/Sinθ

Two-Joint Muscles

Muscles that pass across two joints are called two-joint or bi-articular muscles. This arrangement provides another type of human muscular coordination in the use of body levers. The action of these muscles on the levers is similar to that of a pulley; the muscles act at each joint over which they pass. For example, the rectus femoris causes flexion at the hip and extension at the knee; the gastrocnemius helps flex the lower leg and the plantar flexes the foot; the hamstrings cause flexion at the knee and extension at the hip. In addition, the flexors and

extensors of the fingers might be called multijoint muscles, since they pass over the wrist and at least two joints of the fingers. The complexity of such action is evident.

One outstanding characteristic of these muscles is that they are not long enough to permit a complete range of action simultaneously in the joints involved because of their location on two joints. ROM is limited either because the antagonist muscles prevent full range of action on these joints, or because antagonistic action occurs in the two joints (flexion in one and extension in the other). If the rectus femoris contracts, causing flexion at the hip, and at the same time the hamstrings contract to cause

MINI-LABORATORY LEARNING EXPERIENCE

Action of Biceps Brachii in Forearm Flexion. The action of the biceps brachii is illustrated in Figure 4.19, in which the muscle is shown supporting a weight resting in the hand. The drawing might also be visualized as a "flash" representation of a phase of upward movement of the weight. If the movement starts with the upper arm and forearm at the side, and if the upper arm is held in that position as the forearm moves forward and upward, the forearm moves through the sagittal plane. The axis of movement will be a line perpendicular to the plane of movement and, in this situation, one that passes through the elbow joint. This line will lie in the transverse and frontal planes, since a line may lie in two planes, and both of them are perpendicular to the plane of movement—the sagittal. The rigid bar includes the ulna and radius and the bones of the wrist and hand. The effort arm is that section of the radius and ulna that lies between A and the attachment of the muscle (approximately 3 cm in length). The resistance arm includes the bony mass extending from A to the center of the weight, including the total length of the radius and ulna, the wrist and metacarpals, and a portion of the proximal phalanges, approximately 20 cm in length. The lever is not a simple, continuous mass but consists of several bones bound together by muscles, tendons, and ligaments. The weight of the forearm and hand is not included in the analysis. The arrangement is A-E-R, a third-class lever since the attachment of the biceps brachii lies between the axis and the resistance.

Because we know that if the weight is to be supported, the length of A-E times the amount of muscular force must equal the length of A-R times the weight of the supported object, the amount of muscular force must be more than six times the weight of the object. For example,

$$E \times 3 \text{ cm} = R \times 20 \text{ cm}$$
$$E = R \times 6.67$$

For a resistance of 10 N, the muscular force must be 66.7 N. If the object is to be moved, the force must be even greater.

Note that in identifying the lever elements, we need to consider only the muscle attachment to the

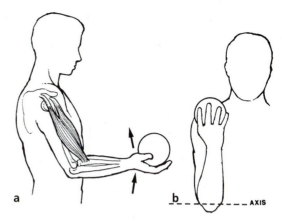

FIGURE 4.19 Action of biceps brachii in forearm flexion. (a) Sagittal plane; (b) frontal plane with axis of rotation shown.

moving segment. It is the point at which energy is applied to the lever. The muscle must have another point of attachment, but that attachment is not part of the lever, although it is an essential part of the total machine. Under certain circumstances for the biceps brachii, the upper arm is the moving lever, as in executing a pull-up. In most instances, the forearm is the moving lever, as in lifting an object.

Use your own values for the loading and/or moment arms of Figure 4.19 and estimate required muscle force.

---

flexion at the knee, the pull of the rectus is increased at the hip because the muscle does not shorten as much as it would if extension took place at the knee. Consider this example. If there is a downward pull on a rope that passes over an overhead pulley, the tension will be transmitted in a reverse direction to the rope on the other side of the pulley. In the case of the flexors and extensors of the fingers, although the joints move in the same direction, the principle of pulley action is evident. Note the limited range of motion in the fingers as you try to make a fist while the wrist is already in full flexion. One of the main advantages of using the two-joint muscles is that they maintain tension without complete shortening. This advantage is not enjoyed by one-joint muscles, which lose tension as they shorten.

Concurrent and Countercurrent. Fenn (1930) and Steindler (1955) have discussed two different patterns of action of two-joint muscles. These patterns are called concurrent and countercurrent. The simultaneous action of flexion (or extension) at the hip and knee is an example of a concurrent pattern. As the muscles contract, they do not lose length and, therefore, are able to maintain tension. In extension at the hip and knee, the rectus femoris muscle's loss of tension at the knee is balanced by an increase in tension at the hip. At the same time the hamstrings gain tension at the knee and lose it at the hip.

During certain phases in the kicking pattern there is a countercurrent two-joint muscle pattern. If flexion occurs at the hip simultaneously with extension at the knee, there will be loss of tension in the rectus femoris and gain of tension in the hamstrings. Thus, while one muscle shortens rapidly in an action, the antagonist lengthens to the same degree and maintains tension at both ends of the attachment. The result is an effective and coordinated movement.

This discussion does not minimize the importance of one-joint muscles. In a single-joint action, they provide the needed force but expend more energy than do the two-joint muscles in the same action. On the other hand, when two joints are involved in the act, the two-joint muscles are more efficient. Elftman (1940) found that in running, although one-joint muscles could do the job, two-joint ones were more efficient. The expenditure of 2.61 hp (1945 watts) by the two-joint muscles was less than the expenditure of 3.97 hp (2962 watts) if single-joint ones were used.

Action of Greater Psoas Muscle in Thigh Flexion. The attachment of the greater psoas muscle to the femur is shown in the left side of Figure 4.20. If this illustration is considered a phase in flexion at the hip, the femur is shown moving through the sagittal plane; the fulcrum of the action is on an axis passing through the hip joint in the transverse and frontal planes. If the weight of the leg is 95 N, the muscle must oppose this force. However, the resistance arm is that section of the femur that extends from the axis to the center of gravity of the leg (approximately 36 cm), and the effort arm is only 6 cm. The effort arm is measured along the section of the femur that extends from the axis to the muscle attachment, since the leg is estimated to be horizontal.

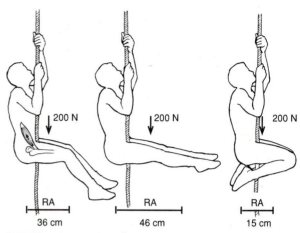

FIGURE 4.20 Action of greater psoas muscle in thigh flexion. Legs in partial flexion (RA = 36 cm). **Calculate the muscle moment required with legs extended** (RA = 46 cm) **and legs in a tight tuck position** (RA = 15 cm).

In Figure 4.20 the angle of pull of the muscle is estimated to be 45°. Since the sine of 45° equals 0.707, the muscle force in the vertical direction is equal to:

$$E \times EA = R \times RA \text{ (for equilibrium)}$$
$$E \times EA = 95 \text{ N} \times RA$$
$$E(6 \text{ cm}) = 95 \text{ N} \times 36 \text{ cm}$$
$$E = \frac{95 \text{ N} \times 36 \text{ cm}}{6 \text{ cm}}$$
$$E = 95 \text{ N} \times 6$$
$$E = 576 \text{ N of vertical force}$$

To determine the total muscle force acting at a 45° angle, divide the vertical force by the sine of the angle. Thus, the muscle force always will be greater than that required when the muscle acts at an angle normal to the bone (90°):

$$\text{Total muscle force} = 576 \text{ N} \times 0.7$$
$$\text{Total muscle force} = 823 \text{ N}$$

In these calculations, the 823 N of muscle force required to support a leg weighing 95 N is equivalent to approximately 183 pounds of muscle force supporting a leg weighing less than 22 pounds. The muscle must exert a force greater than 8 times that of weight of the leg. You can estimate how much force would be

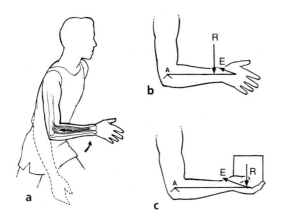

FIGURE 4.21 (a) Action of brachioradialis in forearm flexion. (b) Brachioradialis in a is diagrammed as part of a second-class lever system with the center of gravity of the forearm/hand as the resistance (R), the muscle as the effort (E), and the elbow as the axis of rotation (A). (c) Brachioradialis is part of a third-class lever system when a heavy load is carried in the hand; RA now becomes longer than EA.

required if the legs were held in a tuck position, with the center of gravity of the legs approximately 15 cm from the axis. If the legs were fully extended, as recommended for maximal difficulty, the resistance arm would be 46 cm. Is it any wonder that many people cannot elevate their legs to the horizontal and maintain this position? (This analysis is limited to only one muscle to simplify the mathematic processes.)

Action of Brachioradialis in Forearm Flexion.

Figure 4.21 illustrates flexion of the forearm resulting from contraction of the brachioradialis. The forearm moves through the sagittal plane, and the axis, passing through the elbow joint, lies in the frontal and transverse planes. The fulcrum is on that axis and lies within the joint. The lever includes the radius and the ulna; the effort arm includes the length of the bone extending from the axis to the point of attachment of the muscle, a length of 15 cm. Since the center of gravity of the forearm-plus-hand lies closer to the axis than does the site of the muscle attachment, this is an example of a second-class lever system. This system could be one of great strength, except for the fact that the brachioradialis has such a small angle of pull that there is virtually no movement component to this shunt muscle.

Since the mechanical advantage of the brachioradialis is low, this muscle usually acts to stabilize a fast flexion or movement of a large load in which such stabilization is of prime importance. If a weight were suspended at the center of gravity of the segment, the arrangement would remain an E-R-A lever, that is, a second-class lever. If, however, the weight is moved to the hand, the arrangement could become an A-E-R lever, that is, a third-class lever. It would be necessary to calculate the position of the center of gravity of the system (for example, arm plus hand plus weight) to determine the common resistance arm.

It is clear that a performance may require either great muscle effort or very little muscle effort. The key is adjusting the placement of external weights on the body and by adjusting the position of the limb in space. For efficient movement the forearm and hand should be brought closer to the body, thus decreasing the moment arm for the resistance. Can you explain why this is true?

Action of Rectus Femoris in Leg Extension.

A major joint action in kicking is leg extension. The action of the rectus femoris in kicking is illustrated in Figure 4.22. The leg is shown moving through the sagittal plane; the fulcrum is in the knee joint on an axis that lies in the frontal and transverse planes. The rigid bar includes the tibia and fibula and those tarsal and metatarsal bones that are firmly attached to the leg bones from the ankle joint to the point of ball contact. The effort arm is that section of the bone that extends from the axis to the attachment to the tibia, a length of 12.7 cm (5 in.). The resistance arm includes those bones that extend from the axis to the center of gravity of the leg-plus-foot, a length of 35 cm (13½ in.).

Since the limb is not horizontal, components of the forces perpendicular to the moment arm are described as follows: (1) weight of leg times the sine of angle of leg with the vertical; and (2) effort times the sine of angle of muscle with the forearm. At the point of contact with the ball, the weight of the ball will produce a resistance moment of force in addition to that created by the weight of the leg. The lever now includes the complete length of the body segment, since the ball acts at the distal end of the segment. In previous calculations in which no external forces existed, the resistance arm was measured only to the center of gravity of the body segment, almost as if the remainder of the lever did not exist. When objects are struck or projected, the entire

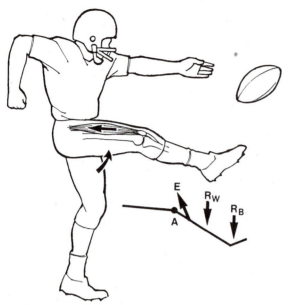

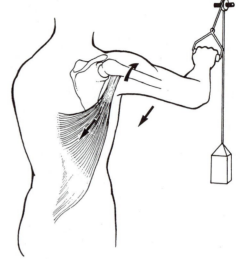

FIGURE 4.22 Action of rectus femoris muscle acting as part of a third-class lever system in leg extension. The axis (A) is at the knee, the effort is at an ineffective angle of pull (E), the resistances consist of the weight of lower leg (R_W) and weight of ball (R_B). Note position of patella at lower leg near extension.

FIGURE 4.23 Action of latissimus dorsi in adduction of humerus. Note the large size of this muscle and its effective role in adduction, extension, and medial rotation of the humerus.

lever, from an anatomic perspective, must be used in the calculations. This concept will be discussed in subsequent chapters. (See Appendix B for sine and cosine.)

Single-Muscle Levers in the Frontal Plane

Action of Latissimus Dorsi in Adduction of Humerus. The humerus in Figure 4.23 is depicted as starting from 90° of abduction and the forearm from 90° of flexion, pointing directly forward. As the latissimus dorsi contracts, the humerus adducts and moves to the side of the trunk through a frontal plane. This shoulder action moves the forearm, although no action occurs at the elbow joint. The forearm also moves through a frontal plane, a concept that some students find difficult to visualize. You may find it helpful to perform the action; note that as the distal end of the upper arm moves through a frontal plane, the proximal end of the forearm moves through a frontal plane parallel to that through which the upper arm moves. The distal end of the forearm and the hand move through frontal planes that are parallel to those through which the upper arm moves.

The fulcrum lies within the shoulder joint on an axis that is in the sagittal and transverse planes. The rigid bar of the lever includes the humerus, the radius, the ulna, the carpals, and the metacarpals. The actual resistance arm is the length of the upper arm, since the forearm and hand are the line of application of force passing through the elbow and are parallel to the axis at the shoulder. This moment arm, therefore, is a perpendicular line from the axis at the shoulder to the line of application of force. The effort arm is that portion of the humerus between the axis and the attachment of the muscle.

This analysis has dealt only with adduction of the arm. Since the latissimus dorsi also causes medial (inward) rotation, there will be a moment of force about an axis passing through the shoulder joint in the lateral-horizontal plane, and the humerus will move in the sagittal plane. A separate analysis of this movement or lack of movement, which is caused by the resistance of other muscles to this action of the latissimus dorsi, could be done.

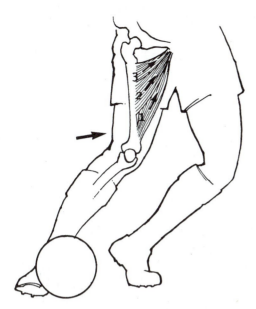

FIGURE 4.24 Action of adductors in lower-limb adduction. (1) Adductor magnus; (2) adductor longus; (3) adductor brevis. The size of these muscles usually is greater than that of the abductor muscles acting at the hip joint.

Muscle-Group Levers

Effort Arm for the Action of Muscle Groups. When more than one muscle contracts to move a segment, the point of application of effort is difficult to determine. Figure 4.24 depicts three muscles, and the effort arm for the action of each is described. If the three muscles contract and pull on the femur at the same time, the amount of force that each exerts, as well as the point of attachment of each, must be known to determine the effort arm for the combined action. The amount of force each exerts is not known, and to describe the effort arm and its length is difficult. It often requires highly sophisticated techniques, such as magnetic resonance imaging. This is true for all situations in which the joint action is caused by the contraction of more than one muscle.

Action of Adductors in Lower-Limb Adduction. The action that occurs in moving a soccer ball to the left of the body is shown in Figure 4.24. As the adductors contract, the lower limb moves through the frontal plane on an axis passing through the hip joint in the sagittal and

transverse planes. The lever includes the femur, tibia, fibula, tarsals, metatarsals, and that portion of the phalanges that extends to make contact with the ball. The lever bones and length will be the same for the magnus, longus, and brevis muscles. However, the length of the effort arm will differ for the three. If each muscle is considered separately, each effort arm will include that portion of the femur that extends from the axis to the point of attachment of the muscle under consideration. The effort arm for the magnus is longest, and that for the brevis is shortest. In all three situations, the resistance arm will include the bones and will be the same length specified for the total lever.

Muscle-Bone Lever Systems, Muscles, and Physiological Cross-Sectional Area (PCSA)

The muscles illustrated in Figure 4.25 are expressed as a percentage of physiological cross-sectional area (PCSA) of one muscle, the vastus lateralis. It is easy to compare

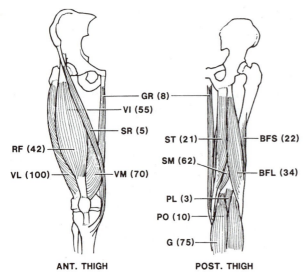

GR (8)
VI (55)
SR (5)
ST (21) — BFS (22)
SM (62)
RF (42)
BFL (34)
VL (100) — VM (70)
PL (3)
PO (10)
G (75)

ANT. THIGH   **POST. THIGH**

FIGURE 4.25 Muscles acting across the hip and knee, expressed as percentage of physiologic cross-sectional area (PCSA) of vastus lateralis (VL) the largest muscle. Several muscles are biarticular, crossing either hip or ankle, as well as knee. Relative effectiveness of each muscle may be estimated from PCSA values and attachment sites (direction of force and length of effort moment arms). VI, vastus intermedius; VM, vastus medialis; PO, popliteus; SR, sartorius; RF, rectus femoris; GR, gracilis; SM, semimembranosus; ST, semitendinosus; PL, plantaris; BFS, biceps femoris, short head; BFL, biceps femoris, long head; G, gastrocnemius.
(Modified from Mastropaolo, J. 1975. *Kinesiology for the public schools*, Paramount, CA: Academy Printing and Publishing Co.)

the relative effectiveness of these muscles acting across the knee and hip, since PCSA is an indicator of the strength of an individual muscle. Note that the vastus intermedius has only 55% of the PCSA of the vastus lateralis. The rectus femoris, a muscle many assume to be the major quadriceps force-producer, has only 42% of the PCSA of the vastus lateralis.

Although the vastus intermedius and the vastus lateralis have larger cross-sectional areas, their angles of pull are very low. The rectus femoris pulls at a much higher angle, producing a more effective force at the knee joint.

The angle of pull of some muscles is increased by anatomic pulleys. The patella increases the angle of pull of the quadriceps muscles, thus increasing the effectiveness of the muscles' forces. Calcium deposits, which accumulate at the site of attachment of some

muscles as a result of excessive use, can also increase the angle of pull. Further information concerning these muscle-bone lever systems is listed in Table 4.1. Since individuals may increase the cross-sectional area of selected muscle groups because of intense, habitual, and long-term exercise of a particular action, the data in Table 4.1 will not coincide with data obtained from individuals. The table does, however, provide a basis for identifying the most effective—that is, the strongest or fastest—muscle-bone lever systems of an average, or normal, human body. The position of the moving body part in space and the plane of movement will determine which of these muscle-bone lever systems are potentially in a position to function. Knowledge of the anatomy of these systems will enable a person to select the most effective movement pattern. You can obtain additional anatomic data from an anatomy textbook and apply it to movement patterns.

Advantages of a Third-Class Lever System

As illustrated in many of the figures in this chapter, the majority of muscles have their distal attachments near the joints. Therefore, the body levers operate primarily as third-class lever systems. Since the muscle effort required in such a third-class system is always greater than the resistance to be overcome, the body has a mechanical disadvantage when performing activities requiring the lifting of heavy loads. The mechanical advantage, *MA*, of a lever system can be easily calculated using the formula

$$MA = EA/RA$$

Note that in third-class levers, *EA* is less than *RA*, so *MA* is less than 1.00, which is a low mechanical advantage. Second-class levers, on the other hand, have longer effort arms than resistance arms, so *MA* is equal to or greater than 1.00, which results in a mechanical advantage. We make many adjustments in our everyday lives to increase our mechanical advantage. To gain more power in prying with a crowbar, we get a longer crowbar, which increases the length of *EA*, thus increasing the mechanical advantage. When carrying a heavy load, we hold it close to our bodies, which decreases the length of *RA* and thus increases the mechanical advantage.

TABLE 4.1 Physiological cross-sectional areas (PCSA) of the largest muscles acting at the major body segments.

Figure	Body Segment	Muscle	PCSA (cm₂)
7–13	Foot	Soleus	47.0
7–14	Shank (lower leg)	Vastus lateralis	41.8
7–15	Thigh	Gluteus maximus	58.8
7–16	Trunk (spinal column)	Levator scapulae	35.5
7–17	Hand, fingers	Flexor digitorum profundus	10.1
7–18	Forearm	Triceps brachii, long head	14.1
7–19	Shoulder girdle	Levator scapulae	35.5
7–20	Trunk (respiration)	Diaphragm	35.8
7–21	Upper arm	Subscapularis	19.8

Modified from Mastropaolo, J.: Kinesiology for the public schools, Paramount Calif., 1975, Academy Printing and Publishing Co.

MINI-LABORATORY LEARNING EXPERIENCE

Can you think of other examples in daily life of how we adjust to increase the mechanical advantage of our lever systems?

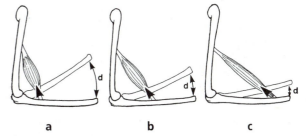

FIGURE 4.26 Given an equal amount of muscle shortening, the effect of length of effort arm on movement of distal end of moving segment can be estimated (d = movement arc of distal end). **Relate these findings to spurt and shunt concepts and to speed and strength concepts.**

The arrangement of the muscle fibers into a featherlike structure compensates for mechanical disadvantage. This kind of arrangement increases the number of fibers in a given bulk, and since the strength of a muscle depends on the number of contracting fibers, the potential strength of the muscle is increased. With the increased strength, we are able to move heavier and longer resistance arms.

There is an important advantage in possessing third-class levers, namely speed. Given the same amount of shortening of a muscle and the same amount of time to produce this shortening, muscles that have the shortest effort arms will produce the greatest distance of travel of the distal end of the lever. (See Figure 4.26.)

Muscles with short effort arms usually have an angle of pull that is mechanically more advantageous than that of muscles with long effort arms. The design of the human body enables us to move our limbs rapidly, providing the resistance is not great.

In the sports world, teachers and coaches have capitalized on this human body design by adding to the length of the body lever some external levers of various lengths, primarily of little or negligible weight.

The effect of this additional external lever, e.g., a badminton racquet, is illustrated in Figure 4.27. The outer end (the hand) of the shorter radius (38 cm), as it moves 90°, will travel through 59.6 cm ([2 × 38 × 3.1416]/4). (*Note:* we divide by 4 in each case because the illustrated distance is one-fourth of a circle.) If the movements were made in the same length of time, the linear velocity of the end of the longer arm will be twice that of the smaller, while the angular velocity is virtually the same. Naturally, the angular velocity will not be precisely the same for the two conditions. However, the decrease in angular velocity caused by the added weight of the badminton racquet is minute compared to the gain in linear velocity.

Adding additional segments and/or fully extending the joints increases the length of the resistance arm, resulting in greater linear velocities at the end of the

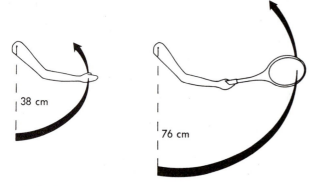

FIGURE 4.27 Effect of length of lever on angular displacement, and therefore on linear velocity of distal end of lever with and without an implement. **Compare this figure to Figure 1.5.**

TABLE 4.2 Angular speeds of body segments reported in biomechanics literature.

Action	Rad/Sec	Degrees/Sec
Flexion at wrist	477	3000
Flexion at wrist with tennis racquet in hand	318	2000
Flexion at shoulder during standing long jump	255	1600
Extension at hip, knee, and ankle during standing long jump	236	1480
Transverse rotation at left hip in overhand throw (right hand)	115	720
Wrist flexion with forearm rotation during badminton smash	952	6000

levers. Individuals with longer limb segments therefore have an advantage in some activities. Baseball pitchers are usually tall with long arms, which helps them throw faster. Tall, long-legged football kickers also have an advantage. There are times, however, when we may wish to increase the angular velocity of the limb(s) at the expense of the linear velocity. Choking up on the baseball bat allows the batter to swing more quickly against a fast pitcher. Can you think of other situations in which someone shortens the resistance arm to gain angular velocity?

Body Segments

Speed of Body Segments

Research on the speed with which body segments can be moved is limited. Hill (1927), the English physiologist, states that in the human body the speed with which each segment moves is related to its length: the longer the segment, the slower its possible speed. This, says Hill, is a safety factor, and he compares these limits to the speeds with which glass rods can be oscillated. A short rod can safely be moved rapidly at a pace that would break a longer one. This relationship of speed to size is seen in the reported number of wing-beats per second of various birds. Hummingbird strokes are as fast as 200/sec; sparrow, 13; pigeon, 8; parrot, 5; stork, 2. The same relationship is shown in the rate of mastication

(contractions per minute) of animals, reported by Amar (1920): ox, 70; human being, 90 to 100; cat, 162; guinea pig, 300; white mouse, 350.

Persons who have observed films of human action know that the wrist action is faster than the action of other joints acting during gross movements. The hand often is not visible without blurring as it is moved very rapidly by flexion at the wrist. Less information exists concerning the rapid movements of the fingers playing musical instruments, particularly the flamenco guitar. The speed of various joints given in Table 4.2 represents some of the reported data. The fastest movement is that of an internationally ranked badminton player.

Velocity of Distal End. Linear velocities of distal ends—and therefore of any object projected or struck from the distal end—will be directly related to the length of the lever. One can expect high angular velocities from rotation about the wrist. But linear velocities of the fingers and of balls projected by means of this action will be low. Conversely, low angular velocities from rotation about the shoulder produce high linear velocities of the hand and of balls projected by means of this action. These relationships are shown in Table 4.3, which represents attempts by physical education students to project a ball as rapidly as possible either by using different

TABLE 4.3 Relationships of moment arm (MA), angular velocity (ω), and linear tangential velocity (V_τ).

Axis	MA (meters)	Distance of Projection (meters)	V_τ (m/sec)	ω(rad/sec)
Hip	0.99	0.66	5.9	6
Shoulder (extended arm)	0.76	0.56	5.3	7
Shoulder (flexed arm)	0.36	0.36	5.0	14
Wrist	0.20	0.20	4.8	24

levers or by modifying the effective radius of a hinged lever (consisting of several joints, as in the arm). The moment arms were measured, and the range of motion was predetermined. The ball was released in a horizontal direction, and the distance of projection and height of ball at the time of release were recorded. Since gravity causes the ball to drop to the ground at a known acceleration, the time of flight of the ball could be calculated by using the following formula:

$$t = \sqrt{\frac{2(\text{height})}{\text{gravity}}}$$

(This is a rearrangement of $H = \frac{1}{2}gt^2$)

Linear velocity of the ball was then equal to the horizontal distance of projection divided by the time of flight. Assume that the linear velocity of the ball is equal to the linear velocity (tangential velocity) of the hand. We determine the angular velocity of the hand, as well as of the other angular velocities of the other levers used, by means of the following formula:

$$\omega = \frac{V_\tau}{r}$$

where r = moment arm, V_τ = ball velocity, and ω = angular velocity.

Body Segment Positioning

A change in the length of the radius is illustrated by a change in the position of the forearm when the hand is moved by medial rotation of the humerus, a joint action that occurs frequently in throwing and striking skills. To understand these changes better, go through the following movements. First, take a position in which the forearm is fixed in 90° of flexion and the upper arm is abducted 90° and laterally rotated, so that the forearm, pointing directly upward, is vertical. From this starting position, rotate the humerus medially so that the forearm is rotated forward and downward in the sagittal plane. The action of the humerus is more difficult to see, but it is also rotating in the same direction and in the same plane as the forearm. The axis is a line passing through the shoulder joint and extending in the same direction as the humerus, roughly along its middle. The radius line must pass through the hand (the point of application of force) to the axis. Thus, the radius is perpendicular to the humerus. The length of the radius will be approximately equal to the length of the forearm (possibly 25 cm). Next, take a starting position in which the upper arm is in the same position as in the first movement but the forearm is fully extended and the hand is facing upward. Now rotate the humerus medially so that the hand faces forward and then downward; try to eliminate any pronation of the forearm. The radius will now pass through the hand to the axis line, which must be extended through the forearm and hand as well as through the humerus. The length of the radius (represented by half the diameter of the hand) will be 2.5 to 5 cm (1 to 2 in.). If the same angular velocity of medial rotation of the humerus is used in the two situations, the linear velocity of the hand would differ (refer to previous equation). The hand in the first movement would be moving ten times faster than in the second movement since the radii are in a ratio of 10:1. Flexion at the elbow can vary from 0 to approximately 140°. The linear velocity of the hand will be least in the instance of no flexion; velocity will increase as flexion occurs. Velocity will be greatest at 90°, and beyond 90° velocity will again decrease.

Medial Rotation. Because medial rotation of the humerus is an outstanding element in the human overarm pattern, because its angular velocity is one of the fastest of the joint actions, and because beginning biomechanics students often fail to recognize it, special efforts should be made to develop the ability to identify this action of the humerus in complex skills. To identify relative positions of upper arms and forearms as medial rotation occurs is also important. This rotation of the humerus on its long axis is usually accompanied by pronation of the forearm.

In studies measuring the contribution of various body levers to the total force, the point chosen for observation has been the release in throws and the point of impact in strikes. All segments between that point and a moving joint are parts of the resistance arm. In a throw, the resistance arm for hip rotation includes the pelvis, the spine, the shoulder girdle on the right side (for the right-handed performer), the humerus, the bones of the lower arm, wrist, and hand, and the bones of the fingers up to the center of gravity of the projectile. In spinal rotation, the resistance arm would include the same segments except for the pelvis; the shoulder joint would include the segments moved by spinal action except for the spine and shoulder girdle. For all joints acting in the throw, the point of application of force is the center of gravity of the projectile; for all strikes, it is the point of impact.

Moment Arm Length. The length of the moment arm for any lever and the speed with which it is moving will change during the force-developing phase, for example, in the forward swing in throwing and striking. However, the direct contribution is a result of the length and speed at the time of release. At that instant, each acting joint can be considered a separate lever. For example, pelvic rotation will move the hand, as may spinal rotation and all other joints between the hand and the hip. The linear velocity of each can be determined, and if the measures are accurate, the sum of these linear velocities should equal the velocity of the object projected. (See Figure 4.28.) This method of evaluating (measuring) the contributions of each lever will be illustrated as specific skills are analyzed in later chapters.

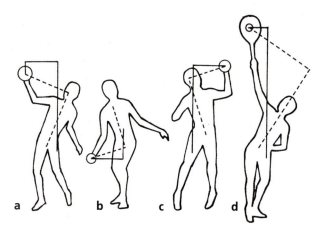

FIGURE 4.28 Length of moment arms in various patterns of joint action. (a) Football pass; (b) underarm throw; (c) shot put; (d) tennis serve. Hip moment arm is shown by unbroken horizontal line from hip axis to center of ball. Spinal moment arm is indicated by broken horizontal or diagonal line from spinal axis to center of ball. Wrist moment arm (not shown) can be drawn from the horizontal line through the wrist to the center of ball. **How does the performer increase linear speed of the hand and racquet by means of other body segments?** The student measures the above moment arms on a scale of 1 cm = 40 actual inches.

Anatomic Differences

As is well known, individuals differ in length of skeletal parts. A child's bones are shorter than an adult's, the average woman's are shorter than the average man's. Even individuals with equal total body heights may have varying arm and leg segment lengths.

■ If all persons can move segments at the same angular speeds, those with longer limbs will have greater linear velocities.

Some authors have suggested that the distance of the muscular attachment from the joint differs in individuals. The greater this distance, the longer the effort arm. But the advantages of this length depend on the relationship between the lengths of the effort and resistance arms. If the forearm were 24 cm long and the attachment of the biceps 2 cm from the fulcrum, the ratio of resistance arm to effort arm would be 12:1. If in longer segments the effort arm, although increased in length, remained in the 12:1 ratio, no advantage would be gained. However, an individual in whom the length of the effort arm is proportionately greater than the total length of the arm and whose muscle strength ratio is also 12:1 will be able to lift heavier weights. Possibly, this gain in ability to lift weights because of a proportionately longer effort arm will be accompanied by a decrease in angular velocity. If, when the effort arm is longer, the muscle shortens to the same degree and for the same length of time as when the effort arm is shorter, the distal end of the bone will be moved a shorter distance in the same time, with a resultant decrease in angular velocity. Little information on individual differences in proportionate lengths of effort arms is available. But the possibility of such differences suggests the need for investigations that might explain differences in strength and speed of joint actions.

MINI-LABORATORY LEARNING EXPERIENCE

Moment arm lengths for the hip, spine, and wrist are illustrated in Figure 4.28, with tracings of the body position at the time of release or impact in (a) an overarm throw such as a football pass; (b) an underarm throw; (c) a push such as the shot put; and (d) an overarm pattern such as a tennis serve. These tracings also illustrate changes in body levers because of different relative positions of segments.

On each tracing, a vertical line has been drawn through the left hip joint to represent the axis of rotation in that joint. In all four cases, that rotation includes in the resistance arm the pelvis, spine, right clavicle, humerus, radius and ulna, and the bones of the wrist, hand, and fingers. In the tennis serve, the racket, as an extension of the hand, is also included. The moment arm lengths differ, depending to a minor degree on the length of the individual's segments, but much more on the position of the segments at the time of release or impact. Horizontal lines perpendicular to the line of flight have been drawn from the axis to the center of the ball. The line of flight is assumed to be directly forward. Although the picture sizes differ to a small degree, assume for this analysis that all are the same: 1 mm on the tracing equals 2.5 cm of actual measure. Measure the moment arms in each picture. Discuss the significance and effect on performance of these measured moment arms.

References

Adrian, M. J. 1981. Flexibility in the aging adult. In *Exercise and aging: The scientific basis,* ed. E. L. Smith and R. C. Serfass. Hillside, NJ: Enslow Publishers.

Amar, Jules. 1920. *The human motor.* London: Routledge.

Atha, J. 1981. Strengthening muscle. *Exercise Sport Science Rev.* 9:1.

Basmajian, J. V. 1973. Electromyographic analyses of basic movement patterns. In *Exercise and sports sciences,* vol. 1, ed. J. Wilmore. New York: Academic Press.

Basmajian, J. V. 1979. *Muscles alive: Their functions revealed by electromyography,* 4th ed. Baltimore: Williams & Wilkins.

Bosco, C., and Komi, P. V. 1982. *Exercise and sport biology.* Champaign, IL: Human Kinetics.

Chapman, H. E. 1985. The mechanical properties of human muscle. *Exercise Sport Science Rev.* 13:443.

Crouch, James E. 1982. *Essential human anatomy.* Philadelphia: Lea and Febiger.

Elftman, H. 1940. The work done by muscles in running. *Am. J. Physiol.* 129:672.

Evans, F. G. 1971. Biomechanical implications of anatomy. In *Selected topics in biomechanics,* ed. J. M. Cooper. Chicago: The Athletic Institute.

Fenn, W. O. 1930. Work against gravity and work due to velocity changes in running. *Am. J. Physiol.* 93:433.

Gans, C. 1982. Fiber architecture and muscle function. *Exercise Sport Science Rev.* 10:160.

Gray, Henry. 1989. *Gray's anatomy,* 30th ed. Philadelphia: Lea and Febiger.

Herzog, W., Guimaraes, A. C., Anton, M. G., and Carter-Erdman, K. A. 1991. *Medicine and Science in Sports and Exercise* 23(11): 1289–96.

Hill, A. V. 1951. The mechanics of voluntary muscle. *Lancet* 2:947.

Hill, A. V. 1965. *First and last experiments in muscle mechanics.* Cambridge, MA: Cambridge University Press.

Hubbard, A. W. 1960. Homokinetics: Muscular function in human movement. In *Science and medicine of exercise and sports,* ed. W. Johnson. New York: Harper & Row.

Huxley, H. E. 1958. The contraction of muscle. *Sci. Am.* 199:67.

Kulig, K., Andrews, J. G., and Hay, J. G. 1984. Human strength curves. *Exercise Sport Science Rev.* 12.

Leyshon, Glynn. 1974. *Programmed functional anatomy.* St. Louis: Mosby.

Luttgens, K., Deutsch, H., and Hamilton, N. 1992. *Kinesiology: Scientific basis of human motion,* 8th ed. Dubuque, IA: Brown & Benchmark.

Nordin, M., and Frankel, V. H., ed. 1989. *Basic biomechanics of the musculoskeletal system,* 2nd ed. Philadelphia: Lea & Febiger.

Perrine, J. J. 1986. In *Human muscle power,* ed. N. L. Jones. Champaign, IL: Human Kinetics.

Radin, E. L. 1986. Role of muscles in protecting athletes from injury. *Acta Med Scand supp* 711:143.

Schotellius, B. A., and Schotellius, D. D. 1978. *Textbook of physiology,* 18th ed. St. Louis: Mosby.

Soderberg, G. L. 1986. *Articular mechanics and function.* Baltimore: Williams and Wilkins.

Spence, Alexander P. 1987. *Human anatomy and physiology.* New York: Harper & Row.

Steindler, A. 1955. *Kinesiology of the human body under normal and pathological conditions.* Springfield, IL: Chas. C. Thomas.

Stetson, R. H., and McDill, J. A. 1923. Mechanism of different types of movements. *Psychol. Monogr.* 32:18.

Tortora, Gerard J. 1990. *Principles of anatomy and physiology.* New York: Harper & Row.

Travis, L. E., and Hunter, T. A. 1927. Muscular rhythms and action currents. *Am. J. Physiol.* 81:355.

Twietmeyer, Alan, and McCracken, Thomas. 1986. *Regional guide to human anatomy.* Philadelphia: Lea and Febiger.

Viitasalo, J. T., Komi, P. V., and Bosco, C. 1984. Muscle structure: A determinant of explosive force production? In *Neural and mechanical control of movement,* ed. M. Kumanmoto. Kyoto, Japan: Yamaguchi Shoten.

Yoshihuku, Y., with Herzog, W. 1990. *Journal of Biomechanics* 23(10).

Zernicke, R. F. 1986. Movement dynamics and connective tissue adaptations. In *Proceedings of the symposium on future directions in exercise/sport research.* Champaign, IL: Human Kinetics.

5 Activation of the Muscle-Bone System*

This chapter describes how the central nervous system and related areas affect human movement and control. It is important to understand the adaptations that occur to produce the harmony of all the body systems.

Understanding joint actions and the resulting lever actions is the foundation for improvement and refinement of motor skill. The performer, teacher, coach, therapist, and industrial engineer try to weave the desired actions into behavior. These actions, created by muscular contraction or relaxation, are triggered by signals referred to as nerve impulses. Nerve action transmits information from the brain to the muscles (as in conscious voluntary movement), from the spinal cord to the muscles (as in reflexive movement) and even from one part of the body to another. Muscles respond to electrical signals and if these signals are organized in an exact pattern the desired action will result. Sage (1977) states:

> The observer of a smoothly coordinated motor performance usually does not realize that the performance represents a fantastically complex integration of many parts of the nervous system to produce the postures and movement patterns. In performing a basketball jump shot, a football forward pass or an intricate dance routine, the complete movement patterns consist of

reflexes, simple movements, and complex movements with precise spatial and temporal organization, meaning that the appropriate muscles are selected and employed at just the right time. (p. 123)

When we consider the details of the control of muscles by the nervous system, keep the general structure of this system in mind. For convenience in discussion, the nervous system is divided into central and peripheral portions. This division does not imply a separation in function, but only in location.

Central Nervous System

The **central nervous system (CNS)** and the spinal cord are well protected by the surrounding bones (the skull and the vertebrae, respectively). All communication among the nerve cells takes place within the CNS.

■ The central nervous system (CNS), which includes the brain and the spinal cord, is the nucleus of the body's communication network.

Brain

The brain, protected by the skull, includes the parts of the nervous system that are the bases of voluntary muscular control, as well as many parts that control reflex behavior. The major portion of the brain consists of the

*Contributed by Joy Hedrick.

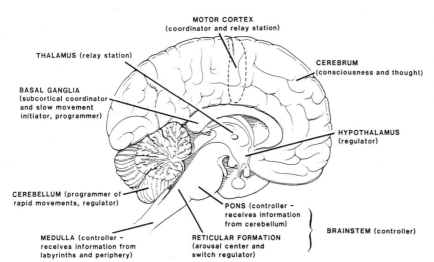

FIGURE 5.1 Human brain. The function of each area appears in parentheses. Note both the specialization and the integration of the different areas of the brain. We now know that the brain (and nervous system) has a high level of plasticity, enabling it to adapt activity in one area to losses in other areas.

cerebrum, the upper portion, which is divided into a left and right hemisphere (Figure 5.1). The surface of this portion, called the **cerebral cortex,** is composed of gray matter that consists mainly of cell bodies rather than nerve fibers. The activity in these cells is the basis of consciousness and thought. Beneath the cerebral cortex are nerve fibers and also other groupings of cell bodies, such as the thalamus and hypothalamus, and mixtures of white and gray matter, such as the reticular formation. Connecting these parts of the brain with the spinal cord are the pons and medulla, parts of the **brain stem.**

A portion of the cerebral cortex located just anterior to the central sulcus is the motor cortex. Within the motor cortex is the **motor map,** which is a topographic representation and nerve center of the location of the muscles within the body. Although the motor cortex is not responsible for designing movement patterns, it is one of the last supraspinal stations for conversion of the instruction to the motor program. It therefore serves as the coordinator or relay station for the information from other parts of the central nervous system. Researchers have recently suggested that the motor cortex is responsible for control of the amount of muscle force (Evarts 1975) and the direction of the force (Georgopoulos, Schwartz, and Kattner 1986).

At the rear of the brain and beneath the cerebrum is the *cerebellum,* which has an important function in movement. The cortex of this section, like that of the cerebrum, is composed of gray matter, while the interior

is made up mainly of the white matter of nerve fibers. The cerebellum is the regulator of muscle tone, coordination, timing, and learning (Rosenbaum 1991).

The **basal ganglia,** which is a group of nuclei located in the inner layers of the cerebrum, receive information from the reticular formation and motor areas of the cerebral cortex and transmit the information to the thalamus. It is responsible for initiating and executing slow movements as well as facilitating and inhibiting a wide variety of movements. Some diseases that result from damage to the basal ganglia include Parkinson's disease and Huntington's disease.

■ The brain is often considered to be the computer or central processor of the human body.

The brain also can be likened to the railroad station or air traffic control tower where flow of traffic is regulated. Events are placed on hold or moved rapidly, interconnections are made, modifications in processing result, and all activity proceeds or is stymied by the station's competence.

It is only natural that sometimes the human body does not move as well as possible or does not move consistently from day to day. Fatigue, nutritional deficits, lethargy, and other factors influence the brain's functioning. Conversely, the functions that occur frequently, such as walking, often appear to be performed without any effort by the brain. It is as if a memory program is activated automatically when walking is produced.

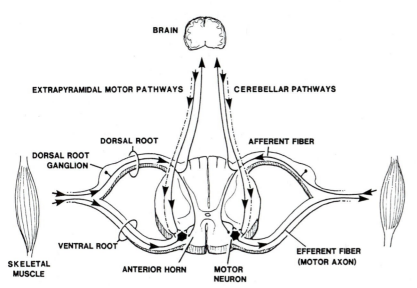

FIGURE 5.2 Cross-section diagram of spinal cord with afferent and efferent fiber connections to the muscle. Single monosynaptic reflex loops involve entry and pathways. More complicated reflex and volitional loops require use of these vertical pathways.

According to Schmidt (1988), complex neural circuits, called spinal generators, may exist within the spinal cord and may be responsible for simple automatic rhythmic actions such as gait.

The brain must interact with the peripheral muscles so that the bones can be moved. This is possible by means of the spinal cord, which can be likened to the super highways and airways of the world. The messages from the brain travel to the muscles, via the spinal cord through the alpha motor neurons. The result is contraction or cessation of contraction (relaxation) of the muscle fibers.

■ Much of what is known about the function and interaction of the many brain centers is a result of studying the various diseases and injuries that affect specific areas of the brain.

While scientists know a great deal about how the brain is involved in movement, there is still much more to learn. Researchers in the areas of artificial intelligence and neural science are providing us with new information.

Spinal Cord

Continuous with the medulla of the brain stem, extending through the spinal canal, and terminating at the upper border of the second lumbar vertebra, is that portion of the central nervous system known as the *spinal cord*. Unlike the arrangement of the brain, the gray matter of the cord is in the interior section, in a configuration resembling the letter "H" (Figure 5.2). The ends of the "H" are referred to as the *anterior and posterior horns*. Surrounding the gray matter are the white nerve fibers connecting various parts of the brain with the cord cells and connecting cells within the cord. The nerve fibers are grouped into tracts. The names of these tracts, such as the spinocerebellar and the corticospinal tracts, often indicate the connected areas and also the direction in which nerve impulses are conducted.

Neurons

Each cell body with its fibers is known as a **neuron** (see Figure 5.3). Those fibers that conduct impulses away from the cell body are the efferent fibers, known as **axons;** those which conduct impulses toward the cell body are the afferent fibers, known as **dendrites.** Rarely does a neuron have more than one axon, and this single axon is usually longer than the dendrites; some axons are as long as one meter (39 in.) in length. Often one neuron has several dendrites; near the cell these may be thicker than any axon, but they taper rapidly and branch repeatedly, forming a network of fiber at no great distance from the cell. Impulses do not pass from one neuron to another except at the point where the axon of one cell body is in close contact with the dendrites of another. This connection, known as the **synapse,** is found

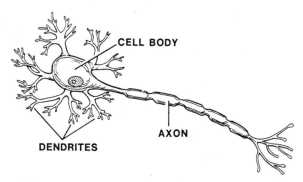

FIGURE 5.3 A typical neuron with its parts labeled. Think of this as a nerve tree analogous to the lung tree and arterial tree, with potential interaction with many other neurons via a synapse, also known as the traffic intersection of the nervous system. The richness of the dendrite tree may well be the key to recovery from neurological traumas.

TABLE 5.1 Cranial nerve identification.

Number	Name	Innervation Site
I	Olfactory	Nose
II	Optic	Eyes
III	Oculomotor	Eyes
IV	Trochlear	Face
V	Trigeminal	Face
VI	Abducent	Eye
VII	Facial	Face (tear ducts, tongue, and ears)
VIII	Vestibulocochlear	Inner ear
IX	Glossopharyngeal	Tongue, Pharynx, Larynx
X	Vagus	Tongue and Neck
XI	Accessory	Neck
XII	Hypoglossal	Tongue

only within the central nervous system. These synapses occur at each level of entry into the spinal cord and throughout the brain.

■ Nerve fibers and cell bodies are not separate units, since each fiber arises from a cell body.

Peripheral Nervous System

The **peripheral nervous system** includes the cranial and spinal nerves and the peripheral portions of the autonomic nervous system (Table 5.1). The latter controls the action of the viscera, glands, heart, blood vessels, and smooth muscles in other parts of the body and is not directly involved in the movement of skeletal parts. The 12 pairs of cranial nerves and 31 pairs of spinal nerves control the action of striated muscle and are thus directly involved in joint actions. The cranial nerves connect the muscles of the face and head and the central nervous system. They carry impulses to the central nervous system from the receptors of the special senses—the visual, auditory, olfactory, and gustatory senses. They also carry impulses from the more widely spread receptors of pressure, tension, pain, and temperature located in the face and head.

The spinal nerves are most directly involved in movements of the trunk and limbs. The 31 pairs are classified according to the area in which each enters the spinal column: 8 cervical, 12 thoracic, 5 lumbar, 5 sacral, and 1 coccygeal (see Figure 5.4). Each group is numbered from the head downward. In general, the shoulders, arms, and hands are connected with the central nervous system by the fifth, sixth, seventh, and eighth cervical nerves and the first thoracic nerve. The trunk is connected by all the thoracic, lumbar, and sacral nerves. The hips, thighs, legs, and feet are connected by the second, fourth, and fifth lumbar nerves and first and second sacral nerve.

Each spinal nerve connects with the spinal cord by an anterior and a posterior root as previously depicted in Figure 5.2. The posterior roots (afferent nerves) conduct impulses from the sensory receptors of those parts of the body with which the nerves are connected, and the anterior roots (efferent nerves) conduct impulses to the muscles from the central nervous system. Lesions and partial damage to the spinal cord results in loss of muscle function and/or control specific to the level of damage. For example, damage to the sacral nerve may result in loss of function in the feet (Refer to Figure 5.4).

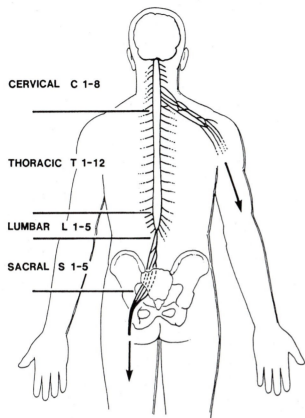

CERVICAL C 1-8

THORACIC T 1-12

LUMBAR L 1-5

SACRAL S 1-5

FIGURE 5.4 The spinal nerves: C, cervical; T, thoracic; L, lumbar; and S, sacral. Note the body part innervated by each nerve. Dysfunction of a specific nerve causes dysfunction in movement coordination and control of the body part innervated by the nerve. Note also that lesions at the spinal cord destroy all spinal nerves arising from the spinal cord caudal to the lesion. **Where could a lesion be and which nerves are damaged if a person were a paraplegic? State the same for quadriplegia.**

Motor Units

Each efferent (motor) fiber in the spinal nerve arises from a cell body in the anterior horn and is connected with a muscle fiber in some part of the body. The majority of skeletal muscles have thousands of muscle fibers, but each is not supplied with a separate nerve fiber. Instead, the axon of the motor neuron divides into many collaterals just before and after entering the muscle. Each collateral connects with a single muscle fiber, all of which contract simultaneously when an impulse is

sent from the anterior horn cell. The entire neuron and the muscle fibers that it innervates are called a **motor unit.** By this arrangement, part of the fibers in one muscle are able to contract while the remaining ones (comprising other motor units) remain at their relaxed length. This arrangement, for partial contraction of a single muscle, is further facilitated by different degrees of strength in the stimulus needed to excite a neuron.

■ A stimulus that is just strong enough to excite the most sensitive fiber is called a *threshold stimulus;* one that is just strong enough to excite all the fibers is called a **maximal stimulus.**

Logically, a given muscle should be able to develop as many different degrees of strength (because of the contraction of fibers in a unit) as there are motor units represented in that muscle. If 100 motor units were present, 100 different degrees of tensions would be possible if progressive summation occurs. A variety of recruitment patterns, however, may be elicited. Therefore, seemingly infinite magnitudes of tension can be produced by a single muscle. The flexor pollicis is one example of a muscle with such infinite graduations of response. The ability to recruit repeatedly and precisely optimal tension is a function of skill.

Since some muscle fibers are innervated by more than one motor unit, the strength of several motor units contracting simultaneously will not equal the sum of the strength of contraction of the individual units. The number of fibers innervated by a single axon varies with the precision of movement required by contraction of that particular muscle. It has been estimated that there is a ratio of 1775 fibers to 1 motor unit in the medial head of the gastrocnemius (which is responsible for large, gross movement). In the tibialis anterior the ratio is 609:1, and in the eye muscles the ratio is 5:1, since very precise movements are needed for effective vision. Generally, the fewer the number of muscle fibers in the motor unit, the more precision it allows.

Stimulation of Motor Units

If the muscle fibers in a motor unit are to contract, they must be stimulated by a nerve impulse from the cell body in the anterior horn cell. This cell, in turn, must be stimulated by impulses that come to it via its short

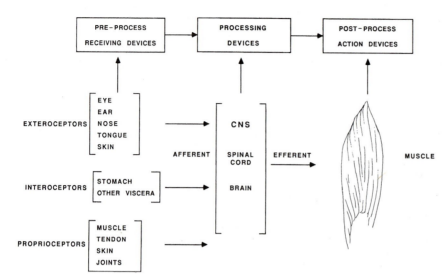

FIGURE 5.5 Schematic of the receiving, processing, and action devices of the nervous system. Stimuli (signals) are received (picked up) by various receptors, often by more than one simultaneously, and sent via the afferent network to the central nervous system for sorting, planning, and programming. The designated response message is sent via the efferent network to the muscle for action. Note that the muscle appears as the action device as well as the receiving device. **Which substructures are specialized in the action part and which in the receptor? See Figure 5.6 for answer.**

dendrites. The dendrites, in turn, must receive impulses through the synapse that they make with many nerve fibers, both afferent (sensory) and efferent. These multiple connections make the motor mechanism of the central nervous system highly complex. If the intention to move originates in the cerebral cortex, then, at the time the nerve impulses from the cortex reach the anterior horn cell, the impulses from the cerebellum from nerve cells in the brain below the cortex and from the afferent fibers arising in other muscles and joints are also likely to be received.

Although recruitment of motor unit firing for gradation of muscular force varies, recruitment occurs in an orderly fashion. A popular theory is that motor units are recruited by size. According to the "size principle" (Henneman 1981), the smaller motor units (small force, slow twitch muscle units, and those innervated by small motor neurons) fire first and the larger motor units (larger, faster muscle units, and those innervated by larger motor neurons) fire last. Lower thresholds exist for the smaller motor neurons. Others say selective recruitment occurs; motor units are recruited according to the task, in effect controlled by biofeedback. Rate coding is yet another variation; motor units change their firing rate, increasing it for increased force demands.

■ It is suggested that recruitment and rate coding are concurrent processes and that the extent of the involvement of each appears to be muscle-dependent (Enoka, 1988).

Receptors

Some comprehension of the complexity of the pathways by which a nerve impulse may reach a motor unit can be gained from considering the source of impulses. An impulse originates in the endings of nerve fibers that are specialized and excited by a specific change in the environment. These endings, known as **receptors,** are each specialized to respond to certain stimuli only. Those ending in the eye respond primarily to light, those in the ear to sound, those in the mouth and nose to chemical changes, and some near the body surface to pressure. Impulses resulting from these changes may reach the cerebral cortex, and the excitations caused there have become known as sight, sound, taste, smell, and touch. The average person is unfamiliar with the many other nerve impulses originating in other types of receptors. They are (1) *interoceptors,* those located in the visceral organs; (2) *exteroceptors,* those responding to stimuli arising outside the body, such as sight, sound, smell, and external pressure; and (3) *proprioceptors,* those found in muscles, tendons, and joints, which respond to mechanical changes within the body. (The latter are of special interest in the study of movement.) A schematic of the role of receptors and central nervous system is presented in Figure 5.5.

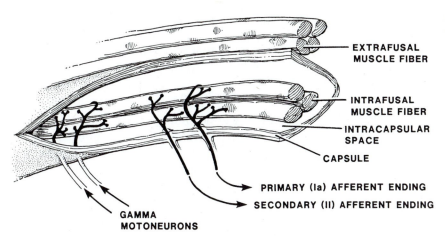

FIGURE 5.6 Schematic representation of a muscle spindle with relevant movement control parts. Note the efferent pathways for the muscle to receive the nerve impulse (message) from the central nervous system and the afferent pathways for the muscle to send messages to the central nervous system.

Proprioceptors

Impulses originating in the proprioceptors may travel to the motor unit (via the spinal cord) and be responsible for joint actions that are not consciously directed. They can be the basis for reflex actions, inherent patterns, adjustments made during performance, and learned skills.

■ Proprioceptors are referred to as our "sixth sense" receptors. This "sixth sense" is termed **kinesthesia**, awareness of one's body in space.

Scientists have identified several of these proprioceptors. They are discussed in the following paragraphs.

Muscle Spindles

As long ago as 1850, it was found that within muscles there are small groupings of fibers that differ in structure from surrounding fibers in the same muscle. These groupings were later given the name *muscle spindle.* Some investigators thought that the muscle spindle might be the specialized receptor in which nerve impulses would be initiated by changes in the degree of contraction in the muscle. In 1894, Sherrington demonstrated that a nerve fiber from the spindle carries impulses to the spinal cord. We now know that the major role of the muscle spindle is to monitor muscle length (Enoka 1988) and that the spindle is a two-way device, both receiving and transmitting impulses.

Figure 5.6 is a schematic representation of a muscle spindle. These receptors lie between and parallel to the muscle fibers. Within a connective tissue sheath, or capsule, there are a number of muscle fibers known as intrafusal fibers. Other fibers in the muscle and not within the capsule are known as extrafusal fibers. Intrafusal fibers are much smaller and consequently produce much less force than the extrafusal fibers. Contraction of all the intrafusal fibers within a given muscle will not produce enough force for movement to occur. They do, however, have a very important function within the muscle spindle. This function is to adjust the bias or gain of the stretch receptor (explained later in this section). The center region of these fibers contains the nuclei (in a nuclear bar or nuclear chain fashion) and is noncontractile. Two types of nerve fibers are in the muscle spindle: (1) efferent, which carry nerve impulses from the spinal cord to the intrafusal muscle fibers; (2) afferent, which carry impulses from the muscle spindle to the central nervous system.

There are two types of afferent fibers. They differ in diameter (the larger transmit impulses more rapidly than the smaller) and in type of ending on the intrafusal fiber. The primary (Ia), or annulospiral, ending of the larger type rarely branches as it approaches the intrafusal fiber; its ending winds around the fiber in the rear of the nuclear sac much like a coil or spring. The secondary (II), or flower-spray, ending of the smaller afferent fiber also connects with the intrafusal fiber in the region of the nuclear sac, but it is farther from the middle than is the primary ending. There is only one primary ending on a fiber. There may be as many as five secondary endings, although only one is most commonly found. Whenever the nuclear bag area is stretched, nerve impulses are initiated in primary and secondary endings and transmitted to the spinal cord. The muscle spindle then, is a type of **stretch receptor.**

Efferent nerve fibers incorporated in the spindle, known as gamma motoneurons, are small in diameter. They connect with the intrafusal fiber above the nuclear sac area, where the muscle fibers have contractile ability. When the gamma efferent nerve impulses reach the intrafusal fibers, the latter contract, stretching the central nuclear sac area. Since the number of intrafusal fibers is small compared to the number of extrafusal fibers in the muscle, this contraction appears to make little or no contribution to movement. Its function is stimulation of the spindle afferent fibers, which now can be seen as sensory, or at least afferent, receptors. Firing of the gamma efferents acts to set the bias on the stretch receptor, adjusting its sensitivity, much like eliminating the "play" in a steering wheel. The muscle spindle can, therefore, be activated one of two ways: (1) stretching the nuclear bag region by muscle stretch; and (2) stretching the nuclear bag region by influence of the gamma efferents.

When afferent impulses are initiated in the spindle and transmitted to the spinal cord, they have the possibility of reaching many parts of the body via the complex synaptic connections and nerve pathways in the cord. Some may be carried to the extrafusal fibers in the same muscle in which the impulses originated (**homonymous** muscle). Some may influence the contraction of other muscles acting on the same joint, bringing into action assisting prime movers and synergistic muscle (see Chapter 4). Some may inhibit the action of antagonist muscles. Such afferent impulses may also activate anterior horn cells in many parts of the spinal cord and thus affect the movement and position of many segments. Some may initiate activity in the nerve cells of the brain stem, subcortical brain areas, and cerebellum. Afferent impulses are the basis for the numerous possibilities for complex reflex acts and for the involuntary joint actions that are a part of voluntarily initiated motor acts. These possibilities support the statement that the mind orders an act and leaves the details of execution to lower levels of the nervous system.

■ Without question the muscle spindle plays a major role in movement; by responding to contraction in the active muscles it serves as a coordinator throughout the action.

Golgi Tendon Organs

Another type of proprioceptor, the Golgi tendon organ (GTO), is found in the tendons close to their muscular origin and in the connective tissue of the muscle. The end of an afferent nerve fiber is surrounded by layers of tendon fibers enclosed in a connective sheath. Within this encapsulated mass the nerve ending branches. When the tendon or connective tissue is stretched, the pressure on the nerve ending initiates impulses that will be conducted to the central nervous system. The GTOs are also stretch receptors, however. While the muscle spindle responds to stretch due to muscular stretch, the golgi tendon organs respond to stretch in the tendon produced by excessive muscular contraction.

■ One role of the GTO is to act as a protector mechanism.

The GTOs help to avoid tearing of the muscle as a result of a forceful contraction. The resulting action of GTO firing, by a series of neural connections via the spinal cord, is relaxation (cessation of contraction) of the homonymous muscle. For example, to relieve a "charley horse," a person attempts to stretch the muscle that is cramped. Since the cramp is a result of an excessive muscular contraction, applying a force to stretch the muscle results in stretching the tendons. The result is relaxation of the cramped muscle.

■ Another role of the GTOs is to provide information of body position since they are located very near the joint capsules.

Pacinian and Ruffini Receptors

Pacinian corpuscles are widely distributed in the fascia of muscles, especially beneath the tendinous insertion of muscles at the joints. They are also found in the deeper layers of the skin. The nerve ending is surrounded by concentric layers of fibrous tissue, within which the nerve branches. Pressure is exerted on the nerve endings due to joint positions and when muscles contract or are stretched. Pacinian corpuscles only respond for a very brief period of time; therefore, they are a source for information on rapid changes of position. **Ruffini endings** are also located in the joint and also respond to pressure. These receptors, however, are slow in adapting and thus are a source for information on continuous states of pressure.

■ Combined information from the Pacinian corpuscles and the Ruffini endings is used to "feel and know" the movement and position of the limbs of the body.

Cutaneous Receptors

Cutaneous, or *skin receptors,* which respond to touch and pressure, are also activated by changes in joints and muscles. They respond to changes in the amount of pressure on the skin and in the area of the movement. Since these receptors respond to a mechanical deformation of the skin, they are also referred to as *mechanoreceptors.* The nerve fibers connected with these receptors reach the spinal cord by way of the posterior branches of the spinal nerves. They branch as they enter the spinal cord, conducting impulses to anterior horn cells at the same level or to higher or lower levels of the cord. These impulses may result in reflex or subconscious movements. Some impulses may be conducted to the cerebellum and may influence the coordination of movements initiated by efferent impulses originating in this section of the brain.

Volitional Contribution to Motor Action

Motor acts are often initiated by a decision (activity originating in the cerebral cortex). That decision does not include conscious, detailed direction of the joint actions that will be needed. Studying motion pictures of our own performance we often observe movements that surprise us. We were not aware of them at the time.

■ The mind orders "whole," and the details occur without conscious direction.

For example, you may decide to sit in a chair. The exact muscles involved, the sequence of the muscles, and the timing of muscular contractions is subconsciously programmed to achieve the task. The

neuromuscular system selects its own methods of achieving the goal set. It is through practice with feedback from many sources that learning occurs. According to Burke (1986),

> The ability to perform at the limit of physical capacity is the essence of competitive sport. This must involve training not only the muscles, which are marvelously adaptable, but also the nervous system, which is no less so. Optimum usage of muscles may well require strategies of usage for which the usual sequence of recruitment is poorly adapted.

Recent work by Grimby (1986) and many others shows that motor units are recruited differently and in different patterns based on the task. If our motor system is to learn the new skill, we must practice it accurately.

■ It is important that individuals practice new skills, or skills they wish to improve, at the same speed and under the same conditions as the performance will require.

A national women's golf champion was asked what she thought about as she prepared to take a shot. She answered, "I see the shot, then feel it, and then I do it." (Further questioning revealed that "seeing" meant visualizing the needed height and distance.) A basketball coach of national repute was asked how he helped his players develop skill in shooting free throws. His reply was identical to the golfer's. He asked the players to visualize the high point of the shot and feel it before beginning the movement. A British scientist believes that it is more important to know what to do than how to do it and suggests that the less a performer knows about the details of the act, the more efficient that act is likely to be.

There is much experimental evidence to support the notion of motor programs. Stored within our brain are a variety of generalized motor programs of actions we have learned (e.g., overarm throwing action, kicking action). Schmidt (1978) suggests that these programs are represented as schemas (abstract representations). The programs include some invariant features such as the order, phasing, and relative force of the events. Specific information, such as the environmental conditions and the desired outcome, is inputted into the program. Specific muscles are not part of the generalized motor program. A simple example to support this can be seen by signing your name on a small piece of paper and then on a large chalkboard. Although you used different muscles to generate each signature, the two signatures will look very similar. Motor control researchers have developed (and are still refining) many models in an attempt to explain the many facets of movement and timing. The proper execution of any motor act involves the closely synchronized action of many brain centers in order to arrive at the precise timing and proper force production of many thousands of muscle fibers throughout the body. When you stop to think about it, it is a wonder that we can move at all!

Involuntary Details of Motor Behavior

We can attribute the involuntary details of common human motor behavior to reflex action and inherent motor patterns. Researchers in the area of motor development have observed different phases within the human life span. In the earliest stage, the reflexive stage (beginning approximately at the third fetal month and continuing until about six months after birth), the nervous system is not fully developed and atavistic (primitive) reflexes dominate movement. As the infant matures (by six months), the reflex action gradually comes under voluntary control and appears as part of a volitional act overriding most of the primitive reflexes. The stepping actions that an infant two to three weeks old makes when held upright with the feet contacting a surface continue to operate reflexively in voluntary walking. The weaving of reflex patterns into voluntary movements could well explain the involuntary details of volitional movement patterns. Many reflexes continue to exist throughout life, such as the Babinski reflex to stroking the sole of the foot.

Stretch Reflexes (Myotatic Reflex)

The knee jerk, **patella-tendon reflex,** is perhaps the most widely recognized human reflex. A sharp blow on the tendon at the knee results in a sudden stretch in the knee extensor muscles and initiates a nerve impulse in the afferent nerve fibers of the muscle spindles. The nerve impulse travels to the spinal cord and then to the

gray matter of the anterior horn cells where the afferent fibers synapse with the dendrites of motor neuron in the anterior horn. The impulse is then conducted via the axon of the motor neuron to the muscle fibers of the knee extensors (the homonymous muscle), and as these contract, the leg is rapidly extended. This type of response also occurs when the pressure on the tendon is a steady pressure rather than a sharp blow.

MINI-LABORATORY LEARNING EXPERIENCE

Try to elicit the patella-tendon reflex by tapping the knee, just below the patella, with the ulnar side of the palm of the hand. Begin with light taps. Once the response is elicited, gradually increase the force of each tap. Is there a change in the magnitude of the response? Now instead of tapping the tendon, exert a steady pressure. Do the muscles respond with a steady contraction?

The voluntary concept and the reflex can be visualized by holding a weight in the hand with the forearm flexed 90°. The intent of the performer is to maintain this angle, with the mind ordering the act in its entirety. The stretch on the elbow flexors (caused by gravity applying a downward force on the hand and weight) signals to the muscle the number of motor units needed. If the weight is increased or decreased, reflex information via the muscle spindle provides the needed adjustment in strength of contraction. The sensitivity of this response can be adjusted with the gamma efferents in the muscle spindles. When a person is aware that the weight will suddenly change there will be little change in the elbow flexion due to the high sensitivity of the stretch receptors. By consciously adjusting the sensitivity of the muscle spindle by firing the gamma efferents, the sensitivity is increased to just below the threshold. Once the slightest amount of stretch is placed on the muscle, the muscle spindle fires. However, if weight is added when the person least expects it, the response will be slower and the change in elbow angle will be much greater. This is because there was sufficiently more stretch needed within the muscle spindle that had to be taken up prior to reaching the threshold.

Have a partner hold a weight in the hand. While the partner watches, add more weight to the hand. Now ask your partner to close both eyes while you add more weight. What happens? Explain. What receptor is involved?

■ The stretch reflex is widely distributed in the body and is especially well developed in anti-gravity muscles.

In the description of the mechanical aspects of standing, the center of gravity of the body is normally positioned in a vertical plane in front of the ankle joint. Gravitational force would pull the body forward, causing ankle flexion. The resulting stretch on the ankle extensors initiates the nerve impulses that control the amount of contraction needed to maintain the position that the performer intends. If the forward lean approaches the limits of easy balance, stretch increases and the stimulation to the ankle extensors increases. The increase in muscle contraction pulls the body back. The intent to stand keeps the ankle joint within a range of flexion that is not consciously controlled. This is termed *gamma bias.* With high-heeled shoes, the amount of stretch in the ankle flexors must be adjusted to accommodate the changed position. This slack is taken up by the gamma efferents in the muscle spindles (Eldred 1967).

Another loop within the stretch reflex involves connections to the antagonist muscles. To assist with the muscle spindle's objective of minimizing the stretch that led to its activation by exciting the homonymous muscle, a message is also sent to relax the antagonist muscles. This response, referred to as *reciprocal inhibition,* serves to reduce muscle co-activation, which would result in stiffness of the joint. In the tendon tap, the knee flexor muscles relax to allow the knee extensors freedom to extend the knee.

One additional part of the reflex circuit involves what is called *recurrent inhibition.* Within the spinal cord, messages from branches of the alpha motor neurons connect with another type of neuron, the *Renshaw cell.*

The purpose of the Renshaw cell is to inhibit the motor neuron that excites it. An interesting effect of the Renshaw cells is that they can be controlled by supraspinal centers. We can therefore control the level of excitation of the motor neurons.

If the intent is to walk, run, or jump, the degree of flexion at the ankle is increased, as shown in Chapters 9, 15, and 16. Flexion is permitted to the extent necessary for the specific act. The angle at the ankle joint may be held stationary as the foot is lifted and later the change in angle is at an angular rate that exactly parallels that of the metatarsophalangeal action. These joint actions are basically the same in the unskilled and the skilled performer. Some mechanism common to both must be in control. This mechanism is the stretch reflex.

Hold your arm horizontally abducted. Slowly swing the arm backward. Note what happens at the end of the swing. Repeat this action progressively swinging faster and faster. Note the response. Explain the mechanism responsible for the response.

In throwing and striking patterns, it is likely that the rapid backswing, by means of the stretch reflex, produces contraction of muscles needed for the forward swing. Based on observations of muscle action, we know that the muscles responsible for the forward swing begin their contractions before the limit of the backswing is reached. These contractions not only stop the backswing but also increase the number of nerve impulses initiated by the stretch and thereby increase the speed of the forward movement. This sudden activation of the muscle spindle results in a more forceful, yet sometimes jerky, contraction. For skills requiring more precision, a slow backswing and/or a pause at the end of the backswing will reduce or eliminate this phasic response. This can be seen in the execution of the golf putt where a slow, controlled backswing is used.

The myotatic reflex is the simplest of those observed in humans, since often only two neurons are involved. (It is referred to as a monosynaptic reflex, since there is only one synapse in the reflex arc.) Other, more complex reflex actions that involve action in more than one level of the spinal cord have been observed. These may result in movement of more than one joint and in some cases movement in a contralateral (opposite) limb. A painful stimulus applied to the foot or hand activating the pain receptors, will result in withdrawal of that limb by flexion of more than one joint. This reflex, which occurs when we touch a hot stove, is termed the *flexor,* or *withdrawal reflex.* This action also initiates impulses that contract extensors in the opposite limb, which are needed to maintain balance (the *crossed-extensor reflex*). For example, a person stepping on a nail will flex that leg and simultaneously extend the other leg to keep from falling.

Righting Reflexes (Labyrinthine Reflex)

The reflexes that act together to maintain equilibrium are known as the *righting reflexes.* They act in normal standing when the adjustments are barely noticeable and also when there is greater threat to balance. When balance is threatened, many body parts, especially the arms, may be seen moving vigorously and widely. These efforts to bring the body's center of gravity over the feet, needless to say, are not always successful. A righting reflex is the response of the head to a loss in its upright position as a result of body movements changing the orientation of the head. For example, this reflex results in a lifting of the head when novices attempt a forward dive into a swimming pool.

Tonic-Neck Reflex

An interesting concept can be drawn from observations reported by Hellebrandt et al. (1961). When a weight was lifted by hand flexion and hand extension, they observed that under stress other segments of the body were moved and that head movements resembled those of the tonic neck reflex. This reflex is noted in children and usually is volitionally controlled in adults.

■ The tonic neck reflex is a response of the limbs to a rotation of the head.

The turning of the head to the side is accompanied by movements in the upper and lower limbs (Figure 5.7). On the side toward which the head is turned, there

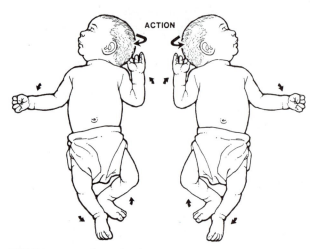

FIGURE 5.7 Tonic neck reflexes. The turning of the head is an action that elicits a response of the upper and lower extremities as shown by unlabeled arrows. Can you see why the turning of the head away from a working arm would increase the strength output of that arm? **Although you can volitionally repress this reflex, can you think of ways you might want to allow it to happen to enhance a performance?**

is adduction at the shoulder and extension at the elbow in the upper limb and flexion at the knee in the lower limb. On the opposite side, there is abduction at the shoulder and flexion at the elbow in the upper limb and extension at the knee in the lower limb.

The resulting position is that seen in the fencing lunge (lower limbs) and thrust (upper limbs). After observing the appearance of the head movements, Hellebrandt and coworkers found that voluntarily turning the head to the working side increased the work output and turning the head to the opposite side decreased the output. The head position evidently affected the number of nerve impulses sent to the wrist muscles. Thus, it is evident that the position of segments other than those acting in a given pattern can affect performance.

■ The neck and **labyrinthine reflexes** are among the most important reflex mechanisms in sport and gymnastic skills. For example, divers and gymnasts use head movements to facilitate body spin, to flex or extend the limbs and trunk when these movements are desired in a stunt, and to attain correct position at the finish.

Reflexes may facilitate or inhibit volitional movements. For example, the tonic neck reflex inhibits the forward tuck somersault motion because cervical flexion causes the lower limbs to extend. This same reflex facilitates the backward tuck somersault because cervical extension causes the lower limbs to flex. When the head is turned to the side away from the striking arm in racquet sports, the tonic neck reflex causes arm flexion, which causes the person to miss the ball. The old adage "Keep the eye on the ball" is well founded.

Gardner (1969) also states that understanding reflex mechanisms is valuable when successful performance requires voluntary inhibition of the associated joint actions, such as pivoting in the golf swing without swaying. She makes this point succinctly by saying, "One must inhibit 'what comes naturally.' "

Inherent Motor Patterns

Although reflex actions are inherent patterns, we will distinguish those that have a conscious purpose from those that are reactions to stimuli that arise in some part of the nervous system other than the cerebral cortex. Withdrawal from intense heat occurs without conscious intent; the withdrawal is often said to occur before one is even aware of the pain. A reflex response does not vary, while a purposeful inherent pattern, characterized by basic similarities, is not stereotyped. If the human overarm throw is an inherent pattern, the details of performance may differ in individuals and in the same individual at various times. But basic similarities will be present. These responses are not learned; they appear without learning, and may be referred to as inherent action or behavior pattern. An action pattern is as typical of a particular species as is the physiological structure of the animal, and species may be identified by their action patterns.

Inherent Motor Patterns in Human Beings

As we study human throwing, striking, and locomotion patterns, common elements are evident. Of course, these elements could be learned, but we see them in the performances of young children who have had no instruction. Even children who have an opportunity to observe

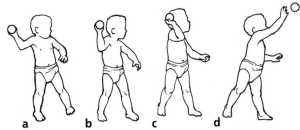

FIGURE 5.8 Tracings based on film of overarm pattern of boy 33 months of age who had no instruction. Joint actions and their sequences resemble those of highly skilled performers and are thought to be an inherent basic pattern of movement. **Analyze the spatial characteristics of this throw with respect to axes of rotation, planes of segmental movement, and sequencing of segmental movements.**

skilled performers would not be aware of details of action. Figure 5.8 shows selected tracings taken from a detailed study of the overarm throwing pattern of David, a 33-month-old boy. He had no instruction in throwing, yet the elements of skillful performance are present. In Figure 5.8a he is seen as forward movement begins. The weight is on the right foot, the left is lifted from the floor, the pelvis is rotated to the right over the supporting foot, and the head faces in the direction of the throw. In b the left foot has been placed forward to facilitate rotation of the pelvis over that limb; the position of the throwing arm has changed little. In the 0.23 second between b and c, lateral rotation in the left hip has turned the torso in the direction of the throw, and rotation of the humerus has carried the elbow ahead of the ball. This is an intriguing instance of timing—forward rotation of one segment and simultaneous backward rotation of another. It is interesting to speculate what the actions would be if they were attempted by conscious direction. Two elements that would be seen in a more skillful performer are lacking: (1) no vertebral action is in evidence—the torso acts as a unit, and (2) the humerus has not held its position in the transverse plane but has been adducted. The position at release is shown in d, 0.03 second after the action shown in c. Rotation of the torso has continued, the humerus has rotated medially, the elbow has extended slightly, and the hand has undoubtedly flexed. The observer can only marvel at the coordinations that result from the intent to throw. This boy and other boys of preschool age have also demonstrated mature underarm and sidearm patterns.

Locomotion patterns (walking, running, jumping, and leaping) are performed by young children. As everyone knows, the complicated coordinations of walking and running develop without maturity and instruction. Detailed observation leads us to believe that the young child's nervous system controls movements within the limits that ensure balance. When running movements first appear, at no time are both feet off the ground. The forward foot is on the ground before the rear foot leaves it. With experience the flight phase develops, and as skill is improved, the proportion of time of the flight phase increases. As when young children attempt a two-footed takeoff for a jump, their nervous systems refuse to allow the center of gravity to move forward unless one foot is moved ahead to receive the weight. This tendency can be seen at all ages, perhaps because of lack of experience in attempting a two-footed takeoff. This pattern reappears with older persons (70- and 80-year-olds) who are asked to run and have not done so for many years. Projecting the body from one foot seems to be the natural, innate pattern.

Another tendency to preserve balance has been observed in the use of the arms in the standing broad jump. Effective use consists of a forward swing in the sagittal plane on takeoff and a backward swing during flight, followed by a forward swing on landing. Researchers using film have shown that elementary-school children and college women whose jumps are shorter than those of their peers do not swing the arms in the sagittal plane (Wickstrom 1983). Instead, the arms are held at horizontal abduction throughout the jump. This resembles the action patterns of birds, whose wings are stretched to the side as they take off for flight and also during landing as the legs reach forward. Young children also exhibit unlearned joint action. A child under three years of age was observed as he jumped from a height equal to his own body height. The legs had been fully extended on takeoff, yet during flight the legs flexed to bring the feet forward for landing. This was not a learned movement; it was his first experience in that situation. What but inherent patterning could be the basis for the action? Lorenz (1950) has stated that undoubtedly animals in general inherit behavioral traits. To suggest that human behavior follows a different pattern would be illogical.

Behavior differs from individual to individual because of the human capacity to modify details of motor inheritance in various ways.

Learning Motor Patterns

If motor patterns are innate, we might logically question the need for learning. There are at least two apparent reasons for learning motor patterns. One is that even innate patterns improve with practice. In addition, if patterns are not practiced during the time at which they appear naturally, they will never reach their full potential. Riesen (1950) reports that newly hatched chickens kept in darkness for 14 days after hatching failed to peck at spots on the ground when brought into the light. He concluded that prolonged lack of practice can interfere with the development of instinctive reflex behavior. He also reports that vision in chimpanzees will not be normal if the eyes are not exposed to light for an extended period after birth. Hess (1958) has shown that the instinctive following of a moving object, characteristic of the young of many animals and known as imprinting, is most strongly developed in mallard ducks if the experience occurs within 13 to 16 hours after hatching.

Since children at an early age, certainly before six years, have the basic patterns of throwing, striking, and locomotion, it is possible that if these patterns are not experienced at the time the nervous system is ready for them to be experienced, they may never reach their full potential. Ranson and Clark (1959) suggest this possibility when they state that although the neurons of an adult human's nervous system are arranged in a hereditary pattern, many of the details of the nervous system are shaped by the individual's experiences.

The second reason for learning is that basic human patterns can and should be modified for specific situations. If the individual is aware of success or failure after performance, the pattern can often be modified without any conscious direction of joint action. This can be illustrated by experience with the 33-month-old-boy. The boy had a running pattern, and researchers attempted to modify the run into a leap. They did not try to verbally explain how to do a leap. Instead, they placed a rolled mat in the runway and asked the boy to clear it as he ran. In the first attempt he took off from a running step and landed with both feet on the mat. No comments were

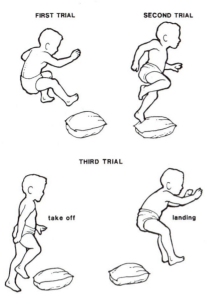

FIGURE 5.9 Motor adjustments made by boy 33 months of age as he attempted to clear obstacle. Although given no instruction he succeeded on the third trial, after first landing on the obstacle and next striking the obstacle during the takeoff phase. On all trials he used a pattern common to that of long jumpers taking off on one foot and landing on both feet.

made, and he attempted a second trial. This time he took off from the mat; he had moved the takeoff too far forward. The third trial was successful; he cleared the mat and landed on both feet (Figure 5.9). They then asked him to continue running after clearing the mat. He then achieved a one-footed landing, which initially was not in balance, but which improved with successive trials. He had in mind a definite purpose as he made these adjustments. That intent was sufficient to modify joint action when he was aware of his failures. His mind had ordered a "whole," but had left the details of execution to those parts of the central nervous system below the level of consciousness.

Perception of Movement and Position

People can usually describe accurately the position of various parts of their own bodies, even with closed eyes. The skilled basketball player knows as soon as the ball is released whether the free throw movements felt right and if the ball is likely to enter the basket. The same can be said of the bowler who knows at the moment of ball release that a strike will result. A skilled performer "feels" the action before executing it. This concept has been used in teaching through visualization and mental practice (also referred to as mental imagery). A number of motor-learning researchers have shown that skill can be improved with mental practice, that is, by recalling the feel of the action and substituting successive recalls for physical practice. These recognitions of position and feel are examples of memory of previous motor experience and of recalling activity in the cerebral cortex that accompanied motor acts and cerebral activity initiated by proprioceptors. Recently, commercial learning packages have been developed based on this concept. These packages consist of repetitions of skilled performances that can be visually imaged and used as a supplement to physical practice of the skill.

Types of Memory

Many kinds of memories are developed from cerebral activity—memories of sounds, sights, smells, touch sensations, and tastes. Each type of memory results from activity stimulated by a nerve impulse from a corresponding type of receptor. Memories of sound develop from impulses initiated in audio receptors. Visual memories are recalled from those initiated in vision receptors. Yet, as far as we know, the nerve impulse initiated in one type of receptor does not differ from that initiated in any other type, as the impulse travels nerve pathways. The difference in recognition in the cerebral cortex results from the location in which the activity occurs. Cerebral activity initiated by visual receptors is in the lower rear of the cortex. Impulses from proprioceptors arrive in the cortex in a fairly large area that extends from the upper middle surface downward.

For example, the area that receives stimuli from the thumb is as large as that representing the trunk. The cortical representation parallels the density of sensory innervation from that part. When movement occurs, impulses are sent to that part of the cortex that represents the moving segments. The resulting cortical activity becomes associated with a specific movement, is recognized as accompanying the movement, and is the basis for memory of the act.

Scientists do not know whether impulses initiated in all types of proprioceptors reach the areas of the cortex as expected. When Sherrington demonstrated in 1894 that a nerve fiber from the muscle spindle conducted impulses to the spinal cord, it was thought that these impulses would reach the brain and be the basis for the cerebral activity that resulted in perception of movement and motor memory. We now know that impulses from the spindle do go to the spinal cord; but we question whether they stimulate activity in the cortical area in a given way. Researchers believe that on reaching the spinal cord, these impulses may be directed to many muscles involved in the act, including the muscle in which they originated. In other words, these impulses coordinate the movement rather than develop memory or awareness.

Memory and awareness develop from impulses that originate in the proprioceptors found in tissue surrounding joints—ligaments, joint capsules, and adjacent connective tissue. As impulses from these receptors enter the spinal cord, they travel on fibers that extend up the posterior portion of the cord and terminate in the medulla, where they synapse with dendrites of cell bodies located in the medulla. The fibers of this second neuron cross to the opposite side of the brain as they ascend, conducting impulses originating in the right side of the body to the left side of the brain and vice versa. These fibers terminate in the thalamus and synapse there with a third neuron, which conducts the impulses to the brain areas shown in Figure 5.6. Feedback information regarding the position of body parts and movement is known as *kinesthesis*. In addition to aiding us in maintaining balance, this feedback is the basis for how we learn motor skills. Without proprioceptive and other feedback information, development of accurate motor programs (learning) would not be possible (Schmidt 1978).

Reaction Time and Movement Time

Many sports rely on the ability to respond as quickly as possible in a given situation. Examples are reacting to the gunshot at the beginning of a race or responding to the movement of an opponent or sport object. Much research has been conducted on **reaction time (RT),** the time from the presentation of a stimulus to the beginning of the overt response and the movement time, the time needed to complete the action. A study of one without the other is not very practical. For example, responding to an oncoming car requires reacting to visual stimuli *and* moving the body out of the way.

Reaction time is composed of several components: sense organ time (time needed for the sense organ to perceive the stimulus); nerve conduction time (time needed to conduct the impulses to and from the spinal cord); brain time (time needed for receiving, translating, and interpreting the message); and muscle development time (time needed for the muscle to develop the force needed to cause movement to occur). Brain time is the longest time interval and has the most variation depending on the situation.

Many factors affect reaction time. There is an optimal foreperiod (time interval between the presentation of a warning stimulus and the presentation of the stimulus) of between one and four seconds. If the stimulus arrives too quickly, the person is unprepared; if it arrives too late, readiness fades. Reaction time also varies with different sense modalities. Visual reaction time is slower than auditory and kinesthetic, or proprioceptive, reaction time (due to additional neural connections of the former). There are some problems in comparing different modalities, however, due to the different scale and different intensities of the signals. There have been some attempts to compare them on an equal scale (Beehler & Kamen 1986). Reaction time increases with increased intensity of the stimulus. There are obviously many factors that affect the ability to react, and in order to obtain the best reaction time, optimum conditions must exist.

In addition to factors that affect the reaction time within an individual, there are other factors that affect RT between groups. Researchers have shown that groups varying in gender and age have different reaction times. The reaction times for males tend to be faster then for females, although the difference is slight. Additionally, with increased age up to late teens and twenties, reaction time improves. The time needed to react to a stimulus during adulthood tends to increase with age. Since active people tend to react slightly faster than inactive people, we would expect that the increase in RT with age could be counteracted the more active a person stays throughout life. Researchers have shown this to be true (Rikli and Edwards 1991).

MINI-LABORATORY LEARNING EXPERIENCE

Using an ordinary ruler and the force of gravity, you can easily measure your own reaction time. Have a partner vertically suspend the end of the ruler between your thumb and forefinger. Have your fingers close to, but not touching the ruler. Without warning, the partner is to drop the ruler so that it slides through your fingers. Pinch the ruler as quickly as possible as it drops. Record the distance (*D*) of the drop in centimeters to the nearest millimeter. Using the following formula calculate your RT in seconds:

$$RT = \sqrt{\frac{2(D/100)}{9.8}}$$

For a more accurate measure of RT, take the average of three trials. An average college student's simple visual RT is approximately .18 seconds. Compare the reaction times of both your left and right hands with this average. To measure the foot's reaction time, have your partner hold the ruler against the wall, with the end suspended between your foot and the wall. When your partner drops the ruler trap it against the wall.

Points to Ponder

What are the typical reaction times required in various situations in daily life? Certainly, sport situations are replete with quick reaction requirements. In daily life, however, there are frequent times when we need to catch falling objects to prevent breakage, stop a movement to prevent injury, or recover our balance in order to land on our feet. Measure the time it takes for a served volleyball to arrive at the receiver. How much time do softball batters (slow pitch and fast pitch) and baseball batters have before they must initiate their swing? How much time does a soccer or field hockey goalie have to respond to a penalty kick or stroke at the goal?

With respect to movement time, can one run faster backward than forward? Is the foot faster than the hand? Relate hand and foot speed to applying bicycle brakes. Should we block a blow with the right arm or the left arm? Is it faster to stop a stopwatch with the thumb or forefinger? Will practice improve any of these reaction times?

■ Knowing reaction time and movement time abilities and capabilities is important to optimize learning and improve skill, as well as to generate safe movement situations.

Neural Adaptation

Neural adaptation refers to possible changes occurring within the nervous system that allow strength and power production to be enhanced. According to Sale (1986),

> Strength and power performance is determined not only by the quantity and quality of the involved muscle mass, but also by the extent to which the muscle mass may be activated by voluntary effort. Strength and power training may cause changes within the nervous system that allow an individual to better coordinate the activation of muscle groups, thereby effecting a greater net force even in the absence of adaptation within the muscles themselves.

Electromyography has provided important information concerning tension-load and tension-velocity relationships, fatigue, strength development, learning, and responses to training. For example, there is a positive linear relationship between muscle tension and load, as well as between tension and velocity (see Chapter 4). Thus, various motor units and muscle fibers may be in a state of tension, depending on the speed and strength necessary to perform the movement.

Tension to produce a movement with the right arm will show irradiation to the contralateral arm. Contraction of one muscle to lift a very heavy object will require tension in many other muscles designed to stabilize body parts. Tension in a beginner will differ from that in a skilled performer.

Initial strength gains in strength training occur much too quickly for any adaptation within the muscle to occur. Increased voluntary strength in untrained limbs has also been found.

■ The effects of strength training result in increases of voluntary strength largely specific to the types of contractions used in the training.

As strength increases, as learning occurs, and as proficiency develops, the amount of tension and number of muscles producing tension will be reduced. Since these changes are not accounted for solely by physiological changes in the muscles, the concept of neural adaptation has been proposed. The nervous system adapts the muscular contraction patterns until the most efficient one is found. Thresholds to illicite various responses, such as in golgi tendon organs, are adjusted. In GTOs the firing can limit functional strength by firing prematurely, causing the muscles to stop contraction too soon. Patterns of muscle tension in the prefatigued and fatigued state are unique to people during activities requiring endurance. The relationship of each pattern to the actual endurance-time performance has not as yet been determined.

Proprioceptive Neuromuscular Facilitation

A popular type of stretching exercise that uses the neural circuitry and the muscle spindles is **proprioceptive neuromuscular facilitation (PNF)**. These procedures, developed by Dr. Herman Kabat in the 1950s, are widely used by physical therapists, athletic trainers, teachers and coaches to increase range of motion (see Chapter 4). PNF is defined by Voss, Ionta, and Myers (1985) as "methods of promoting or hastening the response of the neuromuscular mechanism through stimulation of the proprioceptors."

Three basic PNF techniques improve flexibility (Enoka 1988). The first, the *hold-relax* (HR) technique, involves an isometric contraction of the muscle to be stretched, followed by relaxation and then a stretch of the muscle. This method is based on the observation that following successive excitations, motor neurons are inhibited. Therefore, after holding an isometric contraction, the alpha motor neurons in that muscle are least excitable when they are then put under stretch.

The second technique, the *agonist-contract* (AC) technique, involves a subcontraction of the agonist muscle while simultaneously stretching the antagonist muscle (in this case, the muscle to be stretched). This method uses the reciprocal inhibition effect. While contracting the agonist muscle, there is a reciprocal inhibitory effect (relaxation) on the antagonist muscle. A submaximal contraction of the agonist muscle is used since a maximal contraction (or near-maximal) usually brings on co-contraction.

The HR and AC methods can be joined to arrive at a third PNF procedure (HR-AC), which combines the reciprocal inhibition effect with the post-activation inhibition of the motor neurons. The subject isometrically contracts the hamstrings against a resistance applied by a partner (HR). After relaxing the muscle, the partner applies a force to stretch the hamstrings while the subject simultaneously attempts a submaximal contraction of the quadriceps (AC). Many researchers have found these PNF-based stretching techniques superior to other stretching techniques (e.g., static or ballistic) in increasing range of motion about the joints (Wallin et al. 1985; Etnyre and Abraham 1986).

Plyometrics

A form of training that uses the stretch reflex to improve strength is **plyometrics.** This type of training is effective in developing explosive strength, or power (also referred to as speed-strength). Plyometrics involves an initial eccentric contraction (resulting in muscle stretch), followed immediately by a forceful concentric contraction.

In an example of plyometrics known as depth jumping, the athlete drops off a block followed by a jump immediately after landing on the ground. Plyometrics uses the stretch reflex mechanism as well as the elastic restoring properties in the muscle to generate a greater muscular force than can be achieved volitionally (Hatfield 1989). By putting the muscle under stretch (eccentric contraction), the muscle spindles become excited, activating the stretch reflex, which in turn results in contraction of the homonymous muscle. By volitionally contracting the muscle at the same time, a more forceful contraction results.

Two important features about the effectiveness of plyometrics deal with eccentric strength and speed. It is widely known that athletes can resist much greater force eccentrically than they can concentrically. By incorporating a maximum eccentric contraction, athletes are putting the muscles under greater resistance. Secondly, in most athletic movements (with the exception of power lifting), the speed with which an athlete moves is just as important (or even more important) than the force of the movement. Under traditional weight-training conditions, as one increases the amount of weight moved, the speed of the movement decreases. The neuromuscular system, therefore, is learning slowness, not quickness.

■ By utilizing a sudden concentric contraction after an eccentric contraction in plyometrics, the athlete is not only training more forcefully but also moving more quickly.

Many types of plyometric exercises can be used to apply this training method specific to one's coaching needs. One-legged hopping, two-legged jumps over boxes, high-knee skipping, and medicine ball catches and throws can be used by many track athletes (jumpers, hurdlers, runners, throwers), football linemen, soccer players, and others to increase power in the legs and/or arms (Freeman and Freeman 1984; Radcliffe and Farentinos 1985). Jumping from a higher height or adding additional weight to the body, as long as the speed of movement is not sacrificed, will increase intensity.

■ Since many areas of research in neural adaptation are relatively new, one can only speculate that the training of the nervous system may be the most important discriminator of the highly skilled performer of movement.

According to Sale (1986):

> A question that is often raised in connection with neural adaptation to strength and power training is why humans are designed so that some motor units are so difficult or impossible to activate fully unless diligent training is performed or a crisis situation is faced. The answer usually given is that protection is provided by inhibitions that prevent the making of truly maximal contractions frequently and at a whim.

If ways can be found to increase concentration and effort in training so that complete neural activation of the muscle is possible, coupled with mechanically accurate execution of the movement, highly skilled performers will be able to achieve all that they are capable of achieving.

References

Beehler, P. J., and Kamen, G. 1986. Responses to auditory and electrocutaneous stimuli. *Research Quarterly for Exercise and Sport* 57:298–307.

Burke, R. E. 1986. The control of muscle force: Motor unit recruitment and firing patterns. *Human Muscle Power*, ed. N. L. Jones, N. McCartney and A. McComas. Champaign, IL: Human Kinetics: pp. 97–106.

Eldred, E. 1967. Functional implications of dynamic and static components of the spindle response to stretch. *Am Journal of Physical Medicine* 46:129–40.

Enoka, R. M. 1988. *Neuromechanical basis of kinesiology.* Champaign, IL: Human Kinetics.

Etnyre, B. R., and Abraham, L. D. 1986. Gains in range of ankle dorsiflexion using three popular stretching techniques. *Am. J. of Phys. Med.* 65:189–96.

Evarts, E. V. 1975. Changing concepts of central control of movement. The Stevenson lecture. *Can. J. Phy. Pharmacal* 53(2):197–201.

Freeman, W., and Freeman, E. 1984. *Plyometrics.* Ames, IA: Championship Books.

Gardner, B. 1969. Proprioceptive reflexes and their participation in motor skills. *Quest* 12:1.

Georgopoulos, A. P., Schwartz, A. B., and Kattner, R. E. 1986. Neuronal population coding of movement direction. *Science* 233: 1416–19.

Grimby, L. 1986. Single motor unit discharge during voluntary contraction and locomotion. In *Human Muscle Power,* ed. N. L. Jones, N. McCartney, and A. McComas. Champaign, IL: Human Kinetics.

Hatfield, F. C. 1989. *Power: A scientific approach.* New York: Contemporary Books.

Hellebrandt, F. A., Rarick, G. L., Glassow, R., and Carns, M. L. 1961. Physiological analysis of basic motor skills. *Am. J. Phys. Med.* 40:14.

Henneman, E. 1981. Recruitment of motoneurons: The size principle. In Motor unit types, recruitment and plasticity in health and disease, ed. J. E. Desmedts. *Prog. Clinic Neurophysical* 9.

Hess, E. 1958. Imprinting in animals. *Sci. Am.* 198:81, March.

Lorenz, K. A. 1958. The evolution of behavior. *Sci. Am.* 199:67.

Radcliffe, J. C., and Farentinos, R. C. 1985. *Plyometrics: Explosive power training,* 2nd ed. Champaign, IL: Human Kinetics.

Ranson, S., and Clark, S. L. 1959. *Anatomy of the nervous system,* 10th ed. Philadelphia: W. B. Saunders.

Riesen, A. 1950. Arrested vision. *Sci. Am.* 183:16, July.

Rikli, R. E., and Edwards, D. J. 1991. Effects of a three-year exercise program on motor-function and cognitive processing speed in older women. *Research Quarterly for Exercise and Sport* 62:61–67.

Rosenbaum, D. A. 1991. *Human motor control.* San Diego: Academic Press.

Sage, G. H. 1977. *Introduction to motor behavior,* 2nd ed. Reading, PA: Addison-Wesley.

Sale, D. G. 1986. Neural adaptation in strength and power training. In *Human Muscle Power,* ed. N. L. Jones, N. McCartney, and A. McComas. Champaign, IL: Human Kinetics, pp. 289–305.

Schmidt, R. A. 1978. *Motor control and learning: A behavioral emphasis,* 2nd ed. Champaign, IL: Human Kinetics.

Voss, D. E., Ionta, M. K., and Myers, B. J. 1985. *Proprioceptive neuromuscular facilitation,* 3rd ed. Philadelphia: Harper & Row.

Wallin, D., Ekblom, B., Grahn, R., and Nordenborg, T. 1985. Improvement of muscle flexibility: A comparison between two techniques. *American Journal of Sports Medicine* 13, 263–68.

Wickstrom, R. L. 1983. *Fundamental motor patterns,* 3rd ed. Philadelphia: Lea and Febiger.

6 Mechanical Principles Related to Human Movement

The movements of human beings are governed to a great extent by certain physical laws and principles. Proper use of these laws and principles is one of the goals of the performer and analyst.

Since we live on earth, and anything we encounter in space will be evaluated in terms of our environment on earth, it is vital that we understand the laws governing motion on earth. These laws are usually referred to as Newton's three laws of motion. This type of mechanics is referred to as Newtonian mechanics, also known as classical mechanics. Newtonian mechanics is the physical science that encompasses movement or motion of material bodies of ordinary size moving at speeds that are slow compared to the speed of light. Quantum mechanics, the physical science that evolved from Einstein's theory of relativity, may be applicable to human movement in future years, but will not be included in this book.

Readers with a strong background in mechanics will need to rethink the mechanical principles of rigid, nonliving bodies when applying these principles to anisotropic, living bodies, such as human beings. Likewise, readers with a strong background in biology, especially anatomy, will need to view biology from a mechanical perspective. The mechanical perspective includes both the **kinematics** (temporal and spatial aspects) and **kinetics** (force aspects) of mechanics.

There is one fundamental concept that is the essence of mechanics: *Forces cause predictable and measurable responses of the human body and objects interacting with the human body.*

These responses are movements, deformations, resistive counter-forces (to avoid movement), and breakage. The characteristics of these forces and the characteristics of the human body and the objects involved determine which responses occur. We can predict the responses if we know and can measure the following:

magnitude of the force

point of application of the force

direction of the force

masses of the bodies

form, shape, stiffness, hardness, texture, etc., of the bodies

location of the centers of mass of the bodies and their parts

It is a complex and difficult task to know, and be able to measure, all the characteristics of the interacting bodies. Accuracy in predicting responses is directly related to the amount of information known. Since humans have the ability to generate forces internally and use a variety of strategies in responding to external forces acting on them, we must consider the uniqueness of the human being when studying the principles of mechanics.

TABLE 6.1 Mathematical constructs of Newton's laws of motion.

Law	Movement-Force-Construct	Equation Linear	Rotary
I. Inertia	No force = no movement	$\Sigma F = 0$	$\Sigma M = 0$
II. Acceleration	Force positively related to acceleration	$F = m\alpha$	$M = I\alpha$
	Acceleration is rate of change of velocity	$Ft = mv$	$Mt = I\omega$
III. Interaction	A force creates a counter force	$+F = -F$	$+M = -M$

MINI-LABORATORY LEARNING EXPERIENCE

1. Observe a person striking a ball with a bat, racquet, or other striking implement. Identify the objects that experience contact forces (force caused by two objects in contact with each other). Describe the characteristics of these objects. Estimate the direction of the force from the perspective of the direction of the ball or human body part. Qualitatively assess the magnitude of the force as strong, moderate, or low.
2. Discuss the relationship of these observations and flight of objects.

■ **We must view human movement as more than rigid body dynamics.**

The human body is not a machine. Although it acts according to Newtonian mechanics, it has the ability to dampen or dissipate forces, transfer forces from one body part to another, and to add nonlinear forces to the system of motion. This is why we initially focus on the forces that create motion and the masses involved with the motion. Often motion is dependent on the person and is tempered, restrained, or facilitated by the external forces. For example, two people may move in the same space and use the same duration, but each may produce different force patterns. Level of skill is not necessarily reflected by the performance score.

■ **Forces are anything that causes or could cause motion.**

There are two types of forces: *external forces* and *internal forces*. Typical external forces include gravity (body weight or g's); inertia; friction; ground reaction; fluid resistance (especially water and air), e.g., drag and lift and buoyancy; push (from another body); and moment of force (torque, *M*). Typical internal forces include ligament pull; muscle pull; tendon pull; joint reaction force; elastic force; and moment of force.

■ **Internal forces are not easily measured, but have been derived from cadaver experiments, by assessment of forces on prostheses, and through computer modeling.**

In addition, we consider the concepts of motion to be forces: momentum; kinetic energy; work; potential energy; and impulse. These concepts are derived from Newton's laws of motion as seen in the mathematical representation of the laws in Table 6.1.

Forces are quantities that have both magnitude and direction. Therefore, forces can be represented as vectors, the length of which is representative of its magnitude with a spatial direction. The resulting motion, acceleration and velocity are also vector quantities and can be represented by vectors during analysis procedures.

Understanding the Variables of Mechanics

When discussing forces, accelerations, momentum, and other variables used in mechanics, it is necessary to define each variable with respect to units of measurement.

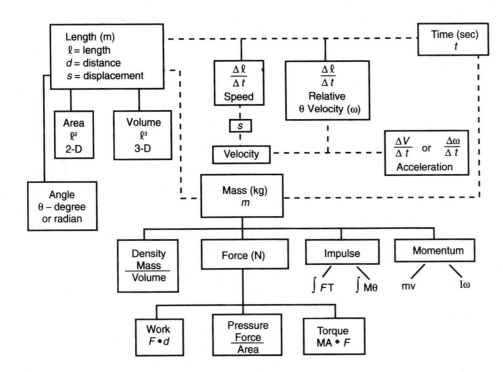

FIGURE 6.1 Fundamental variables of the mechanics of motion.

For example, distance can be measured in feet, meters, and other units. Time is usually measured in seconds, minutes, and hours. A common system of symbols also exists to further define these variables of mechanics. In addition, these variables have been categorized into scalar, vector, tensor, pulsar, and quasar quantities. Most of our human movement analysis will be concerned with scalar and vector quantities.

■ **Scalar quantities** are single element, e.g., speed (magnitude). **Vector quantities** are double elements, e.g., force (direction + magnitude).

The base units and important variables of mechanics are graphed in Figure 6.1. There are three fundamental variables from which all other variables are formed: length, mass, and time. Length is the space variable. Time is an independent variable, and mass is the constant invariant with time that a particle possesses. Further descriptions of the variables in Figure 6.1 appear in Appendixes B and D.

Understanding the Vector Quantities

Among the kinematic variables, **velocity** and **acceleration** have both direction and magnitude. All forces are vector quantities and as such, the simple arithmetic processes used with scalar quantities are not applicable. For example, the scalar quantity of distance can be added, subtracted, multiplied, and divided. The values for two or more forces or velocities at different instances in time cannot be added unless all are acting in the same direction. Body weights can be added since these forces act vertically, while the forces of five people pushing against a huge ball (cageball) at different sites of contact cannot be added arithmetically.

■ Vectors must be added vectorally or algebraically.

Vectoral Addition

There are two common methods of vectorally adding forces: the trigonometric method and the graphic method. These methods also are commonly used to investigate the effect of one or more forces on a body. The fundamental concept of both methods is that of resolving the force vector into two components, each of which can then be compared to any other resolved force vector. Based on a spatial frame of reference, vectors are resolved into vertical and horizontal force components, if the force acts in one plane. If the force acts in three-dimensional space, "cutting through two or more planes," the vector is resolved into three components: one vertical and two horizontal, all of which are orthogonal to each other.

Based on an anatomical reference frame, forces are resolved into normal and tangential components. The normal component acts at right angles (normal) to the body part, such as a headwind striking the body. The tangential component acts parallel to the body (shearing or tangential), such as the force of friction during sliding activities. Since most forces act at angles to the normal/tangential or vertical/horizontal, vector resolution techniques are required to identify optimum magnitudes and directions of forces. Most researchers and movement analysts assume two-dimensional force vectors and resolve the force vector into two components. In many cases, the assumption that the component in the third plane is negligible is a valid one. Three-dimensional vector resolution is best performed with the aid of computer algorithms.

Trigonometric Method.   The trigonometric method is based on the principle that right triangles of various sizes with identical angles will be proportional to each other. This means that the ratio of one side of the triangle to another side will always be identical among such triangles. Therefore, the equations for determining the components of a force acting at a known angle are as follows:

$$H = F \text{ cosine } \theta$$

$$V = F \text{ sine } \theta$$

H is the horizontal component (the tangential component in the anatomical reference frame and frame of interacting surfaces).

V is the vertical component (normal force in the anatomical reference frame and frame of interacting surfaces).

F is the force (the resultant component, also commonly referred to as *R*).

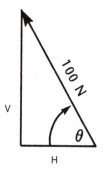

If magnitude (100 N) and direction (θ) are known, look in trigonometry table:

H = 100 N cosine θ

V = 100 N sine θ

FIGURE 6.2   Trigonometric resolution of vector components perpendicular to each other. **Measure the angle and use the trigonometry table in Appendix B to solve for the vertical and horizontal components.**

Refer to Figure 6.2 and calculate the horizontal and vertical forces of the two-dimensional portrayal of a 100 N force acting at a particular angle.

The sines, cosines, and tangents of angles and a review of basic trigonometry appear in Appendix B.

MINI-LABORATORY LEARNING EXPERIENCE

1. Calculate the resultant force (total or actual force) of a karate blow delivered at a 20° angle. The force transducers on the target measured 4000 N normal to the target. Hint: rearrange the equation $V = F \text{ sine } \theta$ to solve for *F*.
2. Compare the normal and tangential forces in the following situations:
   a. a force of 600 N is applied to a football by the foot striking it at a 45° angle.
   b. a force of 600 N is applied as above except at a 78° angle.
   c. a force of 600 N is applied as above except at a 25° angle.

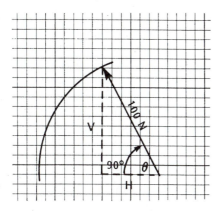

If trigonometry table is
not available:

1. Draw vector of 100 N
   magnitude at angle θ
   with the horizontal

2. Construct right triangle

3. Determine H and V by
   measurement

FIGURE 6.3 Graphic resolution and measurement of vector components perpendicular to each other. **Compare your answers to those you calculated for Figure 6.2.**

3. Calculate the distance run on the hypotenuse of a triangular race course with a distance of 100 meters on the east side and 80 meters on the north side.

4. If a sailboat is being pushed by the wind at a speed of 50 m/sec at 90° to the shoreline, but is experiencing slippage in the water at a 10° angle from the push of the wind, what is the resultant velocity of the sailboat?

Graphic Method. The graphic method of vectorally adding forces consists of diagramming the force vector on graph paper, as depicted in Figure 6.3. A scale is selected, such as one graph unit equals 10 N. Horizontal and vertical lines are drawn and the 90° angle of intersection marked. At some point from the horizontal line, the angle of the direction of the vector is drawn using a

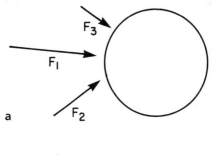

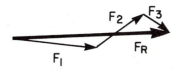

FIGURE 6.4 Graphic determination of resultant force (F) when several forces act on a body. (a) Three forces drawn according to direction and magnitude: F_1 = horizontal force (0°) of 150 units (these can be newtons or pounds); F_2 = 40° directional positive force of 100 units; F_3 = 35° directed negatively of 50 units. (b) Geometrically summing the three forces and drawing the resultant force (R) of 275 units at a 10° positive angle. **Compare your answer using trigonometry to solve for the resultant force and for the horizontal and vertical components.**

protractor. Along this line, beginning at the intercept with the horizontal line, the vector is drawn to scale. For example, in Figure 6.3, 100 N equals 10 graph units. Measure the horizontal and vertical components (from the 90° angle to the intercepts of vector).

MINI-LABORATORY LEARNING EXPERIENCE

Use the trigonometric method and compare your results with the graphic method for Figure 6.4.

If two or more forces act on a body, the forces must be vectorally added to determine the resultant magnitude and direction of the summed force. We do this graphically by drawing the vectors as shown in Figure 6.4. The tail of the vector is placed at the arrow of the other vector, and each is oriented in the prescribed direction.

The resultant (summed) force is drawn from the arrow of the last force vector to the tail of the first force vector. It is measured with respect to magnitude and orientation.

An alternate method, of course, is to separate each force vector into its components. For example, all normal force vectors are added together; all tangential force vectors are added separately. These two component vectors are drawn tail to tail, forming a 90° angle. The resultant force vector is then the hypotenuse of the right triangle drawn by connecting the arrows of each component vector.

Displacements with Respect to Time

When movement occurs, the most readily identifiable parameter is displacement: how far the body or body part was moved and in which direction, whether linear or rotary, the movement occurred. Pertinent measurements of angles and distances are shown in the following examples:

1. Length of stride during walking: is the stride too short or too long for efficient movement?
2. Direction of foot angle with direction of locomotion: can the foot exert the muscular forces effectively with the measured angle?
3. Height of jump: is the jump average, below average, or above average according to achievement norms?
4. Direction of arm movement during throwing: did the arm move toward the target?
5. Relationship of lean of trunk, position of legs, and other body parts: are the distances and angles the same as those seen in highly skilled performances?

Displacement analysis, however, is not enough, since it ignores forces and, therefore, accelerations. For example, two balls may be thrown a distance of 9 m (30 ft), but one may take half the time to travel the distance than the other ball takes. Using the following examples, we could conclude that the faster ball projection is effective while the slower is not:

1. The faster ball, if thrown to first base, will arrive to cause the batter/base runner to be out.
2. The faster ball cannot be stopped by a soccer goalkeeper.
3. The faster ball cannot be intercepted by an opposing basketball player.

Displacement with respect to time is more important than displacement alone. For example, it is important that a pedestrian be able to cross the intersection before a traffic light changes. Speed is the change in position (displacement) with respect to time if the displacement is not given a direction. If the direction is specified, the displacement with respect to time is called velocity. The equation for determining the magnitude of either is the same:

$$\text{Velocity} = \text{Change in position/Change in time}$$
$$= \text{Displacement/Time}$$

We may refer to the speed of a racehorse, a sprinter, or a sailboat as being a certain number of kilometers per hour or meters per second. The velocity would be in these same units, but in the horizontal direction, or at an angle of 20° with the vertical, or in some other system denoting direction.

Knowing the speed or velocity of the movement does not include information about the forces that created this speed or velocity. The rate of change in velocity, however, equals the acceleration, from which one can calculate force:

$$F = ma$$

The equation for determining the acceleration of a body is as follows:

$$\text{Acceleration} = \text{Change in velocity/Change in time}$$
$$= \frac{\Delta V}{\Delta t}$$

The relationships of displacement, velocity, and acceleration with respect to angular motion appear in Figure 6.5.

The following are known relationships of displacement, velocity, and acceleration, whether angular or linear:

1. When the amount of displacement increases from one time period to the next, the velocity increases.
2. When the displacement remains constant from one time period to the next, the velocity is constant and the acceleration is zero.
3. When there is a reversal of direction in displacement, the velocity will be zero at the instant of reversal.
4. At the instant of maximum velocity, the acceleration is zero.

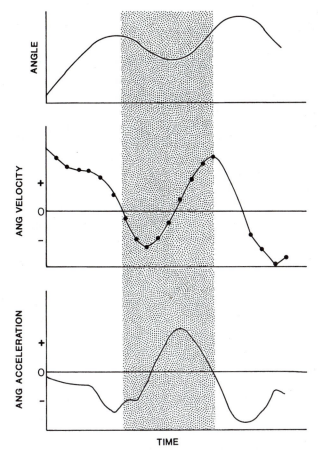

FIGURE 6.5 Computer plots of film data. When angular displacement is maximum or minimum value, angular velocity is zero. When angular displacement slope is greatest, angular velocity is maximum and angular acceleration is zero.

These relationships are seen readily in an analysis of the track start in running. The displacement of the body from the first stride to the fifth increases as the time for each stride becomes less. Thus, the velocity increases, and since the velocity is not constant, positive acceleration occurs. At some point in time, the length of stride and the velocity become constant; the acceleration ceases and becomes equal to zero. Minute changes probably occur in all forms of locomotion at the instant of foot plant and pushoff, but we will disregard these. The runner may maintain a constant velocity, with zero acceleration (after sprinting 60 m in a 200 m race) until the end of the race. At the end of the race, acceleration (change in velocity) might occur. But deceleration usually occurs.

Analysis of the kinematics of projectiles is easy if we consider all forces to be negligible except the force of gravity. The acceleration of any projectile then becomes the acceleration of gravity (9.8 m/sec^2 as an average value) in the vertical direction. A convenient equation for determining the kinematics of a projectile is

$$s = \tfrac{1}{2}\, at^2$$

where s = distance in the vertical direction, a = the acceleration of gravity, and t = time. Although the formula $s = vt + \tfrac{1}{2}\, at^2$ can be applied more universally than $s = \tfrac{1}{2}\, at^2$, there is always some point during the flight of the projectile, whether a ball, human body, animal, or another object, at which the vertical velocity equals zero and the descending flight pattern begins. Since the vertical velocity is equal to zero, the term vt in the equation is also zero.

If the descent of the projected object is timed, we can calculate the maximum vertical distance of projection. For example, if a ball requires one second to fall to the ground from its highest elevation from the ground, this elevation is equal to 4.9 m.

When objects are projected horizontally, with zero vertical velocity, we can measure the height above the ground at the time of projection. Time is equal to the square root of $2s/a$, that is:

$$t = \sqrt{2s/a}$$

The velocity of the projectile in the horizontal direction can be determined, since the horizontal distance traveled, divided by the air time, equals the horizontal velocity. The horizontal distance is easy to measure. Concepts and examples of projectile motion appear in Appendix C.

Useful Equations of Motion

There are known general kinematic relationships between displacement, velocity, time, and acceleration. In the motion of a free-falling body, the initial velocity is zero and the acceleration is a constant (gravitational). These equations are useful for instances of airborne actions when we can assume that gravity is the major force, such as the flight of the body during jumping and the flight of balls during ball sports. There will always be some point during the flight of the projectile at which the vertical velocity is zero and the descending portion of the flight begins.

The following equations apply to the discussion in the previous paragraph:

$$s = vt$$
$$s = \tfrac{1}{2} at^2$$
$$v_f - v_i = at$$
$$v_f^2 - v_i^2 = 2as$$

s is displacement

v is velocity, final and initial

a is acceleration

t is time

f is final

MINI-LABORATORY LEARNING EXPERIENCE

Rewrite the equations assuming the initial velocity is zero. Now rewrite the equations to solve for t.

These displacements with respect to time provide insight into the kinetics of movement. As shown in the equations, we can estimate the forces acting on the body by measuring the acceleration of the body and multiplying this value by the mass of the body. If the force is known (measured by means of dynamographic devices), we can estimate the resulting acceleration of the body. In this way, we can assess or predict the outcome of the performance or the effectiveness of the muscle coordination.

Relationship of Newton's Three Laws of Motion to Translation

Whether or not motion occurs is directly related to the magnitude of force. Newton's first law, the law of inertia, states that a body at rest will remain at rest until some force of sufficient magnitude to overcome its inertia acts

MINI-LABORATORY LEARNING EXPERIENCE

1. Select a smooth-surfaced plank 3 m long and set it on an incline.
2. Place a smooth-surfaced ball at the top of the incline and release the ball without applying force.
   a. Using the stopwatch or an automatic timing device, record the number of seconds from release of ball until it rolls the 3 m.
   b. Repeat the test until reliability is satisfactory.
   c. Measure the angle of inclination of the plank.
   d. Measure or calculate the height of descent (H) of the ball. This can be determined trigonometrically by the following equation:

$$H = \sin \theta \; (3 \text{ m})$$

   which is the same as that explained in Appendix B: Opposite side = $\sin \theta$ (hypotenuse).
   e. Using all these data, show that gravity is a constant force producing a constant acceleration of 9.8 m/sec^2. Remember the following equation:

$$s = \tfrac{1}{2} at^2$$

   or

$$a = \frac{2s}{t^2}$$

   f. Repeat the test, using two different angles of inclination of the board. The same results should occur.

on the body. This law also applies to bodies moving at a constant velocity. We will explain this law first with respect to translatory motion in the vertical direction. The inertia of a body is known as its mass. Mass (body weight divided by gravitational acceleration) is measured in kilograms (newton-second^2/meter or (Nsec^2/m) in the International System of units (SI), also known as the metric system, and in slugs (lb-sec^2/ft) in the English system. A small letter m is used to denote the existence of mass in equations.

Vertical Motion

An upward movement can occur only if the force (f_y) acting on a mass is greater than the weight of the body (w). This can be proved by the application of Newton's second law, which states that the acceleration, and therefore the motion of a body, is directly related to its mass. In equation form, this principle is written as follows:

$$F_y = ma_y$$

where force (F) in the y direction equals the mass times the acceleration (ma) in the y direction.

In the case of more than one force, the symbol Σ is used with the above equation to indicate the "sum of all the forces." Stationary bodies standing on a floor have the acceleration of gravity acting downward on them. If a person stands on the ground, the ground exerts a force (measured in newtons [N]) equal to the force of gravity (w), but opposite in direction. This is in accordance with Newton's third law, called the law of interaction or the law of action-reaction. The former title is preferred because the latter implies a difference in time between the actions (forces), when in fact the reaction occurs simultaneously with the action. Imagine a person standing on the floor. Since the two forces are acting in opposite y (vertical) directions, and since the forces are of equal magnitude, no movement will occur.

Linear Motion in Any Direction

It is evident that linear acceleration will not occur and will not produce translation of the body if the $\Sigma F = 0$. Since movements occur in three planes, or in a three-dimensional world, the forces may be identified as F_x, F_y, and F_z, according to the Cartesian coordinate system discussed in Chapter 4. All these forces must equal zero for translation equilibrium to exist. If F_z and F_y equal zero, but $F_x = 200$ N acting on the body, then a body weighing 490 N will be accelerated laterally in the direction of F_x at a rate of 4 m/sec². The process of determining this is as follows:

Step 1. Always draw a free-body diagram (FBD), that is, depict the body in some simple shape and draw all external forces acting on it. Draw the vectors to scale—large forces are longer than small forces (Figure 6.6).

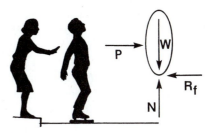

FIGURE 6.6 Depiction of life situation by means of free body diagram. Forces acting on body are represented by force vectors. This method provides convenient identification of probable effects on body. (P, force of push; W, body weight; N, normal force; Rf, friction force.) The friction force equals 10 N and the pushing force equals 210 N. **Therefore, what will happen?**

Step 2. Determine in which of the directions—x, y, or z—the sum of the forces equals zero. Note: If diagonal forces exist, resolve these forces into F_x, F_y, and F_z.

Step 3. Determine which sum is not equal to zero and solve the equation:

$$\Sigma F = ma$$
$$F_y = 0 \; F_z = 0 \; F_x \neq 0$$
$$F_x = ma_x$$
$$F + R = ma_x$$
$$210 \text{ N} + (-10 \text{ N}) = 490 \text{ N}/9.8 \text{ m/sec}^2 \times a_x$$
$$200 \text{ N} = 50 \text{ N sec}^2/m \times a_x$$
$$4 \text{ m/sec}^2 = a_x$$

The acceleration is forward in the x direction.

This basic law of motion, expressed as $F = ma$, indicates that a body will experience linear acceleration when the F does not equal zero. For example, during the act of jumping, the reaction force is greater than body weight because muscle force is causing the body to accelerate upward. By calculating the acceleration, we can use the preceding equation to determine the unknown reaction force. The difference between the body weight and the reaction force is equal to the effective muscle force. The greater the muscle force, the greater the acceleration and, therefore, the greater the vertical distance of the jump. Furthermore, if two persons of different masses exert equal amounts of muscle force, the person of lesser mass will be able to create greater acceleration than the person of greater mass. This is known as the inverse relationship of body mass to acceleration. Note the examples of different people above and the basic equation used. $F = ma$ summarizes only the external forces. Internal reactions, causing deformations of body tissues or resistance at joints and muscle forces, are not considered.

MINI-LABORATORY LEARNING EXPERIENCE

Calculate the accelerations of the following jumpers:

> Jumper A exerts a force of 1000 N to jump upward, body weight = 400 N.
>
> Jumper B exerts a force of 2000 N, body weight = 500 N.

Which person will jump higher?

Calculate the force applied horizontally by the sprinters leaving the starting blocks:

> Sprinter A accelerates 200 m/sec^2, body weight = 600 N.
>
> Sprinter B accelerates 150 .m/sec^2, body weight = 700 N.

Which person applied the greater force?

Discuss the significance of your results and state a biomechanical principle concerning the two situations.

Relationship of Laws of Motion to Rotary Motion

When the Newtonian laws of motion are applied to rotary motion, moment of force is substituted for force, and moment of inertia is substituted for inertia in the equation $F = ma$. With the acceleration no longer linear but angular, the equation becomes:

$$\Sigma M = I\alpha$$

where M = moment of force, I = moment of inertia; and alpha (α) = angular acceleration. Moment of force (M) is defined as the product of the force and its moment arm, that is, the shortest distance from the axis of rotation to the point of application of force. (For a review of these concepts, see Chapter 4.) Moment of inertia (I) is

defined as the rotary inertia or resistance to rotation. It is calculated by multiplying the mass by its radius (distance from the axis of rotation to the center of mass). The units are as follows:

> M = newton meters
>
> I = newton sec^2/meters
>
> α = radians/sec^2

Note the radian is a dimensionless unit and will not be retained.

■ **Determining whether rotary motion will occur is directly linked to the question of whether the point of application of force is other than through the center of gravity of the body.**

In the preceding examples of translation, we assumed that (1) the forces were acting through the center of gravity of the body, or (2) any moments that might have existed were being ignored. In Figure 6.7, however, the forces act distances d_1 and d_2 from the turning point, which is both the center of gravity of the object and the axis of rotation of the object. The forces produce a turning effect, which is termed a moment or identified as torque. Since in Figure 6.7 the sum of the forces is equal to zero, no translation occurs. If d_1 and d_2 did not exist—that is, if the force acted through the center of gravity of the object—the sum of the moments would also be equal to zero, since the moment is calculated by multiplying the force by its perpendicular distance of application from the axis of rotation (center of gravity). Although the concept of moments of force is thoroughly discussed in Chapter 4, the fundamentals are presented in the following solution to Figure 6.7.

If the moment of inertia of the object is determined to be 4 Nsec^2/m, then the angular acceleration of the object will be 10 rad/sec^2. This is determined by the following equation and solution:

$$\Sigma M = I\alpha$$
$$40 \text{ Nm} = 4 \text{ Nsec}^2/\text{m} \times \alpha$$
$$40 \text{ Nm}/4 \text{ Nm/sec}^2 = \alpha$$
$$10 \text{ rad/sec}^2 = \alpha$$

Note: since the radian is a dimensionless unit, it is written after the value of alpha. One radian is equal to 57.3° or 360° divided by 2π. Thus 10 rad/sec^2 is equal to 573°/sec^2.

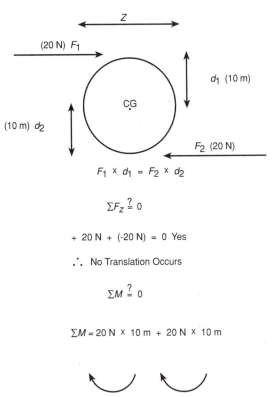

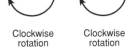

$F_1 \times d_1 = F_2 \times d_2$

$\Sigma F_z \overset{?}{=} 0$

$+ 20 \text{ N} + (-20 \text{ N}) = 0$ Yes

∴ No Translation Occurs

$\Sigma M \overset{?}{=} 0$

$\Sigma M = 20 \text{ N} \times 10 \text{ m} + 20 \text{ N} \times 10 \text{ m}$

Clockwise rotation Clockwise rotation

Moment = 40 NM clockwise

FIGURE 6.7 Use of free body diagram to determine whether or not translation, rotation, or both translation and rotation would occur for a given situation. In this situation, a clockwise rotation will occur but no translation will occur.

This example of two equal and opposite forces that act at equal distances from a point but produce the same direction of rotation is called a force couple.

The internal reaction forces are not considered in this free-body diagram of external forces. For example, the interaction between the force and the surface of the object is not considered. We are assuming that no force is lost (absorbed, converted into heat, etc.) in the act of pushing. The force represents the net force after any lost force is subtracted.

Internal forces must be considered whenever forces act on the human body since different body parts respond depending on the site of application of the force.

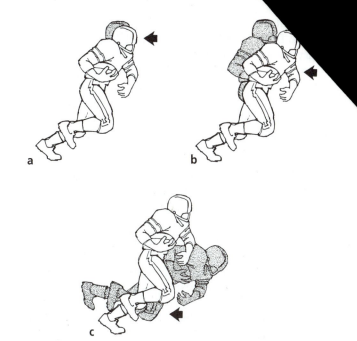

FIGURE 6.8 Identical forces acting on different parts of body produce different moments of force. Straight-line vector is point of application of force. Shaded body part is resultant rotation of body parts caused by moment of force. Note that either the joint caudal to force or the center of gravity of entire body acts as axis of rotation for moment of force.

For example, in football the tackler may apply the force at the head, chest, center of gravity of the body (hips), thighs, or ankles of the ball carrier (Figure 6.8). If the force is at the crown of the head, the head is accelerated backward with rotary motion, producing a reaction force at the atlas (rotary point of head). Although there is little effect on the rest of the body, there is a high potential for neck or spinal cord or column injury. If the same force is applied at the chest, the ball carrier experiences rotation of the body above the lumbar region. Since the mass of these body parts is greater than the mass of the head, the acceleration is not as great as with the head. The reactive moment of force, however, occurs in the vulnerable lumbar region of the spine, which again produces a risk of injury to the body. In both cases, since the feet are in contact with the ground, there may be little or no movement of the lower body. Application of this same amount of force through the center of gravity of the body will produce backward translation of

Mechanical Principles Related to Human Movement **115**

, with no rotary accelerations of body
~~ce~~ is applied to the thighs or ankles, ro-
~~h~~ again occurs. In this case, the feet are
~~contact~~ with the ground, and the body ro-
~~center~~ of gravity.

Changing the Moment of Inertia

A given force acting on a body to produce rotation can
create varying magnitudes of angular acceleration
merely by adjusting the body segments to create varying
magnitudes of rotary inertia. Since the moment of inertia
is dependent on the distance of the center of gravity of
the mass from the axis of rotation, this distance can be
shortened by changing the angles at the joints. For example, angular acceleration is greatest when the leg is
swinging forward and the angle at the knee is as small as
possible. Conversely, angular acceleration is least when
the leg is swinging forward with no flexion at the knee.

This concept is important because nothing comparable occurs with linear motion. The mass is usually a constant when linear acceleration is being produced. **The
moment of inertia,** however, can be changed, allowing
a body part of constant mass to be rotated at a faster rate
of speed even though the same amount of force is applied at the same point on the body.

Linear and Rotary Acceleration Principles

Here are some basic principles covering linear and rotary acceleration:

1. Linear acceleration of a body will not occur unless
   the sum of the forces acting on a body is greater
   than zero.
2. Rotary acceleration of a body will not occur unless
   the sum of the moments of force acting on the body
   is greater than zero.
3. As the force (or moment of force) acting on a body
   increases, the amount of linear acceleration or
   angular acceleration of that body will also increase.
4. If the same force (or moment of force) acts on two
   body masses, the larger mass will experience less
   acceleration.
5. The net result of all forces and all moments of force
   must be added vectorally to determine whether
   acceleration is produced.

Although we can easily determine the total body
kinematics for a runner, determining the kinematics of
the body segments is more problematic. Positive and
negative (popularly referred to as deceleration) accelerations of the limbs continue to occur even when the total
body moves at a constant velocity. Since limb accelerations are angular in nature and derived from angular velocities, there are two components of angular acceleration that are defined in linear terms: tangential and
radial. Their directions are the same as those described
for tangential and radial velocities.

Angular velocities provide information concerning the
ability to perform somersaults and move body parts fast
enough for a given task. There is an interrelationship between linear and angular velocities. One example is:

$$V_t = r\omega$$

Angular velocity can be resolved into two components. One component, parallel to the path in the arc at
the instant of viewing, is the tangential velocity (V_t)
since without the second component (radial velocity),
the movement would continue on a tangent to the arc, in
a straight line. The radial component is directed inward
along the radius at each instant of time to maintain the
circular path of the limb.

Given the same angular velocity, the tangential velocity will increase as the radius increases. This definition of V_t is very important in throwing, kicking, and
striking activities and will be discussed in Chapters 17
and 18. It is also important in the swinging activities of
gymnastics.

Centripetal and Centrifugal Forces

A unique force in all rotary movements is centripetal
force. This force maintains the circular path of the body
or body part in motion. The force is directed radially,
that is, toward the center of rotation. The calculation of
centripetal force is derived, once again, from the basic of
equation $F = ma$. Since centripetal force (C_p) represents
a radial acceleration force, the force can be determined
as follows:

$$C_p = mr\omega^2$$

where m refers to mass, r refers to radius of the arc to
the center of mass, and ω refers to the angular velocity.

We can also calculate centripetal force using the relationship between linear and angular motion:

$$C_p = m \frac{V_t^2}{r}$$

where V_t is the tangential velocity of the arc of movement. This latter equation is more commonly used to explain the phenomenon of gymnasts "flying off at a tangent" and balls being released tangent to the arc of motion. The absence of sufficient centripetal force causes the objects to move in the instantaneous path of motion rather than maintaining the circular motion. Although the cause of this action is actually V_t, centrifugal force is popularly considered to be the cause of this action. Centrifugal force is computed in the same way as centripetal force and may be considered the counterforce of centripetal force.

Table 6.2 includes estimates of centrifugal forces acting at the shoulder joint of a softball pitcher. The pitcher throws five different speeds of pitches. The force increases as the speed (angular velocity and linear velocity) increases.

Here are some observations on the movement skills of recreational sports performers:

Bowlers swing their arms and roll the ball at speeds too fast to produce the required "pin action" for consistent strikes.

Tennis serves and volleys are executed with moderate speed of arm swing.

Softball players throw the ball without explosive force.

Runners in certain track events do not always run "all out," depending on the length of the race and the speed of the opponents.

Although many reasons may account for such low speeds, one major reason is unconscious, or conscious, fear of injuring the joints. Did you ever stop to think what forces are acting on joints due to high accelerations and velocities? We do know that high centrifugal forces result in numbness in distal segments and pain in proximal joint structures. Conduct the following force-of-motion experiment and identify the specific sites and causes of numbness and pain.

■ The ability to tolerate high centripetal forces during throwing and other high-acceleration actions is possible because the forces are of very short duration, often less than 50 ms.

TABLE 6.2 Estimated centrifugal force during softball pitching (pitcher's arm is 0.6 M and the ball has a mass of 0.6 kg).

Speed of Ball		
m/sec	ft/sec	Centrifugal Force (N)
7	20	49
13	40	169
20	60	400
27	80	729
33	100	1089

3. Graph the forces as a function of speed and as a function of mass or weight of the object. Derive a principle based on your graphs.

Controlling centrifugal forces is paramount in gymnastics. The gymnast uses special built-in finger flexion gloves to produce gripping force to combat centrifugal forces. Failure to do so may result in falling from apparatus.

MINI-LABORATORY LEARNING EXPERIENCE

Study the equation in the previous Mini-Laboratory Learning Experience and determine who is at greater risk of flying off the high bar, all other factors being equal: a six-foot-tall or four-foot-tall gymnast? You might wish to use a hypothetical constant tangential velocity and velocities proportional to the height difference (3:2 ratio).

Impulse-Momentum

Although the external forces, such as gravity, that act on living bodies frequently possess constant magnitudes, rarely do any of the forces produced by the living body in motion have a constant magnitude. Each force acts for a period of time ranging from short to long. Muscle forces required to maintain a static position may be of the same magnitude over a short period of time. But there is almost always variation in muscle force during movement of a body segment. This variation is due to such factors as the angle at the joint, the speed of movement, the length of the muscle, and the position of the limb in space at each particular point in time. Furthermore, most human and animal movements require more than one contracting muscle or group of muscles. Therefore, several forces are created when different body parts move in a prescribed sequence and with a specific speed. This use of several body parts in time is called coordination, which also may be referred to as a summation of forces, development of momentum, or creation of kinetic energy.

Summation of Forces

The principle of summation of forces is: the force produced during movement of one body segment will be added to the force produced by the next body segment, and so on until the final action. The most effective timing of these forces has not been investigated thoroughly for all movements of humans and animals. Evidence, however, is conclusive that each force should occur at the time of maximal velocity of the preceding action during sequential summation. The following example investigates the velocity of motion.

A girl of elementary-school age creates muscle force for a short duration of time to accelerate her leg. The foot of her swinging leg contacts a soccer ball and applies force to the ball for a very short period of time. This causes the ball to accelerate, which creates velocity and displacement.

This physical phenomenon can be depicted as a cause-and-effect relation by using the equation $F = ma$ and modifying it to represent the force acting over a period of time (t):

$$\int Ft = \Delta mat$$

■ The product Ft is called impulse, or impulse of force, and its units are newton-seconds (Nsec).

Since velocity equals the product of acceleration and time (at), the equation can be rewritten as:

$$\sum \int Ft = \Delta mV$$

The product mV is termed linear momentum, and its units also are newton-seconds. This equation is known as the impulse-momentum equation; a given impulse will create a given momentum.

In actuality, the equation is more complex, since acceleration represents a change in velocity with respect to a change in time, not merely the relationship $a = V/t$. Readers acquainted with calculus will recognize the following rewriting of the equation as the integral Ft being equal to the change in momentum:

$$\int Ft = m_f V_f - m_i V_i$$

The subscript f refers to final momentum, and the subscript i refers to initial momentum. The integral (Ft) merely means the area under a force-time curve is a graphic representation of the amount of force occurring at each point in time over a selected period. Figure 6.9 depicts three such curves. The areas of the rectangles of force-time can easily be determined by multiplying the length of time by the magnitude of force. In Figure 6.9a, the force was a constant 100 N for 0.4 second. In Figure 6.9b, a greater, but still constant, force was applied for 0.2 second. The situation in Figure 6.9c is the more common force-time curve seen with human and animal movements and is the more difficult area to measure. The areas of all three situations are identical in that the person applied an impulse of 20 Nsec to the ball.

■ Despite differences in maximal force production during different situations when impulses are identical for these different situations, the resulting velocities will be identical.

The product of force and time of application of the force determine the amount of momentum achieved. The human body makes a compromise between the development of maximal force and maximal time of application of force. If the person allows too much time, such as using a full-squat position before jumping, maximal force cannot be achieved because the muscles are in a disadvantageous angle for exerting force upward. The time of execution of the propulsive action of leg extension will be too long. In long jumping, the jumper must have enough time on the takeoff board to complete the leg extension. Too short a time will be ineffective. Too long a time will cause the jumper to decrease horizontal speed acquired during the run and, therefore, decrease

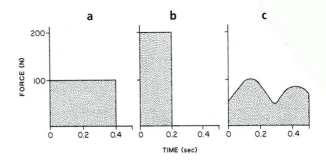

FIGURE 6.9 Theoretical identical impulses of 40 Nsec, but with different amounts of force and different durations of application of force. Most human and animal production of impulse resembles the variable magnitude of force application depicted in c. This is one reason human movement analysis is more difficult than analysis of motions of machines and other inanimate devices.

the force. The ability to generate maximum impulse depends on anatomical considerations such as muscle strength and length and position of limbs as well as the ability to coordinate the movements (neurologic integration). Maximum impulse is achieved by the best, or optimum, combination of force and time of application of force. Impulse creates velocity in a particular mass. Since a certain impulse will create a certain momentum, the greater the mass, the less the velocity.

■ All the principles applicable to $F = ma$ are also applicable to the impulse-momentum equation.

The development of both the force platform and computerized cinematographic analysis have made it possible to analyze the impulse and momentum of performances and, from the point of view of safety, the impulse and momentum of impacts, or collisions.

Conservation of Momentum

Linear Momentum

Impacts, or collisions, of two bodies result in a change in momentum for each of the two bodies. This phenomenon has been called a transfer of momentum. But is better defined as a *conservation* of momentum, which is simply a rephrasing of Newton's third law, the law of interaction (action-reaction). The law of conservation of that when two or more objects collide, ım after impact is equal to the total ّmpact. For example, when a bowling ّsec and weighing 98 N strikes a sta- ; 9.8 N (these higher-than-normal ease of subsequent computations), ‫ں‬ of the ball and of the pin after impact ‫ں‬ce equal to the momentum of the ball and the pin before impact. The pin, being the lighter of the two masses, will have the greater velocity after impact, but the ball will not experience much loss of velocity after impact, since its mass is 10 times that of the pin. As an illustration, if the pin acquired a final velocity twice that of the "before-impact" velocity of the ball, the changes in momentums and ball velocity would be as follows:

Before impact momentum = After impact momentum

$$m_{b1}V_{b1} = m_{b2}V_{b2} + m_pV_p$$

$$\frac{98 \text{ N}}{9.8 \text{ m/sec}^2} \times 7 \text{ m/sec} = \frac{98 \text{ N}}{9.8 \text{ m/sec}^2} \times V_{b2} + \frac{9.8 \text{ N}}{9.8 \text{ m/sec}^2} \times 14 \text{ m/sec}$$

$$70 \text{ Nsec} = 10 \text{ Nsec}^2/\text{m} \times V_{b2} + 14 \text{ Nsec}$$

$$56 \text{ Nsec} = 10 \text{ Nsec}^2/\text{m} \times V_{b2}$$

$$5.6 \text{ m/sec} = V_{\text{ball after impact}}$$

The ball velocity decreased by 1.4 m/sec, while the pin velocity increased 14 m/sec. The momentum of the ball was 70 Nsec before impact and 56 Nsec after impact.

Since velocity is a vector, we assumed that the collision of the bowling ball and pin was a head-on collision and that all velocities were additive, that is, along the same line. If the impact had been at an angle, the momentums would have been resolved into two components (planar motion) or into three components (three-dimensional motion) to calculate the angles of deflection of both objects after impact. Because of the conservation-of-momentum principle, both objects will be deflected from their original line of motion because the impact will have a component parallel (shear force) to the object's original motion, as well as perpendicular (normal).

Success in billiards, racquetball, handball, squash, and other games in which balls rebound from surfaces depends on the performer's ability to judge both the ball's angle of rebound and its speed of rebound. Although trial and error as well as experience may be prime factors in acquiring such judgement, the ability to solve the conservation-of-momentum equations and to explain the concept may provide the analyst with a means of shortening the trial-and-error method. The necessary skills will be thoroughly treated in Chapter 18. In addition, any spin force, friction force, and deformation of the two bodies during impact will introduce factors that affect the measured velocities after impact. The bowling ball-bowling pin impact is as nearly a perfectly elastic situation as can be found in any sport.

■ An elastic situation is one in which no energy is dissipated in heat energy to deform the materials.

The effect of not so perfectly elastic situations, such as when two human bodies collide or a tennis ball collides with a racquet, will be discussed in the work-energy section of this chapter.

MINI-LABORATORY LEARNING EXPERIENCE

1. A spiker strikes the volleyball with a force of 1000 N acting for a period of .018 seconds. Determine the speed of the ball if the ball has a mass of .05 kg. Assume total transfer of force from the hand to the ball and assume no spin has been imparted.
2. Discuss the effect on the velocity of the ball if spin had been imparted.
3. Discuss the effect on the velocity of the ball if the ball absorbed 20% of the force.

Angular Momentum

Moments of force also act over a time period. The momentum created from the product moment of impulse (Mt) is termed **angular momentum** and is written as $I\omega$. The moment of inertia (I), or the resistance to rotation or turning, is measured as the mass of the object multiplied by the radius squared of the rotating body. The ω refers to angular velocity.

■ Since mass rarely changes within a movement, the importance of the radius in the determination of I is primary.

The same principles of linear momentum are applicable to angular momentum. We need to consider the special case of conservation of angular momentum because this phenomenon is often seen in the angular motion of dancers, skaters, divers, gymnasts, jumpers, and other people involved in airborne athletics, as well as in any person or animal using rotary movements. For example, a diver will tuck the arm and legs, an action that concentrates the mass closer to the axis of rotation and thus decreases the moment of inertia of the body about this axis, in order to rotate faster. Since angular momentum can be altered only by external couples or eccentric (off-center) forces, and since the tucking of body parts is due to internal forces, angular momentum is not affected and does not change. Thus, angular velocity increases to maintain the constant angular momentum and allow the diver to execute a turn in a shorter time. The diver can then complete the dive well above water level, increasing the chances of a nearly vertical and controlled entry into the water. In another example of conservation of angular momentum, the ballet dancer and ice skater will start a slow-spinning motion with the arms held horizontally and then will bring the arms quickly to the chest area to increase the angular velocity of the spin. The reverse action with the arms will be used to slow the spin and initiate another movement.

■ By changing the length of their body segments to redistribute their masses, athletes are able to cause changes in their angular velocities (ω) because of the conservation-of-angular-momentum principle.

The momentum remains the same, but the overall movement appears different to the viewer and performer because of the change in ω. These changes in ω produced by movement of body parts will vary with the body segment involved, as well as with different individuals. For example, because the leg has a greater mass than the arm, movement of the leg will produce a greater change in ω. Long-limbed and heavy-boned individuals will be able to produce greater changes in ω than will individuals with short limbs or lightweight distal segments. If a person attempts to perform rotary movements with weights either held in the hands or strapped to different body parts, a more dramatic change in angular velocity will be noted with a redistribution of these weights than without weights, since there will be a greater change in the moment of inertia.

MINI-LABORATORY LEARNING EXPERIENCE

1. A diver has an angular momentum of 400 Nsec with the body in a layout position. The moment of inertia is decreased by one-half. What is the change in angular momentum?
2. A skater is rotating at 5 rads/sec. She begins to rotate 10 rads/sec. What has she done to make this possible?

Angular momentum is further discussed in Chapter 23.

Principles Related to Impulse/Momentum

Here are some basic principles related to impulse/momentum.

1. Greater impulses of force applied to stationary objects produce greater changes in momentum and greater final velocities.
2. For the same impulse, the greater the mass of the stationary object the less its final velocity, since the momentum remains constant.
3. Given the same force, an increase in time of application of force will impart greater velocity to a body. In striking activities this may be possible and is referred to as "hitting through the ball."
4. Maximum impulse can be created by maximizing the force, by maximizing the time of application of force, or by combining optimum force with optimum time. The latter strategy usually is preferred for movements involving locomotion or pumping.
5. Momentum is conserved in the collision of two or more objects; large masses will have lower velocities than small masses after the collision.
6. Angular momentum is conserved within a body by an increase in the angular velocity as a result of a decrease in the moment of inertia, and vice versa.

7. Since a moving body possesses momentum, an impulse or force will be required to stop or reduce the speed of the body.

8. A body in motion would require no force to keep it moving in a vacuum. However, since friction or some other resistance always exists to some extent to reduce the velocity of a body in motion, equal and opposite impulses of force are required to counteract these resistances and maintain the momentum of the body. These impulses are minute compared to the impulse required to develop the existing momentum.

9. To capitalize on the momentum of one's body or body part, one must make each subsequent application of an impulse of force before the momentum has been reduced appreciably by resistances such as friction. Skilled swimmers apply this principle, as do other persons displaying what is termed rhythm, grace, and coordination.

MINI-LABORATORY LEARNING EXPERIENCE

1. Using a twist board, piano stool, or revolving chair, turn a person on the device. Record the number of revolutions for the following positions:
   a. Arms held at sides while standing
   b. Arms held at sides while standing; move arms to shoulder level while standing
   c. Order of step b reversed
   d. Weight placed in the hands and steps b and c repeated
   e. Twice the weight used in step d placed in hands, and steps b and c repeated
   f. Select other positions of your choice.
2. Estimate the changes in the moment of inertia (I) by calculating the angular velocity (ω). Remember that the angular velocity must be expressed in radians: rad = revolutions per second $\times 2\pi$ (pi).
3. Draw conclusions concerning angular momentum and movement of body parts.

Work-Energy

The work-energy approach is a way of viewing the kinetics of motion from a different perspective than the impulse-momentum approach. The product of force and of the distance over which this force acts represents the work done by the force on an object. Our concern is with the distance rather than with the time of force application. When work is done, a change in energy results.

■ **Potential energy (PE)** is the capacity to do work, but no motion exists. **Kinetic energy (KE)** is the energy of motion.

The work-energy equation is:

$$\int Fd = \tfrac{1}{2}mV_f^2 - \tfrac{1}{2}mV_i^2$$

and the units are newton-meters (joules). The two velocities represent final (V_f) and initial (V_i) velocities.

Potential energy of an elevated body is *mgh,* that is, the product of the body weight and the elevation of the center of gravity of the body. Therefore, the *Fd* (*mgh*) will be equivalent to the KE ($\tfrac{1}{2}mV^2$) when the body falls. The following experiment is an application in horizontal work and energy.

MINI-LABORATORY LEARNING EXPERIENCE

1. Place a ball on the floor, holding your hand in a position to push the ball forward.
2. Maintain contact with the ball for 10 cm, pushing with a constant force.
   a. Note the apparent speed of the ball.
   b. Record the distance the ball travels and the time of travel.
   c. Calculate the velocity of the ball.
3. Repeat step 2 but apply the force for a distance of 20 cm.
4. Weigh the ball.
   a. Calculate its mass: N/9.8 m/sec^2 = weight/gravity.
   b. Calculate the kinetic energy for each situation: $\tfrac{1}{2} mV^2$.
   c. Calculate the force: $F = KE/d$ (in meters).

5. Interpret the data: What was the effect of doubling the distance of force application? Did you hold the force constant?

Work is done by each moving segment of the human body. We can investigate the mechanical efficiency of the human body using segmental-total body work and energy analysis.

■ Each body segment creates its own kinetic energy independent of and interdependent with other body segments.

The work-energy approach is useful in analyzing weightlifting and for analyzing and ranking movement tasks with respect to mechanical work and power. Collisions in which deformations are an important component of the interactions of two bodies, as in trampoline bouncing, are also better analyzed from a work-energy approach than from an impulse-momentum, or simple $F = ma$, approach.

■ The work-energy approach is as applicable to rotary motions as it is to linear motion. We can explain the principle of conservation of energy in much the same way as the conservation-of-momentum principle. Conservation of mechanical energy does not always occur, however, since friction is a nonconservative force. Heat energy always results in situations in which friction exists.

Although more applications will be discussed in Parts II and III, one of the most revealing applications of the work-energy concept involves the downward swing of an object, for example, a gymnast on the uneven parallel bars. Figure 6.10 shows a taller person and a shorter person beginning a downward swing from a horizontal position. The taller person will take longer to reach the vertical position because gravity is a constant force accelerating the body downward. Since the center of gravity of the body of the taller person must drop 1.3 m to reach the bottom of the swing, the shorter person will

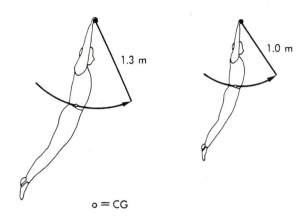

FIGURE 6.10 Different arcs of swing and vertical drops of center of gravity (CG) of two persons of different stature. If both body weights are equal, or if the taller person has greater body weight than the shorter person, the taller person will do more work and develop greater kinetic energy than the shorter person. Vertical drop (radius) multiplied by body weight equals work. **Assuming the shorter person weighs 400 newtons, calculate the potential energy prior to the drop (PE = mgh). Calculate the velocity at the greatest kinetic energy (zero PE).** Remember that the change in energy equals the work done.

reach the bottom sooner. Work done by the taller person will be 1.3 m × body weight; that of the shorter person will be 1.0 m × body weight. Potential energy exists at the start of the movement; therefore, initial $\frac{1}{2}\,mV^2 = 0$. Since the final kinetic energy is equal to the work done, if both persons were of equal mass, the taller person would experience greater downward velocity during the swing than would the shorter person, since greater work was performed.

Since work was performed in different durations of time, we often describe performances by the rate at which the person does the work. This is known as power. Detailed discussion of work and power as related to strength exercises appears in Chapter 10.

Potential and Kinetic Energy of Collisions

Characteristics of Elasticity

When two objects collide, the forces exerted on both objects tend to deform both objects.

■ The property that enables a body to recover its original shape or volume is called **elasticity** and is measured as the ratio of stress to strain, called Young's modulus of elasticity.

Stress refers to the amount of force per unit area of collision, and strain is the amount of distortion (deformation) with respect to original size.

A look at the elastic properties of certain types of materials will help make clear the kinetics of collisions. Rubber, for example, is not perfectly elastic; it does not return to its original shape if distorted to the maximum. In fact, high-tempered steel and spring brass are much more elastic than is rubber. All gases are perfectly elastic substances; for example, gas (air) is used in pneumatic tires. Liquids are also perfectly elastic, but difficult to compress. The inside of the best golf balls has a liquid core. When place-kicking, the toe of the shoe of the kicker often distorts the football as much as one-third of its original shape. The baseball is temporarily flattened against the bat as much as one-fourth. A golf ball may be distorted as much as one-tenth or more and a tennis ball up to one-half of its original shape.

Deformations are noted in shafts of long-handled implements such as rakes and hockey sticks, but are not so noticeable in shafts of hammers and other short-handled implements. Some plastic used in the manufacture of sports and game equipment for elementary-school-age children deform readily but may not easily regain their original shape. When used as striking implements, these plastics are ineffective because the striking implement deforms to a greater extent than does the object it strikes. The ball does not acquire sufficient velocity for the child to experience success.

The characteristics of elasticity can be used to explain why a small boy can hit a tennis ball using a tennis racquet farther than he can a baseball using a bat. The tennis ball can be compressed to the point at which it is considerably distorted. It acquires potential energy. The tennis ball and racquet remain together for a greater time (achieve greater impulse—ft) and for a longer distance (achieve greater work—Fd). In addition, the mass of the ball will not deflect the racquet backward to any measurable extent.

The work done by the boy on the baseball, however, will not be sufficient to distort it and "carry" the ball. The greater mass of the ball also will resist the movement more than did the lighter tennis ball. These concepts are recognized by golf instructors, who recommend that some women and small men not purchase golf balls with a liquid center because the ball cannot be compressed to the same extent as a ball with a rubber center.

Coefficient of Elasticity

The coefficient of elasticity is a number that represents the characteristics of a collision between two objects. It is not a measure of the elastic properties of either material, but of the interaction of the two materials. This coefficient of elasticity of two objects colliding with each other can be determined by the following experiment:

1. Drop a ball from a known height.
2. Measure the height of the rebound.
3. Calculate the coefficient of elasticity (e), using this equation:

$$e = \sqrt{\frac{\text{Height of rebound}}{\text{Height dropped}}}$$

A second method is to measure the velocity (V) of the rebounding object before and after impact. The energy lost during the collision will be represented by the loss in velocity. The equation is:

$$e = \frac{V \text{ after impact}}{V \text{ before impact}}$$

Racquetball, handball, and squash players increase the coefficient of elasticity (also called coefficient of restitution) between the ball and the rebounding surfaces by heating the ball. "Never play with a cold ball" is an adage to be followed, since a cold ball does not rebound as far, as fast, or as consistently as will a hot ball. Different playing surfaces also alter the rebound of balls.

Plagenhoef (1971) studied the characteristics of balls interacting with different surfaces in terms of both coefficient of friction and coefficient of elasticity and found a variety of values with the same ball under different conditions, including different speeds of the ball as it enters the collision.

Handball players sometimes follow a procedure that has a bearing on this discussion. They soak a "stale" handball in hot water. The heat causes a rearrangement of molecules inside the handball, which will then bounce (for a while) as much as when it was new. Handball players also sometimes soak their hands in hot water to help prevent bruises. The fluid in the hands comes to the surface and helps the skin to withstand blows.

The concept of stored energy because of easily deformed materials used for landing surfaces is an important one in some sports, especially in springboard diving, pole vaulting, and in trampolining. The material used has the potential to do work on the performer because of the distance through which it has been deformed. As the material is regaining its original shape, the potential energy of the system is transformed into kinetic energy and the person rebounds from the surface. Divers adjust the fulcrum of the diving board, changing the distance through which the board will deform. The result is more or less kinetic energy and a corresponding change in the height of the dive.

MINI-LABORATORY LEARNING EXPERIENCE

1. Determine coefficients of elasticity for balls interacting with various surfaces. Use the following equation:

$$e = \sqrt{\dfrac{\text{Rebound height}}{\text{Drop height}}}$$

2. Test environmental factors such as:
   a. Heated ball
   b. Cold ball
   c. Underinflated ball
   d. Ball with attached padding

Friction

Friction is the resistance that opposes every effort to slide or roll one body over another.

■ **Friction may be a hindrance or a help in sports and work performance.**

Here are some general facts about friction:

1. Static, or starting, friction is greater than moving, or sliding, friction.
2. Although many factors are involved, friction generally depends on the velocity, load, condition, and nature of the two surfaces interacting with each other.
3. In most practical sports situations, friction tends not to depend much on the velocity of the sliding surfaces.
4. Friction depends on the nature and condition of the contacting surfaces because:
   a. Friction is less when the surfaces are smooth and hard.
   b. With dry surfaces, friction is approximately the same regardless of the size of the area of contact.
   c. Friction is approximately proportional to the area of contact with well-lubricated surfaces.

A simple equation to calculate friction and the coefficient of friction is:

$R = B \times F_n$

R = friction force, B = coefficient of friction, and F_n = normal force.

Another way to present this is as a ratio: the force pressing the surfaces together is represented by N (normal force) and R (force needed to overcome friction). Therefore, $R/N = B$ where B is the coefficient of friction. The smaller B is, the less friction is created. On the other hand, the larger B is, the more the surfaces cling together, and the larger the force required to cause slippage.

■ **Sometimes it is advantageous to produce surfaces that have a high coefficient of friction; at other times it is advantageous to do just the opposite. Therefore, the concept of optimal friction is an important one.**

A performer must select the two materials that will interact according to the needs of the situation and goals of the performance. Each situation has an optimal amount of friction that enables optimal performance. Some coefficients of friction have been calculated for shoe-playing surfaces, (e.g., .4–1.5), but much of what is known about friction and the world of human and animal movement has been obtained through trial and error. Here are some examples of player and equipment adaptation to the element of friction.

1. Ashes are put on automobile tires when driving on snow to increase friction so that sufficient traction against the snow can be secured.
2. In wet weather, a small amount of silica sand on the hands of a passer may facilitate throwing the football more accurately because the coefficient of friction will be increased. However, wet, wrinkled socks inside a football player's shoes do the same thing and are likely to cause blisters.
3. Basketball players attempting to play on a floor that has been covered with wax for a dance may require the soles of their shoes to be irregular with indentations. This way, there is sufficient friction between the soles and the floor surface to enable them to move adeptly.
4. Table tennis paddles that have a rough, irregular surface enable players to put more spin on the ball because of the increased friction.
5. Surfaces such as the new, nonsmooth cement rings used for shot putting and discus throwing prevent the performer from slipping too fast when moving across the ring. Cleats and spikes on athletic shoes have the same effect. Moreover, the placement of the cleats and spikes affects the amount of friction created.

When the problem of slippage is too great and the surfaces cannot be changed, the performer must keep the center of gravity more nearly over the base of support. The performer will have to take short steps, avoid too much body lean, and drop the center of gravity as low as possible by squatting. In this way, the athlete will be able to remain in a playing posture and to perform at reasonable efficiency.

Because of the condition of a surface (for example, slick and wet), it is possible to "spin the wheels" too fast. In such cases, the coefficient of friction will be insufficient for the object, such as a car or a person, to move forward successfully. The two surfaces must be in contact with each other long enough for traction to take place. Moving at a slower speed enables this to occur.

■ Friction Concepts

a. The greater the friction, the greater the muscle effort needed to oppose it.
b. The greater the friction, the greater the reduction of speed in a human body or object.
c. Friction in one movement can be used in a successive countermovement.

MINI-LABORATORY LEARNING EXPERIENCE

1. Experience the effects of friction in the following ways:
   a. Roll down a ramp using a wheelchair, skateboard, coaster, rollerblades, rollerskates, or a scooter. Place different surfaces, such as a rubber mat or carpet, on the ramp and repeat the experiment.
   b. Glide down a snow-covered hill on skis in the cold morning (frozen snow) and in the mid-day sun (slushy snow).
   c. Push a cart or piece of furniture across the room on a tiled floor, then repeat in a room with a carpeted floor. Try a low-pile, smooth-surfaced carpet and deep-pile, uneven-surfaced carpet.
   d. Slide on a smooth surface (linoleum, tile, heavily waxed wooden floor, or marble) with leather-soled shoes. Select three other kinds of shoes with different surfaces.
   e. Devise an experiment to determine friction between implements held in the hand.

For each of the above experiments, state how you might estimate the magnitude or the relative difference in friction among the various conditions and surfaces. Calculate these using the previously presented equation.

Measuring Frictional Aspects

If one surface can be tilted to produce an incline, the angle at which the second surface slips (slides) on this incline can be measured. You can determine the tangent of the angle by referring to Appendix B. This tangent value is equal to the coefficient of friction value. Then determine frictional force using the formula previously given, $R = B \times F_N$.

You can also find the frictional force directly by measuring, with a spring scale, the force required to cause one surface to slide on a second surface.

MINI-LABORATORY LEARNING EXPERIENCE

1. Place a rubber-cleated shoe with a weight inside on a wood surface and determine the frictional force and coefficient of friction by attaching a spring scale to the shoe and exerting a horizontal force on the scale. The highest value of the scale reading will be the limit of static friction. Note that the kinetic friction is slightly less than the static friction, which terminates as soon as slippage occurs. Calculate the coefficient of friction using

$$\frac{R \text{ (friction force)}}{N \text{ (weight)}}$$

2. Repeat the experiment using different surfaces.
3. Repeat the experiment using shoes with different soles.
4. If a spring scale is not available, place shoes on a board that can be tilted. Slowly increase the angle of inclination of the board until slippage occurs. The tangent of the angle at which the shoe slips is the coefficient of friction. To calculate the friction force, you must find the normal force by calculating $N = \text{Weight} \times (\text{cosine of the angle of inclination})$.
5. Compare results from 1 and 4.

Forces in Air and Water Environments

As a body applies a force to, or interacts with, air or water, the particles of air or water are disturbed and experience a change in speed and direction in direct proportion to their resistance to the body. This resistance, which is in keeping with the law of interaction, produces what is termed a **drag force.** The amount of resistance of the fluid depends on its energy, which is influenced by pressure, velocity, and position with respect to the body encountered by air or water. The basis for understanding the human body's interaction with the fluid, whether air or water, is Bernoulli's principle, which states that fluid pressure is decreased whenever speed of flow is increased.

Drag force exists with all bodies of all shapes and sizes, traveling through air, water, or other fluid. Rough, deformed, or less streamlined bodies experience greater resistance than those bodies said to be "aerodynamically designed."

We discuss the effect of a fluid environment on the human body and objects in Chapter 21, aquatics and Chapter 22, cycling. Information for analyzing ball flight in activities such as ball-throwing, striking, and kicking activities is presented in Appendix C and Chapter 19, basketball. The hydrodynamics of the aquatics chapter can also be applied to aerodynamics of ball flight. For example, in the case of a golf ball, backspin imparted to the ball by the golf club helps to create high- and low-pressure areas and, consequently, a drag-lift differential. This effect has also been called the Magnus effect, after a German engineer who is credited with first noting the curved path followed by a cannonball to which spin had been imparted before it became airborne. This rotation, seen in many projections of objects used in sports, is usually created by striking or otherwise exerting a force eccentric to the object. This creates rotation about an axis within the ball, and the ball veers right or left, up or down, or diagonally. This phenomenon is explained by the fact that as a body rotates, it tends to have the fluid next to it move with it, and the air or other fluid just beyond this so-called boundary layer is influenced. As the object travels through a medium such as air and meets the oncoming air, a high pressure is then developed on the side of the direction of the spin and a low pressure on the opposite side. The ultimate result is an increase in the fall or rise of the ball. The aerodynamics of ball flight is described in Appendix C.

References

Barham, J. N. 1978. *Mechanical kinesiology.* St. Louis: Mosby.

Daish, C. B. 1979. *The physics of ball games.* London: English Universities Press.

Hochmuth, G. 1984. *Biomechanics of athletic movement.* Berlin, Germany: Sportverlag.

Hooper, B. G. 1973. *The mechanics of human movement.* New York: American Elsevier.

Merzkirch, W. 1979. Making fluid flows visible. *Am. Sci.* 67:330–36.

Plagenhoef, S. 1971. *Patterns of human motion: A cinematographic analysis.* Englewood Cliffs, NJ: Prentice-Hall.

Rodgers, M. M., and Cavanagh, P. 1984. Glossary of biomechanical terms, concepts, and units. *Physical Therapy* 64:1887–1901.

Schench, J. M., and Cordova, F. D. 1980. *Introductory biomechanics,* 2nd ed. Philadelphia: F. A. Davis.

Townsend, M. S. 1984. *Mathematics in sport.* New York: Halsted Press/John Wiley.

Tricker, R. A., and Tricker, B. J. K. 1967. *The science of movement.* New York: American Elsevier.

II

Tools for Human Movement Analysis

7 Tools for Assessment, Improvement, and Prediction of Movement

T echnology with the attendant sophisticated tools is the state of the art in research in human movement.

As might be expected, the tools used in the study of biomechanics of human movement determine the types of analyses that are possible. The nature, type, and magnitude of data are limited by the tools we select. Quantitative force data, for example, is impossible to obtain through visual perception. Limited qualitative inferences concerning force, however, may be possible. The eyes "record" only temporal and spatial changes, and the brain translates these into a perceived essence of movement, tension, force, and even feeling.

Many tools are available at varying costs. Some tools are more sophisticated than others and require more training. But even the least-sophisticated tool requires training if valid data and maximum analysis of these data are to be achieved. Common tools (including instrumentation systems) and what they measure are:

1. Human eye and other senses: spatial and temporal descriptive data of movement as discussed in Chapter 1
2. Timing devices: temporal data
3. Artificial optical devices, such as single-image photography, stroboscopy, cinematography, videography, and magnetic resonance imaging: linear and angular kinematic data and derived kinetic data when supplemented with inertial information
4. Goniometry and electrogoniometry: joint kinematic data, static positions, and dynamic action
5. Electromyography: muscle action potentials data
6. Dynamography: force and impulse data
7. Accelerometry: acceleration data
8. Modeling and simulation: computer manipulation of the human body for prediction of kinematic and kinetic data and overall performance

We will define, explain historically, and describe in detail each of these tools or systems. You will then be able to select the best tool or tools for your specific biomechanics analysis project. Additional resources are listed at the end of the chapter. In addition, a series of six instrumentation video tapes is available from the publisher of this book. These tapes include information about electromyography and electrogoniometry, high-speed cinematography, digitizing, force platform analysis, force insoles with telemetry, and optoelectronic computerized systems.

Timing Devices

A variety of timing devices (chronoscopes), including stop watches, counters, digital timers, switch mats, photoelectric cells, real-time computer clocks, and laser tubes are now used to record speeds of the human being and its body parts. We can easily assess the outcome of movements (simple, complex, and sequential). A chronoscope is started at a preselected instant in time,

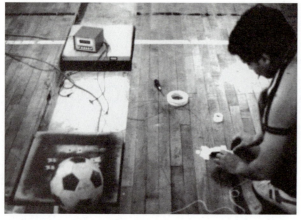

a

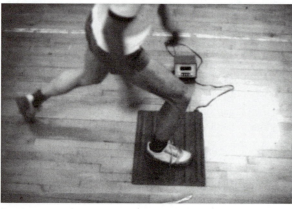

b

FIGURE 7.1 Timing of the soccer kick. (*a*) Speed of the ball is recorded by fabricating a start clock switch when the ball leaves its resting position and the string attached to the ball stops the clock after the ball travels a preset distance. (*b*) A switch mat is used to record the duration of foot contact.

(Compliments of Lafayette Instrument Company, Lafayette, IN.)

evaluations of many movements, in particular the limb movements required in sports and dynamic balance times. Note the intricate system in Figure 7.1 to measure soccer performance.

An even simpler device to use is a radar gun for instant speed display. Radar guns were originally used by law enforcement officers to track motor vehicles. Later they became useful to clock the speed of the baseball pitcher's fast, slow, and curve ball pitches. Now the radar gun is used in many sports, but it is sometimes difficult to position the gun for small balls and balls that travel upward or sideward. Usually the objects must be traveling faster than four to five meters per second.

Photography and Cinematography

Since the flicker response of the human eye is 10–12 frames per second, it cannot see the particulars of a fast motion. Furthermore, since the eye doesn't retain the total motion, investigators turned to various devices to provide permanent images of movement.

A French physiologist, Étienne Jules Marey (1830–1904), was so interested in human movement that he developed photographic means for use in biological research. In his works *Du Mouvement dans les Fonctions de la Vie* and *De Mouvement,* he explained and illustrated how this could be accomplished. Some of the translated works include the history of chronophotography and lectures on the phenomenon of flight in the animal world. Marey was convinced that movement was the most important human function and that it affected all other activities.

Eadweard Muybridge (1830–1904), through his photographic skill, brought a new tool to kinesiological investigation. He was motivated by the work of Janssen, an astronomer who had been successful in taking sequential pictures of stars. Among the numerous Muybridge publications was an 11-volume work, *Animal Locomotion* (1887). A later publication called *The Human Figure in Motion* contains much of his original work. Using 24 fixed cameras and two portable batteries of 12 cameras each, Muybridge was able to take pictures of animals (Figure 7.2) and people in action. By using the zoopraxiscope he could mechanically move the pictures fast enough to simulate the actual movement. As an illustration of how an idea may be developed, Muybridge modified

usually the initiation of the movement. At another instant in time, the chronoscope is stopped. Speed of movement is calculated by dividing the chronoscope time by the known displacement of the movement.

Many of these timing devices have been fabricated by researchers, coaches, and athletes. The electronics can be as simple as two microswitches and two LEDs (light-emitting diodes). We use computer interfacing to record, store, and retrieve multiple-trial and longitudinal

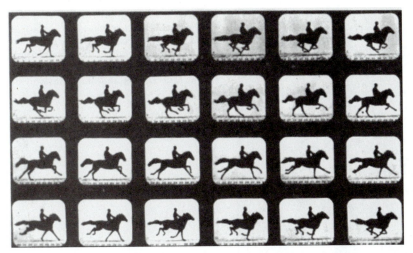

FIGURE 7.2 Motion of a running horse. This is a classic pseudo-cinematographic product of Eadweard Muybridge in the late 1800s. The horse is Phryne L, whose length of stride was reported to be 6 m, 2 cm (19 ft., 9 in.). (Courtesy of the Stanford University Museum of Art, Muybridge Collection 13932.)

this device by mounting transparencies made from a series of his photographs on a circular glass plate. When he rotated the plate, individual transparencies could be projected by a projection lantern in the usual manner. A major refinement of the device was the addition of a second plate made of metal and mounted parallel to the glass plate on a concentric axis, but turning in the opposite direction. The metal plate was slit at appropriate intervals. When the two plates revolved, the metal plate served as a shutter. The persistence of vision between each slit gave the viewer the illusion of motion as each individual picture in the series was projected. As many as 200 transparencies could be mounted on a single plate, and the wheels, or plates, could be revolved endlessly, "a period limited only by the patience of the spectators."

Photography has become more sophisticated since those 19th-century experiments. Many investigations of human and animal movements are conducted with movie cameras (35mm or 16mm) capable of filming at rates up to 500 images per second, which is approximately 50 times the number of distinct images the human eye can detect. Other cameras operating at 40,000-plus filming rates are used in collision and other impact studies of body deformation and destruction.

Single-Image Photography

A single-image camera (126, 35mm, portrait, etc.) is appropriate for analyzing selected positions during a movement pattern. For example, the posture used to ad-

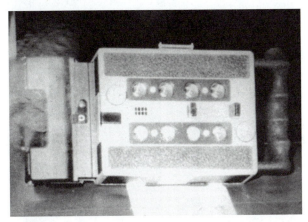

FIGURE 7.3 Graph sequence camera. This is an inexpensive way to obtain eight photographs at set time intervals. Newer 35mm cameras with rapid sequence advance cannot achieve the short time interval of this multiple lens camera.

dress the golf ball, to operate a typewriter, to get ready to swing an axe, or to prepare to lift a 900 N (202.5 lbs) barbell can be photographed and compared to other postures. We can obtain a series of photographs of one movement pattern with devices such as a graph sequence camera or an automatic rapid advance 35mm camera (Figure 7.3).

Another common type of still photography, with the illusion of motion, is stroboscopy or intermittent light photography. Figure 7.4 shows the results of such a technique.

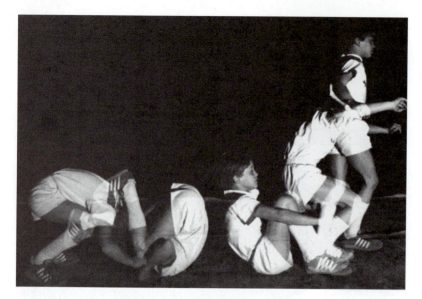

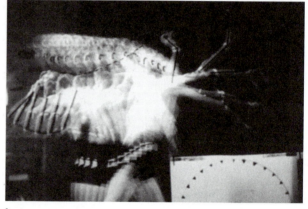

FIGURE 7.4 A stroboscopic photograph. Note the five distinct images taken at equal increments in time. Speed can be deduced by the position of the hair on the third image. **Study the images and determine distances of travel and angles at joints that can be measured.**

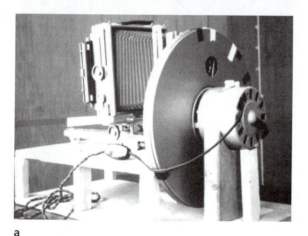

a

b

FIGURE 7.5 An inexpensive intermittent light photography system made from a portrait camera, a disk with one or more slits, an empty film reel canister, and a motor to rotate the disk. The camera shutter is opened for the entire time of filming and light enters only when the slits of the disk rotate in front of the shutter. An example of a photo obtained from this system is included. Contrast this with Figure 7.4.

Stroboscopic photography uses multiple exposures on a single negative, which may be exposed to a brightly lighted or a dark background, and to a subject. In the first case, the exposures are determined by the opening of the camera shutter at a set rate. An inexpensive technique for achieving a simulated shutter opening/closing sequence is to fabricate an external rotating shutter, as shown in Figure 7.5.

In this case, the shutter remains open, and light illuminates the negative at intermittent intervals. For example, small electric light bulbs can be attached to points on the body. These lights may be illuminated continuously, resulting in a line of light on the photograph, or they may flash at a set rate, resulting in a series of dots on the photograph, as in Figure 7.6.

134   Tools for Human Movement Analysis

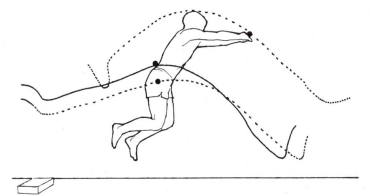

FIGURE 7.6 Light bulbs attached to joints of a performer and filmed with stroboscopic techniques creates a sequence of points and one body image at a light flash. The person carries a small battery pack to power the light bulbs.

A stroboscopic light (true stroboscopy) may illuminate at set intervals (frequencies) the subject or reflective markers placed on the subject. This is by far the most expensive method, since a large power supply is required to trigger the strobe light at successive short intervals of time. An interesting and comprehensive description of the history of high-speed stroboscopy by the "father of stroboscopy", Harold Edgerton, can be found in *National Geographic,* October 1987. The color photographs alone are worth the trip to the library.

Movie Cameras

Although home movie cameras exist, they have been superceded by home video cameras. The home movie camera can usually be operated at 16–24 frames per second. The home video camera has the equivalent of 30 frames per second (Figure 7.7). The movie film, however, can be projected on any wall, screen, plate of glass, or other clear matter, making it easy to trace data from the projected image at varying sizes, even lifesize. Despite the advantage of image size capabilities, the filmed images from these low-speed cameras are usually blurred with most fast movements.

Moderate-speed 16mm cameras are relatively inexpensive and can be operated at 64–128 frames per second to eliminate the blurs of movements slower than, or equal to, brisk walking. Such operating speeds and shutters of 1/64th to 1/128th of a second are adequate for analysis of many activities of daily living and work tasks.

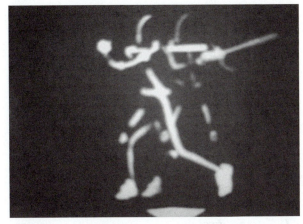

FIGURE 7.7 Photographic images taken from a video monitor in playback pause mode. Note the two images representing the two fields of the image.
(Image taken from Sybervision.)

High-speed cameras (Figure 7.8) however are common and required, though expensive, tools for sports biomechanics. Many sports activities can be filmed at 80–150 frames per second if the shutter exposure time is short enough to reduce or eliminate the movement blur. If it is required to capture specific instances within the movement pattern, the camera will need to operate at rates between 150–300 frames per second. Such applications, for example, include filming the contact of a softball bat with a softball and the initial responses of the foot and leg to impact during the contact phases of a

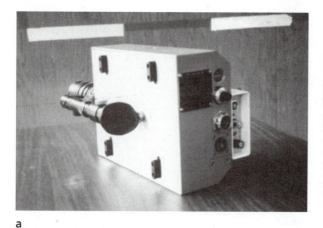

a

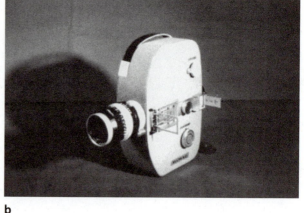

b

FIGURE 7.8 High-speed cameras capable of operating at 500 images per second (LOCAM) and at higher rates (PHOTOSONICS). These cameras have built-in timing devices and can be phase-locked with other cameras for synchronized multiple image filming and synchronized with other data-collection instrumentation systems, such as force platforms and electromyography.

triple jump. Filming rates of 300–500 frames per second are required to precisely capture collisions of two objects moving at high speeds, such as deformation of ball and tennis racquet strings during contact.

Filming rates are often expressed in units of Hz (cycles per second, derived from electricity). So, 128 frames per second is 128 Hz (128 cps).

3-D Cinematography

Since most naturally performed human movements require a three-dimensional (3-D) analysis, instrumentation systems have been devised to capture, simultaneously, two or more views of the performance. This is possible via one camera and one or more mirrors or prisms, or via two or more cameras. The following set-ups are most common:

1. One overhead mirror and one camera
2. Stereophotogrammetry using two cameras in parallel with overlapping fields
3. Two orthogonal cameras
4. Three orthogonal cameras (Figure 7.9 shows the views derived from three orthogonal cameras.)
5. Multiple cameras placed nonorthogonally and/or tilted

The two-orthogonal-camera method frequently consists of the major plane-viewing camera operated at a higher speed than the minor plane camera. For example, a sagittal-view (side-view) camera would be the major plane camera in the system of one frontal-view and one sagittal-view camera operating to film a long jump performance. Sometimes one or more stationary cameras are used with a panning camera. This latter camera tracks the total movement of, for example, the triple jump, and the stationary cameras are used to film only the takeoff phases.

■ Precise calibration is required to obtain valid quantitative 3-D data.

Cineradiography

Another form of photography used to film internal biomechanical research data is cineradiography. This technique consists of synchronizing a camera with a radiograph machine (x-ray) or fluoroscopic machine. The bones are filmed in motion. Note the extreme position of the patella in Figure 7.10.

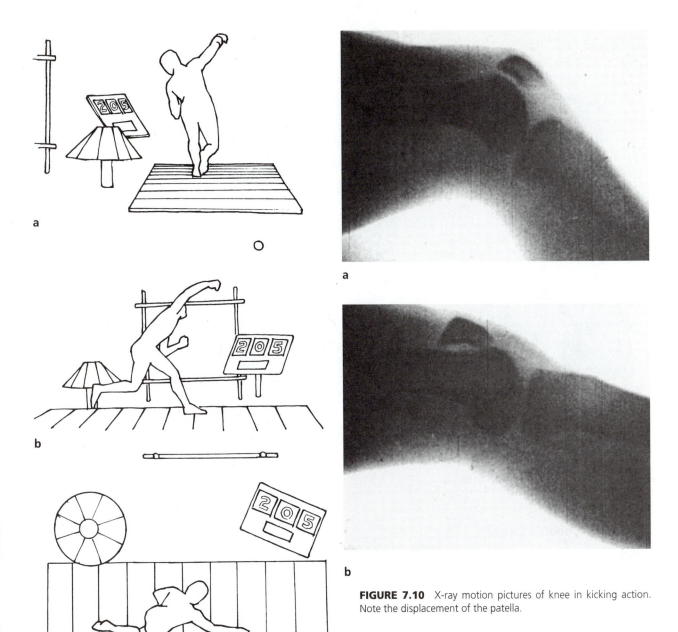

FIGURE 7.10 X-ray motion pictures of knee in kicking action. Note the displacement of the patella.

FIGURE 7.9 Rear, side, and overhead views taken to study an overarm throw. Number 205 identifies subject and trial in series. Note presence of the cone-shaped timing device, as well as uprights and crossbars that establish vertical and horizontal lines to aid in measurement.

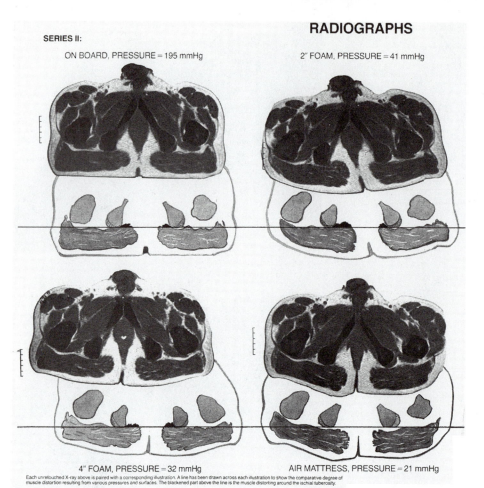

RADIOGRAPHS

SERIES II:

ON BOARD, PRESSURE = 195 mmHg

2" FOAM, PRESSURE = 41 mmHg

4" FOAM, PRESSURE = 32 mmHg

AIR MATTRESS, PRESSURE = 21 mmHg

Each unretouched X-ray above is paired with a corresponding illustration. A line has been drawn across each illustration to show the comparative degree of muscle distortion resulting from various pressures and surfaces. The blackened part above the line is the muscle distorting around the ischial tuberosity.

FIGURE 7.11 Magnetic resonance images of pelvic soft tissues and compression during sitting on an EHOB seat cushion and a wood surface. (Courtesy of EHOB, Inc.)

Magnetic Resonance Imaging

The most recent tool to investigate the tissues and internal movements of the body is known as magnetic resonance imaging (MRI). This is very expensive, but will become a major tool for computer modeling research. The exact position and status of a joint, for example, can be measured so that a "best-fit" prosthesis can be developed. Color is an important component of MRI and has been used extensively to identify positions and displacements of internal body organs and tissues. Excellent color images can be found in the SOMA articles discussed later in this text. An example of the tissues at the lumbar region or pelvis is depicted in Figure 7.11.

Computerized Cinematography

Although we can analyze single-image films or movie films by physically tracing and measuring displacements of one image at a time and then calculating other motion variables from these displacements, since the late 1960s, researchers have used computerized film-analysis systems. A digitizing tablet is interfaced with a computer so that an almost infinite amount of data can be obtained in a short period of time, if the appropriate software is available. These systems have processing components for numerically and graphically printing displacement, velocities, acceleration, moments of force, centers of gravity, etc., as well as statistical data.

Videography

Taking advantage of advanced technology is possible without a great deal of training or money, since video systems are inexpensive and readily available to the practitioner, technician, and general consumer. The advantages of videography over cinematography are

1. the ability to synchronize two images on one screen, which is possible by means of a split-image, special-effects generator.
2. the direct and immediate transmission of the image to a computer, eliminating the human operator required in photographic analysis.
3. the direct playback capability, to provide immediate feedback to both analyst and performer.

In the past, the major disadvantage of videography was the low resolution of video tapes, much lower than that of the highest-quality movie film. Recently, this disadvantage has disappeared with the availability of the SVHS and Hi8 formats in camcorders. These camcorders also have inputs to computers and frame-by-frame forward and reverse playbacks.

Does high-technology videography exist? Oh, yes! As with cinematography, recent changes in videography have been dramatic. Unknown prior to the 1950s, videography has nearly equalled or outdistanced cinematography in computerization, filming rates (20,000 Hz), and interfacing capabilities with other tools. Interfacing videography with a microcomputer is the least expensive high-tech system for analyzing movement. The computer digitally "grabs" an image and the human computer operator then digitizes the selected anatomical markers.

Computerized Optical Systems

A more expensive system consists of electronic digitizing, that is, nonhuman automated digitizing. The camera picks up signals from devices of contrasting intensities that are electronically identified and located in space. From the camera, the images are inputted directly into a computer. A nonvideo image results, for example, only the markers (identifiable signals) are seen by the camera.

The identifiable signals may be reflective tape illuminated by a bright light, light-emitting diodes, prisms of glass, tiny light bulbs or merely contrasting colors. The types and amount of data generated from these signals are limited by the size of the computer and by the data-analysis software. Examples of some of the high-tech video systems now available are in Figure 7.12.

■ The human movement specialist can maximize the analysis of movement through knowledgeable selection of video components.

Cost of these systems, however, may be too high for teachers, coaches, and non-medical researchers. These systems may be found at gait laboratories in rehabilitation centers or hospitals, many universities, and national sports associations.

Split-Screen Videography

We can capture two planes of a movement on the same image of a video monitor with a special effects generator and two cameras. Three cameras can capture three orthogonal planes. The generator has horizontal and vertical sectioning capabilities. An example of a 3-D setup for video taping exiting and entering a mock automobile is shown in Figure 7.13.

Low-Cost Video Cameras

A color camera capable of indoor and outdoor use without extra lighting will be the most versatile. A shuttered camera, to eliminate the blur of regular video camera images, is invaluable for sports movements, but not always necessary for most activities of daily living and work-skill analyses. Such shuttered cameras, however, usually require extra indoor lighting. Images obtained with a regular video camera and a shuttered camera (1/500th-second exposure) are shown in Figure 7.14. High-speed video cameras with capabilities of more than 120 images per second are available but not commonly used in biomechanics of human movement. The 60 fields/second and 120 fields/second cameras have only recently become viable cameras for sports biomechanists.

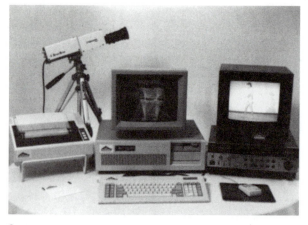

a

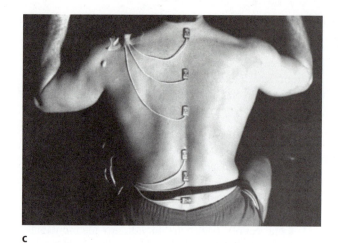

c

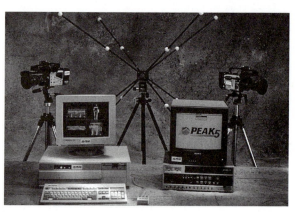

b

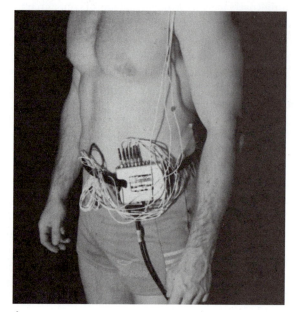

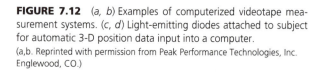

FIGURE 7.12 (*a, b*) Examples of computerized videotape measurement systems. (*c, d*) Light-emitting diodes attached to subject for automatic 3-D position data input into a computer.

(a,b. Reprinted with permission from Peak Performance Technologies, Inc. Englewood, CO.)

d

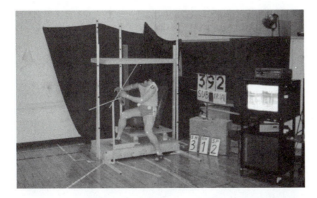

FIGURE 7.13 Split-screen videography: person entering a mock-up of a car door opening. Two video cameras interfaced with a signal-effects generator capture two images on a single screen. (Courtesy of Josef Loczi, University of Illinois at U-C.)

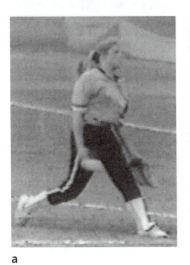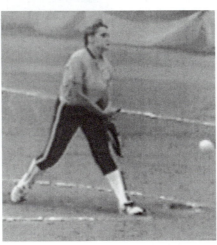

FIGURE 7.14 Reproductions of video images taken with regular video camera, (a), and high-speed shutter video camera, (b).

a   b

Microprocessors are standard equipment in many video cameras. Accessories also are available as add-ons. These add-on devices title segments of the tape, identify events, and imprint a time-generated code on the tape. The images in Figure 7.15 have time codes.

Video Playback Units and Videotape Recording

It is absolutely necessary to be able to still-image and image-by-image advance and reverse the videotape in the playback mode if time-effectiveness with data analysis is sought. Any other recorder will involve too much trial-and-error and frustration to be efficient in selecting the appropriate images to analyze. There are 30 images per second on the commonly available recorder/playback units. Recently 60 fields per second (the ability to grab each of the two fields of each image separately) and 120 fields per second playback units have become available to the researcher. SuperVHS and Hi8 tapes are available with approximately twice the horizontal lines of standard tapes. This new technology has vastly improved the resolution of the images.

Goniometry and Electrogoniometry

Goniometers usually measure static positions of limb segments with respect to the ROM at a joint (minimum and maximum anatomical angles). Goniometers are based on the protractor concept and gravity concept.

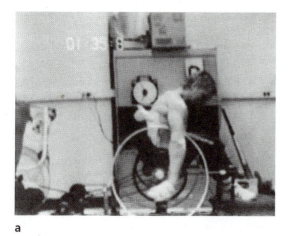
a

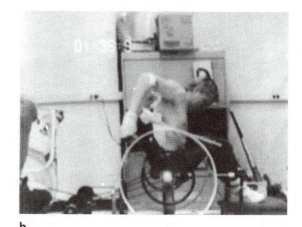
b

FIGURE 7.15 Video prints with time-generated code imprinted on sequenced images.

Sizes of goniometers vary, depending on the sizes of body segments being measured. See Figure 7.16 for examples of goniometers.

MINI-LABORATORY LEARNING EXPERIENCE

1. Carefully position the goniometer along the longitudinal axis of the two body segments forming the joint, with the focal center of the protractor at the joint axis.
2. Ask the subject to move the distal segment to its limit of ROM. Record the angle at the joint.
3. Compare different individuals and/or right and left limbs of the same individuals.

Observing changes in angles at joints is easier with the electrogoniometer (also termed "elgon"), devised by Karpovich in the late 1950s. Essentially a goniometer with a potentiometer substituted for the protractor, an electrogoniometer is a device to measure (*meter*) angles (*gonio*), and consists of a potentiometer placed at the joint center, with two extensions attached to the body parts forming the joint (see Figure 7.17). A potentiometer is a device similar to the volume control on a radio that changes the resistance to the flow of electric current in a circuit. The degrees of movement in the joint to

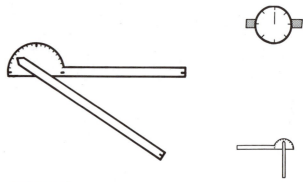

FIGURE 7.16 Goniometers for measuring static anatomical angles at different body sites.

which the device has been attached can be read continuously and directly from an oscilloscope, recording paper, or a computer, eliminating laborious measurement of each image of a photograph. The device has been used with other methods of recording movement; it is especially useful combined with electromyography. For comprehensive description of the elgon and its application see Adrian (1973).

Three-dimensional electrogoniometers have been used in gait analysis in rehabilitation centers and laboratories and on the sports field. The advantages of electrogoniometry include the ability to record the action at the joint when it is not visible to the observer, such as during swimming and twisting movements. Another advantage is the instantaneous portrayal of angular displacement

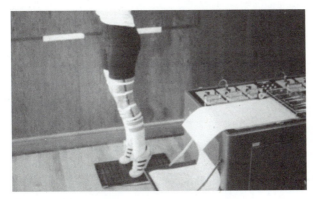

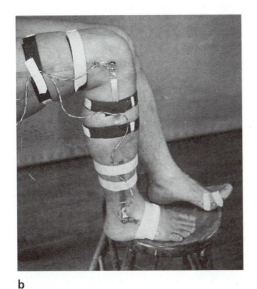

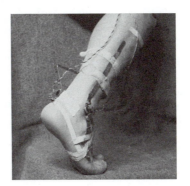

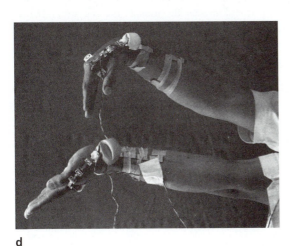

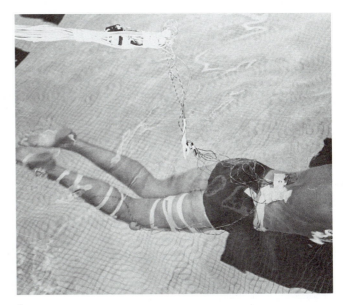

FIGURE 7.17 Electrogoniometers (elgons) for recording continuous angular displacements at the joints to which they are attached.

Tools for Assessment, Improvement, and Prediction of Movement   **143**

with respect to time. Researchers can also link the electrogoniometry system to a computer to obtain angular velocities and accelerations. The use of a telemetry system (transmitting device and receiver with no wire connections, such as with radio and television systems) has been used to monitor joint angles of subjects from racehorses to swimmers to football players.

The goniogram, however, does not convey any spatial orientation of the limb, but solely the angle at the joint, the anatomical angle. There are other disadvantages, common to all devices attached to the body. The elgons must be lightweight, fit the contours of the body, and not interfere with movement. They must be attached to the average axis of rotation at the joint being studied and validated for proper placement for each joint. If many joints of the body are being investigated, the person will appear to be wearing an exoskeleton.

Newer types of electrogoniometers, based on a strain concept (strain of the material is calibrated as change in angle), record two-dimensional angular motion. This is especially useful for studying the spine.

Electromyography

Muscle analysis based on anatomic position of muscles is not definitive of the action that occurs in the living, moving body. The fallacies of analyzing muscle action on the basis of anatomic position were demonstrated by Duchenne in the middle of the nineteenth century. On the basis of electrical stimulation of muscles, combined with observation of partially paralyzed subjects, he described the movements resulting from contraction of specific muscles as they functioned in living subjects. Unfortunately, his findings were not widely used in the United States, since they were published in French and were not readily available until translated in 1949 by Kaplan. By that time, investigators in the United States had begun to observe muscle action in living subjects by recording the electrical changes in muscular contraction. This technique of recording, known as electromyography, has been greatly refined and, as complex motor acts are studied, will provide valuable information for the kinesiologist. The major current contributor to this development is J. V. Basmajian; his book *Muscles Alive,* (1979) is a classic.

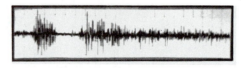

a

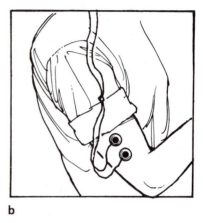

b

FIGURE 7.18   Electromyography. (a) Electromyogram; (b) surface electrodes attached to performer.

Electromyography is the process of recording electrical changes that occur in a muscle during or immediately before contraction. Necessary equipment for electromyography includes a device for picking up the electrical activity, a means of conducting the electrical impulses, and a device for translating them to visual form. The pickup devices are metal disk electrodes placed on the skin over the muscle (see Figure 7.18) or fine wires inserted into the muscle to be observed. Insulated wires then conduct impulses from the pickup to the translating devices. Among the latter are ink writers, electromagnetic tape recorders, computers, and oscilloscopes, from which photographs are made during the activity. The final form is a record, an electromyogram (EMG), similar to that shown in Figure 7.18.

Since the action potentials resulting from muscle contraction do not necessarily occur precisely when muscle contraction is produced, caution is needed in interpreting the EMG. For example, the EMG signal always occurs before movement and is earlier in phasic than in tonic movements. Phasic movements show fast-twitch muscle

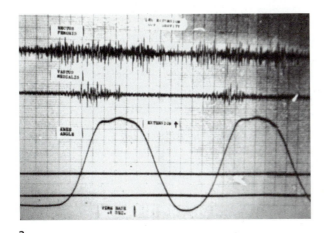

a

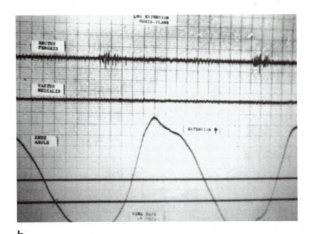

b

FIGURE 7.19 Electromyograms from identical muscles with body limb in two positions. (*a*) Extension of lower leg is against gravity. (*b*) Extension is in the horizontal plane. Note how gravity influences the role and tension produced in the muscle. The top tracing is an electromyogram of the rectus femoris muscle, the electromyogram beneath is of the vastus lateralis muscle, and the lower tracing is the angular displacement at the knee. Extension is represented as an upward trace.

fibers to be active, while slow-twitch muscle fibers are active during tonic movements. Thus, the magnitude of the EMG sign will be proportional to the velocity of the movement, since the magnitude of fast-twitch fiber action potentials is greater than that of slow-twitch fiber action potentials. In addition, the EMG magnitude also is directly related to the resistance to be overcome, or the amount of contraction used for static loading situations. For these reasons, the amount of tension in the muscle is not exactly defined by the EMG.

Furthermore, to interpret an EMG, it is necessary to know several things: which body segments have moved; in which joints actions have occurred, at what rates, and in what sequence; which muscles pass over these joints; and to which bones these muscles are attached. It is also necessary to know whether other forces were acting on body segments, especially gravitation force.

Note in Figure 7.19 that the action of muscles differs during identical changes at the knee joint with a change in limb position with respect to gravity. Since EMGs do not provide kinematic information, other techniques of data collection are used at the same time. For example, researchers use photography (biplane is recommended) data to show limb and muscle position in space and electrogoniometry (elgon at the joint being investigated) to show angle at joint. In the hands of a competent, trustworthy investigator, electromyography is a vital tool for muscle function analysis of postures and movement of all types and in all situations in life. His or her special technical skills include the ability to select and use the best equipment for each study and to interpret the EMG intelligently.

Dynamography

Although dynamography has been used in industry and by engineers for many decades, there was virtually no use of this technique for analysis of human forces produced during sports situations prior to the 1960s. Dynamography is a technique for measuring the forces produced during an activity. In the measurement of strength, primarily peak static strength, dynamography consisted of spring devices and cable tensiometers (Figure 7.20).

Since the last decade, resistance sensors, (strain gauges), pressure sensors, and capacitive sensors have been placed on such devices as canoe and kayak paddles, athletic footwear insoles, ladders, bicycle pedals, and uneven parallel bars to determine the effectiveness of force production by performers using these devices. Strain gauges are considered force transducers since

Tools for Assessment, Improvement, and Prediction of Movement

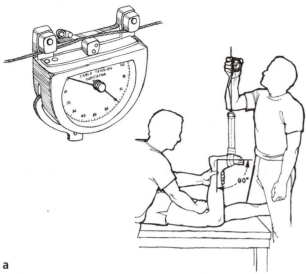

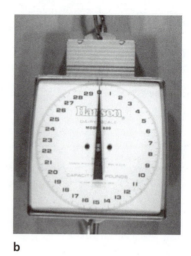

FIGURE 7.20 Mechanical devices to measure forces. (*a*) The cable tensiometer is a versatile device used extensively for several decades by numerous researchers, including H. H. Clarke. (*b*) The spring scale is not only useful for determining body weight and frictional force, but also as a strength-recording device.

they receive power from one system (power supply) and transfer their power (changes in force) to another system (a recorder). These devices are small, lightweight and adaptable to any purpose. A metal ring equipped with four strain gauges, for example, has been used to record the pulling forces of a performer being towed in water and to measure forces in a wire from which a metal ball was attached. (See Figure 7.21; the device in A was used in the hammer throw athletic event.)

Force Platforms

For the collection of large ground reaction forces, a more permanent, nonportable tool has been designed, the force platform. Force platforms have been built in many sizes, shapes, and designs, incorporating strain gauges or piezoelectric crystals to record force-time histories in three planes during such diverse activities as running, jumping, swimming, walking, and other locomotor patterns of human beings as well as cats, dogs, horses, and other animals. Movements of athletes engaged in pole vaulting, shot putting, sprinting starts, golf, and gymnastics, among other sports, have also been measured by dynamographic techniques. Studying

walking down stairs and ramps and performing industrial tasks are other uses of the force platform. An application is shown in Figure 7.22.

The force platform, although hailed as early as 1938 as a tool for analyzing the gait of a cat walking on a treadmill, became the most exciting analysis tool of the sports world of the 1970s. It is now standard equipment in gait laboratories, mainly of a clinical nature, as well as sports biomechanics research laboratories. Improvements and modifications of the force platform concept have been made since its conception. We describe some of the more common innovations below.

Foot Plates

Force insoles (Figure 7.23) have been placed inside shoes in order to circumvent the problems of subjects not striking the platform and not maintaining a natural locomotor pattern. Such portable devices, however, have not been perfected for 3-D recording; at this time, only vertical force measurements are practical. Similar uses are common in the animal world with instrumental horseshoes to investigate gaits of racehorses and injured horses.

The use of anatomically placed sensors on the feet was developed and termed clinical electrodynography.

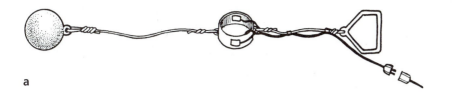

FIGURE 7.21 Strain gauge transducer used in the hammer throw (a). Force-time history of the tension on the cable (b). Notice the cyclic and incremental increase in force during the throwing sequence.

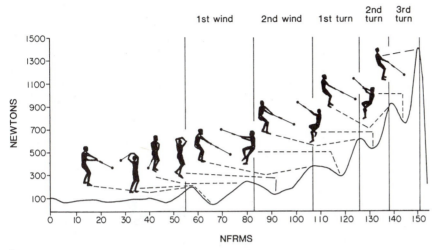

b

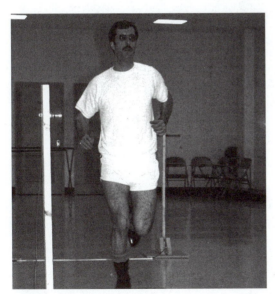

FIGURE 7.22 Subject running over Kistler force platform in experiment to analyze ground reaction forces during foot contact. Three forces are amplified and recorded on magnetic tape for later computer processing.

(Courtesy of Pennsylvania State University, The Center for Locomotion Studies.)

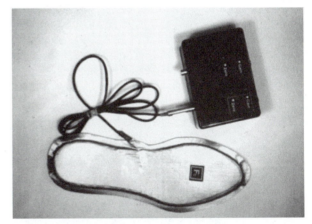

FIGURE 7.23 Force insoles to record vertical forces while worn in shoes constructed at Moss Rehabilitation Center. A videotape is available from Brown & Benchmark.

Tools for Assessment, Improvement, and Prediction of Movement   **147**

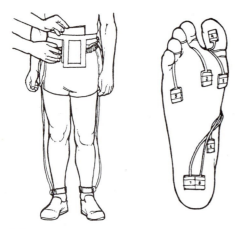

FIGURE 7.24 Electrodynography.

It is a diagnostic tool to identify function and dysfunction of the feet. The EDG force sensors are placed on the plantar surfaces of the feet at six locations (Figure 7.24). The sensors must be validated with respect to reliability and carefully calibrated.

Multiple Force Transducers in Plates

A series of thousands of transducers in one platform has been developed to record minute changes in pressure on the foot. Needless to say, this highly sophisticated technology is expensive and requires complex software development and research know-how. Recently other systems have become available at more reasonable prices. (See Figure 7.25.) Pictorial representation of data from such sophisticated technology may become commonplace in the future and be used for clinical assessments.

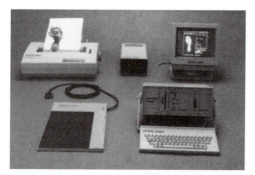

a

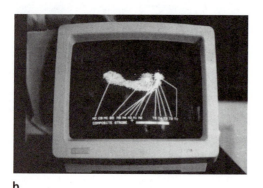

b   c

FIGURE 7.25 Other multisensory devices to record pressures throughout the surface area of weight bearing include the following: (a) EMED-System (Courtesy of Novel gmbh, Germany); (b) Atlantis Scientific Corp. Indianapolis; (c) Footprint. (Courtesy of Pennsylvania State University, The Center for Locomotion Studies.)

Summary of Force Recording Instrumentation

The direct analysis of forces is not today widespread; it remains in the laboratory since it is not practical in natural settings of human movement. There is, however, a need to know the nature of forces that occur during—and actually producing—a movement, especially their implications for strength training and for general safety. In addition, force-time histories (continuous force recordings with respect to time) are an important tool for differing between mechanical and anatomic factors of performance. For example, Figure 7.26 consists of incorrect and correct application of force during two vertical jumps. Incorrect application of force, however, produces greater velocity and a higher jump than that of a mechanically correct jump. Why? The reason is simple and relates to the proportion of a muscle mass and body mass. The performer in Figure 7.26a did not have a muscle strength–body mass ratio high enough to produce an adequate impulse (product of force and time of application of that force). Consequently, the velocity of projection was lower than that of the person weighing half as much, with almost the same amount of muscle strength. This is only one example of the many ways in which dynamography can be used to help the human movement analyst to better understand a performance and interpret the movement.

Accelerometry

The use of accelerometers, devices to measure acceleration, is an indirect measurement of force. Multiplying the mass that is accelerated by the acceleration value yields the force produced or experienced by the mass. Accelerometers can be attached to the human body segments or to tools used, but placement and charting of the position of these accelerometers is crucial to the interpretation of data. An accelerometer can be placed in a fencing foil guard. Then, impact recordings can be

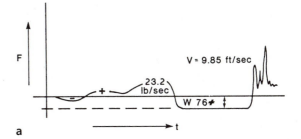

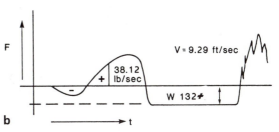

FIGURE 7.26 Force platform recordings of two persons performing the vertical jump. (a) Unskilled, but lighter weight jumper produces greater effective impulse (as evidenced by greater velocity of projection) than skilled overweight jumper (b).

made as a result of the foil striking flesh over muscles and flesh over bone. The muscle impact site recording is shown in Figure 7.27.

Modeling and Simulation

Researchers have combined mathematic modeling of the anatomical characteristics of a living body with simulation techniques for the purpose of predicting performance achievements and developing new performance techniques. Expertise in mathematics, anatomy, physics, and computers is required to fully exploit these theoretical tools. Figure 7.28 shows examples of simulations. (Others appear in chapters on specific sports.) Note how the figures have been graphed as geometric objects to depict volume and mass. The three-dimensionality is also readily apparent.

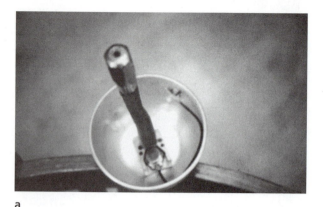

a

FIGURE 7.27 (a) Accelerometer placed in guard of fencing foil to measure G forces; (b) Recording of impact on pectoralis major muscle.

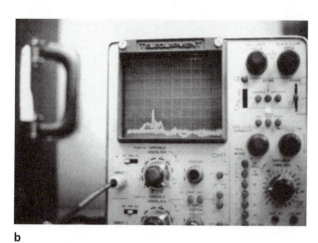

b

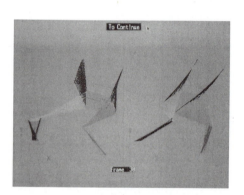

a

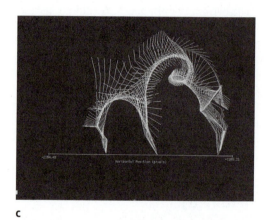

c

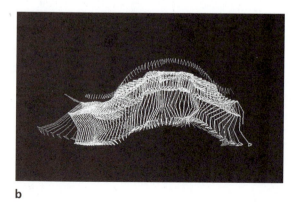

b

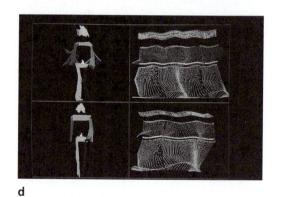

d

FIGURE 7.28 Computer-generated simulations of movement.
(a Courtesy of Josef Loczi, University of Illinois at U-C; b, c, d. Reprinted with permission of Peak Performance Technologies, Inc., Englewood, CO.)

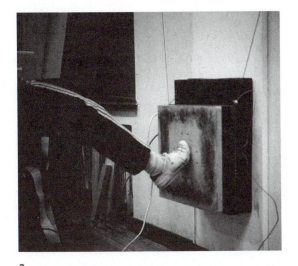

a

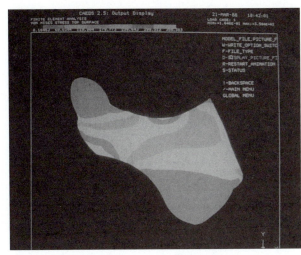

c

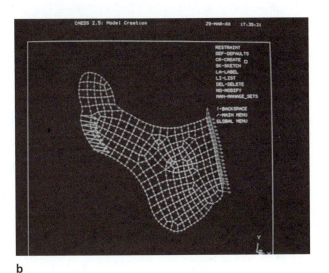

b

FIGURE 7.29 Models constructed using the computer-aided engineering design programs. Karate kick against force platform. (Courtesy of Josef Loczi, University of Illinois at U-C.)

Experimental data collected with the tools of cinematography, videography, dynamography, electrogoniometry, electromyography, and accelerometry are the foundation of the development of the model. Researchers enter the values for relevant parameters and their boundaries (possible ranges) into a computer. Algorithms of motion (equations for calculations) are used in the simulation, in which the movement can be varied with respect to speed, timing, ROM, etc. The movement pattern can then be simulated with the changes in variables to determine if performance is enhanced or if safe limits are exceeded.

Commercially available software packages perform simulations and derive the biomechanically optimized mode. In addition, CAD/CAM, CAEDS, and other commercially available computer-aided design programs perform stress analysis. An illustration of model images is shown in Figure 7.29.

General Guidelines for Use of Tools

It is important that students and researchers of human movement select the tools necessary to solve their questions. In many instances, less-sophisticated tools will be adequate for deriving the answers. Analysis is paralysis if instrumentation is an "overkill." If, however, more sophisticated equipment is required, there are several choices:

1. Purchase more sophisticated tools.
2. Rent tools.
3. Rent investigators with their tools.
4. Become a part of someone else's data bank or research network and let them collect the data for you to analyze.
5. Read the literature and conduct your own research on another question.

■ The sophistication of instrumentation is rapidly improving, but old instruments will always have value for some research studies.

References

Adrian, M. 1973. Cinematographic, electromyographic, and electrogoniometric techniques for analyzing human movements. In *Exercise and sport sciences reviews,* vol. 1, ed. J. H. Wilmore. New York: Academic Press.

Amar, J. 1972. *The human motor.* New York: Irvington Publishers.

Aristotle. 1945. Parts of animals, movements of animals, and progression of animals. Cambridge, MA: Harvard University Press.

Atwater, A. E. 1973. Cinematographic analyses of human movement. In *Exercise and sports sciences reviews,* vol. 1, ed. J. H. Wilmore. New York: Academic Press, pp. 217–58.

Basmajian, J. V. 1973. Electromyographic analyses of basic movement patterns. In *Exercise and sports sciences reviews,* vol. 1, ed. J. H. Wilmore. New York: Academic Press.

Basmajian, J. V. 1979. *Muscles alive: Their function revealed by electromyography,* 4th ed. Baltimore: Williams & Wilkins.

Carlsoo, S. 1972. *How man moves: Kinesiological studies and methods.* London: William Heinemann Ltd.

Chaffin, D. B., and Andersson, G. 1984. Bioinstrumentation for occupational biomechanics. In *Occupational Biomechanics.* New York: John Wiley.

Dainty, D. A., and Norman, R. W. 1987. *Standardizing biomechanical testing in sport.* Champaign, IL: Human Kinetics Publishers.

Duchenne, G. B. 1949. *Physiology of motion.* Philadelphia: Lippincott.

Edgerton H. 1987. Biomechanics instrumentation videotapes. *National Geographic,* December.

Hirt, S., Fries, E. C., and Hellebrandt, F. A. 1944. Center of gravity of the human body. *Arch. Phys. Their.* 25:280.

Hudson, J. L. 1991. The value of visual variables in biomechanical analysis. In *Proceedings of the 1990 symposium of the International Society of Biomechanics in Sports,* ed. C. Tant.

Journal of Physical Therapy. 1984. Special issue on Biomechanics Instrumentation: 64, December.

Karpovich, P. V. 1930. Swimming speed analyzed. *Sci. Am.* 142:24, March.

Kluth, M. E. 1971. The effect of starting block height on the racing dive. Ph.D. dissertation, thesis, Washington State University.

Marey, E. J. 1874. Animal medrauism: A treatise on terrestrial and aerial locomotion. New York: D. Appleton.

Miller, D. I. 1971. Modeling in biomechanics: An overview. *Med. Sci. Sports* 11:115–22.

Muybridge, E. 1955. *The human figure in motion.* New York: Dover.

Newmiller, J., Hull, M. L., and Zajac, F. E. 1988. A mechanically decoupled two force component bicycle pedal dynamometer. *J. Biomech.* 21:375–86.

Seireg, A. A. 1986. *SOMA: Engineering for the human body.* Baltimore: Williams and Wilkins.

Terauds, J., ed. 1979. *Science in biomechanics cinematography.* Del Mar, CA: Academic Publishers.

Vaughn, R. 1984. Computer simulation of human motion in sports biomechanics. In *Exercise and sport sciences reviews:* pp. 362–416.

8 Qualitative and Quantitative Assessment

Data analysis may range from general, subjective, descriptions to the most complex numerical and graphical portrayals of multitrial, multisubject, and multi-instrumental data. Movement analysts are only limited by their imagination and ingenuity in the manipulation of data.

Researchers assess human movement with the sophisticated tools described in the previous chapter or with nothing more than the human eye and brain. Assessment, therefore, may range from a rather superficial and grossly defined explanation of the movement pattern to a precise, analytically detailed numerical evaluation of each aspect of the movement. Although teaching, coaching, clinical diagnostics, and other field situations have usually relied on the eye and brain, advanced technology is becoming a common part of these situations. Highly sophisticated tools of research are now at the disposal of practitioners, and can be used after a short learning period. As discussed previously, there is an interrelationship between tool selection and data acquisition.

The desired types, precision, and amounts of data needed, not the tool available, should dictate the selection of tools. There is a continuum of analysis based on the broad categories of qualitative and quantitative analyses and contingent on the sophistication and amount of data that can be acquired, not which data are better (a value judgment). These two categories are not actually dichotomous; analyses from the qualitative to the quantitative are actually a continuum in which the one merges into the other. The *nature* of the analysis depends on the *goal* of the analysis, and, therefore, on the *problem to be solved*. (See Table 8.1.)

Qualitative Analysis

This type of analysis can be subdivided into behavioral and relative analyses. The former uses nonconcrete or abstract data (information) such as: did the person move, sit, swing a hammer, lift a sack, throw a ball underhand, push a wheelchair, or remain immobile? Such investigation consists of categorizing performances into *yes/no, successful/unsuccessful, with difficulty/without difficulty,* or similar descriptor cells. The type of movement is described in terms such as circular, three discrete actions, and cyclic in nature.

When using relative analysis, researchers compare elements such the performances of two or more individuals or an individual performance and a standardized individual performance. For example, was the performance faster or slower, was it performed at an angle to the vertical, or did it require a movement greater than 90° of flexion? Relative qualitative analysis consists of nonprecise quantification of movement performance.

TABLE 8.1 Analysis descriptors of dance movements based on three systems of analysis: Laban's effort/shape analysis, Hunt's movement behavior analysis, and quantitative analysis. Descriptors can be changed to relate to any type or portion of a movement pattern.

Descriptor	Laban/Qualitative	Hunt/Relative Qualitative	Precise Statements/Quantitative
Time	Irregular	Slow	.2 second
Personal space	Forward	Shoulder to knee	2 meters
Environmental space	Curved	Large	2 m. radius
Force	Exists in legs	Strong tension	80% max. Isometric
Postural/gestural	Stately	Hands more staccato than legs	Hand flex. 20°, .1 second

Quantitative Analysis

The more sophisticated type of analysis is quantitative. It requires the researcher to measure factors of the movement and ascribe numerical values to these factors. For temporal factors, the analysis might include the duration (in seconds) of the preparation phase of the movement, the time difference between one preparation phase of the movement and another phase, or the time difference between one body part beginning to move and another body part ceasing to move. For spatial factors, the analysis might include the direction of the movement, the angle of the forearm with respect to the ground or the hand (in degrees or radians), or the length of the step taken by a softball pitcher (in meters). The typical numerical quantities obtained with optical tools are displacement, velocity, and acceleration. Typical numerical quantities obtained with dynamographic techniques include force, impulse, work, energy, and power. Typical numerical accelerometer data are accelerations or G forces. Numerical values from EMG may be in electrical units such as millivolts or percentages of a criterion. Angular displacement data are obtained with electrogoniometry, with angular velocity and acceleration derived mathematically or electronically. Precise changes, improvements, or dysfunction can be assessed using quantitative data. It is easier to make statistical comparisons with other research data with quantitative data than qualitative data.

Naked-Eye Observational Procedures

Through years of trial and error, the trained teacher or observer of movement learns to recognize many (but not all) skilled and unskilled movement habits. Some habits are sensed; some are recognized. However, only the keenest analyst is able to recognize what a performer does or should do to correct faulty movement or encourage certain movement tendencies for optimum performance. It is almost impossible, without cinematographic or videographic records, to accurately view with the naked eye the distal ends of the limbs in a fast action. Both the starting and terminal positions are seen, but the propulsive phase is almost always a blur. Yet after an observer has had years of practice, some educated guesses are reasonably accurate; these guesses are certainly enhanced by biomechanic knowledge of starting and terminal positions, as well as performance outcome.

To be consistent and reliable both in observing performers learning motor skills and in evaluating movement for practical, diagnostic, clinical, or research purposes (viewed either in life or on film), a researcher must adopt a definite observational plan.

Observational Plan

The plan might include the following steps:

1. View multiple times.
2. View from multiple perspectives (planes).
3. Focus on parts, then whole, then parts.
4. Form a visual-mental image of the performance.
5. Use a checklist. Either construct your own or use one like the one in Table 8.2.

TABLE 8.2   Checklist to qualitatively assess walking. Check the phrases that apply to the evaluated walking pattern.

_____   Head vertically aligned
_____   Head inclined forward (flexion)
_____   Head inclined backward (extension)
_____   Head tilted to side (from front view)

_____   Trunk vertically aligned
_____   Kyphosis
_____   Lordosis
_____   Trunk flexion
_____   Scoliosis (from front view)

_____   Arm swing in opposition to legs
_____   Arm swing less than 45°
_____   Arm swing greater than 45°
_____   Rigid arm swing
_____   Kinematic chain-type arm swing
_____   Hands held in fists
_____   Equal range of motion (ROM) for both arms

_____   Hip remains relatively at the same height (head may be viewed rather than the hip)
_____   Hip bobs up and down (head may be viewed rather than hips)

_____   Shank vertical at initial contact
_____   Shank inclined backward at initial contact
_____   Pushoff with shank vertical
_____   Pushoff with shank inclined forward
_____   Equal ROM for both legs

_____   Thigh remains below horizontal
_____   Thigh becomes horizontal
_____   ROM at knee less than 45°
_____   ROM at knee greater than 45°
_____   Foot held rigid
_____   Foot held in equinos
_____   Foot turned outward excessively
_____   Foot turned inward excessively
_____   Knock-kneed
_____   Bowlegged

_____   Initial contact with heel of foot
_____   Initial contact with flat foot
_____   Initial contact with ball of foot

_____   Weight borne on medial part of foot
_____   Weight borne on lateral part of foot
_____   Weight shifts borne effectively on foot

Using Table 8.2, observe two people and check the items that apply to each person's gait. Place yourself in an appropriate position to set the best view. The changes in angles at the hip, knee, ankle, elbow, shoulder, and knee is best observed when viewed from the side (sagittal plane). The length of step and the changing levels of the body parts also can be estimated. A head-on view is necessary in order to note such movements as toeing-in of the feet, leg alignment at impact and at takeoff, and lateral lean of the trunk.

Observation is best conducted by a whole-part-whole method: view the total body and then each of the major body parts. A videotape that describes this method and applies it to the analysis of locomotor patterns of physically handicapped persons is available from the publisher of this book.

Constructing Your Own Checklists

1. Study other checklists. Refer to specific sports chapters for checklists covering specific sports.
2. Read about the movement to determine what factors are important enough to analyze.
3. List the determinants of skilled and unskilled actions.
4. Arrange your checklist in a scale: e.g., exists or does not exist, or use a numerical/continuum ranking of some type, such as 1–5.

Note the different types of checklists in Tables 8.2, 8.3, 8.4, and 8.5. The first is an exist/not exist type and the other three are a ranking or rating type.

Some common factors that often are included in checklists are:

1. Location of center of gravity with respect to other body parts and base of support
2. The width of the base of support
3. Range of motion and path of movement of various body segments
4. Sequencing of body segment movements
5. Angle of projection of objects released or struck
6. Total perception of the movement's effectiveness, rhythm, awkwardness, etc.

Acoustical Analysis of Rhythmic Pattern of Movement

The rhythms of human beings in action are characterized by signs, motions, and sounds made by their bodies or body parts to express themselves in some manner. The word *rhythm* comes from the Latin word *rhythmus*, which was formed from the Greek word *rhéein*, which means "to flow." It also has a musical connotation because of the elements of accent, meter, time, and tempo. Consequently, the loudness of human sounds and tempo of human motions often have an orderly sequence of closely related elements called rhythm, which can be easily identified by listening with eyes closed.

MINI-LABORATORY LEARNING EXPERIENCE

Figure 8.1 identifies common patterns of walking and running with musical notations. Listen to several persons' walking and running patterns and compare their rhythms with those in Figure 8.1. Compare skilled and unskilled sports performances with the selected sports rhythms in the same figure. Can you tell the difference between skilled and unskilled movements? Study the rhythms of other patterns, such as a person walking with a limp.

Changes in acoustical patterns occur as a result of fatigue, illness, psychological stress, and other factors. Computer technology can be a valuable tool to store and compare (categorize or diagnose) patterns. Such analysis may also be valuable for teaching persons who are visually impaired.

TABLE 8.3 Rating scales for throwing mechanics.

Name _____ Sport _____ Date _____

Throwing Mechanics

Mechanics	Rating	Comments
Preparation phase		
Rear hip rotation, extension		
Rear foot ground contact, power		
Front leg plant, counterforce maintenance		
Stride length, consistency		
Weight shift—rear to front		
Spinal rotation; flexion, lateral flexion		
Sequence of joint action		
Shoulder medial rotation; extension, adduction		
Path of ball, flat arc		
Complete follow-through in direction of throw		
Direction of forces, summation		
Balance position-release and follow-through		
Potential injuries		
Medial elbow valgus		
Medial elbow stress syndrome (compression of radial head)		
Elbow olecranon process, osteochondritis		
Shoulder-long head bicep, rotator cuff		

Conditioning needs to include stretching and strengthening, an equal amount of strength, without stressing.

Rating Scale: 4-very good, 3-good, 2-fair, 1-poor

Courtesy of Lois Klatt, Human Performance Laboratory, Concordia University, River Forest, IL.

TABLE 8.4 Rating scales for running mechanics.

Name _____ Sport _____ Date _____

Running Mechanics

Mechanics	Rating	Comments
Frontal/Coronal Plane		
Foot strike (heel, mid, toe)		
Knee and hip flexion		
Knee angle approx. 170° at contact		
C/q over base of support, breaking force		
Midsupport phase—lowest c/g, knee approx. 145 (diff. approx. 25)		
Takeoff (following—highest c/g—diff. 4 inches)		
Extension of driving hip, knee, and foot		
Rear-leg kick-up		
Stride length (longer inc. speed-shorter dec. speed; consistency)		
Length ground contact relative to nonsupport phase (less–greater speed)		
Pelvis posture		
Trunk—straight line (back flat) throughout stride; body lean		
Head erect, no strain anterior/posterior		
Rhythmic leg movement (consistency)		
Arm action; elbow 90°, relaxed; arms working in opposition—balance factor		
Relaxed run; jaw easy; all body parts effortless		
Sagittal Plane (support and nonsupport phases)		
Foot plant relative to midline—foot forces—pronation to supination, heel, outside border, head of metatarsals at time of pushoff		
Ankle pronation/supination (right/left)		
Knee valgus/vanus (right/left)		
Hip inward/outward rotation, pelvis alignment		
Direction of forces		
Head and trunk/spine control, fixed position—arms and legs working independent of trunk		
Rating Scale: 4-very good, 3-good, 2-fair, 1-insufficient		

Courtesy of Lois A. Klatt, Human Performance Laboratory, Concordia University, River Forest, IL.

TABLE 8.5 Means and standard deviations for 71 variables identified in a biomechanical analysis of 16 vaulters performing successful pole vaults above 5.5 meters. These may be helpful in profiling pole vaulters, predicting performance potential, or identifying performance problems. Some variables may be more important than others; variables are interdependent. This compilation represents one of the more comprehensive biomechanical databases on a single skill.

	M	*S.D.*
Approach Run		
Second to Last Step (touchdown to touchdown)		
1. Step length	2.20	0.14 m
2. Velocity	9.43	0.34 m/s
Last Step (touchdown to touchdown)		
3. Step length	2.04	0.17 m
4. Velocity	9.57	0.52 m/s
5. Swing leg thigh angle at takeoff	64.3	6.3°
6. Trunk angle at instant of last touchdown	88.4	3.7°
7. Horizontal distance between center of gravity (CG) and toe at instant of last touchdown	59.0	8.0 cm
Plant		
(the instant when the pole strikes the back of the box)		
8. Pole angle	27.7	1.1°
9. Trunk angle	87.5	4.2°
10. Relative vertical extension of plant arm	89.0	11.2%
11. Horizontal position of takeoff foot toe relative to top hand (indicates behind hand grip)	41.0	14.0 cm
12. Horizontal position of takeoff foot toe relative to box	3.94 m	12.0 cm
13. Total time of support until plant	0.05	.02 sec
Takeoff (t = 0.00 sec)		
(the instant when the takeoff foot leaves the ground)		
14. Horizontal velocity of CG	7.57	0.36 m/s
15. Vertical velocity of CG	2.43	0.20 m/s
16. Resultant velocity of CG	7.96	0.36 m/s
17. Takeoff angle	17.8	1.5°
18. Height of CG	1.28 m	5.0 cm
19. Total mechanical energy of vaulter divided by vaulter mass	45.6	2.8 J/kg
20. Relative amount of pole bend	4.2	1.5%
21. Pole angle	29.4	1.2°
22. Trunk angle	79.0	6.1°
23. Swing leg thigh angle	65.5	11.5°
24. Relative vertical extension of plant arm	77.8	12.6%

TABLE 8.5 *(continued)*

	M	*S.D.*
25. Horizontal position of takeoff foot toe relative to top hand	16.0	9.0 cm
26. Duration of pole support	0.07	.02 sec
27. Duration of takeoff foot contact	0.12	.01 sec

Swing (t = 0.00–0.32 sec)
(from takeoff until the distance from the CG to the box is a minimum)

	M	*S.D.*
28. Minimum distance between CG and box	2.62 m	10.0 cm
29. Horizontal displacement of CG during swing	2.14 m	18.0 cm
30. Vertical displacement of CG during swing	0.82 m	7.0 cm
31. Duration of swing	0.37	.03 sec

Rockback (t = 0.32–0.79 sec)
(from end of swing until hips are above lower hand)

	M	*S.D.*
32. Maximum relative amount of pole bend	30.6	2.4%
33. Minimum effective pole length	3.40 m	13.0 cm
34. Angle of effective pole at instant of maximum pole bend	61.1	2.3°
35. Time of maximum pole bend	0.48	.04 sec
36. Minimum moment of inertia of vaulter divided by vaulter mass	810.0	150.0 g-cm^2/g
37. Time of this minimum	0.60	.06 sec
38. Horizontal displacement of CG during rockback	1.01 m	9.0 cm
39. Vertical displacement of CG during rockback	1.46 m	24.0 cm
40. Duration of rockback	.043	.05 sec

Extension, Pull and Turn (t = 0.79–1.34 sec)
(from end of rockback until top hand release)

	M	*S.D.*
41. Total backward rotation of body from plant	128.9	10.3°
42. Time when backward rotation ends	0.78	.06 sec
43. Maximum pole extension velocity	4.21	0.63 m/s
44. Angle of effective pole at this instant	83.9	2.3°
45. Time of maximum pole extension velocity	0.84	.06 sec
46. Maximum vertical velocity of CG	5.04	0.38 m/s
47. Angle of effective pole at this instant	85.9	2.0°
48. Trunk angle at this instant	69.1	9.9°
49. Distance between CG and pole at this instant (indicates CG behind pole)	11.0	4.0 cm
50. Time of maximum vertical velocity of CG	0.91	.06 sec
51. Pole angle at instant of pole straightening	87.4	2.5°
52. Trunk angle at instant of pole straightening	61.5	10.4°
53. Time of pole straightening	1.09	.11 sec

TABLE 8.5 *(continued)*

	M	*S.D.*
54. Time of lower hand release	1.09	.06 sec
55. Horizontal displacement during extension, pull, and turn	.81 m	19.0 cm
56. Vertical displacement during extension, pull, and turn	2.02 m	25.0 cm
57. Duration of extension, pull, and turn	0.53	.10 sec
Upper Hand Release (t = 1.34 sec)		
(the instant when the upper hand releases its grip from the pole)		
58. Pole angle	89.5	2.7°
59. Trunk angle	46.5	8.2°
60. Distance between CG and pole (indicates CG behind pole)	46.0	14.0 cm
61. Height of CG	5.49 m	17.0 cm
62. Height of CG above top hand	0.87 m	15.0 cm
63. Horizontal velocity of CG	1.49	0.51 m/s
64. Vertical velocity of CG	1.78	0.81 m/s
65. Work done from plant to release divided by vaulter mass	7.2	4.8 J/kg
66. Excess kinetic energy divided by vaulter mass	2.65	1.94 J/kg
67. Time of upper hand release	1.32	.10 sec
Flight and Clearance		
68. Maximum height of CG	5.70	12.0 cm
69. Horizontal position of CG at maximum height	69.0	17.0 cm
70. Difference between crossbar height and maximum CG height	10.0	9.0 cm
71. Time of maximum CG height	1.51	.05 sec

Courtesy of Peter McGinnis.

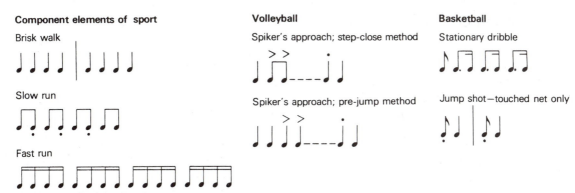

FIGURE 8.1 Rhythmic analysis of walk, run, and skills of selected sports. **Ask a person with musical notation skills to help you beat the rhythms. Next try the movement skills to these rhythms. Does your natural rhythm fit these rhythms?**

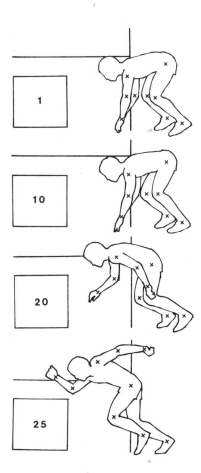

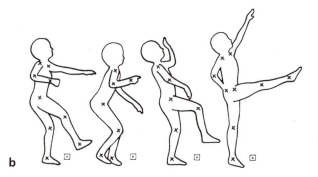

FIGURE 8.2 Two examples of contourograms relative to an inanimate object traced from video images. (a) These were traced on separate transparencies using a felt pen and then retraced on one page. The position of the person is relative to the square. The frame number is in the square. (b) This set was traced directly using the reflection of the video image on a semitransparent digitizing pad (Hi-Pad model 1405).

Videographic and Cinematographic Analyses

Because of high costs, videography has replaced cinematography as a biomechanics tool in the analysis of human movement, except in the area of sports movements. Even in the sports world, however, videography is common, partly because its quality and sophistication have improved considerably. Because of the similarity of the two systems, the analysis methods described are applicable to both.

Qualitative Procedures

There are two types of videographic **qualitative** analyses: observation and tracings. The observation method is the same as detailed in the previous section, Naked-Eye Observational Procedures. Use these procedures as you repeatedly view the video tape or movie film, or look at photographs or stroboscopic photos. Use your checklists to provide a record of your observations.

Tracings are of three types (combinations of these types are common):

1. **Contourograms:** These are whole-body tracings of the performer, similar to a silhouette, but some markings, such as waist, paint, or tape marking at knee, etc., may be drawn.
2. **Point plots:** These are dots of a specific anatomical or object site, such as the knee axis or the center of a ball.
3. **Line segments (stick figures):** These are straight lines drawn between joints and represent body segments, such as a thigh, forearm, etc.

Examples of these types are shown in Figures 8.2, 8.3, and 8.4.

R = RELEASE
C = CONTACT

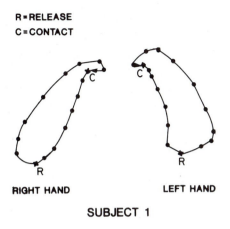

RIGHT HAND   LEFT HAND

SUBJECT 1

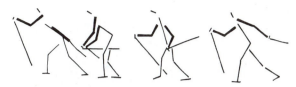

FIGURE 8.4 Example of line-segment tracings of the upper extremities during cross-country skiing. Is it easier to "see the motion" than with the point plots? **What information can you measure?**

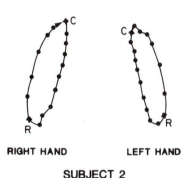

RIGHT HAND   LEFT HAND

SUBJECT 2

FIGURE 8.3 Example of point plots traced from video images. **What information can you glean from these that you cannot from Figure 8.2?**

How to Make a Video Tracing. Affix a clear plastic sheet (transparency) to the television monitor and trace with a felt-tip pen or crayon. Use different colors to depict different frames or different body points or segments. Make movie film tracings by projecting the film onto a smooth-textured white wall or onto a clear glass plate with a reflective mirror. Trace the selected images on white paper or graph paper. (See Figure 8.5.) Tracings, particularly the contourograms, can depict important positions, such as maximum flexion of a limb, most erect position of the trunk, or

takeoff or landing during running. In such instances, however, the time interval between successive tracings will vary depending on the selection. To show real-time patterns, use a constant time interval. For example, trace every image or every third image. To show real-space patterns, do not move the tracing paper from its affixed position; you might also partially or completely superimpose the images on each other. The viewer can readily identify the changes in speed of movement by the amount of superimposition from one tracing to the next. If you wish to avoid this overlapping of tracings, move the paper or place each tracing on a separate sheet of paper. Take care to trace an inanimate object with the performer in the same relationship to this object in each tracing. It will then be possible to make relative and quantitative analyses of these tracings, rather than only pattern descriptions.

Quantitative Analysis

Video and movie film **quantitative** analysis is usually conducted with computerized digitization techniques. Another technique that offers the students a more personal way of learning about movement is to manually measure positions and displacements from the contourogram, point plot, and line-segment tracings. Calculations of other kinematic variables can then be made. By far the most convenient and fastest technique for quantitatively analyzing movement is digitization. There are two forms of digitizing: operator-performed and automated. Two examples of the operator-performed digitizing systems for movie film are shown in Figure 8.5. Operator-performed digitizing of video images may be done with

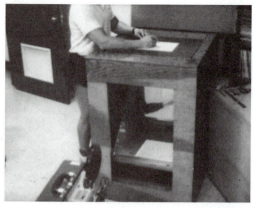

a

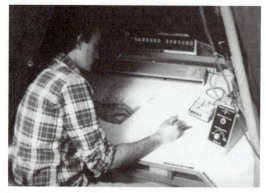

b

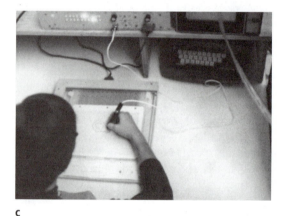

c

FIGURE 8.5 Film analysis systems. (*a*) Using a 16mm L & W projector and mirror box to trace and measure 16mm file images. (*b*) Using a Vanguard 16mm projector head and Numonics acoustic digitizing tablet interfaced with an Apple computer and University of Illinois mainframe computer to obtain spatial coordinates. (*c*) Using a Hi-Pad digitizing tablet interfaced with an IBM computer to digitize film tracings or project the 16mm film to tablet and digitize directly.

video prints (using a video printer) and then placing the print on a digitizing tablet. See Figure 8.6*a* for examples of video prints. The most common digitizing method is a video image-grabbing circuit board connected to a computer. See Figure 8.6*b* for one example.

The Digitizing Process.   No matter which operator-performed system is used, the image is displayed on the digitizing tablet or television monitor. A cursor of some type (pen, glass piece with cross, or computer mouse/cursor) is used to locate the point of interest. When the cursor coincides with the point of interest, a keystroke or other means is used to input the coordinates (*x* and *y* position in space) of the point to the computer. The computer stores all points of each image as position data, and appropriate software smooths the data (manipulates

data to eliminate random errors due to the digitizing process) and calculates displacements, velocities, and accelerations. In addition, by inputting inertial data (mass and moments of inertia) the researcher calculates forces and determines path of center of gravity of the body and its segments. An example of nineteen digitized points and their *x,y* coordinates is shown in Figure 8.7.

Automated "Video" Analysis

We will not explain the automated digitizing systems further because the computerized electro-optical system does all the analyzing. Researchers merely follow the operating instructions, such as "Digitize first 2 frames." The researcher determines what calculations, graphs, and plots are desired.

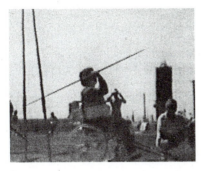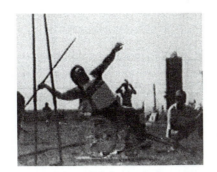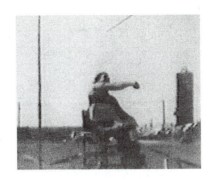

a

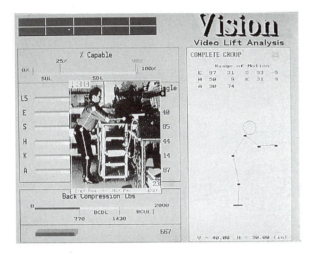

b

FIGURE 8.6 Video images available for digitizing: (*a*) Video image prints of javelin throwing from a wheelchair. These images can be placed on a digitizing tablet for digitizing. (*b*) Video image captured via videotape and video-computer circuit board. (*b*. Courtesy of William DeVries, Vice-President, Promatek Medical Systems, Inc. Vision 3000 video analysis systems.)

■ Researchers are creating their own software. They are also guiding the commercial video systems companies to produce relevent software.

Measurement of Variables. When digitizing, only the position of a point is recorded (measured). Using the computer, the analyst derives all other kinematic and kinetic variables from these position data. **Displacement** is derived directly from position and **velocity** is derived from displacement with respect to time. Acceleration is derived from velocity with respect to time. Kinetic data are derived by inputting known inertial data into the computer.

Linear Displacement. It is important to realize that displacements on film or video are considerably smaller than true size. They must be converted to life size.

Consequently, you must adjust all measurements taken from the picture; use an object of known length in the picture for reference. By comparing the actual size and the projected size, you can determine a multiplier to apply to distances measured on film.

Example 1 Assume that a 1-m measuring stick measures 10 cm (0.1 m) on the screen or tablet. It should be evident that 1 cm on the screen is equal to 10 cm in life. The actual computation of the multiplier is:

$$x \text{ cm on screen} = y \text{ cm in life}$$
$$1 \text{ cm on screen} = y \text{ cm in life}/x$$

or

$$\text{Multiplier} = \text{life size/projected size} = 100 \text{ cm}/10 \text{ cm} = 10$$

Qualitative and Quantitative Assessment   **165**

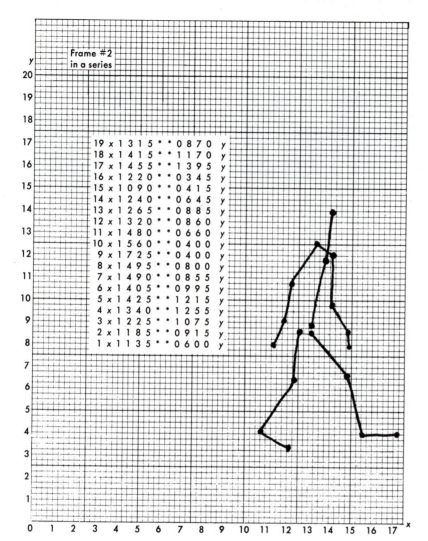

FIGURE 8.7 The x- and y-coordinate system used to analyze movement of a soccer player. Graph paper can be used and measurements made without high-tech instrumentation. Any of the more sophisticated systems in Figure 8.8 can also be used.

Example 2 To compare English measurements, assume that a yardstick measures 3.6 inches on the screen. It should be evident that 1 inch on the screen is equal to 10 inches in life. The actual computation of the multiplier is:

$$x \text{ inches on screen} = y \text{ inches in life}$$

$$1 \text{ inch on screen} = y \text{ inches in life}/x$$

$$\text{Multiplier} = \text{life size/projected size}$$

$$= 36 \text{ inches}/3.60 \text{ inches} = 10$$

Thus, a measurement taken from the film in centimeters or inches must be multiplied by 10 to convert the distance to life-size units of centimeters or inches. (If life-size units in feet are desired, the multiplier is equal to 0.83 to convert screen measurements to feet.)

If a grid screen is provided in the film background, then you can obtain displacement values by simply counting the number of grid lines crossed between frames. For example, assume that you are using grid lines equal to 10 cm in life, and a body segment under study has moved through 16 grid lines. The displacement is equal to 10×16, or 160 cm (1.6 m). To use English measurements, assume that you are using grid lines equal to 4 inches in life, and a body segment under study has moved through 16 grid lines. The displacement is equal to 4×16, or 64 inches (5.3 feet). The use of a grid screen will help reduce the possibility of perspective error.

Angular Displacement. No conversion to life size is necessary in determining angular displacement. But you must be careful that the measurement of the angle is truly within the viewing plane if only one planar view has been obtained. An angle is an angle! Or is it? There are three common ways to measure an angle: anatomical, spatial, and movement.

The anatomical angle is the angle formed by the two body segments, such as the angle at the knee. The anatomical angle may also be termed the *joint angle* or the *inter-body segment relationship angle.*

The spatial angle is also known as the **angle of inclination** or the *body-segment angle* with respect to the vertical or the horizontal. In this case, the segment orientation in space is the variable of interest, not the segment relative to the anatomy.

The movement angle is an abstract commonly used in physical therapy. The angle formed by the starting angle at a joint and the ending angle is measured. This angle is the complement of the anatomical angle.

Other methods of identifying angles have been used and will be created in the future. Researchers have an interest in identifying a system in which angles are referred to as absolute and relative angles. Since all angles are relative to some reference frame, usually space or anatomy, an absolute angle does not exist. The trend, however, is to refer to the anatomical angle as a relative angle and to the spatial angle as an absolute angle.

Time. Ordinary video cameras operate at 30 images per second; the time interval between frames is 1/30th sec. or 0.033 sec. Video players, however, have been interfaced with computer circuit boards that "grab each of the two fields" of an image, creating a 60-frame-per-second camera (higher rates also are possible with direct computer input). Common high-speed movie cameras operate between 60 and 500 frames per second. If a camera operates at 120 frames per second, the time interval between frames will be 1/120th sec. or 0.0083 sec. The time interval is either inputted by the digitizer or electronically selected by the computer in the automated systems.

Velocity. Calculate velocity as follows: displacement/time interval during which this displacement occurs, or

$$V = \frac{\Delta d}{\Delta t}$$

It must be understood, however, that all velocities will be averages of what actually occurs during the time interval. The smaller the time interval, the nearer to instantaneous velocity will be the value. Velocities derived from ordinary video cameras will almost always underestimate the maximum velocity attained during a movement. Whenever velocity is reported for time intervals greater than the smallest time interval recorded during the data collection, the velocity should be identified as average velocity. This concept is true for angular as well as linear velocities.

Acceleration. Calculate acceleration as follows:

velocity change/time change, or

$$a = \frac{\Delta V}{\Delta t}$$

Again the same cautions we described for working with velocity are applicable to acceleration. Another concern with acceleration is the difficulty in obtaining valid data. Since errors in digitizing the position data are magnified when deriving displacement data, and further magnified when deriving velocity data, errors can be very large when deriving acceleration data.

3-D Analysis. Although some researchers have calculated and graphed 3-D displacement, velocity, and acceleration without the aid of computer software programs, 3-D analysis is almost impossible without a total

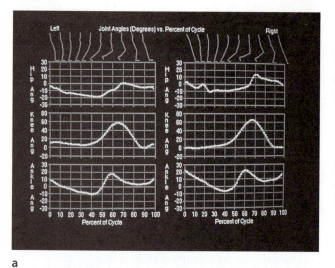

a

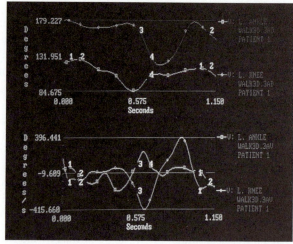

b

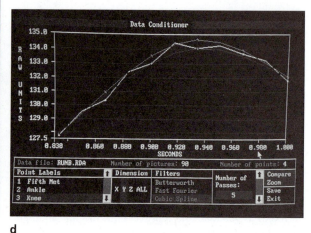

c

d

FIGURE 8.8 Graphics generated via computerized video analysis systems.

(a, Courtesy of Motion Analysis Corp. Santa Rosa, CA; b, c, d, Courtesy of Peak Performance Technologies, Inc., Englewood, CO.)

software digitization system. Automated systems are faster and more precise. In fact, earlier 3-D analyses were actually two planar analyses with only one point, such as the flight of a ball, in true 3-D.

Display of Calculated Data. Graphic portrayals of two-dimensional displacement, velocity, and acceleration with respect to time are shown in Figure 8.8. Other ways of displaying these kinematic data graphically portray two variables with time as the third dimension: angle-angle, angle-velocity (phase portrait), velocity-velocity, and angle-acceleration. An angle-angle plot is shown in Figure 8.9.

Displacement of 3-D data can be graphically depicted as two planes of a stick figure series. (See Figure 8.10).

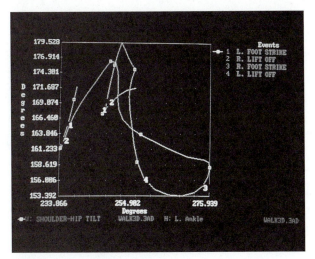

FIGURE 8.9 Angle-angle plots.
(Reprinted with permission from Peak Performance Technologies, Inc., Englewood, CO.)

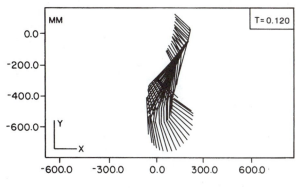

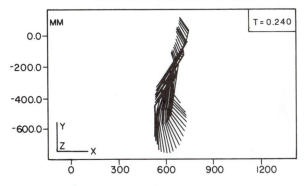

FIGURE 8.10 Computer-generated line segments and angles from the Selspot system. Bicycling with cleats. The computer software has a subroutine to orthogonally rotate the output to any amount required. Some rotations are of greater value for the pattern than for the numerical values.

Until human beings can visualize the 3-D vectors (see Figure 8.11), the technology will continue to be more advanced than the application warrants.

Basic Dynamographic Analysis

Forces recorded with spring scales, cable tensiometers, force platforms, or other displays of force, without respect to time, are expressed as peak forces. If force-time patterns are recorded, as in Figure 8.12, analyses may be a simple qualitative comparison of patterns (i.e., pattern recognition, usually an individual pattern compared to a criterion pattern). If quantitative analyses are made, these may be quite complete and include measurement of the total impulse (area under the curve), the maximum and minimum forces for each curvature, forces at specific instances in time (as determined by other experimental data), peak forces, duration of total force production, duration of different parts of the force-time pattern, and time at which specific forces occur. In addition, the rise-time (slope of the curve) of force production can be measured.

Another way to analyze forces is to construct a force-force diagram as shown in Figure 8.13. This allows researchers to visualize a 3-D perspective.

Accelerometric Analysis

If the application of force is of short duration, such as during impacts experienced in judo throw landings, jumping landings, and contact of a ball with a bat, an accelerometer may be the best transducer to use. The total peak forces expressed in G forces, as well as the slope of

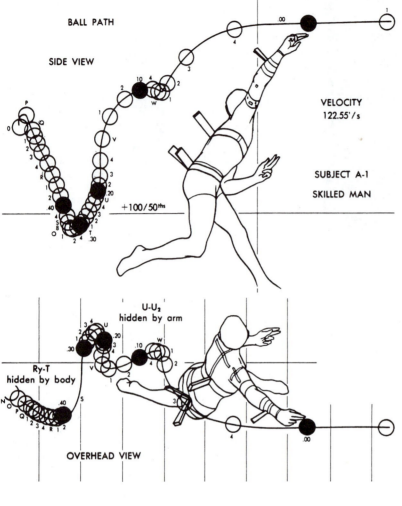

BALL PATH

SIDE VIEW

VELOCITY
122.55'/s

SUBJECT A-1

SKILLED MAN

+100/50ths

U-U₂
hidden by arm

Ry-T
hidden by body

OVERHEAD VIEW

FIGURE 8.11 Tracings from film to show path of ball. Circles represent equal time intervals. Note the fins to track rotations of body segments. Fins are also useful devices when only one camera can be used.

(From Atwater, A. E. 1970. Movement characteristics of the overarm throw, Ph.D. dissertation, University of Wisconsin.)

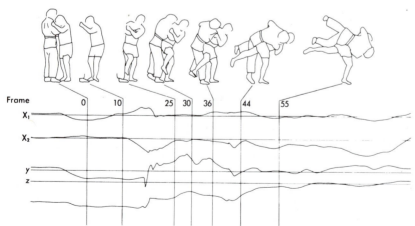

Frame 0   10   25 30 36   44   55

X₁

X₂

y

z

a

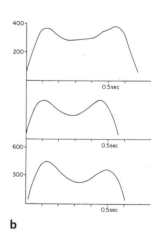

b

FIGURE 8.12 Contourogram and three-dimensional force-time histories of judo throw (a), and walking at different speeds (b). Note how much easier it is to evaluate the kinetics of a cyclic and mostly planar movement than that of a three-dimensional movement, such as a judo throw.

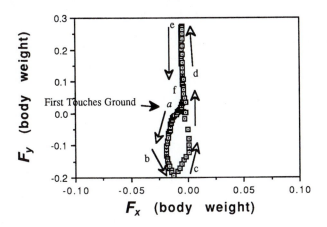

* a-b-c-d-e-f represent foot from heel touching ground till toe-off

a

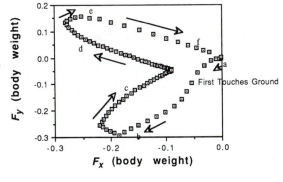

a-b-c-d-e-f represent foot from heel touching ground till toe-off

b

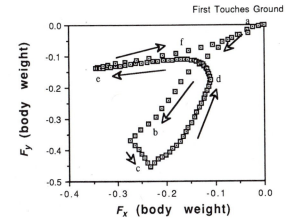

* a-b-c-d-e-f represent foot from heel touching ground till toe-off

c

FIGURE 8.13 Force-force diagrams. (*a*) Walking forward; (*b*) turning at 45° angle to right; (*c*) turning 90° to right.
(Courtesy of Dali Xu. 1984. Masters thesis. University of Illinois of U-C.)

the curve, are common variables to analyze. Based on these variables, researchers at Wayne State University developed a Severity Index as a criterion for potential head injury assessment. Recordings from an accelerometer appear in Figure 8.14.

Electrogoniometric Analysis

Amplitude and duration of angular displacements are the appropriate measurements to obtain from the **goniograms** (recordings from an elgon). Angles at key instances in time are also often measured. Average velocities with respect to selected time intervals can be calculated and accelerations estimated. This helps us

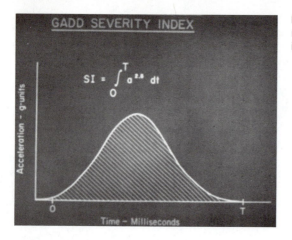

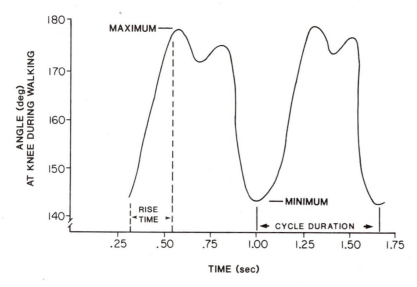

FIGURE 8.14 Measurement of impact deceleration via an accelerometer: rise time, peak G force, total impulse (area under the curve), and severity index (area relative to possible trauma to body).

FIGURE 8.15 Goniogram and analytical process. The maximum and minimum angles are determined, the rise time is measured and angular velocity calculated, and the angles at key instants in time are measured.

identify patterns of changes of angles at the joint with respect to consistency and the norm. Appropriate measurement techniques are identified in Figure 8.15.

Muscle Analysis

We can analyze the active muscles during a movement using electromyography, deductions from anatomical knowledge, and deductions from experimentally obtained kinematic data. Although none of these three methods is error-free, analysis of the electromyogram is the most objective and least error-prone. It is, however,

necessary to separate the artifact from the action potentials; Waterland and Shambes (1969) described this process quite well.

Analysis of the Electromyogram. The basic analysis determines whether the muscle is contracting and estimates the magnitude of contraction. We can compare two muscles, a flexor and an extensor muscle acting antagonistically to each other, by observing the electromyograms in Figure 8.16. Then we can assess relatively changes in the amplitude of the spikes of the electromyogram: none, slight, moderate, or marked.

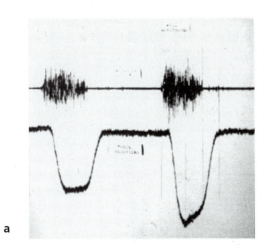

a

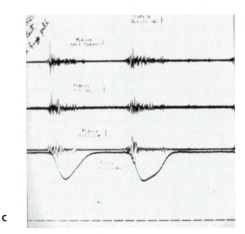

b

c

FIGURE 8.16 Is the muscle contracting or relaxing? How often is there marked moderate and slight contraction? This is the most qualitative method of analyzing electromyograms. They allow us to compare force generated (recorded from a force transducer) and muscle activity.

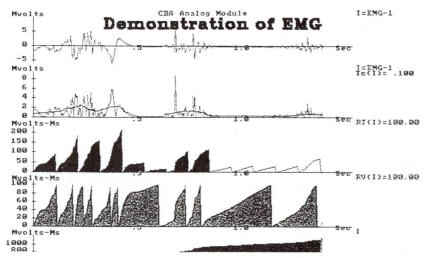

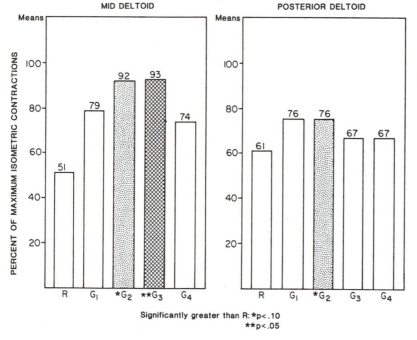

Significantly greater than R: *p<.10
**p<.05

FIGURE 8.18 Graphic portrayal of estimated muscle involvement during five styles of rope jumping. The graphs show muscle action potentials expressed in percent of maximum isometric contraction of middle and posterior heads of the deltoid muscle respectively. A gyro-style rope with long handles and long rope was used.

Rather than compare raw signals of action potentials of the muscle (EMG), most systems include an integrator so that the output will resemble the force-time curves described previously. There is a continuing summation of the action potentials when the signal is integrated, as shown in Figure 8.17. Another common analysis technique is to compare the EMG obtained during performance with the EMG representing maximum isometric contraction of that muscle. If performances require muscular contractions at low speeds, this type of analysis is appropriate. If the performance produces fast speeds, the EMG values will be greater than 100% of the criterion (maximum isometric contraction). Figure 8.18 shows data using this technique.

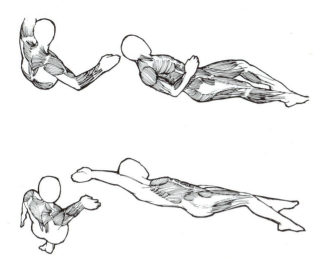

Muscle Figures

The ultimate application of the electromyogram for performance assessment is to create a muscle figure, as shown in Figures 8.19 and 8.20. Figure 8.19 was produced in the 1960s by Mihaly Nemessuri, a well-known Hungarian biomechanist. Figure 8.20 is one of a series of analyses published by the National Strength Coaches Association. This particular set of muscle figures was produced based on a combination of anatomical, cinematographic, and electromyographic interpretation of kayaking. More recently, Pelham, Burke, and Holt (1992) studied the flatwater canoe stroke using a C-I Ergometer and a canoe; they constructed a muscle profile from EMG recordings.

FIGURE 8.19 Identification of muscle involvement during different phases of swimming. **Name the muscles.**
(Reprinted with permission from Nemessuri, M. 1963. *Funktionelle Sportanotomie.* Budapest, Hungary: Akademiai Kiado.)

Composite Analysis

More and more, researchers are combining instrumentation to obtain a comprehensive analysis of a movement pattern. One of the more comprehensive approaches is to investigate movement from initiation in the motor cortex of the brain until completion of the motor act (see Figure 8.21).

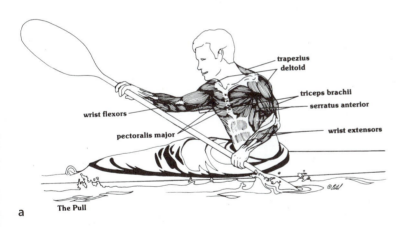

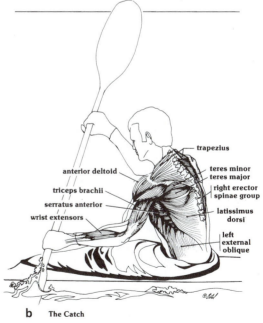

FIGURE 8.20 Identification of muscle involvement during two phases of kayaking. (Reprinted with permission from Logan, S., and Holt, L. 1986. *The Flatwater Kayak Stroke. National Strength and Conditioning Journal 7,* (5):4–11. Illustrations by M. L. Eitel.)

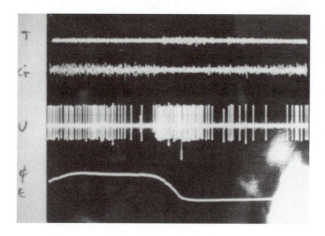

FIGURE 8.21 Multiple data recorded from EEG, electrogoniometry, dynamography, and electromyography. The sequence of onset of each event can be noted. **Try writing a description of the sequence of neuromuscular phenomena from this "picture worth a thousand words."**

References

Biomechanics Instrumentation Video Library. Dubuque, IA: Brown and Benchmark.

Computer Software Movement Analysis Learning Modules. Dubuque, IA: Brown and Benchmark.

Jorge, M., and Hull, M. L. 1986. Analysis of emg measurement during bicycle pedalling. J. Biomech. 19:683–94.

Lanshammer, H. 1985. *Gait analysis in theory and practice.* Uppsala, Sweden: Uppsala University Press.

Pelham, T. W., Burke, D. G., and Holt, L. E. 1992. The flat-water canoe stroke. *National Strength and Conditioning Association Journal* 14 (1): pp 6–8, 86–90.

Physical Therapy. 1984. December issue 4:12.

Waterland J. C., and Shambes, G. M. 1970. Biplantar center of gravity procedures. *Percept. Mot. Skills* 30:511.

Winter, Norman, and Wells, Hayes. eds. 1985. Biomechanics IX-B, section III: Measurement techniques and data processing. Champaign, IL: Human Kinetics Publishers, pp. 185–294.

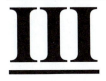

PART

III Movements Across the Entire Spectrum of Life

9 Developmental Biomechanics*

Motor development is a life-long process, starting before birth and lasting until death. Understanding the changes that occur in movement patterns during this life span is essential. This chapter presents some of these changes.

Do 2-year-olds, 20-year-olds and 90-year-olds walk, swing an axe, climb a ladder, or perform other movement patterns in the same way? Of course not. Movement patterns change during a person's life span. Some of these changes occur as a function of growth and development of the human body; others are learned through practice and education. **Developmental biomechanics** *is the study of movement patterns and how they change due to interaction between human beings and their environment.* During the early years, infancy and childhood, sequential and orderly movement patterns emerge at predictable ages. Neurological development and physical development contribute to the nature of these movement pattern changes (and acquisitions). As with other living beings, motor development of human beings has a phylogenetic basis. The acquisition of skill in performing these movement patterns, however, appears to be founded on learning, not heredity theory.

The majority of *early research concerning motor development has focused on children.* These studies have been descriptive in nature, with limited process-oriented experimentation. Since stage theory is the primary analytical model for the study of development, we will describe stages. Our emphasis will be on development of fundamental movement patterns and patterns of activities of daily living.

The second section of this chapter will focus on the aged population. There have been many questions, but few answers, about motor development of adults, especially persons over the age of seventy. Descriptive data, however, do exist; we will use them to develop theories about changing movement patterns among the aged population.

Two other sections in this chapter cover diagnosis for effective teaching and motor control changes with age. Synthesizing the information in this chapter will make you a pioneer in the acquisition of research-based knowledge in developmental biomechanics.

■ Developmental biomechanics is a continuous and lifelong process.

Motor development is one part of the study of human development. In the 1920s and '30s researchers charted the development of twins and children of psychologists. Identification of the movement patterns and *the age and order at which they appeared were reported. Qualitative descriptions of the movements composed the bulk of this research data.*

*Clinical Diagnosis—Lynda Randall
Certain Aspects of Aging—Tonya Toole

Stage-Theory Models

Stage-theory models can be classified into three types: *fundamental stages* (fc); *intratask component stages* (ic); and *kinematic continuum stages* (kc). Although these models have unique interpretations, their goals are identical. All theories include a hierarchical structure to depict progression toward maturation. Here are brief descriptions of the three theories.

Wild (1938) was the first to propose the theory of *stages of development of fundamental movement patterns* (fc). Her treatise on this topic was voluminous and became the foundation for most of the research during the next four decades. Faculty and graduates of the University of Wisconsin have been leaders in motor development with respect to children.

The most advanced stage theory (fc), modified from Wild's stages, is that of Seefeldt and Haubenstricker (1982). They proposed additional stages to more nearly equalize intervals in the progression from one stage to the next. They also used a biomechanical approach to describe each stage. Roberton and colleagues (1976, 1978, 1984) proposed that the changes in throwing, for example, must be divided into substages, that is, each component of throwing has a developmental sequence or series of stages. We propose further that the action of the legs can be charted in stages independently of the action of the throwing arm. Using this concept, there would be fewer stages defined than suggested by Seefeldt and Haubenstricker (1982).

Adrian, Toole, and Randall (1984) proposed that movement patterns in the developmental process be considered a *continuum* rather than *discrete* stages (kc). Here, too, the approach is a biomechanical one. They identify range of motion, planes of motion, and axes of motion. If the goal is maximum speed or distance, then this approach evaluates the level of maturation of the movement pattern by the amount and complexity of space used. In addition, the approach evaluates the temporal aspects and reports the sequencing and speed of the body parts. Again, maturation, the highest stage of development, refers to the fastest and the most effective timing of the body parts. Using stages as a method of defining growth and decline helps envision the whole developmental process from beginning to the end.

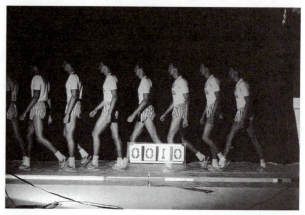

FIGURE 9.1 The walking cycle as depicted in stroboscopic images.

Walking

■ **Walking** is the undergirding ingredient of other locomotive activities.

Steindler (1955) has stated that walking "is a series of catastrophes narrowly averted." First, the body falls forward. Then the legs move under the body and prevent such an accident from occurring by establishing a new base of support with the feet. (See Figure 9.1.)

Walking is a type of reflex action. The reflexes, such as righting and stepping, displayed by the infant are the foundation on which walking is based. Reflexes are the first clues to later voluntary movement. The postural reflexes exhibited by the young child during the first months of life are evident during the standing and stepping actions induced by parents. They are the prelude to the walking action. The adult walking action is the epitome of the horizontal joint action and the synchronization of muscle action into a flowing movement. The action is beautiful to watch, but extremely complex to analyze. It is a remarkable accomplishment, considering the design of the human body, which features a high center of gravity and a small base of support.

The first true walking steps begin between the ages of 10 and 16 months. The young child between the ages of 4 and 7 years usually is thought to walk with adult characteristics. Illness and consequent confinement for a long period of time may cause the walking act to be delayed or, in an adult, to have to be relearned.

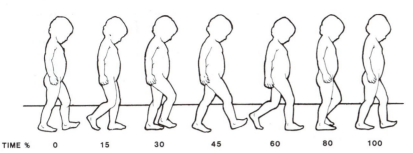

FIGURE 9.2 The walking cycle: support and swing phase and percent of total stride at seven discrete positions. (Child as subject.)

TIME %   0   15   30   45   60   80   100

Some of the phases of walking are altered in injured and permanently disabled persons. Biomechanical researchers are continually trying to develop artificial limbs that enable persons with pathologic conditions to walk as nearly normal as possible.

The bipedal position permits rapid initiation of the motion of walking. The center of gravity is easily displaced in the desired direction because (1) it resides high, at approximately the second sacral segment, over a small base of support; and (2) the greater portion of the body weight is located in the trunk, head, and shoulders, rather than in the lower extremities. This inherently unstable situation necessitates close cooperation of the neuromusculoskeletal systems in the act of walking.

That the center of gravity is located above the main joint of support adds to the instability. The human body is classified as having three effective joints and two effective segments (the lower limbs) for speed and is not considered to have the most effective leg joints and segments for balance. Also, the human body is designed for rapid initial movement in walking and running, but not for sustained speed.

Two Theories. There are two theories explaining the initiation of the step in walking. One involves the displacement of the center of gravity and activation of both the step reflex and the righting reflex. This movement is termed "a falling/catching act," as previously noted. The other theory is that the movement of the center of gravity to its highest position—which is reached when the foot rises onto the toes—activates the gastrocnemius and hamstring muscles. They contract with the pulling of the heel off the ground and, along with the gravitational action on the center of gravity, activate the step.

Phases of Walking. Two phases of walking are depicted in Figure 9.2. The stance (support) phase, composed of heel strike, foot flat, heel off, flexion at the knee, and toe off is approximately 60% of the walking cycle. The swing phase, composed of toe clearance and leg swing, is 40% of the walking cycle. These percentages are changed in the stair ascent and descent, running, leaping, and jumping aspects of motion.

The stance phase encompasses the heel strike, midstance, and push off. The swing phase includes the beginning of the acceleration of the leg as the foot is lifted from the ground and the body weight is centered over the other foot. The swinging of the non–weight-bearing leg and its deceleration in preparation for the heel strike comprise the other portions of the swing phase.

High-Energy Phase. Walking can be described as having a high- and a low-energy phase. The high-energy phase of walking occurs during the stance phase. This is explained by the fact that the descending leg is decelerated just before and at the time of the heel strike, thus preventing injury to the heel. In addition, the shock of the heel as it strikes is absorbed by the lower limb and the entire body, which requires energy. Since the shock absorption enables the body to be balanced during midstance, the energy cost is high. The leg abductors are very active during this time. Finally, the push-off portion of the stance phase initiates the forward propulsion of the body and, therefore, is high in energy requirements.

Low-Energy Phase. The low-energy phase occurs during the acceleration portion (swing phase) of the walking cycle. The hip flexors and knee extensors help keep the heel from rising too high. Dorsiflexion of the toes at

Developmental Biomechanics   **181**

TABLE 9.1 Relationship of cadence and height of person walking at various speeds. There is space for you to add personal data.

	4.02 kmph* (2.5 mph)**	4.82 kmph (3.0 mph)	5.68 kmph (3.5 mph)	6.43 kmph (4.0 mph)
Cadence steps per minute male 1.76 m tall (5'8")	100	112	122	130
Cadence steps per minute male 1.98 m tall (6'5")	92	100	108	115
Cadence steps per minute Reader				

*.067 kilometers per minute or 67 meters per minute
** .042 miles per minute or 220 feet per minute

the midpoint of the swing in preparation for the heel strike prevents the toes from striking first. The hamstring muscles also expend energy to decelerate the leg during the latter stages of the swing. Why is this the low-energy phase? The reason lies in the pendulum action of the swinging leg, which takes considerably less energy than is expended at heel strike, absorption of shock, and push off. Gravity is working in favor of the pendulum swing by pulling the leg mass down toward the ground. The momentum gained at push off helps carry the leg through the swing phase.

It has been estimated that during a portion of the swing phase, the lower leg reaches a velocity of 32.18 kmph (20 mph). In running, this becomes 64.36 to 80.45 kmph (40 or 50 mph).

The most effective walking rate is approximately 70 steps/min for most individuals, but not for all. Amar (1920) has found that at just above 190 steps/min, it is more economical, in terms of energy, to run than to walk. This is true until a speed of just under 250 steps/min is reached.

The number of steps per unit of time varies with the speed of walking and the length of the lower limbs. Data collected by Morton and Fuller (1952) are presented in Table 9.1. Note the differences between the tall man's cadence and the shorter man's cadence.

MINI-LABORATORY LEARNING EXPERIENCE

Test yourself at 100 steps per minute for a time of one minute. Determine your speed of walking: measure the distance traversed in that time and divide that distance by one minute. (Refer to Chapter 5 if necessary.) Convert your answer to mph or kmph and/or convert the speeds in Table 9.1 to feet/min or meters/min.

Can you calculate the average distance of each step? If you calculate distance per step for the two subjects (Table 9.1) and yourself, is there a relationship between body height and step length? Would another anthropometric measurement be a better indicator of predicted step length than body height? If you answered leg length, you are correct.

Anthropometric Influences

Anthropometry influences the preferred or optimum step length and cadence (step rate or frequency of steps) an individual will choose. The step length multiplied by the step rate equals speed of walking. In studying the energy cost for nineteen college women walking on a treadmill electrically driven at 3.2, 4.02, and 4.82 kmph (2, 2.5 and

3 mph), Baird (1959) found the optimum rate (ratio of the amount of work to the oxygen consumption) to be between 4.02 and 4.82 kmph (2.5 and 3.0 mph). Other researchers have hypothesized that human beings will naturally select an optimum cadence for efficient walking.

MINI-LABORATORY LEARNING EXPERIENCE

1. Observe a walk and record the sequences, similarities, and differences in the action made by different people.
2. Using slides, videotape, or film of different walking actions, project the images on a wall or digitizing surface and draw the body segments used in each motion, showing the differences.
3. Have the walkers chalk their bare feet and then execute the motion so that the imprint on the surface can be seen. Compare footprint patterns.

Determinants of Walking

Saunders, Inman, and Eberhart (1953) have discussed the following six determinants of gait (walking). These six determinants continue to be cited in research.

1. Pelvic rotation. The pelvis rotates forward with the swing leg, and the center of gravity rotates forward on each hip as the step is taken. There is a total of 8° of rotation, which reduces the drop of the center of gravity.
2. Pelvic tilt. The pelvis tilts downward during the stance phase of one leg, which tends to shorten the distance from the hip to the ground and keeps the center of gravity from rising too much.
3. Flexion at the knee. Remember that as the heel strike occurs during midstance, the knee is at full extension. When the foot is flat, flexion begins at the knee (5–15°). Then there is extension at the knee and the flexion again at push off. The purpose of this flexing and extending is to prevent the center of gravity from rising unduly.

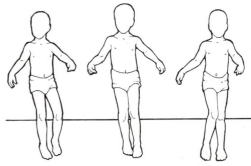

FIGURE 9.3 Walking as viewed from the frontal plane. (Note the changes in shoulder and hip with respect to the horizontal and the adduction/abduction movements of the legs.) This child has cerebral palsy.

4. Foot and ankle motion. The foot and ankle help take up shock and smooth out the path of the center of gravity at heel strike. The foot is in dorsiflexion at heel strike, and as the heel-off and toe-off phases occur, the leg flexes, smoothing out the path of the center of gravity. The foot, ankle, and knee work together as a damper at heel strike.
5. Knee motion. There are two separate actions at the knee during walking. As the ankle rises during the heel-off and toe-off phases, there is flexion at the knee. The flexion at the knee serves as a shock absorber and reduces the degree to which the center of gravity rises.
6. Lateral movement of the pelvis. During walking, the lateral movement of the pelvis is 4.45 cm (1.75 in.) at each step. The femurs are adducted and the tibias are in slight valgus, enabling the body weight to be transferred downward to a narrow base without too much lateral motion (5 cm [2 in.]). (See Figures 9.1 and 9.3.)

If walking starts from a stationary position, the first joint action to occur is flexion at the ankle. The reason is that there is a decreasing amount of tension exerted by the ankle extensors in the standing position when the center of gravity is in front of the ankle joint. When walking is initiated, the ankle extensors permit the center of gravity to move beyond the forward limit that is habitual in standing. The nervous system does not initiate a

Developmental Biomechanics   **183**

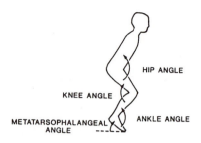

HIP ANGLE

KNEE ANGLE

METATARSOPHALANGEAL ANGLE

ANKLE ANGLE

FIGURE 9.4 Joint actions during foot contact phase in walk of college woman. Time in seconds is shown at bottom: heel strike occurs at zero time, foot flat is at 0.15 sec, rear foot lift is at 0.50 sec, and toe lift is at 0.75 sec. Angles between body segments are shown in degrees at left. Downward slope of lines indicates flexion, and upward slope indicates extension.

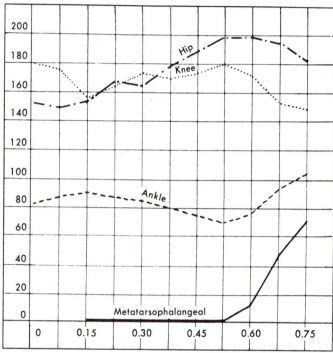

correction because one foot will be moved forward to receive the body weight. As the forward-moving foot is placed on the walking surface, the momentum of the moving body and the push from the rear foot carry the center of gravity over the new support. As each new foot contact is made, the momentum of the body is conserved by adjustments at the joints.

Joint Actions

Joint Actions of Lower Limbs. Joint actions of the lower limbs include those of the supporting limb and the swinging limb.

Joint Actions of Supporting Limb. Movements at the hip, knee, ankle, and metatarsophalangeal joints from the time the heel makes contact with the walking surface until the toes leave that surface are shown in Figure 9.4. A graph such as this one presents detailed and exact information that, if described verbally, would require many times the space taken by the graph. Here we can see the direction of each change in angle at the joint (joint action), its degree in a given time, and the relationship between actions. It is important to learn to interpret such graphs and to visualize the joint actions and body positions shown at each time interval. In the illustration, notice that the heel makes contact at 0 sec in time; then, for the first 0.15 sec, the ankle joint change is an increasing one (plantar flexion), bringing the entire foot in contact with the walking surface. From this point, all joint actions will be reversed muscle actions: a decreasing angle at the ankle (dorsiflexion) inclines the leg farther forward, an increasing angle at the knee moves the thigh, and a decreasing angle at the hip moves the trunk.

Because after 0.15 sec the center of gravity is in front of the ankle joint, gravitational force will flex the lower leg; this action is controlled by the ankle extensors, which lengthen. Extension at the hip and knee will be the result of contraction of the extensors at these joints.

At 0.525 sec, the leg has reached the desired degree of inclination (not consciously determined), and the plantar flexors contract with force enough to resist gravity, which now acts on the metatarsophalangeal joints and raises the foot from the surface. At point 0.60 sec, the other (advancing) foot is making contact. Then the center of gravity is moved over that foot by the forward momentum developed in the time from 0.15 to 0.60 sec and by the final push with the toes and plantar flexors of the rear foot. Note that the flexion is occurring at both the hip and knee in this final phase. We will further explain the function of joint actions in the section on inclinations of the segments.

Joint Actions of Swinging Limb. After contact, the rear foot must be swung forward to establish the new contact. The swing, occupying 0.45 sec, is accomplished by flexion at the hip. From full extension, the thigh flexes 34°, bringing the thigh ahead of the trunk. Just before contact, the thigh extends slightly (3°) to lower the limb for contact.

The angle at the knee, approximately 135° as the foot left the ground, continues to decrease for a brief period—0.75 sec. This action lifts the foot from the ground and also shortens the resistance arm for the hip action, reducing the energy needed for moving the limb forward.

The ankle joint, which was at an angle of 115° as it left the ground, decreases (dorsiflexion) immediately, lifting the forepart of the foot to clear the ground. Dorsiflexion continues until the last 0.75 sec before contact. Then plantar flexion extension begins and continues until full foot contact is made.

Inclinations of Segments of Supporting Limb. In all locomotor and balance activities, a change in angle at any joint in the supporting limb changes the inclination of the segments above that joint. In standing, flexion at the ankle inclines the legs, thighs, and trunk toward the horizontal; extension at the ankle moves these segments away from the horizontal. In most forms of locomotion, simultaneous action is likely to occur in the joints of the supporting limb. This action may counteract the effects of distal joints or increase them. (See the discussion on locomotor patterns on land in this chapter.)

The angle made by each segment with the horizontal in walking is shown in Figure 9.5. The angles are those between a horizontal line drawn through the joint at the distal end of the segment and a line drawn through the segment. All angles are measured from the front except that for the foot, which is measured from the back. Foot measures shown begin at the time the foot is in full contact with the ground, and its inclination is therefore 0° until the heel is raised. At 0.525 sec, the heel leaves the contacting surface, and the angle of inclination changes from 0° to 72° as the final push is made.

Leg Inclination. Leg inclination during full foot contact is changed by ankle action only. As flexion at the ankle occurs, it is paralleled by the change in leg inclination. However, when foot inclination begins to change at 0.525 sec, foot inclination and ankle action affect leg inclination. As foot inclination begins, the change in angle at the ankle is at the same rate as the foot inclines; therefore, the inclination of the leg remains constant. If foot inclination is greater than the extension at the ankle, leg inclination will increase. These changes are shown in Figure 9.5. From 0.525 to 0.75 sec, as a result of a 36°-extension at the ankle and a 72°-increase of foot inclination, the leg is inclined forward 36°.

Inclination of the thigh is determined by the inclination of the leg and by knee action. Extension at the knee moves the thigh toward the front horizontal; forward inclination of the leg moves the thigh in the same direction. From 0.15 to 0.525 sec, 26° of extension occur at the knee and the leg inclines forward 20°. The thigh during this time is moved 46° toward the front horizontal. In the last phase of foot contact, the 50° decreased angle at the knee moves the thigh away from the horizontal as the leg inclines 36°. Thigh inclination during this period decreases 14°.

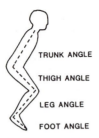

TRUNK ANGLE

THIGH ANGLE

LEG ANGLE

FOOT ANGLE

FIGURE 9.5 Angles of inclination of body segments (expressed in degrees at left) during foot contact phase in walk of college woman. Joint angles are depicted in Figure 9.4. All angles are measured from front horizontal except those of the foot. Note the constant inclination of trunk, resulting from adjustment at hip joint to thigh inclination. Time in seconds is shown at bottom: heel strike occurs at zero time, foot flat occurs at 0.15 sec, rear foot lift occurs at 0.50 sec, and toe lift occurs at 0.75 sec.

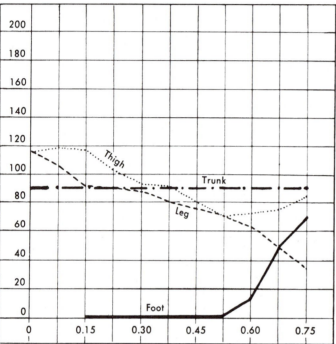

Inclination of the trunk is determined by thigh inclination and hip action. As the thigh inclines forward, the angle at the hip increases at the same rate, keeping the trunk at a constant angle. This is efficient mechanics, eliminating the effort that would be required if the trunk inclination changed.

MINI-LABORATORY LEARNING EXPERIENCE

Using optical techniques described in Chapters 7 and 8, measure the joint angles and body segment angles of inclination in Figures 9.1 and 9.3. Graph these angles and compare the stance phase angles with Figures 9.4 and 9.5.

The joint actions just described provide the major forces in propelling the center of gravity in walking. At the same time, other joints contribute to the total movement. Among these contributions are rotation of the pelvis on the supporting femur due to medial rotation at the hip joint. These actions lengthen the stride. At the same time, the swinging limb is rotated laterally at the hip to keep the foot aligned in the desired line of direction. The torso is also rotated by spinal action to keep the shoulders facing the desired line of progression. As the speed of walking increases, the rotation of the spine is aided by shoulder action, with the right arm moving forward as the left foot advances.

Variations in Stride

Speed. The joint actions and segmental inclinations shown in Figures 9.4 and 9.5 are those of a college woman walking at what she considered her average speed. As the speed of walking changes, the relative duration of the support and swing phases also change. In fast walking, the stance phase and swing phases are likely to be equal. In slow walking, gravitational force contributes less; the inclination of the leg decreases, and the length of the step is shortened. Whatever the speed, the same joints are acting, and each will be making the same type of contribution. However, variations occur in timing, range, and speed of joint actions.

Kinetics of Walking

The action of the muscles in the foot-flat position is a cooperative one in which the quadriceps, femoris, hamstrings, and gluteus medius, as well as the soleus, act during the supporting phase. The rise and fall of the body in a vertical direction is 5 cm (2 in.), and the percentage of body weight alternates between 80% as one foot leaves the ground, and 120% as the heel strike takes place at the time the foot descends. The path of the center of gravity is that of a sinusoidal, or smooth, curve; no sharp braking force is evident. There is side-to-side lateral and medial sway of about 5 cm (2 in.). The physically disabled person has greater rise and fall in a vertical direction (as much as 10 cm [4 in.] than the normal individual).

Backward Force. In addition, there is backward force as the heel strikes the ground during the end phase of deceleration of the leg. When the foot is flat, there is a forward force as the push off commences, as well as a torque as the lower limb twists about the hip joint. The axial rotation of the lower limb is such that it moves, in the swing phase, into internal rotation during the heel strike. At push off the external rotation takes place.

The muscles of the lower limb are busy firing in rapid order during the act of walking. Acting as stabilizers and shock absorbers, they contract over a short period of time and then relax. They cause extension, flexion, and internal and external rotation. They help decelerate and accelerate, and yet they fire in milliseconds and then re-

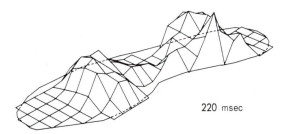

FIGURE 9.6 Pressure pattern under foot of a person during support phase of walking. The largest pressures occur in the mid-heel region and across the metatarsals. Although other people may produce similar pressure patterns, many people will have dissimilar pressure patterns.
(Courtesy Pennsylvania State University Biomechanics Laboratory).

main quiet a great portion of the time. During the last portion of the swing and the first portion of the stance phase, 20% of the major muscle action occurs.

Body Weight. The body weight is centered on the heel, and then it moves forward toward the lateral edge of the foot and diagonally toward the undersurface of the big toe. The effect of moving the body weight in such a manner enables the walker to offset much of the recoil effect. Figure 9.6 shows the pressures on the various parts of a foot during the stance phase. Although similarities can be found among individuals, each pressure pattern is unique to each person.

To understand the contributions that each moving segment makes to the force that moves the body, keep these three important concepts in mind.

Reversed Muscle Action. First, whenever the toes are not free to move (as when they are in contact with the supporting surface and are supporting the body weight), each segment proximal to the toes is moved by reversed muscle action. Metatarsophalangeal joint action moves the foot, not the toes; ankle joint action moves the leg, not the foot; knee joint action moves the thigh, not the leg; hip joint action moves the trunk, not the thigh.

Gravity as a Facilitator. Second, gravitational force is a major contributor to segmental movements in locomotor patterns. When the body's center of gravity is not directly above the ankle joint, gravity tends to initiate movement at that joint. If the center of gravity is in front of the ankle joint, gravitational force tends to flex the foot. If muscles at the ankle contract and prevent such movement, gravity can raise the foot. If the action is moving the center of gravity forward, the heels will be raised. If the action moves the center of gravity backward, the fore part of the foot and the toes will be raised.

Pushing Action-Reaction. Third, locomotor patterns in walking are pushing patterns—pushing against the support surface. Some segments move in a direction other than that of the desired line of force. Counteraction to the undesired movements must occur. In addition, as a segment moves, it carries with it all segments proximal to it. As the leg moves (when the foot is fixed), it also moves the thigh and trunk; as the foot moves, it moves the leg, the thigh, and the trunk. Therefore, the movement and position of a segment are determined not only by action of the joint at its distal end, but also by the movements of the segments distal to it. Before movements of a segment can be described or explained, both the movement of the immediately distal segment and the angle of the segment must be described (measured).

In summary, the main propelling force in the stepping-running-jumping pattern is derived from extension at the knee. To this is added the force of gravity, which rotates the entire body around the metatarsophalangeal joints. Extension at the ankle and hip keep the center of gravity in an advantageous position to move it in the desired direction.

Ground Reaction Forces During Walking

The following information on walking was gathered by the use of a force platform capable of measuring vertical forces and horizontal (forward/backward and medial/lateral) forces.

1. Horizontal and vertical forces are exerted against the platform (ground) during walking; the ground exerts equal and opposite forces against the body.
2. A forward force is exerted on the ground as the heel strikes it. The reaction force is a backward force, braking the forward momentum of the body. This force is approximately 20% of the total body weight.
3. Beginning with heel strike to foot flat, the vertical vector increases in magnitude to 120% of the total body weight.
4. At mid-stance, the vertical force has decreased and is equal to 80% of the total body weight.
5. At mid-stance all horizontal forces are negligible.
6. After heel off, the vertical force rises again to 120% of the total body weight and decreases to zero as the foot is lifted from the platform.
7. From heel off to toe off, there is a backward push against the force platform causing a forward reactive force (propulsive force) of approximately 20% of total body weight.
8. The foot pushes medially on the ground during heel strike and laterally on the ground during flexion at the knee.
9. Vectoral addition of vertical and horizontal forces can be seen in Figures 9.7 and 9.8. The magnitude of the force is represented by its length and the angle of inclination from the vertical represents the rates of vertical and horizontal forces. Note the rather vertically oriented vectors throughout the stance phase.

MINI-LABORATORY LEARNING EXPERIENCE

1. Ask people to walk in response to a metronome, a drum beat, or recorded music (march, foxtrot, rock, jazz). Observe and tabulate limb and body movements for each condition. Use the checklist in Chapter 8 or construct your own.
2. Determine whether there are any differences in gaits of various persons wearing different types of shoes and clothing. Measure or estimate such variables as step length, range of motion at the ankle joint, and speed of walking.
3. Record differences in gait patterns between injured and uninjured individuals.
4. Compare the walking patterns of young children and adults.

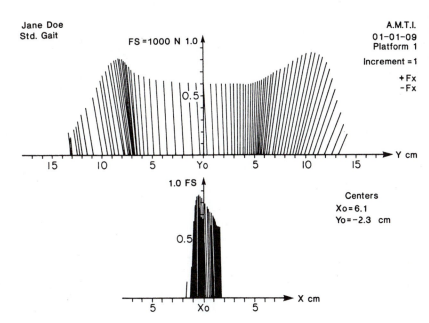

FIGURE 9.7 Vectoral force pattern of support phase of walking. The length of the line represents magnitude of force and the orientation of the line represents angle with the ground.
(Courtesy of Advanced Mechanical Technology, Inc. Force platform—generated data.)

Motor Development of Children

Children's early motor development takes place in a sequential manner, from the reflex actions of the newborn to the more complex actions of the mature person. The first actions of the fetus as well as of the newborn child are reflexive and are primitive and postural in nature (atavistic). Their purpose is survival; that is, they are done for securing food (sucking) or for protection (attempt at righting from a falling action).

There are various ways to classify voluntary movement of children. Gallahue, Werner, and Luedke (1975) list such movements as:

1. Rudimentary movements follow reflexes and, in the opinion of some, build on them. The reflexes begin five months before birth and continue for about two years.
2. Fundamental movements begin at one to two years of age and continue until seven years. They involve walking, running, throwing, and jumping, but are immature.

3. Complex sport skills begin at approximately age seven to ten years and are carried on into adulthood.

The reflexes are the first clues to later voluntary action. The stability patterns of creeping and crawling, followed by walking, and the manipulative patterns such as grasping, reaching, exploring, pulling, and twisting are the real basis for the later rudimentary and fundamental movements. The exact period for learning these skills varies considerably, but there is an age range at which these movements are best learned. They are usually learned in an unvarying sequential manner, regardless of the age range.

Immature Patterns of Fundamental Movements

The next sections describe examples of the immature movements inherent in running, throwing, catching, kicking, and jumping. We have already described walking.

Developmental Biomechanics　　**189**

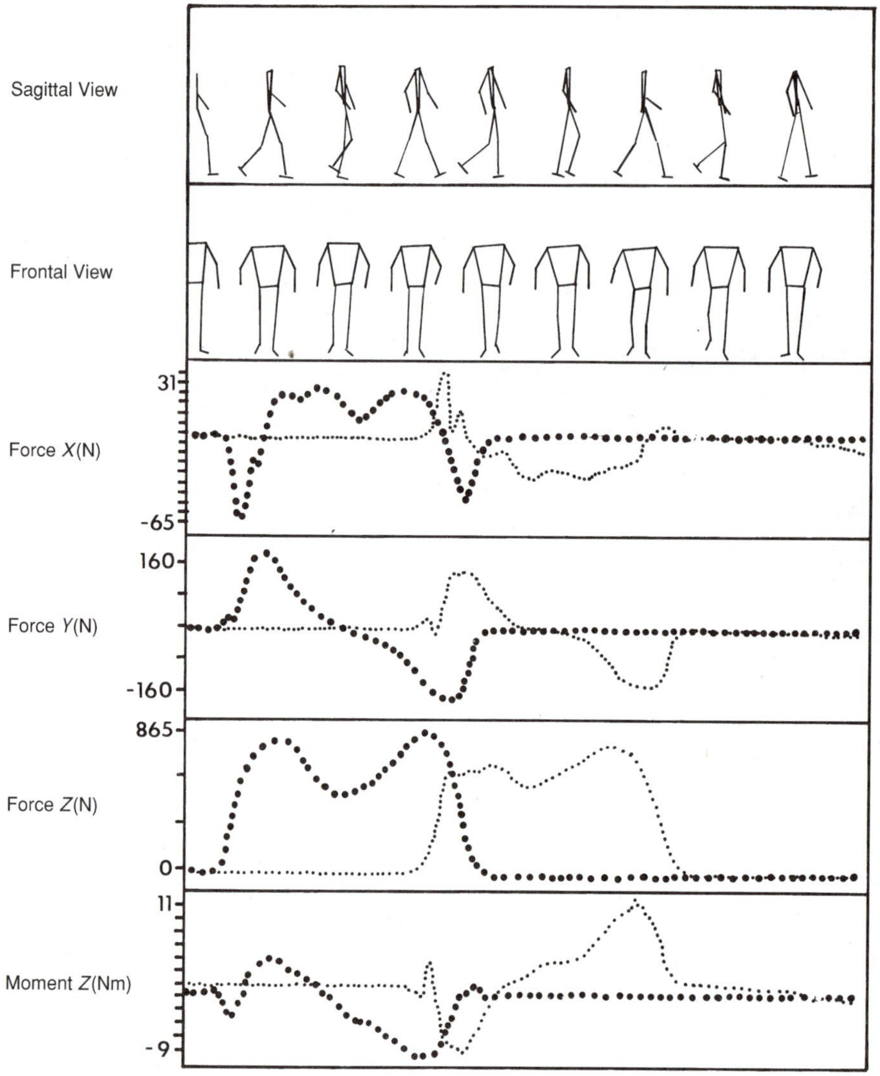

FIGURE 9.8 Walking force-time graphs.
(Courtesy of James Richards.)

Sagittal View

Frontal View

Force X(N)

31

-65

Force Y(N)

160

-160

Force Z(N)

865

0

Moment Z(Nm)

11

-9

Running

During the early learning period for running, there is no observable flight phase, and the base of support is wide. The feet are spread as in Figure 9.9. The feet are rotated outwardly and laterally, and the stride is short. The center of gravity of the body is forward, and the action resembles tiptoeing rather than running. The arm swing is relatively rigid and is more lateral and horizontal rather than vertical. As maturity is gained, there is a definite flight phase with increased stride length and stride frequency.

The support leg is more fully extended at takeoff, and the arms flex, extend, and move more vertically. (See also the discussion of mature running in Chapter 15.)

Throwing

In the early immature throwing action, the movement at the elbow and part of the follow-through are similar to the mature action (Figure 9.10). However, the center of motion is the elbow, with very little action elsewhere. The feet do not move, or at least there is no shifting of the feet

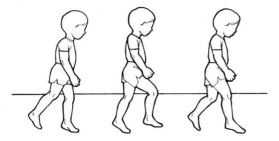

FIGURE 9.9 Child in running pattern. Note "tiptoe" style. There is no flight phase in this early stage of running.

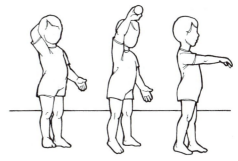

FIGURE 9.10 Immature throwing pattern. There is no step with the leg opposite from throwing arm.

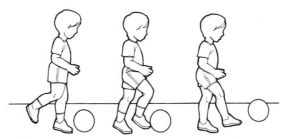

FIGURE 9.11 Immature kicking pattern. Note short backswing of the leg.

into a step as the throw is executed. The axes at the shoulder, opposite hip, and spine are lacking. The throw is accomplished from a fixed, almost rigid position. (See the discussion of mature throwing in Chapter 17.)

Catching

In the early stages of catching, the head remains stationary regardless of the angle and height of the incoming object (ball). The hands remain fixed and slightly flexed and are not adjusted to the height path of the ball. At the point of contact with the ball, the hands have very little "give," that is, the momentum is not attenuated. Mature individuals who catch in this manner are said to have board hands. There is very little, if any, flexion at the knees to help absorb the shock of the ball's velocity. (See the discussion of catching in Chapter 14 and the contourograms of Figure 9.15.)

Kicking

The young child initially makes very little movement of the upper body (arm and trunk) when kicking (Figure 9.11). There is a very low amplitude of backswing, and often there is very little or no follow-through. The arms are kept to the side for balance. The kicking leg contacts the ball while the shank is deeply flexed. (See the discussion of mature kicking and striking patterns in Chapter 18.)

Jumping

The young child initially steps rather than jumps (Figure 9.12). The pattern is a stride up or down as the situation dictates. Gradually the one- and two-foot takeoffs are learned. Frequently, in attempting to jump over a barrier, the young child merely jumps vertically rather than horizontally. The one-foot jump, is next in sequence after the step, and then the two-foot takeoff is learned. A run and a

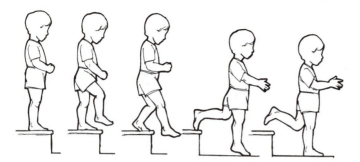

FIGURE 9.12 Child jumping down from step has an immature jumping pattern, since the action is actually a step down. For rising from the floor, see Figure 9.19.

step are combined in the leap. The ability to take off with one foot and land on two feet follows in the sequence. (See the discussion on mature jumping in Chapter 16.)

■ Biomechanical analyses of children's patterns requires an understanding of developmental concepts.

Environmental Constraints

Often the limiting factor in the development of movement patterns by children is the architectural design of the environment for adults. For example, ascending and descending stairs pose problems for three-year-olds. Compare the leg action of the child in Figure 9.13a with the leg action of the adult in Figure 9.13b. Why does the child have difficulty ascending the stairs? Measure the angles at the hip joint and at the knee joint.

Clinical Diagnosis of Skills for Effective Training*

Observation and Analysis of Skills

One of the most important functions of the physical education practitioner is the observation and analysis of motor skills. In observing motor skills, the teacher, clinician, or coach conducts a systematic, visual inspection of the gross and fine aspects of the performance and compares the observed movement patterns to a

---

*Contributed by Lynda Randall

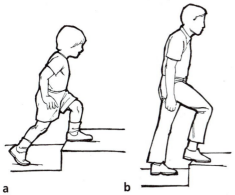

FIGURE 9.13 Ascending stairs: (a) Young child; (b) adult. Compare the angles at the hip and at the knee during initial contact with lead leg. Compare angles at knee, ankle, and metatarsal joints of pushoff leg.

prescribed model or visual image. This process, entailing "decisions made by skill instructors regarding the nature of the learner's performance problems and the factors that give rise to them" (Hoffman 1983, p. 36) has been termed **clinical diagnosis.**

Clinical diagnosis is essential to effective teaching because it has six major functions in enhancing learning. These include

1. evaluation of motor skills by use of process measures.
2. identification of developmental stages in the acquisition of fundamental motor skills.
3. provision of accurate and precise feedback to the learner.
4. development of teaching cues.
5. selection of developmentally appropriate learning activities and design of optimum learning environments.
6. application of clinical diagnosis to coaching contexts.

Each of these functions is described in the following sections.

Evaluation of Motor Skills. Skills tests have traditionally been used to evaluate performance on the basis of product or end-result scores. *Product* measures refer to the description of the outcome of the movement in terms of time, accuracy, or force. *Process* measures involve descriptions of the movement of the performer, or "force-producing actions" (Safrit 1981, p. 155). For example, skill in overhand throwing might be assessed by the number of balls thrown within a given time period, the distance that the ball was thrown, the accuracy of throws aimed at a target, or the velocity at which the ball traveled. These are four examples of product measures.

All of these measurements, however, fall short in the sense that they provide no information about the form of the throwing pattern (i.e., the force-producing motions of the arms, trunk, and legs). With process measures, the observer can determine the level of throwing proficiency displayed by describing the action of the humerus, forearms, and pelvis-spine, as well as the nature of the stepping patterns (ipsilateral or contralateral stepping, length of stride) and the presence or absence of a follow-through. Three stages of throwing proficiency that might be determined by process measurement are outlined in Table 9.2.

MINI-LABORATORY LEARNING EXPERIENCE

Place the throwing performances (Figure 9.14) in the appropriate development level using the scheme in Table 9.2.

One important factor that has limited the application of process measures in assessing motor skills is the unavailability of instruments that could be easily applied. Instruments designed for evaluating fundamental motor skills were designed primarily for research purposes and necessitated the use of sophisticated film-analysis techniques. These instruments did not lend themselves to reliable observations in a live setting. Two investigators, Griffin (1984) and Cozzallio (1986) provided encouragement for the use of process measures in practical settings. In the first investigation, Griffin developed a process measure for throwing, striking, and kicking that was found to discriminate gender and grade-level differences and correlated positively with product measures. In a similar study, Cozzallio developed a gross motor

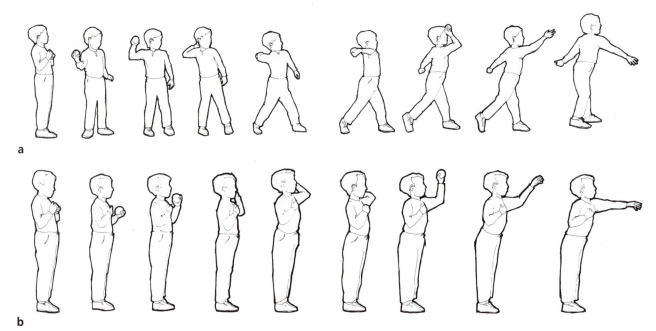

a

b

FIGURE 9.14 Sequential contourograms of throwing performances of two young boys.

(Illustrations courtesy of Steven Barnes, Florida State University, Tallahassee.)

TABLE 9.2 Developmental levels of skill proficiency in overhand throwing.

Body Segment	Level 1	Level 2	Level 3
Arms	a. Primarily a flinging motion from the elbow b. Elbow of throwing arm remains in front of the body c. No forearm lag (elbow extends early) d. Fingers are spread at release	a. Humerus rotates to oblique position as ball is brought behind the head b. Arm swings forward high above the shoulder in delivery c. Cocking of wrist occurs at completion of throw d. Forearm lags behind humerus in delivery	a. Arm swings backward in preparation b. Elbow of nonthrowing arm is extended for balance c. Thumb rotates medially downward d. Fingers are close together at release e. Pronounced forearm lag
Trunk	a. Body faces forward throughout b. Little or no rotation of shoulders and hips (remain facing target)	a. Block rotation of trunk (simultaneous rotation of hips and shoulders in preparation) b. Shoulders turn to face target in delivery c. Forward trunk flexion completes delivery	a. Differentiated trunk rotation (hips-spine-shoulders) in delivery b. Throwing shoulder drops slightly in preparation c. Throwing shoulder faces target in follow-through
Legs	a. No stepping b. No weight transfer	a. Definite shift of weight b. Ipsilateral stepping (same arm and leg move forward)	a. Weight is on rear foot in preparation b. Oppositional stepping (opposite arm and leg move forward)

Note: Children who are in transition between levels of skill proficiency may exhibit intersegmental variations (i.e., different levels of maturity are reflected in the action of the three body segments).

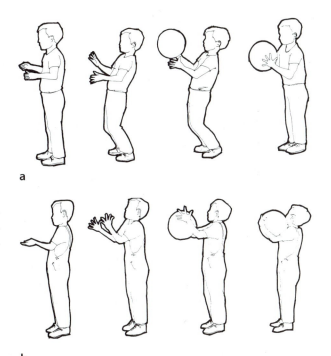

a

b

FIGURE 9.15 Sequential contourograms of catching performances of two young boys.
(Illustrations courtesy of Steven Barnes, Florida State University, Tallahassee.)

screening instrument for kindergarten that was found to be valid and reliable for use by classroom teachers. The instruments used in both of these investigations were checklists, which required the rater to match the observed motor patterns with established criteria. Similar checklists appear in Chapter 8.

Identification of Developmental Stages. Identifying stages in the acquisition of fundamental motor skills is another teaching competency that requires proficiency in clinical diagnosis. A vast amount of literature consists of descriptions of the stages of development through which children pass in acquiring basic locomotor, manipulative, and axial movement patterns. Although most children do pass through similar stages in developing motor patterns, there is a great deal of variation in the rate at which they do so and, thus, in the rate they mature.

Therefore, process measures can provide a useful tool for allowing the teacher to identify children whose level of proficiency (immature to mature) deviates significantly from what is typically observed at a given age level. For example, a nine-year-old child who demonstrated immature patterns of catching (e.g., avoidance behaviors, trapping the ball against the chest) would signal the need for remedial efforts. (See Figure 9.15.)

Provision of Feedback. Defined as "information generated about a response that is used to modify the next response" (Siedentop 1983, p. 7), providing feedback is another essential aspect of effective teaching that is enhanced by critical diagnosis. Sensory and proprioceptive feedback are intrinsically available to the learner and are obtained through visual, auditory, tactile, and kinesthetic cues. When this information is insufficient, however, the learner is dependent upon the teacher to provide augmented or supplementary feedback (Singer 1980, p. 455).

Singer (1980, p. 282) has cautioned that the mere availability of feedback does not ensure improved performance by children. It appears that the "type, form, and receptivity to it" are factors to be considered. A limited amount of research has been conducted in this area, but several researchers (Barclay and Newell 1980; Newell 1976; Newell and Kennedy 1978) indicate that younger children benefit more from general feedback, while precise feedback facilitates the performance of older children. An extension of this finding is that teachers should provide feedback related to gross aspects of the movement pattern to young learners and those who display an immature movement pattern. In contrast, older and more skilled learners are able to cognitively process more precise feedback.

Development of Teaching Cues. In addition to providing a frame of reference for giving appropriate feedback, clinical diagnosis can guide the teacher in the identification of teaching cues. Teaching cues are short phrases that direct the learner's attention to a specific aspect of performance, such as "racquet back, side to the net," as opposed to the product of the movement: "Did the ball pass over the net?" Analysis of movement patterns from a biomechanical perspective results in the identification of scientifically correct teaching cues. No cue is often more effective than a miscue. A correct cue, however, will be most effective.

Selection and Design of Learning Activities and Environments.

Clinical diagnosis is an inherent process in the selection of developmentally appropriate learning activities and the design of optimum learning environments. Rink (1985 p. 191) has emphasized that "a major problem in group instruction is that students function at different levels of ability in most tasks. . . ." Therefore, it is essential to determine the appropriateness of the content and the manner in which it is presented.

Consider, for example, the appropriateness of a game of kickball for a group of first-graders. Prior to introducing the game, the teacher, through clinical diagnosis, observes that many of the children perform at an immature level in the fundamental skills of throwing, catching, and kicking. Demands of performing these skills in a dynamic game situation, with the added stress of competition, produces an environment in which the execution, much less the improvement, of these skills is unlikely. More appropriate tasks would be those in which the children perform the skills under static conditions or without the element of competition (e.g., throwing and catching with a stationary partner or kicking a stationary ball).

Morgan and Garrett (1984) have developed an innovative approach to helping children acquire motor patterns. They used cut-out figures or silhouettes drawn from 16mm film of children performing motor skills to help the children develop a clear visual image of the skill to be learned. By emulating the shape seen in the figure, children attempt to kinesthetically memorize the body position. Children might, for example, work in pairs and provide feedback to each other on the accuracy of their replication of the body position to be assumed in a sprinting start. Additional practice could be gained by asking the children to replicate the shape with eyes closed, or the teacher might provide formative feedback to the children in this manner.

Coaching.

Application of skill analysis to coaching contexts is the last major purpose for developing competence in clinical diagnosis. Effective coaching requires a thorough knowledge of the mechanics of correct performance of given skills and the development of a clear visual image by which to compare observed performance to a theoretical model. This visual image is the basis for error detection and precise and accurate feedback.

MEAP

The Michigan Educational Assessment Program (MEAP) (Michigan State Board of Education 1984) contains a variety of process assessments for fundamental motor skills (locomotor and object control) and body management skills (body awareness, body control, posture). The battery includes a number of product measures as well, in addition to combined process and product assessments of physical fitness (endurance, flexibility, and muscular strength). Researchers at the University of Virginia (Kelley, Dagger, & Walkley 1989) used the MEAP recently in an assessment-based approach to developing fundamental motor skills in preschool children. These researchers found that children in an experimental group made significant gains in six motor skills when qualitative assessment was incorporated in a 12-week instructional program.

Clinical diagnosis is an essential element of effective teaching and plays a significant role in the enhancement of learning all motor skills. Hoffman (1983) has used the analogy of teaching and medicine to emphasize the importance of accurate diagnosis:

> As the physician's decisions regarding medical treatment are contingent upon his/her diagnosis of the patient's ailments, so are decisions regarding feedback, verbal prompts, or the nature of practice experiences contingent upon the instructor's diagnosis of the learner's performance deficiencies. Obviously, then, the teacher's ability to correctly ascertain the learners' problems . . . and allow that assessment to inform subsequent decision about the prescriptive part of teaching would appear to be a major determinant of his/her effectiveness in helping learners attain the skill goal. (p. 37)

■ Biomechanical analysis is essential for clinical diagnosis of skills.

Biomechanics and Aging

Many cardiologists believe that walking briskly at a constant speed of 3–4 mps has great health benefits. The breathing rate is increased noticeably, and 1500–2000

At the age of 66, Hulda Crooks climbed Mt. Whitney. She has climbed that mountain 21 other times, and, at the age of 91, climbed Mt. Fuji in Japan.

calories can be burned in a week by walking two miles four times a week. There is a biomechanically correct way to walk in order to reap the greatest benefits and to reduce the possibility of adverse effects.

Locomotor Patterns and Aging

The stereotypic gait of the older person in American society consists of slow, short, shuffling steps in which there is decreased range of motion at all joints and a slumping of the head, shoulders, and upper trunk. That this pattern is not typical for able-bodied older persons has been shown by Murray (1967) in her extensive investigations of walking patterns of both able-bodied and physically impaired adults. Able-bodied males 60 to 65 years of age, for example, showed no differences in stance, stride width, swing, double-limb support, transverse, or sagittal rotations of the pelvis, hips, knees, and ankles, or movements of the trunk compared to younger men. Shorter steps (3.1 cm), shorter stride lengths, and increased out-toeing (2.7°) were the only significant differences noted. Since this was a cross-sectional study rather than a longitudinal study, one cannot be sure whether these differences were due to the age variable itself or to the sample within each age group. Also, it must be kept in mind that often the most able-bodied are the volunteers as subjects. Results could be distorted.

Since individual differences in cadence, range, and speed of limb movements exist in every age group studied, the older person can be expected to be able to execute a walking pattern in the same manner as young and middle-aged persons. There are long striders and short striders, fast walkers and slow walkers, and persons with varying amounts of out-toeing and limb segment rotations among all age groups. Note the erect posture and "normal" range and stride of the 70-year-old woman in Figure 9.16.

If, however, Parkinson's disease or another pathological condition afflicts the older person, the gait

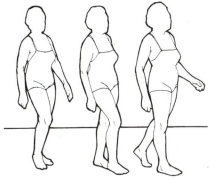

FIGURE 9.16 Normal walking pattern of an able-bodied 70-year-old woman. Note erect posture and normal opposition of arms and legs.

pattern will be impaired. A "Parkinsonism gait" is one with short, unstable, shuffling strides, with the body flexed at the hips and throughout the spinal column. Another type of gait pattern seen among the older population afflicted with labyrinthine dysfunction is a widened lateral stance and lateral sway or lurching of the body during changing of the base of support. Persons with total hip replacement, however, appear to be able to establish a normal walking pattern, as noted by research conducted by Murray (1967).

Running

Although some older persons are competing in senior Olympic racing competition and triathlons, the majority of older people do not include running in their daily lives. An exception would be those who engage in running required for such sports as tennis and softball. The speed of running is low for the average older person. The contourograms depicted in Figure 9.17 represent the running form of women aged 60–80 years who engaged in swimming as a form of daily (or every other day) exercise. Is this a jogging sequence or a maximum speed sequence? The women were asked to, and did, run as fast as they could. When comparing the kinematics of their run to the patterns of university track-team women who sprinted and paced, it was found that the older women ran at the speed the younger women paced. The kinematics were identical. If the older women's performances, however, were compared to

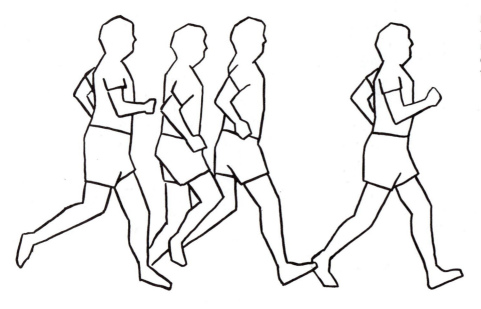

FIGURE 9.17 Sequential contourograms of running performance of an older woman who engaged in swimming program for exercise.

Foot Contact

Midstance

Midflight

Takeoff

the sprint performance, there was little similarity. What conclusions would you draw from these data to answer the question, Can older women run?

Jumping Patterns

Investigations of vertical jumping patterns of older women who had not executed the pattern since high school once again show no evidence of an age-related factor. The only difference noted between data from college-age women and from an older population was in the lack of speed of extension of the leg at the knee joint. The sequencing of limb movements and the force-time histories were similar for both populations. The lack of extension speed may be due to aging, disuse, ratio of slow and fast-twitch muscle fibers, or ratio of muscle cross-section to body weight. More research is needed to better understand the capabilities of older persons.

Age-Related Changes in the Motor Control Systems that Subserve Performance and Skill Acquisition*

This section discusses some age-related changes that effect both performance and skill acquisition of older adults.

Sense Organs. As we know from the changes in ourselves or in older relatives and friends, the eyes and ears change as we age. Close vision becomes more blurred, and we are not able to see as well at night or when the lighting is dim. Our depth vision becomes less precise. Hearing may be impaired as well. Only certain pitches may be inaudible, or all frequencies may be affected. Other sense organs affected by aging include the vestibular apparatus and proprioceptors. As a result, balance is affected in standing and walking, climbing stairs,

*Contributed by Tonya Toole

and turning. Our proprioceptors tell us how far we have moved, how fast our movements were, how much force we used to make the movement, and the positions of our limbs in space. While we do not have specific evidence about the nature of change in these proprioceptors with age, we suspect that they, too, transmit signals to the brain. It has been stated that of the five senses, decrements occur first with sight, hearing next, then smell, taste and touch, in that order.

Central Nervous System. One seemingly natural effect of aging is slowing of responses. Putting the brake on the car very rapidly or catching oneself to prevent a fall when balance is lost are common fast movements that are essential to everyday living. Response to a light and sound stimulus are both slowed with age. Other central nervous system declines include cognitive functions dealing with organizing information, whether it be new or old. A simple task such as organizing the events of the day may be difficult for some older adults. When memory must be used to attend to a specific input or stimulus, many older adults experience difficulties. This specific deficit is called memory-driven attentional selectivity and is typical of the normal aging process. Other normal changes with aging include difficulties in putting new information into memory and retrieving or finding old information, especially if that old information is not so very old. These are deficits in encoding and retrieval and they affect most of us as we age. Storing information for a short period of time is also affected with age. Trying to remember the name of a person you met yesterday is an example of this short-term storage deficit. The older person's memory is also more susceptible to interference from other information stored in memory, as well as from noise or other stimuli in the environment. Many of these central nervous system deficiencies can affect learning and performing motor skills.

Muscular System. The natural aging process also affects the muscular system. There is a decline in muscle fibers, mass and muscular strength. Decreased flexibility also occurs, and stability is affected by this change in the muscular system. Time required for the antagonist muscle groups to relax prior to initiating a movement also increases. All of these changes affect an older person's ability to control movement.

Skeletal System. Whereas females are generally affected more than males by decline in bone mineral content and bone mass, both sexes experience an increased incidence of osteoporosis with the aging process. Thus the bones may not tolerate impact forces, such as occur during walking, gravitational compressive forces, and muscular forces. High incidence of fractures of bones exist in the older population.

Effects of Motor Control Systems' Decline on Biomechanics of Movement and Skill Acquisition*

This section discusses how a decline in the motor control systems of the body affects the biomechanics of movement and skill acquisition.

Sense Organs. Reduced and restricted vision greatly affects balance for the control of movement. This change in the visual system also limits a person's ability to use feedback from the eyes for many daily living skills, as well as for learning new skills. Other less-effective feedback systems must be used to maintain performance and assist in the learning of new skills. Accuracy of performance is greatly affected by visual impairment, whether the task be driving a car, lifting a pan of boiling water from the stove, or hitting a tennis ball over the net. Perceptions of oncoming stimuli (e.g., balls in racquet sports or cars on the road) can be slowed and distorted. Stages of development for skill acquisition must change as a result of these changes in the visual system. The rate of skill acquisition for an open skill (environment-changing) is slowed.

Suggestions for the Practitioner. A restriction in vision need not prevent the older adult from learning new motor skills and performing old ones. Practitioners need to follow a few guidelines in order to assist clients in learning new motor tasks and maintaining optimum performance in spite of visual loss: (1) Learn about each individual's visual impairment. Has it been corrected adequately? If not, deal with each person's problem individually. (2) Slow the stimulus (e.g., the oncoming ball) in practice situations. Response to the ball will be

---

*Contributed by Tonya Toole

delayed, so it is essential that its speed be reduced. (3) Provide auditory feedback to the learner who has visual impairment. For example, "Get your racquet back sooner to hit the ball earlier." (4) Provide other sources of auditory feedback, such as "Hit now!", or "You're lined up to the right for this shot—move your feet to the left by two inches." (5) Use bright stimuli such as orange balls or illuminescent paint or tape on the balls and boundaries of the court. With persons who have an impaired vestibular apparatus that affects balance, the practitioner could suggest brisk walking, stationary bicycling, or swimming for aerobic exercise instead of walking. Since ballistic skills may be impaired by this restricted balance control, encourage these persons to limit their range of motion so that the line of gravity stays well within the base of support. Of course, this may decrease force production but it may provide the performer with increased confidence that balance will not be lost.

Central Nervous System.   Slowing of responses to stimuli will decrease speed of movement in response to stimuli in open tasks (e.g., badminton, tennis, racquetball), necessitating competition with age peers who also have slowed responses. Accuracy becomes a more important component of the task than speed. Daily living skills may also be affected by slowed behavior. Performances of tasks such as turning the head to orient to someone who is speaking, catching a falling object, and braking a car may be slowed and impaired behavior may result.

Cognitive function decline also affects learning and maintenance of performance. For example, memory-driven attentional selectivity decline will impair the ability to attend consistently to a portion of a new skill, such as increasing the range of pelvic rotation in the golf swing. Encoding is also adversely affected with age, and this could potentially slow one's ability to learn new movement patterns for all newly learned motor tasks. Retrieval of previously learned tasks may also be detrimentally affected, since the proper motor program must be located and retrieved from memory each time we perform a task. If the performer has difficulty in retrieving the correct motor program, performance will be inconsistent and error-filled. We cannot expect the consistent performance of youth nor can we expect a once-learned

task (for example, an overarm throw) to exhibit its skillful youthful qualities. Portions of that task could be temporarily affected by lack of complete retrieval, interference from other similar tasks, or from a general decaying condition.

Changes in the central nervous system need not prevent the older adult from participating in physical activity; the benefits of aerobic exercise to the central nervous system are becoming well known. Practitioners need to encourage the older adult to get involved in aerobic exercise and maintain a weekly workout program. Slowing of responding and memory changes may well be reduced by a consistent and vigorous aerobic program that includes maintaining the target heart rate for the recommended time. Slowing of movement is a natural response for many older adults who realize that their response speed has slowed. Encourage the older adult to play a favorite sport with age peers who also have slower responses.

The practitioner needs to be aware that declines in the memory system may affect the older adult's ability to remember events of the day or organize new information. These declines may also affect retention of motor skills. What was once a skillful movement for the young adult may show some inadequacies in old age because of changes in memory. Portions of the skillful motor program may not be retrieved at one certain time, one skillful aspect may decay more rapidly than others, and remembering to attend to one specific cue may be difficult. The practitioner should patiently remind the performer of aspects of the task that need attention. Search for a cue that the learner/performer can more easily remember; this may well be a different word cue for each individual. Teachers also should write cue cards for the performer to use periodically as reminders. When the older adult learns a new skill, teachers need to use a great deal of content repetition and many practice situations. This will tend to reinforce what was taught and prevent the older adult from forgetting essential cues. Using many visual cues will also help the learner to remember better. Provide pictures of the task, repeat demonstrations, and have the performer watch his or her own performance on videotape or in the mirror. The performer should look at body parts that move.

Muscular System. Decline in muscle fibers and muscle mass will limit force-production capability, movement speed, and reaction to a fast stimulus. Strength will be affected, which will, in turn, affect equipment standards and construction. For example, more flexible shafts for golf clubs might be required. Decrease in flexibility will limit the range of motion for most sports skills and many daily-living skills such as reaching for the top shelf, bending for cleaning chores, stretching when gardening. Stability for riding a bus, climbing stairs, and carrying groceries may also be affected by decline in muscle mass. Falls are more prevalent for older adults, and women fall twice as often as men. Is it because of lower strength or poorly designed footwear for walking?

Skeletal System. Due to selective bone-mass loss, the center of gravity will change from younger years. This may place restrictions on motor control and may necessitate change in contemporary motor-skill technique. For example, stride length for brisk walking will have shortened for the person with bone loss in the spinal column and hip/femur area who must maintain a stooped posture.

Changes in the muscular and skeletal systems will necessitate changes in motor behavior. Practitioners should not expect the older adult to produce the magnitude of forces in motor tasks that are achieved in youth. Limb speed (movement time) and total body speed can be enhanced, however. Since a strength training program can increase muscle mass and strength, older persons should be encouraged to participate in a strength training program for their age group. Maintenance of range of motion for daily living skills must be promoted through daily stretching exercises. Changes in the muscular system also affect stability. The older adult should be encouraged to widen the base of support for many daily-living skills. A wider base of support increases safety and effectiveness when, for example, standing at the check-out line at the grocery, standing and talking, standing in the kitchen and then moving to perform tasks. A wider base of support should also be encouraged for motor skills and for other daily living skills in which the base of support is moving, such as in riding a bus. Encourage the use of handrails when they are provided. Wearing lower-heeled shoes will promote better balance for the older person.

Biomechanical Requirements of Movement

In order to better understand the limitations of movement achievements by older persons, it is important to measure the characteristics of movement patterns. What are the temporal, spatial, and kinetic requirements of common movement patterns performed by older persons and of movement patterns not normally a part of these persons' repertoire?

Speed requirements of walking can be related to the minimum required speed to cross a traffic intersection. Based on research by Aniansson, 1.4 m/sec should be the criterion speed for walking. Average speed of "normal, functional walking" by a group of 419 70-year-olds was found to be less than the criterion speed. Aniansson calculated average speeds of 1.2 m/sec for males and 1.1 m/sec for females.

A small group of women age 58–80 were tested on their speed of walking normally and as fast as safely possible. Although this group also did not normally walk 1.4 m/sec or faster, their maximum safe walking speed was 1.9 m/sec, well above the criterion speed.

Klinger et al. (1980) reported on the movement characteristics of twelve women aged 60 years and older who were actively involved in a regular exercise program. Videotapes were recorded during performance of activities of daily living, exercises, and sports skills. In addition, electrogoniometers were placed at the elbow and knee to continuously record movements about those joints. A force platform was used for one of the performances, the vertical jump. The group could be qualitatively divided into a high- and low-ability grouping. The high-ability group members were characterized as moving faster, transferring body weight more easily, and showing a greater range of motion, more erect trunk posture, and better coordination, evidenced by greater continuity of sequencing of movements. The researchers used a Rohler's Index (Wt./Ht. × 10) to determine if this anthropometric measurement correlated with the placement of persons into the two groups. The high-ability group had the lower Rohler's Indices, but one person in the low-ability group also showed a low R.I. The range for the high-ability group was 124–149 and for the low ability group 124–173. The importance of strength and body mass was noted in the inability of some of the individuals to rise from sitting on a low block or the floor, although they were able to rise from a chair.

Effects of Disuse

In an effort to relate the disuse phenomenon to aging changes, comparisons of angular velocities and displacements were made among the three types of activities. Movements at the knee during walking showed 40–60° of flexion and peak angular velocities of 133–360°. Although the sitting and rising activities required greater range of motion, the angular velocities at the knee were less than those measured during walking. Negligible ROM and ω were seen in the other activities of daily living. Vertical jumping, a sports skill, showed a minimum of 400° and a maximum of 800° angular velocity at the knee joint. In addition, the range of motion at the knee almost doubled when jumping. Force-time histories of these jumping patterns were similar to those found with college women. The major difference was in the inability to develop greater leg extension velocity and, thus, greater impulses. For the category ADL, negligible angular displacements and velocities at the elbow were recorded during walking, sitting, rising from a chair, and simulation of putting on pants. Combing hair showed 42–95° of motion and ω of 72–360° at the elbow. Generally, movements of eating required 95° of motion and speed of 200–400° at the elbow. Floor mopping showed approximately 40° of motion at 200°/s at the elbow. Arm exercise patterns produced average angular velocities at the elbow of 500°/s. Additionally, the velocity of forearm extension during some arm exercises was faster than some of the striking or throwing skills. For example, the elbow extensions in the tennis backhand stroke were 300°/s. Typical velocities for throwing, however, were 800°/s of extension at the elbow. The fastest extensions occurred during batting, the overhand badminton stroke, and overarm throwing. These velocities were greater than 800°/s, although they varied greatly from individual to individual. The next fastest velocities occurred in the medicine ball throw and the tennis stroke, which were about 400°/s. The velocities achieved by these older women in these sports skills were much less than the velocities reported for young skilled performers. But it should be noted that one-half of the subjects tested had no sports background, while others had not performed the skills since high school. Even though the velocities were low, they were much higher than those achieved in the activities of daily living.

■ Exercises and sports skills, such as batting, throwing, jumping, and arm extensions, cause the limbs to move with greater velocity and through a larger range of motion than do the activities of daily living.

To withstand strains and maintain a high quality of life, the older person must engage in activities requiring greater ROMs and velocities than necessary for ADL. Some of the implications of this study are: (1) Stress on bones is produced by muscle contractions, the stronger the contraction, the greater the stress. Therefore, if stresses on the bone are less, disuse may be a major cause of early so-called aging changes in bone. (2) Lack of fast movement also reduces stress on the joints and may have implications for osteoarthritis. (3) Due to a lack of fast movements by the elderly, there are no phasic muscle contractions, and fast-twitch muscles may not be used. (4) If the range of motion at the joint is less, a definite loss of flexibility may be experienced over time, which in turn leads to a further decreased range of motion.

MINI-LABORATORY LEARNING EXPERIENCE

1. Time three 60-year-olds in running and walking 30 yards.
2. Time three 18–22-year-olds over the same distance.

Do a similar study using the same subjects ascending twelve stair steps. Why the difference?

ADL: The Foundation of Developmental Biomechanics Related to Aging

The fundamental area of human movement analysis is ADL (activities of daily living). ADL is the foundation for survival and the basis for many work and leisure activities, including sports and dance. A large number of an adult's waking hours are spent in ADL or activities of work. In fact, most people over 60 years of age spend almost all their time with ADL and engage in few, if any, other types of activities.

In general, ADL consists primarily of movements performed at slow to moderate speeds, the majority of movements requiring little muscle effort. When the task is strenuous, people (especially older people) will rest frequently or avoid performing the task.

As one becomes older, the ADL becomes more difficult to perform, especially if these activities have been performed inefficiently—that is, in less than a biomechanically sound manner—in one's youth. The research in this area has been conducted mainly to identify problems of physically disabled persons and dysfunctioning and unsafe conditions. In addition, ADL research is important to the construction of prostheses, braces, and other orthotic devices. However, research on normal ADL analysis is limited.

The six major classifications of ADL are:

1. Locomotion: walking, ascending and descending stairs, stepping into vehicles
2. Changing levels: moving from chair to standing, moving from bed to standing, stooping, kneeling
3. Lifting and carrying groceries, suitcases, and other objects
4. Pushing and pulling: using a wheelbarrow, manual lawn mower, rolling pin, typewriter
5. Working with long-handled implements: axe, hoe, broom
6. Working with small implements: pencil, saw, hammer, knitting needles, eating utensils, hatchet.

Analysis of selected ADL relative to classifications 1 and 2 appear in this chapter, relative to classification 3 appears in Chapters 11 and 12, and relative to 5 and 6 in Chapter 12.

Ascending Stairs

Ascending stairs poses a problem to many persons who have weak leg extensors. The leg is lifted by the contraction of quadriceps femoris and other flexors at the hip, and the foot is placed on the next step, which is usually 23 cm higher than the preceding one. The body weight, then, must be lifted 23 cm, which has been selected as the optimum step height for the average adult. The amount of leg lift and the optimum angles at the hip and knee joints differ for individuals with varying leg lengths. However, all persons show a greater range of motion at the knee, hip, and ankle during stair locomotion than during walking on level ground. Thus, muscle weakness affects the stair-climbing pattern of obese and short people to a greater extent than that of lighter and tall people.

■ Handrails can provide reactive force assistance for persons with weak leg muscles who need to ascend stairs.

Raising the Center of Gravity

Lifting the body requires that the center of gravity of the body be shifted from the rear foot to the new supporting foot and that the rear foot initiate plantar flexion. This plantar flexion will raise the center of gravity of an adult male with a size seven foot approximately eight cm. Thus, one-third of the total distance through which the body weight must be lifted may be achieved by this action. This action is not as effective for people with smaller feet. The ideal sequential timing of extension at the hip and knee of the lead leg with respect to plantar flexion of the rear foot produces a series of acceleration forces caused by these muscle contractions. Thus, the summation of these forces facilitates raising the center of gravity of the body the necessary 23 cm to the next step. In this manner, a person can compensate for weak quadriceps muscles, which are the primary muscles used by many healthy young persons in stair locomotion.

Correct placement of the total foot on each stair tread is important for individuals who have balance problems. Unfortunately, some stairs do not have sufficiently wide treads to allow large persons, who often weigh more than average, to place the total foot on the tread. One must be careful not to place the foot so far forward that the toe catches on the lip of the step as the foot is lifted.

When placing the total foot on the tread, the muscles crossing the ankle joint can relax and the foot is in a neutral position. From this position, the foot dorsiflexes as the other leg enters the swing phase of ascent. From this dorsiflexed position, a person can generate greater force because of the distance through which plantar flexion can be accelerated, compared to the person who uses the ball of the foot during the support phase of ascending stairs.

Another advantage of the neutral position of the foot is that it releases tension in the gastrocnemius, facilitating extension at the knee. This facilitation occurs because the gastrocnemius crosses the knee, as well as the ankle. With the absence of tension in the gastrocnemius, the quadriceps can move the leg with less force than if co-contraction between agonists and antagonists existed.

Critical Speed of Ascent

There is, however, a critical speed of ascent at which most people prefer to use only the ball of the foot rather than the whole foot. Although this critical speed varies with individuals, it represents the speed at which the person rapidly passes through each single-support phase; that is, there is no sensing of a static single-support position. The faster the speed of ascent, the more pronounced the absence of full foot contact. With speed, however, the likelihood of the person's ascending two steps at a time is great. A person may again use the full foot contact, since the height to which the leg must be lifted is lower with a full-foot landing than with any other type of landing. In addition, passive dorsiflexion of the foot can take place, thus shifting the center of gravity of the body forward and upward with little muscle effort.

Descending Stairs

The problem imposed by the act of descending stairs is opposite that of ascending stairs. While ascending stairs results in positive work (the product of body weight and height), descending stairs is negative work, since the muscles eccentrically contract to regulate the speed of descent caused by gravity. Once again, the line of gravity is shifted from one tread to the next via each foot, and greater stability is achieved with contact of the total foot than with the ball of the foot. The ball of the foot, however, usually makes the initial contact with the tread; thus, the body weight may gradually be lowered the final centimeters of the total distance of descent.

People may turn the foot for a diagonal placement if the foot is too long for the tread width. This pattern is noted frequently in persons running downstairs. However, in this case the ball of the foot may be the only part of the foot contacting the stairs. A person using a fast descent allows gravity to accelerate the descent of the body, minimizing the amount of eccentric muscle con-

MINI-LABORATORY LEARNING EXPERIENCE

1. Measure the angles at the knee and hip for people of different heights as each assumes a stair-ascending position with each foot on a different tread. Rank the people with respect to ease of ascent, based solely on the collected data. Give reasons for your ranking.
2. Calculate the work done by four individuals of different body weight when they are ascending one set of stairs, using the following formula:

Body weight × total height of stairs = work done

3. Calculate the maximum power achieved by these same individuals when they ascend this same set of stairs as fast as possible, using the following formula:

Work divided by time of ascent = power

4. Ask one person performing in steps 2 and 3 to perform with a backpack, heavy coat, heavy boots, or other weight attached or carried. Calculate work and power. (*Note:* Body weight now includes the addition of clothing or load.)
5. Discuss the results of steps 2 to 4.

traction. The person has confidence that the end of the stairway will be reached before the acceleration causes lack of body control.

Changing Levels of Movement-Immature and Aging Group

Rising from a bed or chair and lowering oneself to these pieces of furniture involve the same general principles as in locomotion on stairs. Weak quadriceps muscles usually cause the difficulty in rising from furniture. The lower the furniture, the more difficulty the person will encounter, since he or she must perform more work (i.e., raise the center of gravity a greater distance) and will begin the movement at an unfavorable angle of muscle pull. In addition, the type of material and the construction of the furniture seat influence the method of rising. Mattresses and cushions do not provide a sufficiently rigid surface for the generation of reactive forces and therefore pose a greater problem than do rigid chairs.

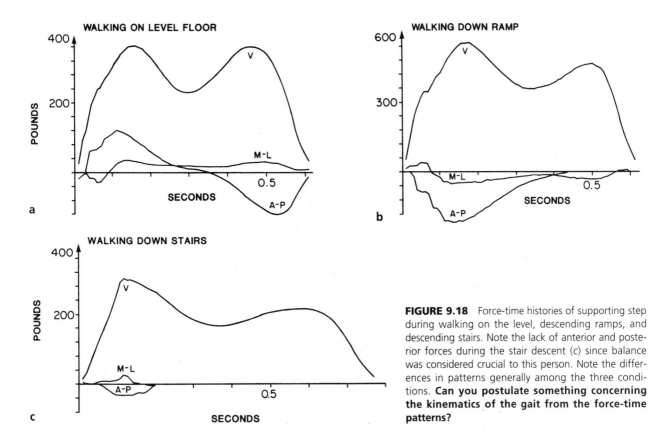

FIGURE 9.18 Force-time histories of supporting step during walking on the level, descending ramps, and descending stairs. Note the lack of anterior and posterior forces during the stair descent (c) since balance was considered crucial to this person. Note the differences in patterns generally among the three conditions. **Can you postulate something concerning the kinematics of the gait from the force-time patterns?**

The following general principles and movement analysis are useful for the improvement of the act of rising from furniture. The first action by the person desiring to rise from a chair is to move the center of gravity near the edge of the chair seat. Next, the person places one foot under the chair and one foot slightly in front of the chair legs. The person shifts the center of gravity over the new base of support, the feet, and stands by means of leg extension. If the muscles of the leg are not strong enough to raise the body weight at the initial angle of execution, the person may accelerate the trunk by alternating actions in the sagittal plane and may use the acceleration (which might be redefined as energy or momentum) of that body part to assist the muscles of the legs to create the necessary force to lift the weight of the body. In addition, the arms can be used to add a counterforce to the body weight by pushing against the chair or against the thighs. The latter action directly aids in extension at the knee joint.

MINI-LABORATORY LEARNING EXPERiENCE

Read (1966) studied the force-time patterns of older women walking on the level, descending stairs, and descending ramps. Typical results are shown in Figure 9.18. Based on these results, answer the following questions:

1. Which environment requires greatest forward or backward push? Which requires least?
2. In which environment is the vertical force greatest?
3. If a person had osteoporosis of the femur, which environment would be most traumatizing?
4. What are the unique problems of each environment?

Another example of the use of momentum of a body part to facilitate the performance of a movement pattern is found in the act of rising from a bed. Since the full length of the body may be distributed on the bed, the legs can be raised from the bed and then allowed to swing toward the floor with the help of gravity. This leg swing then raises the trunk to a sitting position. If the leg swing is facilitated by muscle contraction, the momentum of the leg swing may produce enough trunk motion to propel the person into a standing position with the help of a hand push against the bed. This technique uses both the strong muscles that cross the hip joint and the momentum of approximately one-third of the body mass to compensate for weak muscles crossing the knee.

Other Actions

Stooping, squatting, and sitting on the floor or ground are patterns common to scrubbing floors, placing items in drawers and cabinets, dusting furniture, picking up shoes and other items from the floor, and doing certain gardening tasks. With the advent of many labor saving devices, some of these tasks have been eliminated from daily activity patterns, and others have even been eliminated altogether. There are instances, however, when stooping or sitting on the floor may be necessary and desirable. Most labor-saving tools do not find items that are dropped on the floor, do not clean the corners of the room, and are not worth the cost or effort for such tasks as putting one potted plant into the ground. These activities require greater ranges of motion at the hip and knee joints than walking and stair locomotion. Greater strength is needed to initiate the upward movement from the squat or sitting position on the floor than is required to rise from a chair or bed.

Rising From the Floor

There are numerous ways to descend to and rise from the floor-sitting position. Persons over 70 years of age and young children select methods on an individual

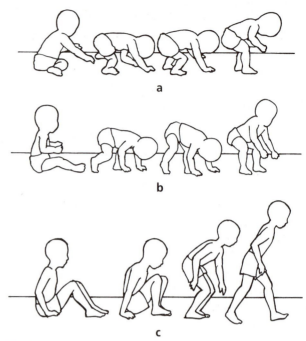

FIGURE 9.19 Three patterns of rising from floor. Depending upon anthropometry, muscular strength, and balance, persons will prefer one pattern over another.

basis. Three patterns of young children are shown in Figure 9.19. Older people use all these patterns. The strength of the quadriceps with respect to body weight, the distribution of body weight, balancing capabilities, and previous experiences with success at the initial learning age are some reasons for the particular method a person selects. Several patterns are nevertheless possible because none requires maximum contraction of muscles. Therefore, persons can be inefficient until the task becomes one of maximum, or nearly maximum, effort because of a physical disability. Then efficiency is sought in the pattern. For example, efficiency is a necessary requirement in teaching a stroke patient to rise from the floor.

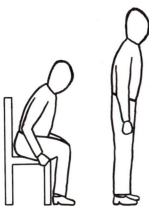

FIGURE 9.20 Kinematic sequence of an elderly man rising from a chair.

Rising From a Chair

Figure 9.20 shows an elderly person rising from a chair. The elderly man has moved his center of gravity forward, made use of his hip flexors, and moved his feet nearer the chair to have his center of gravity under the base of support.

Guidelines for Evaluation of ADL Performances within the Life Space Environment

Use these guidelines to evaluate ADL performers:

1. Is the coefficient of friction optimum for prevention of slipping and generation of force? If not, which surfaces can be changed? Determine how changes can be made.
2. Assess the body weight, specific muscle strength of "acting muscles," postural deviations, and neuromuscular functioning (such as balance) to determine which factors are probable causes of ADL dysfunction. Determine how to modify the pattern or correct the factor.
3. Do imposed environmental conditions, such as carrying packages, interfere with an otherwise skilled movement pattern? If so, use the principles of moments and the assistance of devices to alleviate the problem.

MINI-LABORATORY LEARNING EXPERIENCE

People desiring to perform the squat after not having attempted a squat for some time should test their ability to do so in this way:

1. If possible, perform the movement in water.
2. Assume the squat position while horizontal to check the range of motion and to eliminate the effect of gravity.
3. Assume a semisquat position.
4. With the assistance of a person, chair, or some other aid, assume the squat position.

At the first sign of pain, the movement should be discontinued until strengthening exercises can increase the stability of the knee joint.

References

Adrian, M., Toole, T., and Randall, L. 1984. Presentation at Computer Learning Session at AAHPERD National Convention, Anaheim, CA.

Amar, J. 1920. The human motor. New York: Dutton.

Andriacchi, T. P., Ogle, J. A., and Galante, O. 1977. Walking speed as a basis for normal and abnormal gait measurements. *Journal of Biomechanics* 10:261.

Aniansson, A. 1980. Muscle function in old age with special reference to muscle morphology, effect of training, and capacity in activities in daily living. Ph.D. thesis, University of Göteborg, Sweden.

Armstrong, C. W., and Nash, M. 1983. Performance error identification as a function of visual and verbal training. *Abstracts of Research Papers* 48.

Baird, J. 1959. Energy costs of women during walking. Ph.D. dissertation, University of Southern California.

Barclay, C., and Newell, K. 1980. Children's processing of information in motor skill acquisition. *Journal of Experimental Child Psychology* 30:89–108.

Bates, B. T., James, S. L., and Osternig, L. R. 1978. The use of orthotic devices to modify foot mechanics. *Journal of Biomechanics* 11:210.

Cooper, John M. 1991. Some practical observations regarding the elderly. *Biomechanics in sports IX:* Proceedings of the Ninth Symposium on Biomechanics, Ames, IA.

Cozzallio, E. R. 1986. The development of an assessment instrument for screening selected gross motor skills of kindergarten children, Dissertation Abstracts International 47:118A (University Microfilms No. DA8604166).

Gallahue, D. L. 1990. *Understanding motor development: Infants, children, and adolescents.* Indianapolis: Benchmark Press.

Gallahue, D., Werner P., and Luedke, G. 1975. *A conceptual approach to moving and learning.* New York: Wiley.

Griffin, M. R. 1984. The utilization of product and process measures to compare the throwing, striking and kicking proficiency of third- and fifth-grade students, Dissertation Abstracts International 45:279A (University Microfilms No. DA8427302).

Hoffman, S. J. 1983. Clinical diagnosis as a pedagogical skill. In *Teaching in physical education,* ed. T. J. Templin and J. K. Olson. Champaign, IL: Human Kinetics.

Johnson, V. 1989. The effect of age on the sit-stand patterns in women. Ph.D. dissertation, Indiana University.

Kelly, L. E., Dagger, J., and Walkley, J. 1989. The effects of an assessment-based physical education program on motion skill development in preschool children. *Education and Treatment of Children* 12(2):152–64.

Klinger, A., Masataka, T., Adrian, M., and Smith, E. 1980. Unpublished report presented to AAHPERD Research Symposium.

Morgan, W. R., and Garrett, G. E. 1984. A developmental instructional approach: Learning basic track and field skills. In *Proceedings for the 2nd national symposium on teaching kinesiology and biomechanics in sports,* ed. R. Shapiro and R. J. C. Marett, pp. 97–104, AAHPERD: Reston, VA.

Morton, D., and Fuller, D. 1952. *Human locomotion and body form.* Baltimore: Williams and Wilkins.

Newell, K. 1976. Knowledge of results and motor learning. In *Exercise and Sports Science Reviews,* vol. 4, ed. J. Keough, and R. Hutton. Santa Barbara, CA: Journal Publishing Affiliates.

Newell, K., and Kennedy, J. 1978. Knowledge of results and children's motor learning. *Dev. Psych.* 14:531–36.

Read, K. 1986. Walking patterns of older women on the level, descending stairs, and descending ramps. Master's Thesis, University of Illinois at Urbana, Champaign.

Rink, J. 1985. *Teaching physical education for learning.* St. Louis: Mosby.

Safrit, M. J. 1981. *Evaluation in physical education,* 2nd ed. Englewood Cliffs, NJ: Prentice-Hall.

Saunders, J., Inman, V., and Eberhart, H. 1953. Major determinants in normal and pathological gait. *J. Bone Joint Surg* 35A:543–58.

Seefeldt, V., and Haubenstricker, J. 1982. Patterns, phases, or stages: An analytical model for the study of developmental movement. In *The development of movement control and coordination,* ed. J. A. S. Deslo and J. E. Clark. New York: John Wiley.

Siedentop, D. 1983. *Developing teaching skills in physical education,* 2nd ed. Palo Alto, CA: Mayfield.

Singer, R. 1980. *Motor Learning and Human Performance: An application to motor skills and movement behaviors.* New York: Macmillan.

Steindler, A. 1955. Kinesiology of the human body under normal and pathological conditions. Springfield, IL: Charles C. Thomas.

Wild, M. R. 1938. The behavior pattern of throwing and some observations concerning its course of development in children. *Research Quarterly* 9:20–24.

10 Biomechanics of Exercise

Can exercises be placed into categories? Are there procedures to use in designing and evaluating exercises? We explore and assess different types of exercises in this chapter to provide guidelines to answer these questions.

Biomechanical assessment of exercise can reduce its risk of injury and maximize its benefits. Exercises should be based on biomechanical as well as physiological principles. For example, if the goal of an exercise is to strengthen the pectoralis major muscle, one cannot assume that the posture selected will, in fact, cause the pectoralis major to contract as the primary muscle. The exerciser must scientifically position the body parts in the planes of desired muscle function. Furthermore, the posture selected to perform the exercise must not cause excessive stress to the spine, as illustrated in Figure 10.1. In one of the body postures depicted, the lumbar curvature is increased dangerously.

■ An important, although not often-considered, contribution of biomechanical assessment of exercise postures and movement patterns is reduction of the risk of injury during exercise.

Biomechanical assessment of exercise maximizes the benefits of the exercise. For example, if range of motion at a joint is to be increased, the movement must be performed in the plane of desired increase throughout the entire possible range of motion and with the adjacent body parts positioned to facilitate stretch. This does not happen automatically. One of the most common examples of changes in plane of movement is noted during the exercise to increase range of horizontal extension at the shoulder. The arms begin the movement at shoulder level and usually drop during the backward stretch, rather than remaining at shoulder height. The correct and incorrect executions of this exercise are depicted in Figure 10.2.

■ Biomechanical assessment of an exercise contributes to maximizing the benefits of the performance.

The goals of the exercise should be clearly defined, and the exercise pattern executed in such a way to assure that the goals will be achieved. One common goal is to maximize the benefits and minimize the risks of injury. For example, the movements must be precisely performed and the posture, speed, load, and other aspects of the exercise determined based on the goals. This helps prevent deleterious side effects.

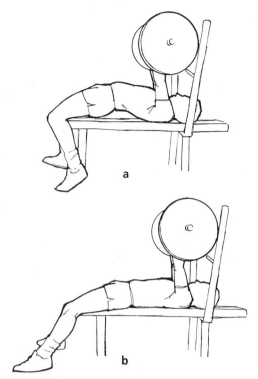

FIGURE 10.1 Two people performing the bench press. Note the excessive lumbar curvature in a. This posture is less safe than that of b. Physical condition influences how the people perform the exercise.

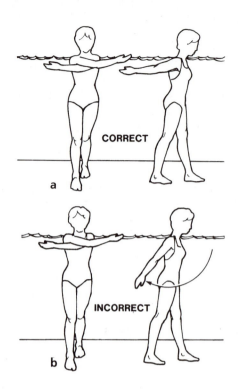

FIGURE 10.2 Horizontal extension exercise performed correctly by (a) and incorrectly by (b). B includes movement in a plane other than the horizontal and does not maximize muscular strength development of the pectoralis muscle or at the shoulder.

Guidelines for Biomechanical Design and Evaluation of Exercises

Today, most people interested in exercising want scientifically designed programs, ways to monitor their effort, and display devices for visual feedback of their achievements. A synthesis of knowledge from physiology, anatomy, physics, and biomechanics is essential, not only to design exercises, but also to analyze performance of the exercises. In addition, cultural, sociological, and psychological aspects also influence the specific exercises people choose. Since several exercises usually elicit similar benefits, performers select the most appealing one.

Basic guidelines for biomechanical design and evaluation of exercise are:

1. **State the goal precisely.** Is the goal to (a) increase strength in a particular muscle, (b) increase range of motion at a particular joint and in a particular plane, (c) increase decision-making skills with respect to type of movement and timing of movement, or (d) enhance kinestheses and balance? Be specific in stating the goal of the exercise. It is not enough to state that the goal is to improve one's ability to play volleyball. What are the necessary physical requirements? These requirements might be greater maximum leg strength or explosive power, increased range of motion at the shoulder, increased hand flexion, etc.

2. **Identify the exercises that could fulfill the goal.** There are numerous sources in which exercises can be found. Select the most appropriate for the population that will perform the exercises. Consider factors such as age, experience, strength, physical condition, and convenience. If no existing documented or published exercises appear appropriate, use biomechanical knowledge to define a beneficial exercise.

3. **Determine the minimum characteristics required of the person for success.** Based on the literature or empirical research, identify the average strength requirement, ROM requirements, and other characteristics a person must possess to perform the exercise. Identify stress to joints and any other potential dangers to the person. If a person has a physical impairment, how can you modify the exercise for safe and effective performance?

4. **Determine the body position required to initiate the exercise.** Define the body alignment and posture necessary to fixate the body parts required to stabilize and facilitate specific movements.

5. **Describe exactly the movement to be executed.** Form a mental image of the sequence of movements.

6. **Identify probable execution problems.** Identify likely problems in executing the required movement. At which instances during the exercise is the person likely to arch the back, lean with the trunk, or rotate a leg or arm in such a way that the benefits are reduced and/or potential for injury is increased?

7. **Evaluate the performance.** Ask the person to perform the exercise and evaluate the performance with respect to safety and technique. Modify performance if necessary.

8. **Determine duration, intensity, and frequency of exercise performance.** Ability to perform and improve performance is based on the triad of exercise prescription: DIF (duration, intensity, and frequency). These three components will be explained in the following section, since they should be used in all exercise prescription. An acronym to remember is that "DIF makes all the difference" between maximizing benefits from exercise or exercising for little or no gain.

Strength Exercises

Strength exercises not only improve the strength of muscles, but may also strengthen the bones, ligaments, and

---

Exercise Categories

It is easier to discuss the biomechanical principles of exercise if we can categorize each exercise into one of four types. The categories are based on the primary body structures affected (changed/developed/enhanced) through exercise. The four categories are:

1. **Strength exercises.** Exercises to improve strength and power of muscles, ligaments, and bones
2. **Flexibility and stretching exercises.** Exercises to increase range of motion at the joints
3. **Neuromuscular exercises.** Exercises to increase neuromuscular functioning, such as agility, balance, and coordination
4. **Cardiovascular-respiratory exercises.** Exercises to improve anaerobic/aerobic capacity

---

tendons. This strengthening occurs since the muscles exert their contractile forces on the tendons and bones directly and the ligaments increase tension as a result of movement or fixation of the bones to which the ligaments are attached. Although we can measure bone strength through densiometry techniques (see Chapter 3), that measurement is usually relegated to the research laboratory. Ligament and tendon strength also are usually not measured in the exercise setting. Thus, we only consider the muscles in this biomechanics of exercise chapter. Muscular strength can be measured by determining the maximum force that can be exerted, such as the maximum weight that can be lifted. Consider also other aspects of muscle development.

Strength exercises consist of exercises to improve strength, endurance, and power. The exercises may be static (isometric contractions of muscles) or dynamic movements requiring concentric or eccentric contractions within various constraints. The effect of these muscle contractions is measured by the following formulas:

1. load (force/weight)
2. work (load × displacement)
3. power (work divided by time to perform the work)

Strength exercises also can be measured according to the torques (moments of force) placed on the joints and subsequent stress to the tissues comprising the joint. Knowledge of moment arms and muscle angles of pull, as well as the ability to estimate their magnitudes, will allow exercise directors and participants to determine the relative difficulty of each selected exercise. They will also be able to determine the safe initial load and starting and ending positions and to progressively increase the load according to the gains in strength. In this way, they can formulate the optimum regimen for improvement of strength. (Refer to Chapter 4.)

Measurement of Load, Torque, Work, and Power

Measuring load, torque, work, and power is easiest if people use free weights or weight machines. In such conditions, the load or torque is known. If people perform exercises involving their own bodies as the loadings, such as when performing push-ups, the calculation of load is more complicated. In this example, the load is a percent of body weight, specific to each exerciser. Likewise, the length of arms determines the displacement variable for calculating work during a chin-up. The anatomy, environment, and movement must be considered when calculating load, torque, work, and power.

■ Differences in anthropometric characteristics result in differences in the work produced by two persons lifting the same external load or performing the same exercise with their bodies as the load.

We determine the intensity of the work performed in an exercise by the amount of muscle effort required to move the external weight through a distance and at a specific speed. A viable method of estimating the intensity of an exercise is the calculation of work performed during the movement. In the leg press, the work performed is equal to the product of the distance the weight is raised and the magnitude of the weights. Work performance with respect to a given exercise usually differs among individuals. For example, the tall, long-legged person might raise a weight of 200 lb (454 N) a distance of one foot (0.28 m), while a short, short-legged person might only raise the weight half that distance. The work done would be only half as great. Total work is equal to the amount of work for each lift multiplied by the number of lifts (repetitions). In the case of the tall and short

person, ten repetitions would be equal to 454 N × 0.28 m × 10 for the tall person and only 454 N × 0.14 m × 10 for the short person. Work is in units of newton-meters, which are equal to joules.

■ Equalizing the number of repetitions for all people in an exercise class does not equalize the work done, but overtaxes some individuals and undertaxes others.

Not only may the distance the body is moved differ, but the resistance (load) differs. A heavier person will perform more work than a lighter person, despite the fact that each executes the same exercise. This difference may be only of slight importance if both individuals have appropriate muscle mass. If one individual has predominantly fat (adipose tissue) and another person has predominantly muscle, the inequality with respect to intensity of exercise is magnified. Without a biomechanical assessment, optimum levels of duration and intensity cannot be achieved. The danger of excessive overload in strength training is high. This is especially true in arm strength exercises, such as pull-ups and push-ups. Pull-ups and push-ups have always been easier for short-armed ectomorphic/mesomorphic individuals to perform. For example, male and female gymnasts are always at the top of arm strength performance scales. Refer to Table 10.1 for comparison of force required and work done by short, medium, and tall individuals (with corresponding arms lengths), both muscular and obese, when performing chin-ups.

MINI-LABORATORY LEARNING EXPERIENCE

Rank the level of muscular fitness of the six people listed in Table 10.1 based on the following different criteria:

1. Number of repetitions performed
2. Work done for one chin-up
3. Total work done
4. Adjusted total work done using the exercise: equalizing equations

Discuss the results.

TABLE 10.1 Work performed by people with different anthropometric characteristics. One chin-up and the maximum number of chin-ups.

Subject	Arm Length (cm)	Body Weight (newtons)	One Chin-Up (newton-meters*)	Repetitions Performed	Total Work Done (NM)
Muscular persons	55	600	330	10	3300
	48	500	240	15	3600
	39	445	174	20	3480
Obese persons	55	600	330	2	660
	48	500	240	3	720
	39	445	174	4	696

*A newton-meter (Nm) is equivalent to a joule.

Exercise-Equalizing Equation

In order to equalize work done, we propose an exercise-equalizing equation. This equation is based on the available muscle mass, the body weight, and the anthropometric lengths of the body. Unfortunately, we can only estimate muscle mass in the exercise situation. This is a limitation of the equation; however, it has greater validity than existing age- and sex-related norms. The exercise equalizing equation is:

Adjusted work = work performed × adjusted lean body weight

Work performed = Number of repetitions × (weight lifted + body segment weight lifted) + displacement of weight

Adjusted lean body weight = equalizing factor percentage lean body weight

The equalizing factor is based on average percentage lean body weight. Thus, people with average lean body mass will have no adjustment in work performed. People with greater lean body mass (more muscular) will "receive credit for less work than actually performed," and persons with less lean body mass (obese) will "receive credit for more work than actually performed." Application of the exercise-equalizing equation to these three cases is:

fat = 20%, Adj. Work = 1.0 × Work (average)
fat = 30%, Adj. Work = 1.1 × Work (obese)
fat = 10%, Adj. Work = .09 × Work (muscular)

MINI-LABORATORY LEARNING EXPERIENCE

1. Using the data from Table 10.1, estimate the work when performing the following:
   a. Pull-ups from leaning position in which two-thirds of the body weight rests on the feet
   b. Push-ups from a knee support position in which one-half of the body weight rests on the knees
2. Assume that the lean body weight is 85% for the muscular persons and 70% for the obese persons. Using the exercise-equalizing equation, calculate the adjusted work for exercises in step 1.

This basic concept of individualized work also has implications when considering the amount of time (duration) spent engaging in a specific exercise and the production of power. If ten repetitions are required of all persons in an exercise class, some people will take longer to perform these ten repetitions than will others. This usually results in the muscles of slower moving and taller people contracting for a longer period of time. Both work and power are affected. These faster actions are performed at the expense of greater accelerations and greater muscle force.

■ Use caution when prescribing exercises that involve body weight as the resistance.

Isometric Exercise

Although isometric exercises produce no actual work, they may be useful in strengthening muscle groups. In particular, people who have broken or sprained a body part will find that isometric exercises are the only possible exercises to prevent atrophy of certain muscles enclosed in a cast. This type of exercise is convenient to perform and appeals to people who do not wish to exert themselves unduly or perspire while exercising. Persons with high blood pressure and certain other heart conditions should refrain from executing this type of exercise. Since occlusion of the blood supply to the muscle occurs, and since people reflexively tend to hold their breath during isometric exercises, the duration of each muscle contraction should be short, preferably less than six seconds. Counting is a useful means of achieving normal breathing during isometric exercises.

Isometric contractions can be combined with yoga exercises and tension-control programs, which will be described in later sections of this chapter. Isometric exercises have the following limitations: (1) Muscle strength improves primarily at the angle at which isometrics are performed, and (2) selected muscle fibers are activated. Thus, it is unlikely that a muscle will be strengthened throughout the range of motion solely by the use of isometric exercises. Neither will all the muscle fibers be activated by isometrics.

Concentric and Eccentric Exercises

Concentric exercise is known as positive work and **eccentric exercise** is known as negative work. When performing exercise the negative work usually is discounted and not calculated. For example, work is calculated for the action of lifting a weight, but no credit is given for lowering the weight. We advocate that exercise credit be given for eccentric exercise, especially when isokinetic machines are used. A popular name for strength exercises in which a constant weight is used is isotonic exercise. When loading varies or remains constant, but the velocity remains constant, the exercise is known as an isokinetic exercise. Both types of exercises will be discussed in this section.

Isotonic exercises, though misnamed since muscular tension is not a constant magnitude throughout the exercise, are the most common. Nordin and Frankel have renamed this type of exercise in which an unchanging external load is applied *isoinertial* exercise. The exercised body part moves through an angular displacement, as when weights are used and in everyday tasks. Quite often, however, when weights are being lifted the starting position is a weak position. Thus, the capability of the muscle at all positions other than the starting position is not even approached during this exercise. Furthermore, the person exercising in this manner is likely to accelerate the weight rapidly after the initial inertia is overcome, causing momentum to be the primary force throughout the remainder of the movement. Because muscle action is necessary merely to begin movement, strength is not developed in other segments of the range of motion to the same degree as at the start of the movement. To ensure maximum benefits from isotonic exercises, the performer should move at a nearly constant velocity rather than allow momentum to vary and facilitate the movement.

The use of free weights, such as barbells in weightlifting competition, is a classic example of the use of acceleration to enable the lifter to succeed. If the timing is exactly correct—that is, if the barbell has begun to accelerate upward—the lifter can change from a position in which the shoulders are above the bar to one in which the shoulders are below the bar. Full arm extension can then be used to lift the weight above the head. In other lifts, the bar may be swung toward the thighs to reduce the moment arm and use the inward swing to overcome the inertia of the stationary bar.

Plyometrics

Isotonic exercises as described in the previous section have been of the concentric contraction type. **Plyometric exercises** take advantage of eccentric contractions of muscles to facilitate performance. The portion of this contraction activated by muscle elasticity and by stretch reflex is not known, but both have been implicated (Kilani 1988). Plyometric depth jumping is the most popular form of eccentric exercise. The person drops from an elevation, lands, and immediately jumps to another elevated platform. The act of landing and preparing to jump again involves eccentric contractions and muscular strength gains. Limitations on elevations and use of weights must be made to avoid injury to the joints. Inability to control the landings is a potential trauma-producing problem and care must be taken to design a safe situation. Start with drops of 2–6 in. and progress to higher elevations. Trauma to the body can be estimated by performing these depth jumps onto a force platform. Other plyometric information appears in Chapters 5 and 11.

Isokinetic Exercises

The concepts of zero acceleration and graphic output of the force applied during exercise was incorporated into strength-conditioning programs in the 1960s. This system of exercising was termed *isokinetics*. Since the limb is not allowed to accelerate, muscle force must be used throughout the exercise. The addition of graphic displays of the force-time curve or force-angle curve ensures that the performer attempts to apply muscle force throughout the exercise rather than "cheat through the move," or "throw the limb."

Isokinetic machines can be set to move at various specified rates for improvement of strength or power. Both the resistance and the speed can be varied, providing a variety of work outputs. Since the same work output may be produced by using either a high resistance (force) with low velocity or a low resistance with high velocity, the product of force × distance × repetitions (total work produced) may be identical for a given time period.

Isokinetic devices have made it possible to assess power quantitatively and exercise in a more scientific manner than was possible previously. However, these devices have limitations in speed; only the very latest machines have maximum speeds (600°/s) approaching those used in sports. Since so many sports movements require power, it is important to construct exercises to improve power. Such exercises are designed to increase the velocity at which loads of varying weights can be moved.

Understanding Muscle Torques

When weights are lifted from a semi-squat or full-squat position, there is a danger of injuring the joints (ankle, knee, hip, lumbar spine) because of the increased moments of force (torques) acting at these joints. You might suppose that the moments of force would increase

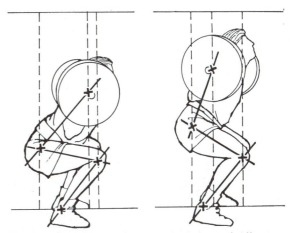

FIGURE 10.3 Squat performances by persons of different anthropometry. The weight line and moment arm from various joints are drawn so that the relative moment at these joints could be estimated. Each weightlifter is 850 N and the scale is 20:1.

proportionately with the increase in weight lifted. But this linear relationship does not always exist with human beings. As the weight changes, the person changes the kinematics of the lift. Furthermore, all persons do not change their kinematics in the same fashion. Hay, Andrews, and Vaughan (1983) found that one lifter, in changing from a weight 60% of maximum to one 80% of maximum, increased the moment of force at the knee two-fold, while another individual showed a *decrease* in the moment of force at the knee.

■ The most important factor for safety *and* improvement is the manner in which a weight is lifted.

MINI-LABORATORY LEARNING EXPERIENCE

Using the information in Chapter 4, identify the moments of force for each of the squat performers in Fig. 10.3. Which joint has the greatest moment? Anthropometric data influence the performers since they shift body segment positions to maintain equilibrium. The scale is 20:1 and each lifter has a body weight of 850 N and is lifting the same weight.

Increasing the resistance may produce different bene-fits or may pose different dangers than are found with the lighter resistance. For example, arm extensions with free weights or attached weights may not increase the strength of the triceps brachii because performers may rotate the arms outward and thus use the strong shoulder girdle muscles (rhomboids) to change the angle at the shoulder. This change in angle may cause the arm to ac-celerate so that the weaker triceps brachii can be assisted in producing extension at the elbow. Other compensa-tions may include rotation of the body along its longitu-dinal axis and the use of the momentum of the body and the stronger arm to begin the arm extension. The weaker arm is therefore bypassed or allowed to extend only after upward acceleration has occurred. Body lean and other kinematic actions can be observed when performers are compensating. EMG studies are useful to determine which muscles *are* active when performing a certain ex-ercise and which *should be* active.

■ When lifting free weights, the number of muscles required to stabilize the body are greater than when the body is fixed in a weightlifting machine.

Torques during Sit-ups.　Since the human being walks on two feet in an upright position, the anterior muscles of the trunk tend to be underdeveloped and weak. The abdominal muscles in particular are usually inadequate for protection of the lumbar curve of the spine during both heavy lifting and carrying a fetus. To understand the role of the abdominal muscles, ask a person to lie in the supine position. When a person is lying supine, the lumbar curve increases, and people usually can place their hands under the curvature without encountering re-sistance. This increased curvature causes an increase in compression at the posterior edges of the disks and the superior/inferior articular facets of the vertebrae. The rectus abdominis muscle can contract to tilt the pelvis and thereby decrease the curve and reduce the stress to the spine. If the abdominal muscle is not strong enough to reduce this stress, there is potential danger of damag-ing the disks during sit-ups and other lifting activities.

One of the most common abdominal strengthening exercises is the sit-up, with its many variations. As the sit-up is initiated, the iliopsoas muscle contracts, tilting the pelvis into an increased lumbar curve and preventing

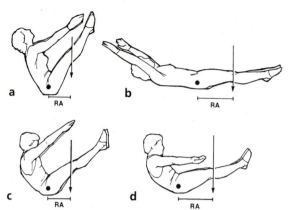

FIGURE 10.4　Differences in moment arms during V-type sit-ups. Arrows represent gravitational force acting on legs (weight of legs); RA, moment arm of resistance (hip to weight vector). The moment of force acting counterclockwise on legs opposing the muscle effort can be calculated using RA = 45 cm (in *d*) and weight of legs = 325 N. Note that the moment arm in *c* is approxi-mately two-thirds of that in *d*. **Calculate the moment in *a*. If the woman weighs 590 N (130 lbs.) and her legs are 40% of body weight, what would the muscle moments for her be?**

trunk flexion. This lack of trunk flexion prevents the shortening of the moment arm of the part of the body being lifted from the floor. Only the anterior ligaments and muscles can oppose this resistance moment. Thus, the rectus abdominis contracts to decrease the lumbar curve, facilitating trunk flexion during the sit-up and re-ducing the stress to the lumbar vertebrae.

Based on the equation of moments of force, a selec-tion of graduated exercises may be made. The differ-ences in resistance moments during various sit-ups is il-lustrated in Figure 10.4. The resistance is equal to the weight of the upper body, that is, from the hip joint to the top of the head, including the arms. The moment arm measured by the distance from the hip joint to the center of gravity of the upper body according to the dis-tribution of the body parts. When an external weight is added to the upper body, the total resistance is the sum of this external weight and the weight of the legs on the resultant resistance moments of force that are illustrated in Figure 10.4.

■ For some individuals, the sit-up is a high overload. These people should not perform sit-ups.

To understand the anatomy of the body it it necessary to know precisely what roles the muscles are likely to perform. In the example of the sit-up, the rectus abdominis does not create flexion at the hip joint or cause the sit-up action. It stabilizes the pelvis in the desired position to prevent injury to the spine, and it facilitates the flexed trunk position. The action of the iliopsoas and other flexors at the hip can be more nearly equalized with that of the rectus abdominis by performing sit-ups; quite often this gain in strength is several times greater than the strength gain in the abdominal muscles. If the trunk is not flexed during sit-ups, little gain in abdominal strength results. Thus, rather than the complete sit-up, persons with weak abdominal muscles might well do head and shoulder raises, static "V" sitting positions, or sit-downs.

Flexibility and Stretching Exercises

Range of motion (ROM) exercises are designed to increase the mobility of all joints of the body in all the planes possible for each joint. For maintenance of ROM, one may exercise faster and less often than if specific movements are to be enhanced. As with strength exercises, care must be taken to prevent an increase in performance in one plane or direction at the expense of performance in another plane or direction. For example, exercises to increase plantar flexion of the foot without concomitant exercise to increase dorsiflexion are likely to cause a foreshortening of the Achilles tendon or triceps surae muscle or both, severely limiting the amount of dorsiflexion possible. Such a condition causes pain in walking barefoot or uphill.

■ Most ROM exercises are designed to improve posture and symmetry of body.

The ROM exercises lengthen certain muscles, increasing ROM at a joint, and attempt to equalize the respective roles of agonist and antagonist muscles. Since the shortened muscle is usually stronger than the lengthened muscle, strength exercises should compliment ROM exercises.

ROM exercises may be performed alone, with the aid of others who produce a force (passive exercise for the exerciser), or using walls, towels, or other devices. In each condition, the movement may be conducted at various speeds and with or without the influence of gravity. Yoga, Tai Chi, and other slow-moving exercises are safe and combine an isometric strength advantage with the ROM benefits. With practice and continual exercising, persons beyond the age of 40 can achieve ROM values not possible for them in their earlier years.

ROM and Speed

There is a potential danger when ROM exercises are performed with high velocities or accelerations. In these situations, either the muscle force or the force of gravity causes a momentum that may override the myotatic reflex, which normally protects the body from injury. Injury then occurs as the soft tissues are extended beyond their length and tear. In other instances, the myotatic reflex is elicited, causing a contraction in muscles that were to be lengthened and defeating the purpose of the muscle lengthening exercise.

Muscle strain or complete separation can result when one attempts to increase the length of the muscle beyond its strain limit. Older people, who have a decrease in the elastic component of the soft tissues, and people who have fibrous tissue or calcium deposits are particularly susceptible to injury if ROM exercises are performed rapidly. Exercises performed while the body is under water are especially safe for these people. Moderate speeds of movement and the use of gravity, under control, sometimes provide a means of attaining ROM goals not possible in slow movements.

ROM Benefits

The importance of biomechanically well designed ROM exercises cannot be underestimated. As with strength, the inability to perform normal ROM exercises at a specific joint may indicate severe restrictions on normal functioning and may prevent performance of some common ADL, work, or sports movements. For example, ROM limitations have prevented many people from putting on and taking off shoes and socks. Lowman (1958) has described numerous postural deviations and shown how each has a deleterious effect on athletic performance. Cardiorespiratory function and endurance, as well as movement efficiency of limbs, have been hampered.

There is evidence that athletic performance may produce postural deviation that must be corrected through appropriate ROM and strength exercises.

■ Asymmetry and postural deviation often occur because of repetition of movements in work, the arts, and sports.

Most ADL and job-related patterns of movement tend to promote kyphosis (contracted pectoralis major muscles) and elevated shoulders. These characteristics also are noted in weightlifters and persons involved in other sports. Through an assessment of ROM restrictions, individualized ROM exercises can correct unique anatomic characteristics.

Programming for ROM

If based on biomechanical principles, any range of motion exercise program would include exercises for every joint in the body, in each of the planes the joint allows an appreciable movement to occur. Assess range of motion required for sport, work, playing a musical instrument, performing basic activities of daily living, and other movement patterns prior to selecting exercises. Identify inadequate range of motion for the task and give priority to exercises that develop adequate ROM for the task. If the movements are high-acceleration sports movements, the exercises should be used to produce greater ranges of motion than the individual is capable of producing without assistance. This implies that another person or safety-controlled device should be used to place a more gradual and slightly increasing force on the body part than that which is possible by the exerciser alone. If this is not practiced, the ROM exercise may never achieve the same ROM that occurs in the sport (since dynamic ROM is greater than static ROM), and damage to the soft tissues could result. The action of another muscle or force will tear a muscle; a muscle cannot tear itself. A muscle is lengthened beyond its capabilities by the forceful contraction of an antagonist muscle, by the force of gravity, or by another person.

Neuromuscular Exercises

Neuromuscular facilitation, or perceptual-motor exercises, involves the development or maintenance of balance, speed, agility, coordination, and other eye-hand or eye-foot exercises. During the early years of life, these exercises are necessary to assist the child in learning to move effectively. Late in life, disuse, pathologic conditions, or the aging process may require people to relearn these basics. Researchers using rats as subjects have shown that exercise increases the size of neurons and facilitates neuronal pathways of the central nervous system, including enhancement of the brain. Therefore, we might speculate that continued practice of coordinated movements might improve, or at least maintain, neuromuscular functioning during the later years of life.

Eye-hand coordination skills, reaction-time skills, movement time in all possible planes of movement, eye-foot coordination skills, and bilateral, contralateral, ipsilateral, and other combinations of upper- and lower-extremity patterns can be selected and made part of a daily exercise program. Additional benefits to strength and ROM will also occur with many of these perceptual-motor exercises.

One other type of neuromuscular facilitation exercise is tension control. Basmajian (1979) states that skilled persons know how to effectively reduce the tension levels in muscles that are not necessary to a movement. The unskilled person cannot do so, and excessive tension from undesirable muscle action interferes with the success of the movement. Woods (1980) has shown that the Jacobson method of tension control is effective in learning to regulate tension levels. Again, the biomechanical principles center on the perception of a moment of force, a quantity of work, or a postural deviation. The ability to recognize and regulate tension in one muscle is the basis for achieving efficiency in movement patterns.

The ability to replicate precisely a previous movement and to determine when and how fast to perform this movement can be evaluated using analysis tools described previously. Integration of this knowledge, together with biomechanical and motor-control theory, can determine whether an exercise incorporates the desired speed, coordination, balance, and agility characteristics.

Cardiovascular Exercise

Why is biomechanical analysis a part of **cardiovascular exercise?** Although aerobic and anaerobic exercises are devised to enhance the functioning of the heart, lungs, and, in general, the respiratory and circulatory systems, the joints of the body cannot be ignored. Aerobic exercise often involves moderate to vigorous movements of a repetitive, and usually cyclic nature; the same body parts move many times in the same manner. The same joints, muscles, tendons, and ligaments are stressed repetitively. Repeated stress, occurring frequently, at short intervals, and with high magnitudes, has been termed the *overuse syndrome*. The body tissues can fatigue in the same way that a person feels fatigued. Such fatigue of tissues may result in tears, fractures, and other injuries. Such overuse has been noted in aerobic exercise, such as aerobics (aerobic dance), jogging, rope jumping, swimming, running, and bicycling. Aerobics now includes a variety of impact levels: high impact, low impact, bench stepping, Jazzercise, etc.

MINI-LABORATORY LEARNING EXPERIENCE

Biomechanical analysis of aerobic exercises is critical to reduce trauma to the body. Think about the movements in three types of aerobic exercises, other than rope jumping, and list the areas of the body most likely to experience trauma. The areas for rope jumping are: feet, knees, back, shins, hip, wrist, and shoulders.

Although the major two reasons for injury, excess repetitions and incorrect technique, are the same for all these forms of aerobic exercise, there is an important difference between aerobics and the other exercises. Aerobics often is a group activity. Other forms of exercise are usually individualized. Thus, aerobics has been chosen as an example of the application of biomechanics to aerobic exercising.*

---

*Used by permission of authors of *The complete encyclopedia of aerobics: A guide for the aerobics teacher* (Klinger, Adrian, and Tyner-Wilson 1986).

1. The greater the body weight, the greater the potential for injury.
2. Airborne activities produce greater forces to the body than do nonairborne activities.
3. Fast twisting movements of arms and upper trunk produce reaction forces in the lower back.
4. Stress is proportional to the surface area of the body receiving the force and to its magnitude.
5. The least amount of stress is placed on the joint if the bones are aligned in a straight line.
6. The knee joint supports the least stress if it is aligned above the foot during all body support phases.
7. Alignment of the trunk above the pelvis provides the greatest potential for a balanced position.
8. The farther the limbs move away from the trunk, the greater the potential loss of equilibrium.
9. The longer the limb that is swinging, the greater the reactive force at the joints.
10. The faster the limbs move away from the trunk, the greater the potential loss of equilibrium.
11. The faster the swinging movements, the greater the reactive force at the joints.
12. The greater the body segment weight, the greater the muscular strength required to perform an activity.
13. The longer the body segment, the greater the muscular strength required to perform an activity.
14. The taller the person, the more time needed to perform the activity; or the taller person compensates using greater accelerations, consequently greater muscle force.
15. Safety can be increased or decreased by modifying the intensity of an exercise.

Water Aerobics

A multitude of water aerobics programs protect the joints of the body and create an environment for safe exercise. The resistance of the water is the load, increasing with the velocity of the exercise. Hand paddles, fins, body segment weights, and other devices increase the load against which the person must work. There is no traumatic impact force, such as experienced on land.

Water aerobics are also appropriate for older people with weak musculature, people with arthritis, people with neurological deficit, especially resulting in equilibrium problems, and people with paralysis or loss of one or more limbs.

Hazardous Exercise?

We believe that no exercise is inherently hazardous. It is the way it is performed, the assumed posture, the mismatching of the exerciser's anatomy, state of health, disability, lean body weight, biological age, body mass, etc., to the exercise, and the inappropriate use of DIF that creates the hazard. Naturally, we realize that all exercises have a potential to produce injury and trauma to the body tissues. But total lack of movement is more hazardous than performing movements based on biomechanical principles. We have addressed potential problems with different styles of sit-ups and modifications made in aerobics and the introduction of water aerobics for safety in other sections in this chapter. The concepts can be generalized to all other exercises and exercise equipment.

■ The older the person, the more likely a traumatized body. Therefore, greater care must be used in prescribing correct DIF.

Jump Ropes

There are various jump ropes designed to develop strength in the upper body. Weights are placed in the handles or the rope itself is heavy and elastic. When the rope is turned the force created by its acceleration creates a pull on the shoulders or wrists. For some people the use of these ropes develops the muscles at these joints, but other people traumatize these muscles. DIF needs to be carefully evaluated. This is difficult, since there is no easy way to determine the forces created by the turning of the rope.

Weight Training

Weight training can be of two types: free weights and weight machines. The use of free weights and various types of resistance machines are more versatile ways of strength development than weight machines. The body is less restrained, and a variety of types, sizes, and magnitudes of weights can be used. Muscles are required to stabilize proximal joints and the trunk and to balance the central mass of the body. The person must learn to adjust to asymmetrical strength variations. Thus, exercising with free weights is often advocated as the "natural exercise." Weight machines, however, have the advantage of reducing the risk of injury due to inability to balance or control weights. In addition, body parts can be supported and muscle groups isolated for strength development.

The general principles of exercising hold true with weightlifting. The position and amount of lordotic curvature must be evaluated. The use of a weight belt to fix the lumbar spine is a safety measure to provide reactive forces against a stable body segment. Increasing the abdominal pressure through respiration— exhaling on the forceful lift—has an estimated 10% benefit to the performer.

■ Modeling of the spine during lifting tasks in industry is applicable to the analysis of weight training and weightlifting. Refer to Chapter 12, Occupational Biomechanics.

Deep Knee Bends

The lower a person squats, the more open the knee joint and the greater the torque. But as noted previously, the torque may be reduced by actions of the trunk as the person assumes the deep squat. We do know that the muscles, tendons, and ligaments adapt to the forces of the action, as demonstrated by the squatting postures assumed during work and rest in many Asian cultures. The problem in suggesting deep knee bends for the U.S. population is that the movement is uncommon in U.S. daily life, the loading is usually too great with respect to scientific progression of loading, and there is risk of loss of balance and subsequent creation of torsion and injury.

A listing of selected exercises and potential problems associated with each appears in Table 10.2.

MINI-LABORATORY LEARNING EXPERIENCE

1. Study Table 10.2.
2. Add other exercises to this list using biomechanical procedures.
3. Create an exercise chart for your own use.

TABLE 10.2 Sample listings of exercises and potential problems with biomechanically incorrect execution of each.

Exercise	Incorrect Action	Potential Problem
Sit-ups	Extended legs Hand pushing against back of head	Create strain to lower back muscles Create strain to neck muscles
Yoga plow	Extended legs touching floor behind head resting on floor	Stress on cervical spine
Windmill (standing alternate toe touches)	Hyperextended legs Fast or bouncing movements	Stress to poplitial muscle Strain to lower back muscles
Hurdler stretch	Flexed leg is medially rotated extended at hip	Strains knee

Exercise Equipment Evaluation

Each year, new exercise products are developed for the public, fitness centers, health spas, and other agencies. Those who create these products need to biomechanically analyze them and the related performance techniques before distribution to the public. If this is not possible, the professional in charge of these products should evaluate them prior to purchasing or immediately after acquiring them. Although standards for testing fitness equipment are almost nonexistent, committees of the American Society for Testing Materials are trying to develop standards. (Contact this national standards writing body at ASTM, 1916 Race Street, Philadelphia, PA 19103.)

Here are some questions to ask about biomechanical evaluation of fitness equipment.

1. Can persons of different sizes use the equipment in a comparable manner? For example, if a bicycle ergometer is being evaluated, can a tall exerciser and a short exerciser adjust the bicycle to enable both of them to move their legs through comparable ranges of motion? See Chapter 12 for more information on this topic and evaluate the position of the short and tall exercises in Figure 10.5.

2. Can exercisers of varying fitness levels use the equipment? For example, if leg strength is low, is the initial resistance loading on the device too high? Conversely, is the highest resistance loading too low for a potential exerciser with strong legs?

3. Is the equipment stable and otherwise safe to use? The equipment should resist pulling, pushing, and deliberate attempts to tip it. For example, will a recumbent bicycle tip if the exerciser grabs the

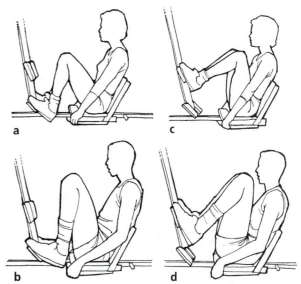

FIGURE 10.5 Two persons performing a leg press on a weight machine. Differences in body segment angles, muscle angles of push, and direction of application of force are shown for each foot plate position and each individual. Drawing a vector through the shank in *c* and *d* best estimates the direction of force application. Note the use of the balls of the feet to change the angle of force through the shank axis.

machine to maintain equilibrium when getting up from the seat?

4. Do safety limits exist, or are guidelines written for safe use?

5. What unsafe postures are likely to be assumed unless the exerciser has guidelines? For example, note the postures in Figure 10.6. Identify the position in which the body parts/tissues are at risk. Hint: compare the

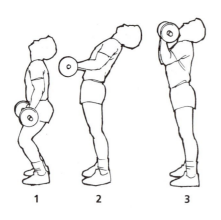

a

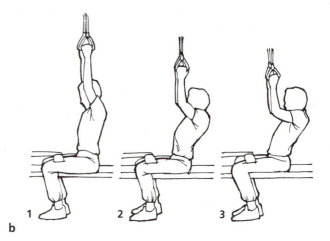

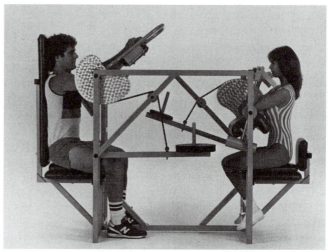

b

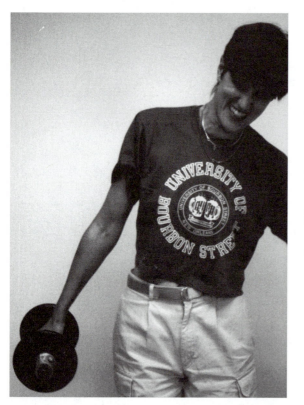

c

FIGURE 10.6 Postures used during exercising. Determine the postures in which the lordotic curvature is excessive, the body alignment is not vertical, or there is a high potential for incorrect posture.

(*d*, Universal Biceps/Triceps machine. Courtesy of Universal Gym Equipment, Inc.)

d

amounts of spinal curvature and estimate the line of gravity of the human body external load system.

6. What specific benefits can be derived from the equipment? Compare the claims of the manufacturer and the actual benefits as deduced from the performance. Identify the planes of motion, axes of rotation, probable muscles involved (strength), range of motion (flexibility), sequences of motion (coordination), and changes in line of gravity (balance).

MINI-LABORATORY LEARNING EXPERIENCE

Study the different fitness machines in Figure 10.7.

1. Describe the adjustments that needed to be made with respect to structure and design for fit of exerciser.
2. Identify the ROM and planes of motion that the exerciser uses.
3. List the probable muscles that would be strengthened by using each exercise machine.

Feedback Devices and Exercise

Almost all commercial cardiovascular exercise equipment has some form of graphic/digital display for feedback of results to the exerciser. Feedback also exists on the more expensive strength machines. Common factors displayed include duration of exercise, rate of stepping, pedalling, climbing, etc., work and/or force, heart rate, and calories burned (estimated from body weight, age, sex, and literature nomograms). Power is not usually a part of the machine displays.

Linking Machines Together. A microprocessor is connected to less expensive exercise machines for home or club use. More expensive machines now have on-board computers and use high technology software, such as Windows, and enhancements such as VGA graphics. Multiple machines, such as bicycle ergometers, can be interfaced to the same video monitor and competitive endurance races can be monitored. (See Figure 10.8.)

Controlling the Machine

Some cardiovascular devices are programmed to reduce resistance if the person's heart rate exceeds the preselected target heart rate. The machines are controlled by the heart rate of the exerciser and the workload is varied accordingly.

Programmable to the Person

Strength machines have been programmed to store prior performance. Force curves are retrieved and compared with current performance. The computer can assign load values for the workout, including specific and different loadings at various angles. Profiles of personal fitness levels and data banks of information on many people are now the state of the art in the exercise world. (See Figure 10.9.)

■ Optimization of exercise effectiveness and safety is achieved through computerized programmable feedback exercise machines.

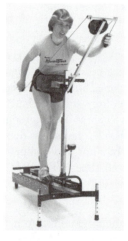

a

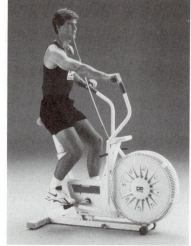

b

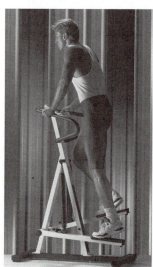

c

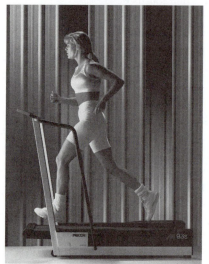

d

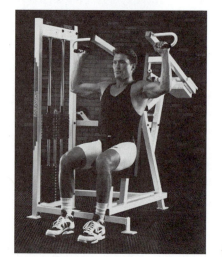

e

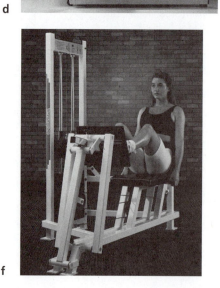

f

FIGURE 10.7 Fitness equipment machines designed for specific purposes. (*a*) Nordic Track Pro designed for aerobic enhancement and strength training of arms, upper back, and legs; (*b*) IP Airgometer for aerobics and arm and leg strengthening; (*c*) Stepper for aerobic and leg strengthening; (*d*) Treadmill with variable speed settings and inclines; (*e*) Power Circuit Shoulder Press Machine with multi-purpose hand positions which change the angle on the muscles for different workouts and also has counterbalanced lift in arm for rehabilitation patients, deconditioned users, and novices; (*f*) Power Circuit Leg Press with large foot rest and inclided seat.

(*a*, courtesy of Nordic Track; *b*, courtesy of Diversified Products; *c* and *d*, courtesy of Precor, Inc.; *e* and *f*, courtesy of Universal Gym Equipment, Inc.)

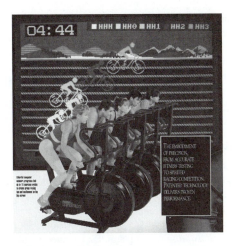

FIGURE 10.8 Bicycle ergometers linked for competitive racing in the exercise room.
(Photo reprinted with permission from StairMaster™ Sports/Medical Products, Inc. from the Windracer™ exercise cycle brochure.)

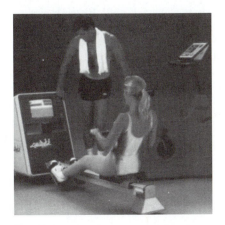

a

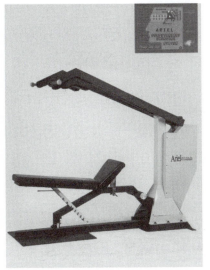

b

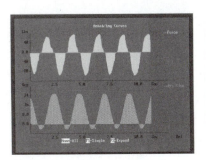

Average Force Curve combines all repetitions into an upstroke curve in the upper half of the screen and a downstroke curve in the lower half.

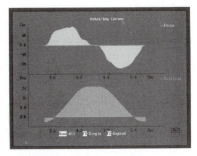

Curve Expansion identifies details of a repetition not otherwise easily distinguishable.

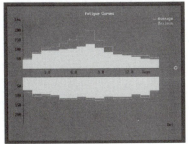

Repetition Display shows performance (upper curve) in conjunction with range of motion (lower curve).

c

Pyramid Curve displays performance as a function of controlled changes in speed or resistance.

FIGURE 10.9 High-technology feedback systems. (*a*) Rowing machine; (*b*) Ariel CES 5000 Multi-Function Strength Machine; (*c*) Functional information provided by the Ariel CES 5000 software. (*a*, courtesy of Life Fitness; *b* and *c*, courtesy of Ariel Life Systems, Inc.)

References

Ariel, G. R. 1978. Computerized dynamic resistive exercise. In F. Landry, and W. A. R. Orban, (Eds.), *Biomechanics of sports and kinanthropometry,* ed. Miami: Miami Symposia Specialists.

Basmajian, J. V. 1979. *Muscles alive: Their functions revealed by electromyography,* 4th ed. Baltimore: Williams and Wilkins.

Bedi, F. J., Cresswell, G. A., Engle, J. T., and Nicol, M. S. 1987. Increase in jumping height associated with maximal effort vertical depth jump. *Res. Q Ex & S* 58:11–15.

Cabri, J. M. H. 1991. Isokinetic strength aspects in human joints and muscles. *Applied Ergonomics* 22(5):299–302.

Flint, M. M. 1965. Selecting exercises. *JOHPER* 35:19.

Garhammer, J. 1991. Biomechanics of weight lifting and training. In *Biomechanics of sports,* ed. C. L. Vaughan. Boca Raton, FL: C.R.C. Press, Inc.

Hay, J. G., Andrews, J. G., and Vaughan, C. L. 1983. Effects of lifting rate on elbow torques exerted during arm curl exercises. *Med. Sci. Sports Exerc.* 15(1):63–71.

Kilani, H. 1988. Stretch-shortening cycle in human muscle contraction: The role of the stretch reflex in force production in various vertical jumps. Ph.D. dissertation, University of Illinois at Urbana-Champaign.

Klinger, A., Adrian, M., and Tyner-Wilson, J. 1986. *The complete encyclopedia of aerobics:* A guide for the aerobics teacher. Ithaca, NY: Mouvement Publications.

Lipetz, S., and Gutin, B. 1970. An electromyographic study of four abdominal exercises. *Med. Sci. in Sports,* 2 (1):35–38.

Lowman, C. L. 1958. Faulty posture in relation to performance. *JOHPER* 29:14.

Madsen, N., and McLaughlin, T. 1984. Kinematic factors influencing performance and injury risk in the bench press exercise. *Med. Sci. Sports Exerc.* 16 (4):376–81.

Miller, B. P., and S. L. D. 1981. Power in athletics through the process of depth jumping. Track and Field Quarterly Review 81:52–54.

Radcliffe, J. C., and Farentinos, R. C. 1985. *Plyometrics: Explosive power training.* Champaign, IL: Human Kinetics.

Ricci, B. Marchetti, M., and Figura, F. 1981. Biomechanics of sit-up exercises. *Med. Sci. Sports Exerc.* 13 (1):54–59.

Terauds, J., ed. 1979. *Science in weightlifting.* Del Mar, CA: Academic Publishers.

Woods, M. 1980. Tension control, Unpublished report, Seattle: Tension Control Clinic.

11 Rehabilitative Biomechanics

In all phases of society, there is a need for rehabilitative procedures. These include such activities as exercise, locomotion using supplemental devices and/or substitute limbs, and ADL training. Biomechanical appraisal of these procedures is essential.

What is **rehabilitative biomechanics?** It is that part of biomechanics applied to the study of movement patterns of injured and disabled persons. Why is it important? How does it integrate with occupational therapists, corrective therapists, physical therapists, and other health services and medical personnel? In general, these specialists identify dysfunctions among the population and design programs to alleviate or compensate for these dysfunctions. The rehabilitative biomechanist can aid the therapist in analyzing movement patterns, predicting forces acting on the joints, designing assistive devices, optimizing performance, and reassessing performance after rehabilitative training. A team approach is required, although some biomechanists may also have therapeutic training, and can work more independently than those without training in both therapy and biomechanics. Some therapists have a basic background in biomechanics, but this background consists primarily of anatomical biomechanics.

Major Goals of Rehabilitative Biomechanics

Rehabilitative biomechanics involves three major areas: rehabilitative exercise, rehabilitative locomotion, and ADL analyses and rehabilitation. In the latter two areas, the evaluation and use of supplementation and substitution devices are part of the biomechanists' concerns.

The goals of rehabilitative biomechanics are:

1. Define the biomechanical characteristics of the patient. Do not assume normal anatomy. Identify anomalies and assess muscle weakness.
2. Evaluate movement patterns and postures of the patient and compare these to normal patterns.
3. Determine whether normalcy of function is a realistic goal. If not, determine the compensatory pattern to be used.
4. Evaluate the exercise and training program developed by the therapist.
5. Evaluate the use of supplementation and substitution devices.
6. Assist with the design of supplementation and substitution devices.
7. Evaluate the workspace environment.
8. Conduct ADL analyses.

Rehabilitation Exercises

Traditionally, the open kinetic-chain system exercise has been used during the major part of rehabilitation exercise programs. An example of an open kinetic-chain system is a lower leg extension with a weighted boot attached to the foot while the injured person sits with the thigh fixed on a table. This system is similar to the simple lever systems described in Chapter 4. The less massive distal segment is free-moving and the more massive proximal segment is fixed.

Although the open kinetic-chain system appears to work well for rehabilitation of the upper extremities, there is some question about its efficacy in the rehabilitation of the lower extremities. During ADL, we do not tend to use our legs as open kinetic-chain systems. Most of the time our legs are used to support our body weight and apply force to the ground. Thus a closed kinetic-chain system exists. For example, in walking, the less massive segment (the foot) is fixed, and the most massive segment, the thigh "pulls the body forward" during the support phase of walking. The functional use of the leg, therefore, is very different from that of the open kinetic-chain system rehabilitative exercise. (For further information of functional use of the leg during walking, refer to Chapter 9.)

Muscle strength and range of motion can be improved using open kinetic-chain system exercise, but the forces acting on the joint may not be identical to those of closed kinetic-chain system exercises. In addition, it is known that the sensory inputs, including kinesthesis, adaptive responses, and multisegmental coordination, are not developed to any extent using the open kinetic-chain system exercise.

Comparison of Open and Closed Kinetic-Chain System Exercises

1. Each system creates different proprioceptor discharges due to differences in torsional, rotational, rolling, gliding, and sliding actions at the joints and different muscular and ligamentous tensions.
2. Open kinetic-chain system exercises generally isolate target muscles and closed kinetic-chain system exercises use stabilizing and accessory muscle groups as well as the targeted muscles.

3. Balance, coordination, and postural adjustments are required during closed kinetic-chain system exercises.
4. Closed kinetic-chain system exercises are specific to ADL functioning.
5. Larger shear forces have been measured during open kinetic-chain exercises than during "comparable" closed kinetic-chain exercises. This often occurs because of the co-contraction of muscles that stabilize the joints.

MINI-LABORATORY LEARNING EXPERIENCE

Study the figures in Chapter 10 and identify which ones are open kinetic-chain system exercises and which ones are closed kinetic-chain system exercises. Remember, the key difference is which segment is fixed and which is free-moving.

Guidelines for Rehabilitative Exercises

Keep the following guidelines in mind when working with rehabilitative exercises.

1. Move the body part slowly in order to reduce acceleration to a negligible value.
2. Allow the muscles to contract throughout the range of motion by maintaining low velocities and, therefore, controlling momentum.
3. Maintain alignment of body parts, since any change in alignment will change angles of pull and lengths of muscles, tendons, and ligaments.
4. Maintain balance of antagonist muscle groups. For example, if the exercise is to strengthen the biceps brachii, also conduct exercises to strengthen the triceps brachii.
5. Use one or more sets of exercises to improve and maintain the integrity of all structures and tissues related to the area of injury. This often includes the joints proximal and distal to the injury site.
6. Develop alternative exercises to reduce boredom and provide versatility for home and travel environments.
7. Maintain or develop aerobic capacity.

Example of Rehabilitative Exercises for the Medial Collateral Ligament of the Knee

It is important that the muscles that flex and extend the shank at the knee be strengthened. Concommitantly, the ligaments must be protected. This is usually achieved by dorsiflexing the foot and locking the knee during certain aspects of the performance of the exercises. Can you explain why?

Because the leg swings from the hip, the muscles crossing the hip joint should be strengthened, as well as the muscles and ligaments crossing the knee joint, when planning an exercise program to rehabilitate the knee. The following section discusses a series of exercises to aid you in biomechanical analysis of the anatomy involved.

The first set is a series in which the load (resistance) is only the person's body part. The number of repetitions is selected based on the severity of the injury and the physical attributes of the injured person. For example, a long-legged, an obese-legged, or a severely injured individual might perform three repetitions, while five would be the usual starting number for average people.

Open Kinetic-Chain System Exercises

1. **Sit and extend.** *Action:* Sitting on a table or chair with the knee at a right angle, the lower leg is slowly extended to the horizontal. The foot is in dorsiflexion throughout, and, at the end of the extension, the knee locks.
   Analysis. All the quadriceps femoris group of muscles contract, and the strong rectus femoris initiates the action.

2. **Long sit leg extension.** *Action:* The person sits on a table or floor with leg to be exercised extended and resting on a surface. The knee is locked and the foot dorsiflexed as the leg is lifted (flexion at the hip) from the table. The other leg is flexed and the foot placed on the table near the knee of the extended leg.
   Analysis. The rectus femorus muscle is virtually eliminated from functioning. The medial collateral ligament is protected as the vasti muscle groups are strengthened.

3. **Prone lying.** *Action:* In the prone-lying position with the foot dorsiflexed, the leg is raised (extended at hip).
   Analysis. To maintain muscle balance, the hamstrings and gluteus maximus muscles are being strengthened.

4. **Prone lying with flexed leg.** *Action:* The leg is flexed 90°, and the foot is dorsiflexed. Extension at the hip (lifting thigh from table) is executed.
   Analysis. The hamstrings are virtually ineffective and the muscles crossing the hip are strengthened.

5. **Side lying leg lift.** *Action:* Person lies on one side, flexes the lower leg, and lifts the injured leg in an abduction movement. The foot is dorsiflexed.
   Analysis. Abductor muscles crossing the hip are being strengthened.

6. **Side lying, upper leg flexed.** *Action:* Person lies on one side, flexes the upper leg and lifts the injured leg in an adduction movement. The foot is dorsiflexed.
   Analysis. The adductor magnus, brevis, and longus muscles crossing the hip are being strengthened.

7. **Stand and lift.** *Action:* In a standing position, the person flexes the lower leg to the horizontal, maintaining a vertical position of the thigh. The foot is dorsiflexed.
   Analysis. The hamstring muscles are isolated as the prime movers.

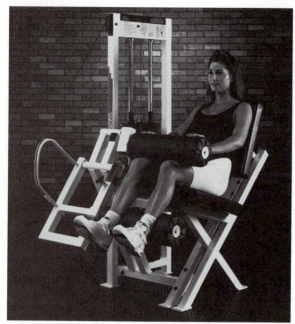

FIGURE 11.1 Power Circuit Leg Curl Machine offers a seated position for greater comfort than the traditional prone position machines. Especially beneficial for pregnant women, rehabilitation patients, and unconditioned users. Has a counterbalance lifting arm for low starting resistance.

(Courtesy of Universal Gym Equipment, Inc.)

All the above exercises can be performed with a one- to two-pound weight added to the ankle. Weight machines can be used as the body tissues become stronger. (See Figure 11.1.) The same progression of DIF described in Chapter 10 is used during rehabilitative exercises.

Closed Kinetic-Chain System Exercises

1. **Walking.** Use parallel bars or other supplementation, such as canes or crutches.
2. **Toe raises on a single leg.** Stand on one foot and lift body weight to ball of foot. This can be done with weight machine.
   Analysis. Contract all muscles crossing ankle, knee, and some of hip muscles.
3. **Bench stepping.** Use a regular stairway step, a bench, or an aerobic exercise stepping bench for stepping up and down.

Analysis. Contract all muscles crossing ankle, knee, and hip, with emphasis on the hamstring/quadriceps strength.

4. **Bicycling.** Use a stationary bicycle or ergometer.
   Analysis. See section on cycling in Chapter 22.
5. **Stepping machine.** Independent or dependent stepper.
   Analysis. Both types have same muscle involvement as with bench stepping. Independent stepper involves more stabilization muscles.

Rehabilitation Locomotion

Evaluation

Prior to locomotion training for rehabilitation, you need to functionally assess the subject. Part of this assessment includes exercise therapy progress, but a major consideration is a biomechanical assessment of walking performance. Various checklists appear in Chapters 8 and 9. Other common clinical methods include the use of electro-optical computerized equipment that have been placed in research gait laboratories. See Chapter 7 for illustrations of such equipment.

Evaluation of pre- and post-surgery performance and general rehabilitation after disease, chronic and acute pain, muscle weakness, spasticity or paralysis, sensory disturbances, illness, and accidents often is complicated by the fact that people compensate for a dysfunction. Because the body is a kinematic/kinetic-chain system, other parts of the body appear to be dysfunctional as they assume compensatory roles. Some effects of muscle weakness/contractures on gait (walking) are shown in Table 11.1.

Validity of prediction of gait anomalies, as well as prediction of muscular weakness or contracture, is investigated by means of biomechanical modeling of the anatomy and planes and axes of movement. The following is a simplified example of modeling.

■ The angle of pull of muscle is always a vector in the plane of the muscle. Muscles lying in the same plane, but on the opposite surface of bones, will become slack as the contracting muscle shortens. Thus, if the posterior tibialis muscle is in constant contracture it will pronate the foot, collapse the longitudinal arch, and produce forefoot varus. The anterior tibialis becomes slack.

TABLE 11.1 Effect of Muscle Weakness and Contracture Upon Gait.

Muscle Weakness	Gait Change
Hamstrings	Hyperextension of leg occurs
Internal rotators	Leg externally rotated outward
Anterior tibialis	Drop foot (foot in calcaneovarus position and toes drag); may walk on toes to compensate

Muscle Contracture	Gait Change
Gastrocnemius	Equinus foot
Adductors	Scissoring of legs; feet will cross
Iliopsoas	Lordosis and trunk lean

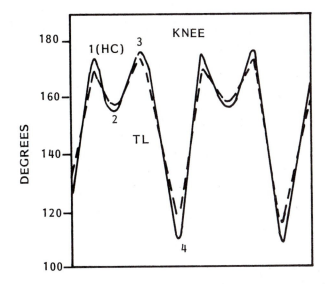

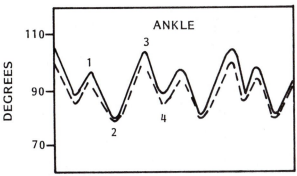

FIGURE 11.2 Compensations made by the non-braced leg to restrictions due to bracing.
(From Taylor, B., Adrian, M., and Karpovich, P. 1967. Effect of restriction of joint movements in one leg upon the action of similar joints of the other leg. *J.A.P.M.R.* Jan–Feb.)

Refer to the anatomical charts in Chapters 3 and 4 and set up other muscle weaknesses and contractures. Predict gait anomalies. Refer also to Steindler (1957).

As we have seen, many changes in gait can result from one part of the body failing to function effectively. Researchers have investigated the nature of compensation and its effects on gait. One such investigation by one of the authors consisted of artificially inducing dysfunction (Taylor et al. 1967). A long leg brace was placed on the leg of an able-bodied male. This brace could be adjusted to produce four constraints at two joints: (1) a rigid ankle; (2) a rigid knee; (3) a rigid ankle and rigid knee; and (4) a reduced range of motion at the knee. Electrogoniometers were placed at the knee and the ankle of the unbraced leg to record the angular kinematics at these joints as the man walked with the previously stated constraints. Changes in the kinematics of the non-braced leg occurred to compensate for dysfunction in the other leg and are shown in Figure 11.2.

Anatomical asymmetry between right and left legs often results in gait problems. For example, Schuit (1988) investigated the effect of leg length discrepancies on ground reaction forces and lower extremity joint angles during the stance phase of walking. Ground reaction force vectors and kinematic data were collected for eighteen subjects wearing recreational footwear. Subsequently, appropriately sized heel lifts were fitted into the shoes of the short leg for each subject and were worn for three weeks. After the test period, kinetic and kinematic data were again recorded. A significant increase was found for maximum vertical force for both legs after the lift was added. A significant increase in maximum medial force was found for the short leg, in both no-lifts and lift conditions. Such medial and lateral differences are an indication of compensatory mechanisms acting to stabilize the body during ambulation. The increase in vertical force was no more than 10% and reflective of the unequal leg-length adjustments. (See Figure 11.3.)

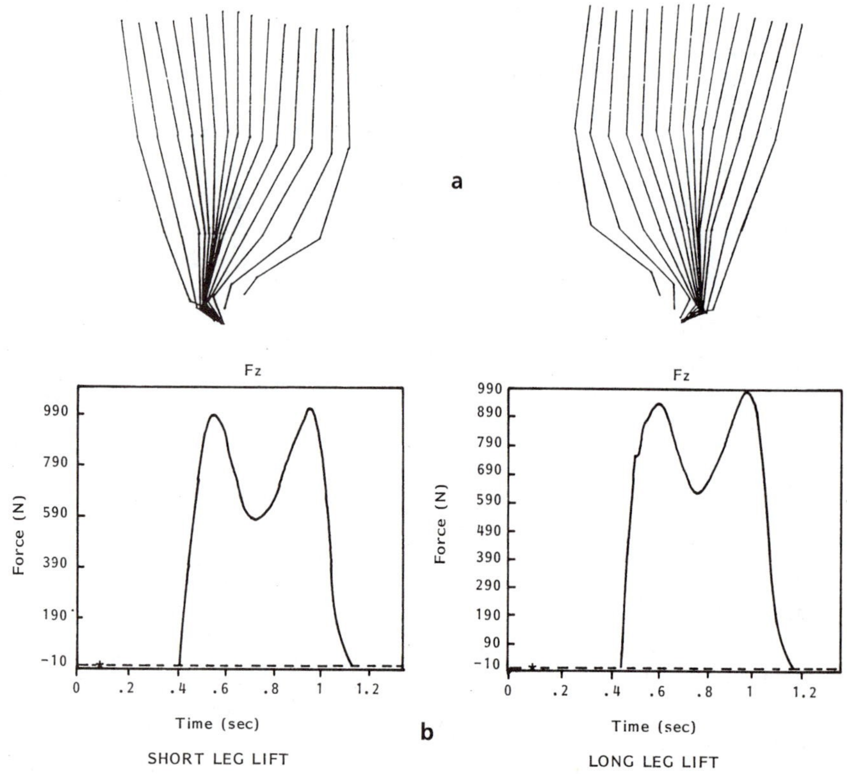

FIGURE 11.3 Data collected from persons with unequal leg lengths. (a) Angle of leg at heel strike; (b) force-time curve. (From Schuit, Dale. 1987. Ph.D. dissertation, University of Illinois at Urbana-Champaign.)

SHORT LEG LIFT

LONG LEG LIFT

MINI-LABORATORY LEARNING EXPERIENCE

Videotape the walking pattern of a person wearing one high-heeled shoe and one sandal without a heel height. If you have access to a force platform, obtain ground reaction forces during the support phase of each foot.

1. Measure the kinematics (e.g., ROM, angles at key phases of the cycle) of each leg, arm, and the trunk during the support phase of each foot.
2. Measure the duration and maximum forces during the support phase of each foot.
3. Determine asymmetries and propose reasons for these differences.

Supplementation Devices

This aspect of rehabilitation refers to assistive devices that are attached to or used by the person as supplementary to the human body. There are two categories: adaptive devices and orthotic devices.

Adaptive Devices

These devices are held by the person and consist of canes, crutches, and walkers. With respect to the upper extremities, they include such devices as adaptive eating utensils, handle grip bowling balls, and computer controlling devices.

The type of ambulation aid to select for use is determined primarily by the amount of weight to be borne by the aid. Common ambulation aids listed in a hierarchy of

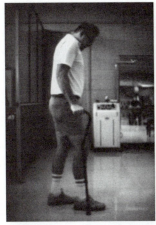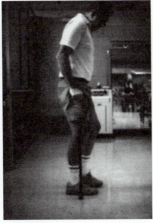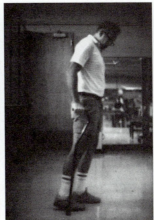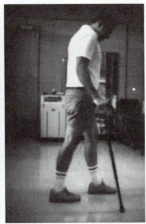

FIGURE 11.4 Walking sequence using cane.

weight-bearing potential are the single cane, aluminum forearm crutch, two forearm crutches, two axillary crutches, and the walker. Canes are mainly used by those who require aid in balance since a cane should bear no more than 20–25% of body weight. Forearm crutches can support 40–50% of body weight. The axillary crutches and walker are used in early rehabilitation and in permanent disabilities in which 80% or more support of body weight is required. Crutches are useful, however, only if the arms can hold the crutches and keep pressure from the radial nerve, preventing crutch paralysis. If the arms are weak it is difficult to walk more than a short distance with crutches. Some people cannot use crutches effectively. Walkers are more appropriate if balance is also a problem.

■ How is the effective and safe weight-bearing pattern executed? How can the pattern be measured? Discuss these questions, and then refer to the hints in the mini-laboratory learning experience after the following section.

Walking Pattern Using Adaptive Devices

This section discusses walking patterns used with the various adaptive devices.

Cane. Step with the involved leg only when the cane and the sound foot are on the ground. Use the cane on the contralateral side of body with respect to the involved leg, in order to relieve compressive forces on the hip of the involved leg. (See Figure 11.4.)

Four-Legged Cane. This has the same use as the single cane, but is used when greater stability is required and the person walks slowly. Fast walking will cause users to execute a rear-front two-point contact pattern with the cane, nullifying its stability potential.

Forearm Crutch. This has the same use as the cane, except it is used when the hand cannot grasp and the wrist is weak. The forearm crutch is also used when the hands cannot grasp because of arthritis.

Two Crutches. This is a three-point gait with the involved leg and both crutches moving as one unit and the sound leg moving independently. (See Figure 11.5.)

Walkers. Walkers have been used extensively with frail elderly people and people who have had an amputation and are learning to walk with a prosthesis. There has been limited research on problems associated with

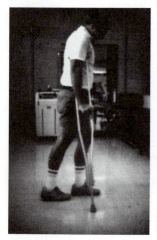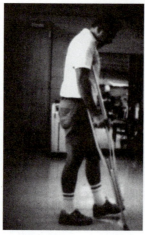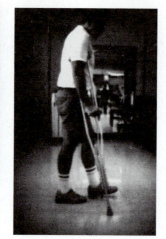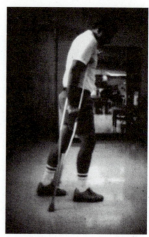

FIGURE 11.5 Walking sequence using crutches.

walkers, but the following have been noted in biomechanics analysis of walking patterns with walkers. Users must lean forward and increase their trunk flexion, thus assuming an abnormal posture when using walkers. The walkers often are too short for the person and excess weight is placed on the walker and, consequently, on the user's shoulders. Walking becomes difficult because the walker cannot easily be lifted for the next step.

Possibly in an effort to counter these problems, designs of walkers have changed in recent years. Wheels, brakes, and other innovations have improved walking performance. More biomechanics research is needed.

Orthotics

Prescription of orthotic devices to be worn in shoes has become common since the running boom of the 1970s. Running injuries were attributed to poorly designed shoes, weak musculature controlling the feet, and bony malalignments. Podiatrists, sports medicine personnel, and advertisers advocated orthotics of all types. Researchers have shown that orthotics can change the orientation of the foot and the kinematics of the foot and leg during running. The primary use of orthotics is to create a neutral subtalar joint to prevent over-pronation of the foot, which creates stress at the medial ankle joint and to the medial collateral ligaments at the knee.

MINI-LABORATORY LEARNING EXPERIENCE

Use a force platform or a standard body-weight scale to record vertical ground reaction forces during walking with and without ambulation aids. Compare the following conditions:

1. Normal walking.
2. Contact the scale or platform with the cane during walking. Place hypothetical disabled foot on scale. Place sound foot on scale.
3. Use a swing-through gait with two crutches.
  . Contact the scale with the sound foot and then with one crutch.

Record the weight of the person, and check whether the reactive force on the cane was acceptable. Do the same for the crutches.

If a person had very little stability and great weakness in the legs, what gait pattern would be substituted for the three-point gait? Explain the sequence of supports and what forces would occur.

Not all people need orthotics, and not all orthotics are beneficial. McPoil (1987) showed that during walking,

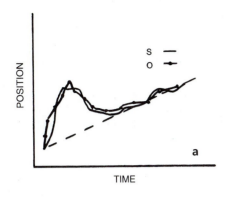

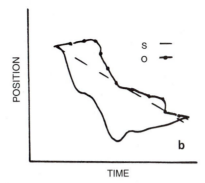

FIGURE 11.6 Force-time pattern during support phase of walking barefoot, with shoes (*s*) and with orthotics inside the shoes (*o*). Orthotics have little value for the person in a. with a forefoot varus problem.

(From McPoil, T. 1987. Ph.D. dissertation, University of Illinois at Urbana-Champaign.)

an orthotic to correct forefoot valgus may have no greater value than a well-designed, well-fitted shoe. See Figure 11.6 for force platform recordings.

MINI-LABORATORY LEARNING EXPERIENCE

1. Walk and concentrate on the pressures experienced on the feet. Do you strike hard or soft on the heel? Do you feel more pressure on the second or the first metatarsal? Record your perceptions.
2. Videotape your feet during walking. Analyze the movement patterns and estimate the muscles acting to cause the movements.
3. Repeat the preceding process with the following conditions. Place wedges of foam or plastic at the following sites of a shoe (either inside or taped to the sole):
   a. Under the big toe
   b. Along the lateral border of foot
   c. Under the medial heel

   Evaluate the results.

An athlete diagnosed with a stress fracture, foot pain, and performance problems was evaluated walking with a forefoot supinating-type orthotic and walking without the orthotic. The paths of the center of pressure during support were generated using a force platform. Important differences were noted in the sites of pressure, especially in the pushoff phase. (See Figure 11.7.)

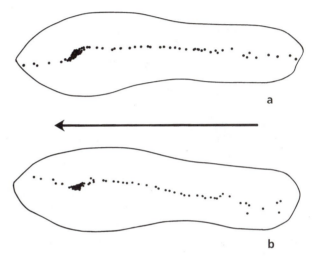

FIGURE 11.7 Lines of pressure during walking with an orthotic (*a*) and without an orthotic (*b*).

Substitution Devices

In this category are replacement body parts, such as leg and arm prostheses for persons with amputated limbs. For those who have further functional disability, wheelchairs and other external forms of transportation are used as substitutes for walking.

Adjustments to substitution devices is far more difficult than adjustments to supplementation devices. This may, in large part, be due to the inability of users to psychologically adjust to "body replacement."

Prostheses

There are two basic categories of lower limb **prostheses:** below the knee (BK) and above the knee (AK). Upper limb prostheses are classified as below-elbow (BE) and above-elbow (AE) prostheses. Based on the biomechanics of motion, the loss of function due to active links in the kinematic chain of motion is directly proportional to the number of links lost. Thus, AK amputees have lost two links (foot and shank) in their kinematic chain, and BK amputees have lost one link. A prosthesis is designed to duplicate normal functioning. This goal, however, depends on the patient's level of general functioning ability, the level of amputation, and practicality. The BK prosthesis may be a single-axis foot attached by single plane hinges to the shank or a single-axis foot attached by single plane hinges to the thigh. It could also be designed to allow inversion, eversion, and torque absorption. Of course, the latter design would not be appropriate for persons with amputations at near-patella level and with weak musculature at the knee level.

The more elaborate and more functional (simulating the functions of the living leg) the prosthesis, the greater the ability of the person to perform ADL and sports activities. So much progress has been made in design, both general and customized, of prostheses that people with lower limb amputation or impairment can participate in any sport including skiing, running, mountain climbing, basketball, and high jumping.

The Flex-Foot is an example of a below-knee prosthesis that stores and releases energy in a manner similar to a coil or spring. It duplicates the heel-toe action of the natural footstep. The flex of the material cushions the impact, stores the energy (through this deformation in flexion), and then springs back (releasing energy and acting as a propulsive force into the next step). It is excellent for running. Dennis Oehler has run 100 meters in 11.73 seconds wearing the Flex-Foot.

Evaluation of Prostheses

The following criteria can be used in the evaluation of the prostheses:

1. Fit: Stump fit and proper sizing are essential to comfort and function.
2. Alignment: The prosthesis should be an extension of the upper leg.
3. Length: The length must be functionally correct.
4. Weight: Optimum weight for amputee to handle depends on musculature.
5. Stability: The prosthesis position must be constant and dependable.
6. Tolerable Pressure: Too much pressure will cause sores, trauma, and complications.
7. Durability: The prosthesis should not break during use.

The process of fitting any prosthesis continues to be a serious problem for amputees. In many cases, if the prosthesis is fitted to the exact length of the other leg, it may be functionally too long or too short for the person using an abnormal gait pattern. For example, if there is instability in the stepping pattern and the trunk compensates for this problem, the sound hip may be carried lower than the other hip during the support phase of walking. The prosthesis, then, is functionally too short. Lengthening the prosthesis may solve the problem for a short time, but as the person becomes stronger and the gait pattern improves, the prosthesis then is too long. Thus, it is necessary to assess the gait pattern frequently. Biomechanics analysis and documentation of the gait pattern is valuable to the rehabilitation staff.

MINI-LABORATORY LEARNING EXPERIENCE

The following sites have been selected for amputation because of accidents, nerve damage, or circulation occlusion: (a) 12 cm above knee; (b) 12 cm below knee; and (c) below maleoli. Describe what functions are lost and what characteristics of a prosthesis would be required to establish near-normal function after amputation at each of the sites.

Transportation Devices

Rowing bikes, hand pedaling bikes, water ski seats, roller sled for ski training and wheelchairs are used for sports or transportation. The most common type of transportation device is the wheelchair. An immense amount of research has been conducted to match the wheelchair to the

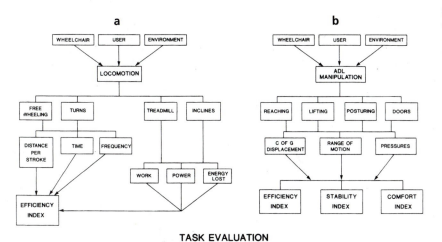

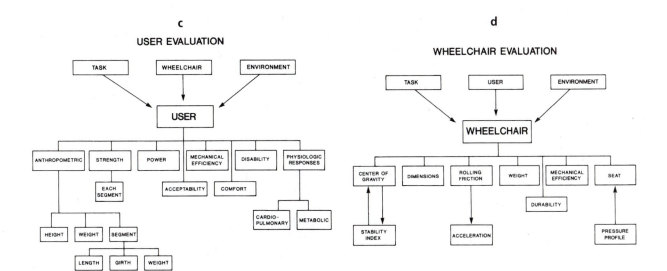

FIGURE 11.8 Model to evaluate wheelchair, task, user, and environmental interrelationships to optimize mobility of wheelchair user.

functional needs of the individual. Recently, the sports world has been the place in which the greatest innovations have been made. The Veterans Administration research and development programs have been a continual source of progress to the ADL wheelchair user.

Wheelchair Research Model

The model presented in Figure 11.8 is a comprehensive approach to determining characteristics of the wheelchair, the person, and the interaction or functional matching of the wheelchair to the user. It is the latter aspect that is the focus of much biomechanics research. Shoulder injuries, ineffective maneuvering of the chairs, increased desire to perform wheelchair sports, and rejection of the traditional chair are some of the reasons for this research.

The relationship of the seat position to the handrim, axle of the wheel, and required movement of the upper arm has been found to be so important that customized chairs are being developed. Power and mechanical work

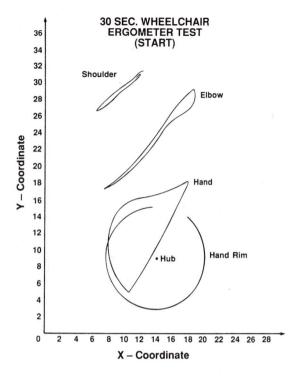

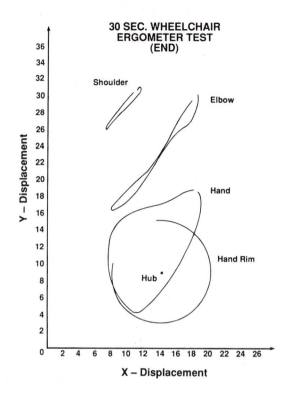

FIGURE 11.9 The kinematics of wheelchair propulsion at the 10 sec point and 30 sec point during a 30 sec anaerobic test to exhaustion.

are measured to determine the best position for optimum performance by athletes. Study Figure 11.9 and describe the movements of the anatomical points observed.

Wang (1991) investigated the interaction between the kinematics and muscle kinetics using 3-D filming techniques. Some of his data are shown in Chapter 24.

Velocity curves of wheelchair propulsion of a sample of paraplegics and quadriplegics were obtained by Gehlsen (1991) and appear as Figure 11.10. Note that the ratio of contact times to recovery times were similar for both groups. These data were obtained by persons using a "push technique." Today the contact times and ratios have been reduced by using a "punch technique."

ADL Analyses and Concerns

ADL consists of locomotor, self-care, management of devices, communication, and home-management activities. The self-care activities include such tasks as dressing, toiletry, and combing hair. Leisure activities comprise a vast continuum of activities ranging from sedentary activities to organized athletics. Performances of all these tasks as performed by the physically disabled have been only qualitatively assessed. The most common method is a five-level ranking: (1) able to perform; (2) able to perform in certain situations (such as afternoon or under optimum friction conditions); (3) can perform with difficulty; (4) can perform with assistance (listing the type of assistance); and (5) cannot perform. Unfortunately, we have only limited analysis of the movement patterns. Little information exists concerning the ranges of motion, strength, and technique requirements for successful performance. There is a need to develop a model for the physically disabled, possibly a number of models to address various classifications of disabilities. Only then will the disabled have an equal chance with the able-bodied to optimize their performance. Analysis of common movement patterns and problems/adaptions of physically disabled persons is presented in the next sections.

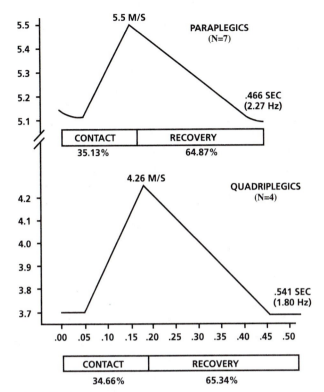

FIGURE 11.10 Comparison of mean speeds and contact/recovery times during wheelchair propulsion by paraplegics and quadraplegics.
(Courtesy of Dr. Gale Gehlsen.)

Physical Disabilities and Ascending Stairs

For the analysis of stair ascent see Chapter 9. Common modifications of people with physical disabilities when they are ascending stairs are of two types: (1) the person uses a handrail; and (2) the person marks time, that is, places both feet on each tread. The use of a handrail not only compensates for balance dysfunction but also provides a reactive surface for the hand. Arm extension produces another force for raising the body and compensating for weak quadriceps.

People who have had a stroke or other trauma that has resulted in the failure of one leg to function as well as the other should lead with the nontraumatized leg when ascending stairs, since muscular strength is vital to lift the body weight. For these people, total foot placement, strengthening of extensor muscle groups, and exact control of the center of gravity with respect to the base of support are important requirements for success in ascending stairs.

Physical Disabilities and Descending Stairs

Stair descent is also described in Chapter 9. Those with physical disabilities should lead with the disabled leg when descending stairs, since maximum stability is required on the upper tread during the lowering of the lead leg. The nondisabled leg can be lowered quickly as soon as the lead leg is supported. This action minimizes the amount of time during which the impaired leg is the sole support of body weight.

■ Certain principles are applicable for both descending and ascending stairs. The person maintains dynamic stability, uses forward and upward momentum, and involves a sequencing of muscle contractions to accelerate the body in the desired path. Modifications are made in the pattern according to anatomic characteristics of the performer and environmental conditions. A coefficient of friction less than optimum reduces horizontal forces and increases vertical forces.

Changing Levels

General kinematics of rising from and lowering to a bed or chair, squatting, stooping, and sitting are also described in Chapter 9.

Since one side of the body usually is disabled after a stroke, the stroke patient should place the foot of the disabled leg close to the hips when attempting to rise from a seated position on the floor. The other leg is raised to a position supported by the knee and shank. The center of gravity is shifted to the foot, and the hands exert a push against the floor. If the leg is not strong enough to extend to the standing position, the person should grasp a piece of furniture to assist with extension of the leg, much the same as the handrail is used in stair locomotion.

■ Transfer of momentum of one body part often is used to compensate for loss of function in another body part.

A major concern of biomechanists is the incidence of injury to the knee as a result of squatting, kneeling, and stooping. As the squat position is achieved, the knee is placed in an open position, or what is sometimes termed a *loosely packed* position. This makes the knee vulnerable to dislocation and rupturing of ligaments or muscles crossing the joint. If these tissues are strong, it is unlikely that an injury will occur. There is, however, a danger of injury because of loss of balance or a deliberate twisting motion that would place excessive stress on the knee. The knee would then be injured because of the torsion, not the separation in the sagittal plane. Obese people, those who discover that they cannot rise from the squat position, and those who attempt to perform movements requiring greater balance and strength capabilities than they possess are the most vulnerable to injury during squatting activities.

Persons desiring to perform the squat after not having attempted a squat for some length of time should test their ability to do so in this way:

1. Assume a simulated squat position while lying to check range of motion and eliminate the effect of gravity.
2. If possible, perform the movement in water.
3. Assume a semisquat position.
4. With the assistance of a person, chair, or some other aid, assume the squat position.

At the first sign of pain, the movement should be discontinued until strengthening exercises can increase the stability of the knee joint.

Transfers

Often, ADL activities, known as transfers, are more traumatizing to the rehabilitative specialist than to the physically disabled person. A transfer involves physically moving from one position to another such as wheelchair to car seat or bed to wheelchair. The primary injury site to the rehabilitative specialist or other medical personnel is the lower back. The common injury site to the disabled person performing a self-transfer is the shoulder.

━━━━━━━━
MINI-LABORATORY LEARNING EXPERIENCE

Qualitatively analyze the three methods of transferring depicted in Figure 11.11, *a*, *b*, and *c*.

Describe the planes of motion, axis of rotation, and major muscles required in the transfer.

Draw force vectors and free-body diagrams for the propulsive phase in each.

Rank the amount of force required by the patient in each figure.

Identify high stress areas to the joints.

Indicate how you might quantitatively measure the forces at the propulsive phase.

━━━━━━━━

References

Baretta, R., Solomonow, M., Zhou, B. H., et al. 1988. Muscular coactivation—the role of the antagonist musculature in maintaining knee stability. *Amer J SpMed.* 16:113–22.

Baumann, J. U. 1991. Requirements of clinical gait analysis. *Human Movement Science* 10 (5):535–42.

Butler, D. L., Noyes, F. R., and Grood, E. S. 1980. Ligamentous restraints to anterior-posterior drawer in the human knee: A biomechanical study. *Jb&JtSurg* 62A:259–70.

Dahle, L. K., Mueller, M., Delitto, A., and Diamond, J. E. 1991. Visual assessment of foot type and relationship of foot type to lower extremity injury. *Journal of Orthopaedic and Sports Physical Therapy* 14(2):70–74.

DeLuca, P. A. 1991. The use of gait analysis and dynamic EMG in the assessment of the child with cerebral palsy. *Human Movement Science* 10(5):543–54.

Deusinger, R. 1984. Biomechanics in clinical practice. *Physical Therapy* 64. Special issue.

Fleckenstein, S. J., Kirby, R. L., and MacLeod, D. A. 1988. Effect of limited knee-flexion range on peak hip moments of force while transferring from sitting to standing. *J Biom.* 21:915–18.

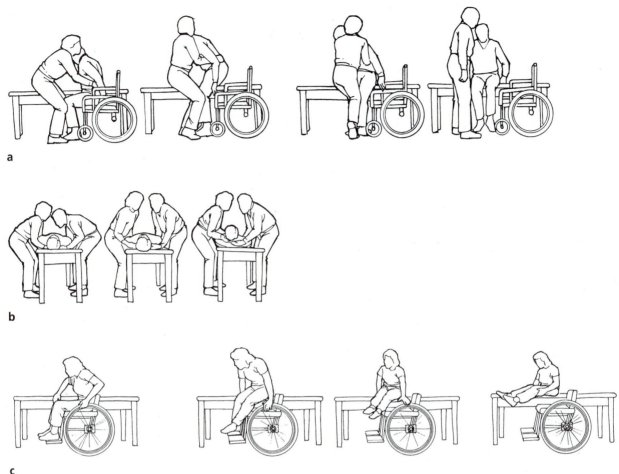

a

b

c

FIGURE 11.11 Three methods of transfers. **Visualize the muscles and angle of push required for each of the types of transfers.**

Gehlsen, Gale. 1991. Unpublished special report. Ball State University.

Grood, E. S., Suntay, W. J., Noyes, F. R., et al. 1984. Biomechanics of knee extension exercise. *Jb&JtSurg* 66A :725–34.

Jebsen, R. H. 1967. Use and abuse of ambulation aids. *JAMA* 199(1):63–68.

Kegel, B. 1985. Physical fitness sports and recreation for those with lower limb amputation or impairment. *J Rehab. R&D*, clinical supplement no. 1.

McKenzie, D., Clement, D., and Taunton, J. 1985. Running shoes, orthotics, and injuries. *Sports Medicine* 2:334–47.

McPoil, T. G. 1987. The effect of foot supports on ground reaction force patterns. Ph.D. dissertation, University of Illinois at Urbana-Champaign.

Moore, S., and Brunt, D. 1991. Effects of trunk support and target distance on postural adjustments prior to a rapid reaching task by seated subjects. *Arch Phys Med and Rehab* 72(9):638–41.

Palmer, M. L., and Toms, J. E. 1986. *Manual for functional training*. Philadelphia: F. A. Davis Company.

Palmitier, R. A., An, K. N., Scott, S. G., et al. 1991. Kinetic chain exercise in knee rehabilitation. *Sports Medicine* 6:402–13.

Pedretti, L. W. 1981. *Occupational therapy.* St. Louis: C. V. Mosby.

Perry, J. 1967. The mechanics of walking: Part of the proceedings of an instructional course principles of lower-extremity bracing. *JAPT* 47:778–815. See also the entire issue.

Peszcznski, M. 1958. The intermittent double step gait. *Archives of Physical Medicine and Rehabilitation* 39.

Schuit, D. 1988. The effect of heel lifts on ground reaction force patterns and lower extremity joint angles in subjects with structural leg length discrepancies. Ph.D. dissertation, University of Illinois at Urbana-Champaign.

Steindler, W. 1957. *Normal and pathological gait.* Springfield, IL: Charles C. Thomas.

Taylor, B., Adrian, M., and Karpovich, P. 1967. Effect of restriction of joint movements in one leg upon the action of similar joints of the other leg. *J.A.P.M.R.* Jan–Feb.

Walker, P. S., Rovick, J. S., and Robertson, D. D. 1988. The effects of knee brace hinge design and placement on joint mechanics. *J Biom.* 21:965–74.

Wang, Yong Tai. 1991. Relationship between kinematic factors and muscle activity during wheelchair propulsion. Ph.D. dissertation, University of Illinois, Urbana-Champaign.

12 Occupational Biomechanics

Most industries are seeking ways to improve worker productivity and, at the same time, eliminate injuries. Workers want to be able to perform without being tired, tense, or exhausted at the end of the day. In this chapter, we concentrate on these concerns.

Occupational biomechanics is not only a subdivision of biomechanics. It is also one component of the broad area of human ergonomics, the study of the interaction of the worker and the industrial environment. While human ergonomics encompasses the physiological, biomechanical, psychological, and environmental aspects of work, occupational biomechanics is limited to the anatomical (including anthropometrical), mechanical, and environmental aspects of the work task as each is related to the other. Worker productivity and work safety are the two most important goals of both the occupational biomechanist and the ergonomist.

■ Occupational biomechanics is enhancing performance without compromising safety.

Methodological Approaches

Chaffin and Andersson (1984) have identified six methodological areas of occupational biomechanics. The functional anatomy and anthropometrical methodologies depicted in Figure 12.1 are the foundation for the other four methodologies: task analysis, mechanical-work capacity evaluation, modeling, and instrumentation.

Functional Anatomy and Anthropometrical Methodologies

Anthropometric tables give mean values and percentile values for such factors as stature, body segment lengths, widths, circumferences, and ratios. Examples of these normative data are Figure 12.2, Table 12.1, Appendix E. Industry uses these data for sizing of furniture and work areas.

■ Anthropometric norms are not always appropriate for the individual worker.

These data used by industry consist of information defining the size, shape, and form of the human body performing the task, as well as the kinematic capabilities of the human body. For example, a biomechanist will determine the range of motion at each joint with respect to space and time and the optimum positioning of the muscle-bone-joint lever system to produce optimum or maximum force to safely, efficiently, and effectively perform the task.

Task Analysis

Analysis of the task itself involves classification and time-prediction methodology. The elements of each task are identified with descriptors such as reach, position, and grasp. The number and types of elements that comprise a

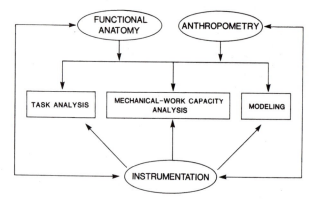

FIGURE 12.1 Relationships of methodological areas of occupational biomechanics.

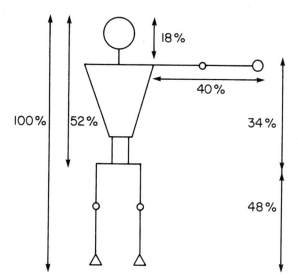

FIGURE 12.2 Proportionality of body segments with respect to total body stature.

task can be tabulated and the predicted time to complete the task calculated. Biomechanists classify tasks to enable comparisons of commonalities and develop hierarchial matrices, both before assigning a worker to a task.

Mechanical-Work Capacity Analysis

The mechanical-work capacity evaluation methodology consists of determining performance levels based on worker characteristics such as strength, stature, and hand size. Although most of this evaluation has been conducted with physiological instrumentation, the amount of work or power produced prior to discontinuance, due to fatigue or exceeding a time limit, is another viable way of evaluating these parameters. Biomechanists compare work and power requirements to muscular strength of the worker. Biomechanical researchers formulate frequency, load, and performance technique standards, based on predicted stress to body tissues.

Modeling

Biomechanical modeling by means of the computer is the most recent investigative methodology. As noted previously, modeling is a safe process for estimating forces acting on the performer and evaluating the potential productivity and risk of injury. Modeling of the worker, the environment, and the task as separate systems and then as one combined system is very productive.

Instrumentation

Instrumentation is required to conduct research in occupational biomechanics. Motion pictures were the basis for most time-motion studies of industrial tasks from the 1920s through the 1950s. Instrumentation now usually includes videography, electrogoniometry, accelerometry, dynamography, electromyography, and computer technology.

Occupational Biomechanical Considerations

Physical tasks require manipulation, often using high intensities of strength, of tools, or objects in the work space. Concern for overexertion in lifting, pushing, pulling, and carrying is paramount. Another occupational task area is that of the person who sits or stands at a workstation performing very low-strength manipulations. In this situation, repetitive trauma is the major concern. In the United States today, the video display terminal operator is thought to be at greatest risk for repetitive trauma.

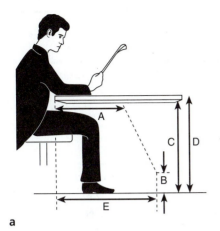

a

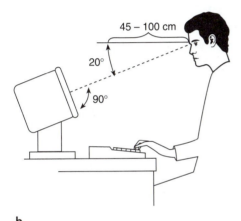

b

FIGURE 12.3 (a) Workstation and relationships of working desk surface and height to worker. A, minimum of 450 mm for working desk, and 300 mm for data terminal table; B, 150 mm; C, minimum of 630 mm; D, 670-780 mm; E, minimum of 600 mm. (b) Workstation and line of vision.

■ Trauma may be caused by a one-time overexertion action or by repetitive low-intensity actions.

Workspace (Workstation)

Biomechanical analyses must include the analysis of the workspace, since it often determines the manner in which the task will be performed. There are three types of workspaces to consider: sitting, standing (including

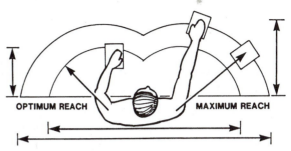

FIGURE 12.4 Normal reach distances for a visual display unit (VDU) workstation are identified as maximum reach and optimum reach.

twisting), and locomotor spaces. Since the advent of the information society, sitting is by far the most prevalent work position. High-technology and computer-related businesses have resulted in less reliance on physical strength to perform occupational tasks. Ultraefficient transportation devices bring objects to the worker's table, bench, or chair. In other cases, jobs require video display terminals and information manipulation. For example, few dentists now stand and twist their bodies as they work. A swivel adjustable chair is used to reduce the possibility of injuries due to twisting. Average, mean, or normative anthropometric data are used to determine the amount of space a worker can easily use and determine the dimensions of the inanimate objects incorporated into the workspace.

Environmental Matching

Examples of pertinent measurements and the biomechanically designed sitting workspace, known as environmental matching, are shown in Figure 12.3 and Figure 12.4.

Forces during Sitting

Let's look at the sitting posture from the perspective of long-term sitting without undue stress to the spine. Did you know that the measured pressures on the lumbar vertical discs during sitting are higher than during standing at rest? The difference between these sitting and standing pressures can be as much as 35% of the lowest measured sitting pressure. Changes in posture and changes in the chair configuration result in changes in

MINI-LABORATORY LEARNING EXPERIENCE

Using the workstation depicted in Figure 12.4, determine the dimensions for your personal anthropometrically correct workstation.

1. Measure your arm length, biacromial width, and chest width and determine the maximum limits of reach and maximum size of an appropriate worktable.
2. Calculate your optimum reach using 65% of your maximum reach.
3. Determine the dimensions of your optimum work table size, taking into account where you would place frequently used and/or heavier objects.
4. Determine muscular strength at 10, 20, 30, 40 and 50% of your maximum reach. (You might attach a strap to a spring scale and place the strap around your wrist. Ask someone to hold the spring scale while you pull against the scale. You can test different muscle groups by changing the placement of the scale.)
5. Graph your results and compare muscle strength with maximum reach and with your answer in step 3.

disc pressure. In fact, a 200% reduction in disc pressure can occur merely as a result of modifying each of three chair parameters: the inclination of the backrest; type of arm support; and the amount of lumbar support. Naturally, researchers cannot do human movement analysis on workers by invasively placing a force transducer in the intervertebral discs of the spinal column to measure disc pressure. This technique, however, has been used in research settings; values appear in Table 12.1.

Pressure on the lumbar discs is determined by the angle at the hip, the lengths of hip muscles at that angle, the tilt of the pelvis, and the weight of the upper body. Chaffin and Andersson (1984) determined that the 135° angle at the hip was the normal position of balanced muscle relaxation. At an angle of 135°, the natural curvature of the lumbar spine is maintained. An angle greater than this angle will increase the lumbar spine curvature, and angles less than 135° will reduce this curvature.

TABLE 12.1 Disc pressure (expressed as percentage of relaxed lean back position) when a person sits in chairs with different configurations and performs different tasks.

Backrest Angle (degrees)	Disc Pressure (%)
90	171
100	129
110	99
120	89

Trunk Position	Disc Pressure (%)
Relaxed lean back (with back support)	100
Vertical	105
Relaxed (slouch)	123
Posterior slouch	125
Anterior lean (straight)	139
Anterior lean (slouch)	157

Task	Disc Pressure (%)
Writing (arms on table)	124
Depression of pedal	124
Typewriting	146
Lifting weight (arms horizontal)	170

(Compiled and modified from Chaffin, D. B., and Andersson, G. 1984. *Occupational biomechanics.* New York: Wiley-Interscience.)

Inclined backrest (110–120° backward) is a position similar to that used in "hog motorcycles" and recumbent bicycles. Unfortunately, many work tasks cannot be performed in this position. Or can they? Could you design a workspace to capitalize on this more efficient sitting position? Specially designed chairs and footrests increase productivity and reduce stress. Different designs are based upon different concepts. For example:

1. Best lumbar curvature, less pressure on femoral artery, and reduction of trunk twisting (Figure 12.5).
2. Best angle for pelvic tilt and balanced thigh muscles (Figure 12.6). However, it is difficult to work at this angle.
3. Feet relaxation, less thigh pressure, pelvic tilt (Figure 12.7).

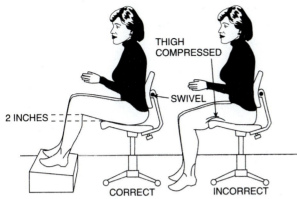

FIGURE 12.5 Biomechanically correct and incorrect sitting position and furniture. The highest point of the seat should be at least 2 in. below the popliteal crease of the worker. If necessary, this must be accomplished by a footrest. The backrest should swivel about the horizontal axis to align with the lumbar curve.

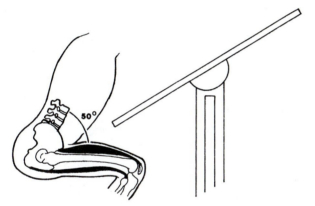

FIGURE 12.6 Sitting position designed for optimum pelvic tilt and balanced thigh muscles.

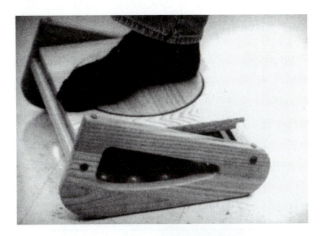

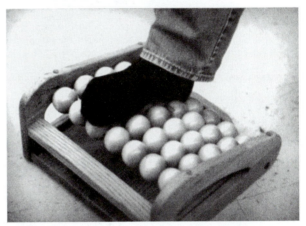

FIGURE 12.7 Footrest that also functions as an exercise and massage device for the feet.
(Courtesy of R&R.)

Nonautomated Materials Handling Limits

Pushing, pulling, lifting, and carrying objects without the aid of automation accounts for almost 90% of industrial overexertion claims made for lower back pain. Although automation will reduce the number of workers performing these handling tasks, many tasks will still not be automated in the foreseeable future. Biomechanists must evaluate the strength requirements of the task, considering such factors as frequency and duration of tasks, weight and dimensions of the object handled, and the geometry of the workplace.

In 1981, the National Institute for Occupational Safety and Health published its *Work Practices Guide for Manual Lifting*. It included its analytical procedures and an equation for calculating the safe lifting loads for two-handed, symmetrical lifting tasks. The general theory on which this equation was based was that "overexertion injury is the result of job demands that exceed a

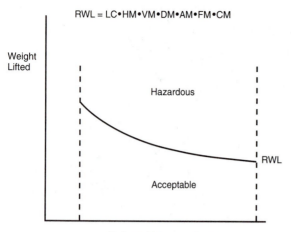

$$RWL = LC \cdot HM \cdot VM \cdot DM \cdot AM \cdot FM \cdot CM$$

FIGURE 12.8 1991 Equation for recommended weight limits during lifting on the job. LC = load constant of 51 pounds; HM = horizontal multiplier; VM = vertical multiplier; DM = distance multiplier; AM = angle multiplier; FM = frequency multiplier; and CM = coupling multiplier.

worker's capacity." Since that time, biomechanists recognized that there was a need to reevaluate the equation and the recommended practices. For example:

1. There continues to be a high incidence of back injuries related to lifting.
2. New factors related to causes of injuries have been identified.
3. Twisting and repetitive motions were not considered in the 1981 equation.

■ **Asymmetric lifting** is more likely to cause injury than symmetric lifting and should be avoided.

Therefore, a panel of experts and experienced users, consisting of safety and health specialists from industry/labor and biomechanists, industrial engineers, physiologists, and psychologists, reviewed the literature, determined the factors of importance, and developed the new equation for a recommended weight limit applicable to all types of lifting activities. The basic concept is shown in Figure 12.8.

The equation is based on a referenced standard lifting load of 51 pounds from a standard position of 25 cm from the ankles and a vertical height of 75 cm. Any deviations from these, as well as increases in asymmetry, frequency of lifts, distance moved, and the ineffective hand-to-object coupling (grip method) will result in a decrease in the recommended weight limit. This equation has to be validated by industrial and laboratory testing and injury data, but, based on preliminary results, it is an improvement from previous guidelines.

MINI-LABORATORY LEARNING EXPERIENCE

Evaluate boxes, bags, and containers with handles and compare with the recommended good hand-to-object coupling norms described below:

1. Optimal handle design—cylindrical shape, smooth and nonslip surface, diameter of 1.9–3.8 cm, at least 11.5 cm length, 5 cm clearance.
2. Optimal hand-hold cut-out—semioval shape, smooth, nonslip surface, 3.8 cm height, 11.5 cm length, 5 cm clearance, and 1.1 cm container thickness.
3. No handles or cut-outs—fingers must be capable of reaching nearly 90° under the container.

Lift several of these boxes and describe differences in perceived effort between those that comply with recommended specifications and those that do not.

Lifting Technique

The proper way to lift objects from the floor or other low positions is covered in most kinesiology and biomechanics textbooks and industrial safety pamphlets because of the vulnerability of the human body to low back injury. Three methods of picking up an object are shown in Figure 12.9. The weight vector of the object and its moment arm from the principal axis of lifting motion can be drawn. Based on these facts, position *a* has the least moment of resistance force and the least stress on the trunk, more specifically the lumbar region. Position *b* primarily needs lumbar extensor muscles to counteract the object being lifted. Depending on the weight of the object, however, either one or the other or both may be acceptable methods of lifting the object. Position *c* is never

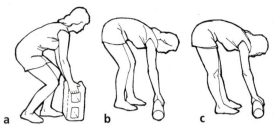

FIGURE 12.9 Three methods of lifting an object from the ground. (a) Least stress on spinal column; (b) acceptable stress on spinal column; (c) undesirable stress on knee and spinal column.

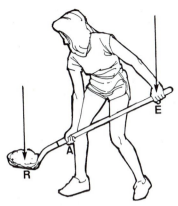

FIGURE 12.10 Lifting dirt with long-handled shovel. This is a first-class lever system. (R, resistance; A, axis; E, effort.)

acceptable because it places stress on the posterior of the knee and stiffens the legs in a position of genu recurvatum (hyperextension at the knee).

If the weight of the object is light, either position *a* or *b* is acceptable, providing the lifter is not so heavy that the musculature cannot control the action of stooping and returning to a stand. The obese person is more apt to stoop rather than squat because the leg strength is probably insufficient for rising from a squat. If the object is heavy, an obese person might not be able to achieve success with position *a* but could swing the object toward the legs, using position *b* in the manner of a weightlifter. The moment arm for the resistance is decreased, and then the object can be lifted with the back. There is danger in such a pattern because the swing may not remain in one plane and could cause twisting of the trunk and vertebral damage. Probably a combination of slight leg flexion and trunk flexion is the most effective and safest method of lifting heavy objects for all workers.

Chaffin and Andersson have shown that there is a direct relationship between the amount of stress in the lumbar region on one hand and the horizontal distance of the object from the person's base of support and the vertical distance the object is moved. Therefore, the safest position is one in which the object is near the center of gravity of the body. This position minimizes the moment arm of the resistance.

Long-Handled Tools. When human beings use long-handled implements such as rakes, hoes, brooms, axes, and shovels, the interfacing of the body size of the implement is an important consideration. For taller-than-average

individuals, the commercially available long-handled implements may be too short for efficient use. The person must assume a stooped posture that promotes excessive tension in the neck and upper back muscles, as well as possible tension in the lumbar region. Taller persons should adapt to the implement by performing the task with increased flexion at the knees and hips to maintain a more efficient trunk position. Shorter-than-average persons must adapt to the average-length implements by adjusting the placement of the hands.

Long-handled implements require the user to establish the most efficient lever system possible, sacrificing movement distance for force improvement in many cases. For example, when using a long-handled shovel to lift a load of dirt, a person separates the hands to produce a first-class lever system. The hand nearer the load acts as the fulcrum (axis of rotation), and the more distant hand exerts a force downward through a long distance (Figure 12.10). Thus, the hand supporting the weight of the shovel and dirt is at or near the balance point of the system. The long moment arm of the handle of the shovel allows movement with a significant mechanical force advantage. Use of the large muscle groups—the leg muscles and the oblique muscles of the trunk—to lift and even support the implement is also a means of using the implement more efficiently.

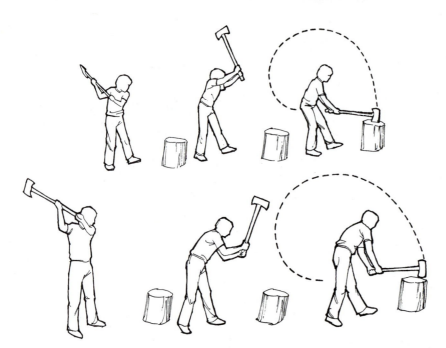

FIGURE 12.11 Movement pattern of axe during wood chopping by two people of different stature. Note arcs of swing.

In some instances, a person will push, slide, or pull the implement to move a resisting material, rather than lift it. These other actions, such as sweeping and raking, require less muscle effort and produce less work (and less energy) than does lifting. The exception is the type of action in which there is an unusually high coefficient of friction for the materials involved, such as shoveling wet, heavy snow.

Chopping wood with an axe resembles many of the actions described in the tennis serve and other overarm patterns used in sports. The use of the implement necessitates holding the handle near the axe head on the upswing to decrease the resistance moment arm and to increase control over the implement. The other hand is placed at the end of the handle. The body counterrotates and the axe is lifted in a curved path above the head. The back hyperextends and the legs flex. On the forward swing of the axe, the body rotates, the trunk flexes, and the legs extend as one hand slides to meet the other hand at the end of the handle. This latter action increases the moment arm and thus the arc and velocity of the axe head as the axe swings forward and downward. Trunk flexion carries the force of the axe through the wood as the muscle force and gravity combine to accelerate the weight of the axe head.

As with sports skills, the greatest acceleration occurs at the instant of contact, and the best performer accelerates the axe head the fastest and through the greatest distance. The taller and longer-limbed person has the potential for creating the greater force. Note the path of the axe head for a tall person and for a short person chopping wood, as depicted in Figure 12.11. However, since multiple levers are acting, the coordinated timing of these levers and the body's neuromuscular speed determine the effectiveness of the act. Thus, shorter people might outperform taller people.

Small Tools. One of the best approaches to the study of work movements with small tools in industry is that of time-motion analysts (human engineers). They have analyzed movements required in industrial tasks, set guidelines, and made modifications in the human-machine task or in the environment to improve the efficiency of the human-machine operation. Because of the financial need of business to obtain maximum production for minimum cost, including minimum cost in human years of productivity, the analysis of industrial tasks is extensive.

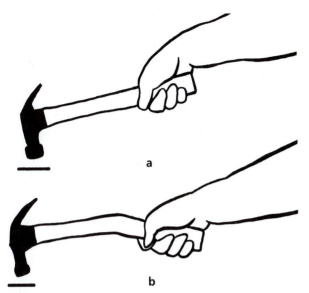

FIGURE 12.12 Hammer handle orientation to reduce carpal tunnel syndrome possibility. (*a*) Regular handle and ulnar deviation of downswing. (*b*) Hand and forearm are aligned (coplanar).

TABLE 12.2 Checklist of factors to consider when investigating repetitive trauma potential.

Postural Aspects	Human-Equipment Interfacing	Anatomical Functioning
Keep elbows down.	Avoid compression ischemia.	Keep forward reaches short.
Minimize moments on spine.	Avoid critical vibrations.	Use work gloves.
Consider strength and any other differences.	Avoid stress concentration.	Avoid muscular insufficiency.
Optimize skeletal configuration.	Keep wrist straight (angle at 180°).	Use curved linear motions.
Avoid head movement.	Use customized chair.	Avoid antagonist fatigue.

Carpal Tunnel Syndrome

Carpal tunnel syndrome and its cumulative trauma disorders have become prevalent among workers using hand tools continually. The radial or ulnar nerve, artery, or the tendons are traumatized through repeated movements, pressures, or extremes in positioning of the hand and fingers.

Since grip span is related to grip strength, tools need to be designed to fit the anthropometry of the hand. Average maximum-grip strength is achieved at a span of 5–8 cm. If, however, a single tool shaft is held, the diameter should be approximately 4 cm. The most important factor, however, is to maintain the hand coplanar with the forearm; if this is done there will be little impingement on the tissues crossing the wrist. A new design in tools and sports equipment is the "bent handle" concept. In Figure 12.12 the hand-forearm are coplanar when striking with the curved handled hammer. This is an improvement over the straight handle, during which there is pronounced ulnar deviation at impact.

Repetitive Trauma

Single high forces, or moments of force (torques) are not the only cause of injury. As in sports, the overuse syndrome occurs. This overuse syndrome is known as repetitive trauma in the workplace. It is a subtle cause of injury, difficult to detect without an analysis plan. Table 12.2 is a checklist of items to avoid or remember.

MINI-LABORATORY LEARNING EXPERIENCE

Use Table 12.2 to evaluate someone using a VDT. Do the same for someone in a factory, home workshop, or simulated industrial assembly-line job.

Vibration

Lower back problems have been attributed to whole-body vibrations experienced by tractor, bus, and truck drivers. Segmental vibrations have been known to cause sudden blockage of blood circulation, most notably Reynaud's syndrome, in which precise movements of the hands are impaired and tactile sensitivity reduced.

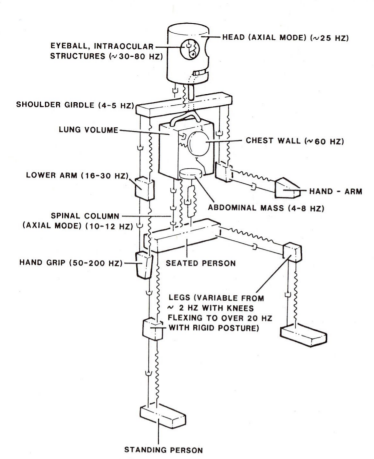

FIGURE 12.13 Mechanical system representing the human body subjected to vertical vibration. Note the highest vibration frequencies are the hand grip, chest wall, and eyeball.

(Adapted from Chaffin and Andersson's [1984] adaption from Rasmussen et al. 1982.)

The human body is modeled as a dynamic mechanical system of springs, attenuators, links, and masses, as shown in Figure 12.13. Resonant-frequency levels vary among body parts when vibrations of 100 Hz or less are applied to the body as a whole. Think of the body as analogous to a bowl of gelatin that is shaken. Stretch reflexes, muscle fatigue, and organ muscle contractions have been documented as responses to whole-body vibrations. Precise effects on the nervous system are largely unknown, although psychological stress reactions, as well as reductions in alertness, have been noted. Determining the limits of tolerance of vibrations and standards for occupations in which vibrations occur are important challenges to biomechanists.

Kinetic Modeling

Kinematic models are used in occupational biomechanics, as described in other chapters. Kinematic models are most useful as templates to compare individual performances, including performances on work tasks. Forces acting on the worker, however, are not treated in kinematic models. The primary purpose of *kinetic* modeling is to understand the stresses to the human body in order to determine risk of injury. Although any part of the body or the total body can be modeled, there are six primary sites of interest in occupational biomechanics: lumbar spine; elbow; hand; knee; hip; and shoulder. The whole body usually is modeled for investigations of

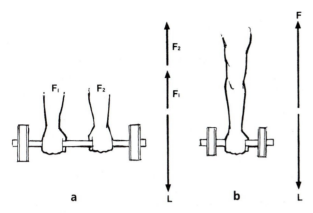

FIGURE 12.14 Load held in one hand and load held in two hands. Free body diagrams are depicted to left of situation. F, muscular force; L, load to be lifted or held.

stresses at the lumbar spine, hip, and knee. One-link models may be adequate for modeling the hand, and one-, two-, or three-link models are used for investigations of stresses at the elbow and shoulder.

Single-link Models

As outlined in Chapter 4, the simplest modeling is the planar static single-link model. In a job-related situation, the hand carrying a load is one of the simplest models to depict. Figure 12.14 represents this model, with the configured drawing and the freebody diagram. The load in *a* is borne equally (note load is held horizontal) with both arms. Therefore, each force is equal to 1/2*L* (half the load). In the case of the one arm carry (*b*), the arm must exert a force equal to the load. This vertical arm carry is without measurable torques and the skeleton may absorb the reactive forces of the load. Muscles may only be required to contract in order to stabilize the joints.

If the hand in Figure 12.14*b* were flexed radially (abducted), the load would be creating a moment of force (torque) around the wrist axis. The moment arm would be equal to the perpendicular distance the weight is from this axis (approximately 8 cm). In this case, the moment of force (8 cm × weight) would be in the clockwise direction for the load and in the counter-clockwise direction for the muscle force.

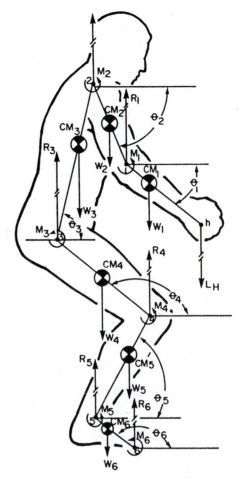

FIGURE 12.15 Six-link free body diagram of forces and moments in sagittal plane in quasistatic position during lifting.

Multiple-link Models

In the preceding examples, we did not consider the weight of the body segment. The joints of the body must always support the weight of the segment or segments that are distal to the support reaction. For example, during standing the hand-segment weight is distal to the wrist, the forearm plus hand are distal to the elbow, and the total upper extremity is distal to the shoulder. The total body reaction will be at the joints of the foot-ankle system. (See Figure 12.15.)

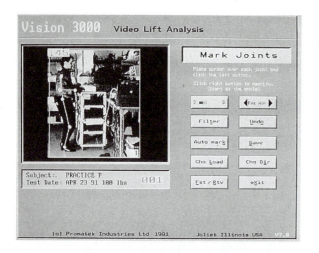

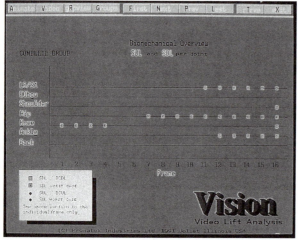

FIGURE 12.16 Video images and analysis of lifting.
(Courtesy of William DeVries, vice-president. Promatek Medical Systems, Inc.)

Note that the body segment weights act at the center of mass of the segment or system of segments (one link). If the support of the body changes, the reactions due to body segment weights will change accordingly.

Computer Modeling (Mathematical Modeling Using a Computer)

When considering accelerations and when movement is multiplanar, it is best to use computer-interfaced digitizing of data and computer software to calculate the forces, moments of force, and stresses to joints, tendons, ligaments and muscles. Researchers can obtain pseudo-3D relatively inexpensively with two video cameras. The planar images from each camera are analyzed separately and moments and forces estimated for each plane. Values low in one plane are considered negligible. Therefore, some movements can be investigated in single planes (2-D). If, however, an individual has large force values for a work task in which the normative data include only low values, this pseudo-3D technique will prove worthwhile. Such an individual is at risk and must be taught to modify the techniques used to perform the task or change jobs. A dynamic model is shown in Figure 12.16.

■ Modeling of occupational tasks has yielded a wealth of knowledge about performance and safety. The greater the information accumulated, however, the more complex the interpretation. For example, based on research on lifting tasks, the compressive stresses are less in the squat-style lift than in the stoop-style lift. The shearing forces, however, are greater in the squat style. What does that mean?

Computer Simulations. Biomechanists use modeling to assess differences in standing and sitting postures and movements at work stations because of anthropometric differences, as well as strength and flexibility differences. They can then suggest changes in the task and/or the environment and conduct computer simulations to determine if the changes would be beneficial or detrimental to worker productivity and safety. The original forces determined experimentally via modeling are used during simulation. Modeling also reduces the risk of injury from trial-and-error adjustments by the worker. The computer simulations in effect become the trial-and-error experimentations. (See Chapter 24 for more on how modeling may be used in the future.)

References

Battle, M. C., Bigos, S. J., Fisher, L. D., Hansson, T. H., Jones, M. E., and Wortley, M. D. Isometric lifting strength as a predictor of industrial back pain reports. 1989. *Spine* 14(8):851–56.

Chaffin, D. B., and Andersson, G. 1984. *Occupational Biomechanics*. New York: Wiley-Interscience.

Easterby, R., Kroemer, K. H. E., and Chaffin, D. B., ed. 1982. *Anthropometry and biomechanics: Theory and applications*. Proceedings of the NATA Symposium, Cambridge, England. New York: Plenum.

Garg, A. 1989. An evaluation of the NIOSH guidelines for manual lifting with special reference to horizontal distance. *Am. Indust. Hyg. Assoc. J.* 50(3):157–64.

Garg, A., and Badger, D. Maximum acceptable weights and maximum voluntary strength for asymmetric lifting. *Ergonomics* 29(7):879–92.

Garg, A., and Saxena, U. 1980. Container characteristics and maximum acceptable weight of lift. *Human Factors*. 22(4):487–95.

Hamilton, N. 1986. A postural model for the reduction of neck tension. Ph.D. dissertation, University of Illinois.

Karhu, O., Harkonen, R., Sorvali, P., and Vepsalainen, P. 1981. Observing working postures in industry: Examples of OWAS application. *Applied Ergonomics* 12(1):13–17.

Karhu, O., Kansi, P., and Kuorinka, I. 1977. Correcting work postures in industry: A practical method for analysis. *Applied Ergonomics* 8(4):199–201.

NASA 1978. *Anthropometric source book* (3 vols.). NASA Reference Publication 1024.

Olsen, R. A., ed. 1981: *Handbook for design and use of visual display terminals*. Sunnyvale, CA: Lockheed Missiles & Space Company.

Ruhmann, H., and Schmidtke, H. 1989. Human strength: Measurements of maximum isometric forces in industry. *Ergonomics* 32(7):865–79.

Snook, S. H., and Ciriello, V. M. 1991. The design of manual handling tasks: Revised tables. *Ergonomics* 34(9):1197–1213.

Tichauer, E. R. 1978: *The biomechanical basis of ergonomics: Anatomy applied to the design of work situations*. New York: Wiley-Interscience.

13

Biomechanics in the Arts*

Many words used in biomechanics, such as stability, inertia, acceleration, leverage, posture, friction, force development and force absorption, are the legacy of arts performers, especially dancers. This chapter will explore how these factors affect dancers and other artists.

In the arts, particularly the performing arts, individuals refine techniques and movements to become more efficient in reproducing patterns in dance, music, theater, and visual art. In these art forms, except for dance, the movement itself is not the product to be evaluated or critiqued. But the artist must be as concerned with the biomechanics of movement as an athlete or dancer. Effective movements and postures are the means by which the performer/artist creates the desired artistic expression. Since the show must go on, it becomes critical to the performing artist that injury or medical complications do not disrupt concentration, practice, or performance.

Dancers, musicians, visual artists, and actors practice and perform very long hours on a daily, weekly, and even lifelong basis. Many artists begin an art form at an early age with the expectation of many years of active participation. Unlike most sports participants and dancers, who are adolescents or young adults when they attain peak performances, it is not uncommon for a talented musician, artist, or stage performer to reach a peak in middle age and continue actively into the final years of life. As in sport, some individuals choose an art form as a career; for others, it is an intensely pursued avocation. Specialization begins at a very young age, following progressions of skill development handed down from teacher to teacher—even when that progression is not biomechanically sound. In progressing from beginner to skilled artist, intensity increases, as does time spent in practice and performance. Sometimes as much as ten hours a day are spent practicing. Such concentrated, repeated movements lead to overuse syndromes in musicians, artists, and dancers similar to the problems of the weekend athlete whose activity is also compressed into a short time period. As one easel artist suggested, his brush arm took as much punishment as that of a major league pitcher (Rowes 1986).

Dedication to improved technique and performance has sometimes been carried to such extremes as to be detrimental. Pianist and composer Robert Schumann rigged a weighted pulley system attached to the ceiling to strengthen his fourth finger. As a result, he permanently damaged his hands because he was not aware of the anatomical constraints of finger extensor tendons, which prevent the fourth finger from working independently (Ortmann 1962).

---

*Contributed by Carol Brink and Lela June Stoner.

To convey their ideas, artists must sometimes perform under very difficult conditions. Frequently, dramatic artists assume contorted postures or wear heavy costumes, headgear, and make-up to convey their ideas. Consider Jose Ferrer in the role of French artist, Toulouse-Lautrec. He performed for long hours with his lower legs strapped to his thighs to portray the artist, whose legs were deformed due to bone-growth disruption in the femur. Mime artists count on the success of their illusion to produce an image of a real event. Marcel Marceau performs a magnificent sequence of walking against the wind. To do this, he assumes a very awkward body position for a person not leaning into an actual wind force. The illusion is complete because he is able to maintain his center of mass aligned over his base of support in the absence of the actual gale force. To lose balance destroys the illusion, yet, in the absence of an actual force, muscles must contract in tense, uncomfortable patterns.

Participants and teachers of an art form share similar concerns: At what age, for instance, should one begin to dance en pointe (in toe shoes)? Are there physical characteristics that facilitate technique, or do they contraindicate successful performance, for example, dental problems that hinder the playing of wind instruments? What is the most efficient way to perform or develop techniques? How can postural tensions be reduced during practice and performance? Which muscle groups control the required movements? How can injury be avoided—especially injury severe enough to stop performance? The latter concern is one typically considered only after a medical problem arises.

As opposed to athletes, who are accustomed to physical training and the body's need for strengthening and stretching of muscles, artists rarely consider the consequences or needs of their body in practicing or performance. For example, take the case of a high school cymbalist whose marching band practiced twenty-two hours over a seven-day period. The young musician complained of painful shoulders much like the bicipital groove, the biceps tendon pain experienced by swimmers—a clear case of overuse without appropriate conditioning or rest periods (Huddleston & Pratt 1983; Lubell 1987).

Recognition of the special needs of the artistic community has resulted in a new medical speciality, arts medicine, which is growing rapidly, as did sports medicine in the last decade. The Miller Health Care Institute for the Performing Arts, located in Manhattan just a few blocks from sites where dancers, musicians, and actors perform nightly, is an example of the new medical centers devoted to the problems of performing artists (Rowes 1986, Van Horn 1987). The institute uses a team approach combining the efforts of physician/orthopedist, laryngologist, physical therapist, and artist to resolve physically debilitating problems. In an effort to keep the artist performing and active, the team analyzes movements as carefully as an athletic teacher/coach, seeking to identify the cause of painful or stiff movements. As a result of their work with artists, Miller clinicians have suggested that a performing artist must engage in warming-up, muscular-strengthening, and stretching regimes similar to those of athletes. Biomechanists have consulted concerning safety, injury prevention, technique, and conditioning for the artist, dancer, and actor. Biomechanical analysis of movements used by artists is as valuable to the performing artist as it is to the person participating in a sport or performing a routine occupational task.

Biomechanical Principles for Artists

The following principles are some of the basic ones described in Chapter 6, restated and reemphasized for their importance to the analysis of artists' movements.

Stability

The body is stable when the center of gravity is maintained over the base of support. The intersection of the line of gravity with the center of the base of support yields the greatest stability. Intersection of the line of gravity near the edge of the base lessens stability but facilitates mobility. Decreasing the size of the base of support or increasing the height of the center of gravity will decrease stability. Postures that align body segments and external implements over the base of support provide stability with less muscle fatigue.

Inertia

The body will continue in a state of rest or uniform motion unless acted on by a force sufficient to disturb this state. Segments or implements can be efficiently maintained in a state of motion when a small force is required to maintain that motion.

Acceleration

The acceleration of the body is directly proportional to the force imparted to it, in the same direction as the force and inversely proportional to its mass.

Leverage

Shorter levers rotate faster. When moving a long lever or implement, apply the force as far as possible from the center of rotation to produce greater muscular control of that implement.

Friction

(Friction is the ease of one surface moving on another surface.) The amount of friction depends on the nature of the surfaces and the forces pressing them together.

Force Development

To maximize force, apply that force directly in line with the center of mass and in the direction of desired movement. When possible, use large muscles to initiate actions and follow sequentially with segments of decreasing mass. Implements and objects concentrated close to the body's center of gravity can be moved or controlled using less force than when objects are held further away.

Force Absorption

The velocity of the body should be slowed gradually over time, especially during landings. The area of the absorption should be as large as possible.

The Dancer

Dance is an art form that uses the body as its instrument of expression. It differs from sport since it is not concerned with movement just as a means of performing some feat, such as scoring points, but is more concerned with the artistic intent and expressive quality of the movement. This aesthetic aspect of dance is of utmost importance and must not be overlooked during biomechanical analysis of dance.

Dance is an arrangement of patterns in space and time, which require varying degrees of force to perform. The properties of movement that a dancer must consider include moving through space using locomotor patterns combining the walk, run, jump, and hop, or moving within a personal space using nonlocomotor movements. The dancer is also concerned with initiating and terminating actions, airborne moves, balances, turns, extensions of the limbs, spatial relationships, rhythmic patterns, force, and energy. The extraordinary physical demands in performance of dance techniques may be comparable to those placed on highly competitive football players (Teitz 1983). When the movements are performed with efficiency, fluidity, and artistic expression, it is understood that there is another important abstract aesthetic quality at work, but which is very difficult to measure.

■ The grace and ease that dancers display use the elements of time, space, and force, as well as an aesthetic abstract quality.

Dance Forms

Many forms of dance have evolved throughout history and in different geographical locations. Each specific dance form (technique) has unique and specific performance characteristics yet is based on the same biomechanical principles as sports and movement in general. Dance (techniques) may be generally classified as either recreational or performance, depending on the goal of the person dancing. These are not exclusive categories because there is almost always crossover between them. For example, a person's main goal may be recreational dance, yet others are often watching, so he or she is also performing. Recreational forms include social, old time, aerobic, folk, square, breakdancing, country-western, etc. Dance forms with performance as their main goal include ballet, jazz, tap, modern (creative), and some forms of ethnic (dances from specific cultures). Each technique has a movement vocabulary that differentiates it from the others; however, there is also crossover in vocabulary between forms.

■ Today, most professional dancers are trained in a variety of dance forms, and sometimes more than one form is mixed in the choreography of a dance.

Performing dance forms—ballet, jazz, tap, and modern—have developed and changed through the years. Ballet movement encompasses a sense of the ethereal—fluidity, harmony, geometry, precision, variety, and a touch of regal elegance—and is based on a classical technique that originated in the courts of Italy in the sixteenth and seventeenth centuries. Jazz dance reflects the diversity of American culture, yet has origins in the rhythms and movements brought to America by African slaves and has been most influenced by social dance and popular music (especially jazz). Forms of jazz dance are found in musical theater, film and television, music videos, and nightclub acts. Tap dance comes from a blend of American cultures and is unique because of the rhythmic sounds made by taps placed on the shoes. It has been influenced by the Irish jig and the African stomp, and has unique styles such as the waltz clog, softshoe, or cakewalk. Modern dance broke away from graceful, ethereal movements of formal traditional ballet around the beginning of the twentieth century and expresses more diverse ideas and emotions. In the beginning of the modern dance movement, there were no particularly exacting techniques. But through the years different styles and training systems have been developed by well-known professional dancers, including Doris Humphrey, Martha Graham, Merce Cunningham, Jose Limon, and others. General principles of movement are the basis of most modern dance techniques, rather than individual, particular steps.

Poses

A dancer moves slowly or quickly through space, creating linear and rotational designs interspersed with balanced motionless poses. Balanced positions may be breathtaking for the audience when the dancer remains motionless in a difficult pose for several seconds. Balance is derived from keeping the center of gravity on a vertical line over the base of support. The center of gravity shifts with every change of position because the distribution of weight changes. To keep in balance when shifting the weight of a body part, a dancer must either shift another body part in the opposite direction or shift the body as a whole so that its center remains over the supporting foot. To regain lost balance, the body can adjust by a shift in the center of the supporting force at the floor; a push horizontally against the floor by the supporting foot; or a shift of the upper body towards the direction of fall, thus creating a force from the floor in the opposite direction. For the dancer, shifts in body positions must be kept small and subtle so that the illusion of motionless balance is not destroyed.

MINI-LABORATORY LEARNING EXPERIENCE

Apply the principles of equilibrium to answer the following:

1. What is the effect of raising the arms from a low position to a position over head while balancing on one foot? Why does this happen?
2. Why is it more difficult to balance in releve (lifted high on the ball of the foot) rather than on flat foot?
3. Why is it difficult to move into a pose quickly?

Turns

We seldom see dance without turns. Variations in turns result from the position of the body, angular acceleration and velocity, and whether it is a one- or two-foot turn. A turn starts with a preparation position followed by a torque (force) exerted against the floor, which causes the angular acceleration and rotational motion. Angular acceleration depends on the amount of torque and the moment of inertia. The moment of inertia is a quantity that depends on the mass of the body and also on how the mass is distributed. When the body parts are close to the axis of rotation, the moment of inertia is smaller than when the body parts are away from the axis. Therefore, turns that are slower generally have body positions with the arms or legs wide. When dancers want to accelerate the rotational motion, they bring the arms and/or legs closer to the body. To slow down again, they widen the body position.

The chaine turn is a two-step turn progressing in a straight line with the body rotating 180° on each step. A sequence of chaine turns are generally performed together.

What effect will occur with the following variations?

1. The arms are out to the side on the first step and the hands move forward and together on the second step of the turn, then back out for the beginning of the next turn, etc.
2. The arms are out to the side on the first step, the hands move forward and together on the second step, and continue to be held together until the end of the turning sequence.
3. The arms are held out to the side during the total sequence of turns.

Partnering

Dancing with a partner brings an added dimension of excitement to a performance. Each dancer must become sensitive to the other person's weight and shape and also the other's use of space, time, and force. A common movement in partnering is a vertical lift. The lift should maximize the effective use of timing, strength and coordination of both dancers and equilibrium principles. The person being lifted should jump with strength, and the lifter should maximize the use of the legs by keeping the back straight, using the arms mostly when they are almost straight at the height of the lift. The beginning or impetus for the lift comes from the jump of the person being lifted. When the momentum from the jump is expended, the strength of the arms and legs of the lifter take over. When a dancer is lifted to a position of stable equilibrium, the masses of both lifted and lifter must be directly over the base of support to achieve balance. On the descent, the motion must be slowed to ensure a gentle landing that does not jar the person and also to create the illusion of effortlessness. The person being lifted has no means to exert a force to help slow the downward motion; therefore, the lifter must use the strength in the legs as well as the arms. If the body of the lifted person is allowed to slide against the partner, friction between the surfaces of the two bodies will also aid in slowing the descent.

The easiest place to hold a lifted person is directly overhead. It becomes increasingly difficult to support a person the farther away from center he or she is. Explain this phenomenon in terms of strength and equilibrium.

Ensemble Dancing

Ensemble (group) dancing demands great precision. This is achieved most easily if the dancers have similar body shapes and sizes including height, weight and body type-ectomorph, endomorph, or mesomorph—and if they have similar inherent movement styles. The size and shape of a dancer affects the height of jumps and leaps, the length of steps, the height of kicks, etc. Each individual dancer must adapt to match the "norm," which usually is the medium sized person. In modern dance, there is now more tendency not to have as much precision in the performances, but to allow individuals to move in a natural way that suits their body and movement style.

All jumps involve forces and vertical accelerations. The height of a jump is dependent on the downward vertical force exerted against the floor and the length of time of vertical distance (d) through which that force is exerted. This downward force comes from the upward phase of the preparatory plie (knee bend). If the ratio of the vertical force against the floor and a dancer's weight is R, then the height of jump (H) is calculated by the formula

$$H = d(R-1)$$

Timing is an important factor in a dance and is dictated by the choreography and the tempo of the music. If precision of a group is important, the time in the air for all persons must be the same. The time in the air for a jump is dependent on gravity ($g = 32$ feet per second) and the height of the jump (H). The total time in the air (T) is derived from the formula

$$T = 2\sqrt{2H/g}$$

Movement-analysis Systems

Several systems that analyze movement performance through observation, description, and recording methods exist. The Simplified Movement Behavior Profile System-atic movement-behavior analysis is one approach to the quantitative study of movement styles and is discussed in Chapters 7 and 8. Three other systems are Benesh Movement Notation, Labanotation, and Effort Shape.

The Benesh system is the most popular in the United Kingdom and is particularly suited to record the stylistic movements of ballet. It is written on a five-line music stave (the lines represent floor level, knee height, waist height, shoulder height, and top of the head), which forms a matrix for the human figure. Movements and postures are recorded using symbols for each part of the body and different types of motion.

Labanotation was first developed in the 1930s and is most popular in North America. It has been used to record industrial time and motion studies as well as dance. The score uses symbols written on a vertical staff where the central column represents the support (usually the feet) with successive columns outward representing movements of the legs, body, arms, and hands. The time duration is indicated by the vertical length of the symbol.

In Labanotation the quality of movement is not notated, so Laban (the creator of Labanotation) developed another system called Effort Shape. Shape is defined as how the body shapes itself in space such as rising, widening, advancing, etc. The Effort components include:

1. **Flow—either free or bound**
   a. free—easy flowing, streaming out, abandoned, ready to go
   b. bound—controlling the flow, streaming inward, holding back and restrained, ready to stop
2. **Space—either direct or indirect**
   a. direct—zeroing in, pinpointing
   b. indirect—encompassing focus, flexible or indirect
3. **Weight—either strong or light**
   a. strong—impactful, vigorous, powerful
   b. light—using fine touch, airy, delicate
4. **Time—either sudden or sustained**
   a. sudden—urgent, hasty
   b. sustained—taking time, leisurely

These effort qualities then are put into combinations to get such movements as dabbing (direct-sudden-light) or punching (direct-sudden-strong).

■ The movement-analysis systems of Benesh, Labanotation, and Effort Shape were the forerunners of computer animation of dance movement.

Dance Physique and Training

The structure and physical condition of the body, the dancer's instrument of expression, is an important consideration for any person selecting dance as an avocation or profession. A preferred physique for those who wish a professional career in ballet is as follows: aesthetically proportioned and thin; total body alignment and symmetry; extraordinary ligamentous flexibility, especially in the knee and hip; rounded toes of medium size with the first two toes of equal length; foot arches capable of development but not flat or too high; and muscular balance, including balance of strength, flexibility, and endurance of opposing muscle groups. Clarkson et al. (1989) examined anthropometric measures of dance students and professional dancers and found that dancers tend to be tall and thin, had relatively smaller upper arms and larger calves and ankles compared with normative data.

Dance training varies by type of dance, sex, and culture, but often starts before puberty. In the American ballet schools, females often begin training at the age of seven, with males entering at eleven or older. Russian ballet dancers, both boys and girls, start at an average age of ten, and in China the age is twelve (Hamilton and Hamilton 1991). Today, dance training has become more intensive and competitive for those interested in pursuing a dance career. Each year 15,000–20,000 dance students audition to train at schools affiliated with American professional ballet dance companies. Approximately 2000 are chosen and only 2 or 3 of those will actually go on to stage careers in ballet (Dunning 1985).

Dance training lasts for eight to ten years for dancers to become proficient in most dance forms. This long training period may affect the dancer's growth and development. Amenorrhea (no menses for three or more months) and a delay in menarche have been found to be common in dancers of different nationalities. Scoliosis is also found to be more prevalent in ballet dancers than in the general population. It has been speculated that bone integrity may be compromised by the early training, leading to scoliosis and stress fractures. Whether scoliosis is

developmental or congenital is unknown. Other causes may be poor nutrition, low body fat, or the retarded onset of the menstrual cycle (Warren et al. 1986). The presence of scoliosis is not a contraindication to taking dance classes, but should be referred to an orthopedist for treatment.

■ Dance training for young dancers may affect growth and development, including amenorrhea, delay in menarche, and scoliosis.

Pointe work (toe dancing) raises the center of gravity of the dancer, decreases the contact area of the shoe on the floor, and makes traction difficult because of the stiffness of the sole. The first two metatarsals bear most of the weight when en pointe. Therefore, these bones begin to remodel so that the cortex of the first and second rays thicken (Schafle 1990). These factors increase technical demands of pointe, which should be reserved for those dancers who wish to pursue ballet as a career rather than recreation.

■ Pointe work should not begin until growth in the feet is complete and adequate strength and control in the feet, ankles, knees, thigh, hip, and trunk is achieved.

Turnout is the ability of a dancer to externally rotate the legs. Dancers strive for a perfect, or 180°, turnout from the hip joint and begin and end most movements from one of the five basic positions of the feet (Figure 13.1). This turnout is considered aesthetically desirable and essential to give the dancer freedom of movement in every direction. Turnout is considered so important in ballet that many professional dance organizations measure the amount of turnout in prospective dancers before accepting them in the dance school. Abduction of the leg is limited by impingement of the greater trochanter on the superior rim of the acetabulum and adjacent illum. But with external rotation the pelvis tilts to the opposite side and the head of the femur assumes a more inferior position, which delays contract and allows a greater range of abduction. Kushner et al. (1990) measured passive hip abduction and lateral rotation using a goniometer and Leighton flexometer and found a positive correlation—the greater the external rotation the more abduction achieved.

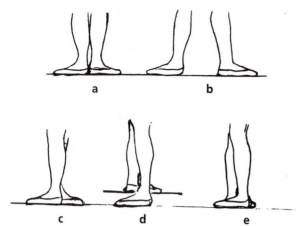

FIGURE 13.1 Five basic dance positions: (a) 1st, (b) 2nd, (c) 3rd, (d) 4th, (e) 5th.

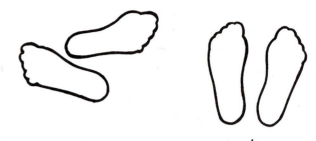

FIGURE 13.2 Position of feet: (a) Start and (b) end of takeoff phase of sissonne.

Turnout, however, is not a biomechanically advantageous position of the takeoff foot (or feet) for forward or backward elevation. A cinematographic study (Brink 1987) showed that dancers did not retain their original turnout in their takeoff phase of the sissonne (a forward jump starting in fifth position, and ending on one foot). They started in a turned-out, fifth position, but shifted to a forward position before leaving the floor (Figure 13.2).

The amount of turnout is influenced by bony, capsule and ligamentous, and musculotendinous factors. The bone limits consist of the depth of the acetabulum and the angle at which the head and neck of the femur are set on the shaft of the femur. The configuration of these bones is an absolute limitation in the range of movement. Turnout will also be limited by tightness in the fibrous soft tissues of the capsule and ilio-femoral and pubo-femoral ligaments. These ligaments may be stretched by careful static stretching during early training, but they are extremely difficult to stretch after maturity. Tightness in the muscles (sometimes after injury) may restrict turnout but can usually be increased by gently stretching.

■ Turnout is aesthetically desirable and essential for freedom of movement by the legs, but is not always a biomechanically advantageous position for elevations. Amount of turnout is governed by anatomical features.

MINI-LABORATORY LEARNING EXPERIENCE

1. Stand with both feet pointed straight forward. Swing the right leg laterally while keeping the body upright and the right knee facing forward. Next, turn the right leg outward so that the knee faces upward when you swing it.
   a. What muscles are lifting in each situation?
   b. In which position were you able to raise the leg higher? Why?

Dance Injuries

Today, the young dancer is faced with demands in both time and effort that may be accompanied by injury. The most common sites of dance injuries are in the lower extremities—feet, ankles, knees, shins, hips, and lower back. Chronic injuries are most common, but acute injuries are also frequent.

Many dancers strive to increase their turnout in deleterious and injury-provoking manners. Forcing the feet beyond the natural line by assuming the perfect turnout position of the feet while the lower legs are flexed, and then straightening the legs, is a common technique error. This faulty technique is generally accompanied by pronating the feet excessively and gripping the floor, "screwing" (twisting) the knees, and/or hyperextension of the back. These situations are discussed below.

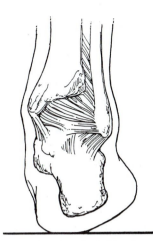

FIGURE 13.3 Excessive pronation with calcaneal eversion (rearfoot view).

In excessive pronation, the subtalar joint allows the heel (calcaneaus) to evert, and the talus is forced to internally rotate and to plantarflex. The foot collapses and the arch rolls in on itself (Figure 13.3). It may also cause the first ray to rotate internally and evert, setting up a bunion formation. The collapsing of the foot also puts excessive strain on the tibialis posterior muscle, which overworks, attempting to "hold up the arch." This strain may cause pain in the dancer identified as a shin splint (Kravitz 1987).

"Screwing the knee" uses the iliotibial band to gain further external rotation of the tibia at the knee. The patellar attachments of the iliotibial band pull the patella into an abnormal position while being subjected to large compressive forces generated during a plie (bending the knee). These strains often lead to medial knee pain (Teitz 1987) and can result in patellofemoral dysfunctional problems (Schafle 1990).

Increasing the hyperextension of lumbar lordosis of the back may increase external rotation of the hip by decreasing the tension on the iliofemoral ligaments. This results in undue strain on the lumbar spine, which, repeated over time, may cause low back pain.

Muscular imbalance, or an unequal capacity for contraction and/or stretch of the agonistic and antagonistic muscle groups, may be structural or caused by consistent patterns of misuse or overuse. A muscular imbalance may cause a snapping or "clicking" in the hip joint with hip flexion, hip abduction, or in the supporting leg when balancing on one leg. The tendons slide over the greater trochanter, or the iliofemoral ligament slides over the femoral head causing the snapping sensation. Other common muscular imbalances in dance include tightness of the hip flexors; increased pelvic inclination; imbalance between the inward and outward rotators of the hip joint; imbalance of strength between flexors and extensors of the torso, pectoralis minor syndrome; and neck and shoulder tension. Often in muscular imbalances, the agonist is tight, but the pain occurs in the antagonist. Corrective exercises may help relieve the imbalance and pain, if both agonist and antagonist are lengthened and strengthened through developmental exercises (Fitt 1987). If left uncorrected, almost every muscular imbalance will result in some type of pain.

Undue strain on the lumbar spine repeated over time will often cause low back pain. Lordosis, or a hyperextended spine, is one form of undue back strain and may be caused by tightness in the anterior hips, weakness of muscle groups (abdominals, gluteals, adductors), swayback knee, weight carried too far back, overturning the feet (turning the feet beyond the degree of turnout available at the hip joint), or arms held too far back. Other causes of lumbar strain may be forcing the spine into a hyperextended position or externally rotating the hip to achieve the desired height of the back leg in the arabesque position. Incorrect lifting and lifting of excessive loads, as in partnering, is another cause of low back pain.

■ Chronic injuries of the lower extremities are the most common dance injuries, usually caused by faulty technique, undue strain, or muscular imbalance.

MINI-LABORATORY LEARNING EXPERIENCE

Place your body into the position shown in Figure 13.4.

1. How can the strain on the lower back be avoided?
2. What other dance activities and daily living skills perpetuate this posture?

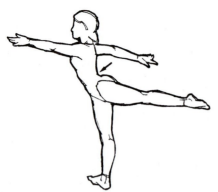

FIGURE 13.4 Strain on lumber spine due to hyperextension. **How can this be avoided? What other dance activities and daily living skills perpetuate this posture?**

Dance Environment

■ The environment—particularly the shoes and floor—in which a dancer performs may contribute to injuries.

The soft ballet shoe has no cushioning, no shock-absorbing material or design features, and no space for orthotics. Pointe shoes have a stiffly constructed box to enclose the front of the foot, which is padded with lamb's wool or other cushioning material. Two areas of concern with dance floors are the hardness and the finish of the floor. Most dancers feel that a suspended floor is important for absorption and resilience for elevation movements. The correct amount of friction with the floor is important to prevent slips and falls, and yet permit the dancer to perform turns with ease. Dancers often use rosin on their shoes to increase friction. Too much friction, however, may also be dangerous. Stage floors may be especially difficult to dance on, and many dance companies travel with their own special stage floor coverings.

Dance Research

Biomechanical research in dance is in its infancy. Dancers have always used the naked eye as a research tool to mimic the performance of other more expert dancers or to analyze the technique of students whom they are teaching. Videotape and film have been used to record movement for historical purposes or to learn the sequences of movements for new dances. Now, dancers

are using more sophisticated tools for skill analysis. The choice of research tools varies depending on the desired hypothesis, or question in mind, and the data needed to examine that hypothesis.

Cinematography and videography systems record the image, project it, digitize it, and provide for data analysis using computer programs. Cinematography has been used to compare the filmed performance of specific dance steps to that described in the dance literature. It has also proved to be a valuable tool in unveiling the hidden worlds of the dancer. Since many dance movements are performed rapidly, the naked eye may be duped into seeing the body doing something other than what is actually occurring. Biomechanical dance research began in 1972 with MacDuff's (1972) study on the grand jete, a favorite dance skill for cinematographic analysis (Koller 1973; Gaffney 1977; Plastino 1977; Ryman 1978). Based on analysis of high-speed film, Hinson et al. (1977) found that subjects began the rotation for the tour jete on takeoff rather than as commonly thought, during the flight component. Gans (1985) studied the relationship between shin-splint pain in ballet dancers and heel contact on ascent and descent from jumps. Her results showed that dancers with a history of shinsplints demonstrated more double heel strikes than the other group.

The electromyogram (EMG) measures the electrical signal, or muscle action potential, associated with the contraction of a muscle. Beale, Scearce, and Moore (1976) used electromyography to study the muscle action potentials of the erector spinae and rectus abdominus muscles during the performance of the demi-plie and grand plie (small and full bend of the knees) in first position and compared dancers at three different skill levels. They found that the more advanced dancers used these muscles in a more efficient manner. Another research study (Ryman and Ranney 1978) demonstrated that different dancers had their own unique patterns of muscle usage in the performance of the grand battement devant (lifting a straight leg forward), even though the dancers had many years of standardized drilling in the performance of the skill.

Force transducers and force plates are kinetic research tools that record the force exerted by the body on an external body. Bejjani, et al. (1988) studied the demands of the percussive footwork of Flamenco dancers

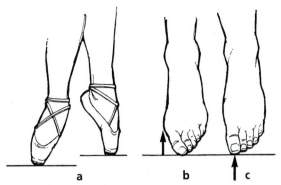

FIGURE 13.5 Relevé en pointe with eversion (*a*); shear pressure at metatarsal-phalangeal joint (*b*); and normal pressure en pointe (*c*).

on the musculoskeletal system using sensors placed on the feet, skin mounted accelerometers, and vibration pressure diagrams. Pressure transducers have been used to study the relative pressures on the toes in pointe shoes. The great toe was found to bear the most pressure, and the pressure on the second toe varied with toe length and shoe padding. An everted position in releve (Figure 13.5) was the cause of increased pressure in the metatarsal phalangeal joint (Teitz, Harrington, and Wiley 1985).

Nonspecific peak torques of female and male dancers were measured by an isokinetic dynamometer and compared to other athletes. Male dancers had similar characteristics to other male athletes, but female dancers were lower in relative force production compared to other female athletes (Kirkendall et al. 1984).

Because the different components of biomechanics are all interrelated, dance research often combines two or more components for a more complete picture of a problem. Micheli (1984) studied the physiological profiles of dancers by measuring cardiovascular response with a modified balke treadmill protocol, assessing endurance with an isokinetic dynamometer, and measuring flexibility with a Leighton flexometer. The results of the study showed that ballet dancers possessed aerobic fitness levels higher than the general population of the same age and sex, but lower than that of endurance athletes. Female dancers had strong lower extremity musculature but relatively weak upper extremity muscles, and they showed a remarkable degree of flexibility.

Often it is difficult for dancers to keep abreast of current trends and advances in technological research techniques, as well as various other aspects of the dance profession. When the artistic world of dance becomes more technologically sophisticated, many questions currently raised may be studied from the biomechanical perspective to identify safe, effective, and efficient dance technique.

■ Collaborating with colleagues who have specialized knowledge and access to various biomechanical research instruments may be imperative to further the dance research.

MINI-LABORATORY LEARNING EXPERIENCE

1. Describe three balance positions used in dance and discusss how the principles of stability influence them.
2. Why does the dancer keep the center of gravity slightly more forward while using a walk movement than in a normal walk?
3. What technique skills does a dancer use in the absorption of the weight of the body on landing from a jump?
4. How can a person being lifted by a partner assist in the lifting process?
5. The body is accelerated in jumps and leaps in dance. What forces cause these accelerations, and what would be considered the mass?
6. How does rosin on dance shoes increase friction?

The Musician

Introduction to music as an art form occurs at a very early age, and it is not uncommon for a musician to remain active very late in life. For example, classical guitarist Andres Segovia performed well into his 90s. Small discomforts that serve as warnings of overuse are frequently ignored because practice and performance is not inhibited. In perfecting the fingering of a difficult passage, the pianist or guitarist rarely considers the possibilities of carpal tunnel syndrome, nor does the violinist respond to temporomandibular dysfunctions caused by tightly pressing the violin between the chin and shoulder. Many musicians are reluctant to seek medical assistance as pain becomes chronic because they fear loss of work or prestige when the problem is known.

Vocal and instrumental musicians use muscles to control air flow, embouchure, fingering, bow action, slide manipulation, and body posture while performing. As they work to perfect techniques handed down from one generation of musicians to another, it is important that they protect themselves against the constant bodily abuse of rapid repeated actions performed with considerable strength and precision—movements that do not fit a natural pattern. Historically older-style instruments, e.g., keyboards, were very heavy and stiff and required a forceful attack in order to produce sound. As the touch of modern instruments became lighter (easier to depress), technique did not always change to accommodate that alteration. Individual differences also fostered inappropriate technique. For example, pianists who used the flattened finger playing style of Vladimir Horowitz soon found fast passages to be disasterous because he was unique in his ability to play rapidly without using a curved finger position, i.e., the shortened lever (Sataloff, Brandfonbrener, and Lederman 1991).

■ A shorter lever moves faster and uses less muscle effort.

Posture

Playing style for the violin changed from being held against the chest to the virtuoso technique of Paganini who held his violin against his chin. As a result of the violin being fixed at the chin, considerable fatigue and pain occurred in the bow arm and lower back of violinists. Sieber (1969) studied the violin bowing arm in an effort to identify problems unique to its use. A recent Swedish invention, a different form of support for the violin, was developed to minimize spine problems. Gamba leg has been described among musicians who attempted to play the viola da gamba (an earlier, violin-type instrument) and who suffered overuse syndrome of the leg as a result of holding the instrument securely

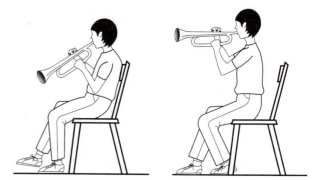

FIGURE 13.6 Slouched and erect postures of trumpeter.

against the chest by using leg pressure (Howard 1982). Of those under the age of 25 who play the violin, 75% suffer back pain (Silverstolpe 1983), which suggests that, at an age when musicians are increasing practice and performance time, back injury is prevalent. Biofeedback during practice has been used to help string and woodwind musicians reduce unnecessary tensions (Levee, Cohen, and Rickles 1976; Levine and Irvine 1984; Morasky, Reynolds, and Clarke 1981).

In controlling their technical performance, many musicians must also manipulate cumbersome instruments that encourage awkward postures or positions because of instrument size or configuration or because of the cramped quarters in which it is played, e.g., the orchestra pit. Musicians who play large instruments such as the double bass, cello, or tuba face the added challenge of moving it from place to place as well as holding it upright to play. Some sit with leg and hip imbalances due to sharing a music stand or manipulate a bow or slide while keeping both the conductor and music clearly in view. A harpist not only maneuvers a large instrument, but faces the prospect of constant tuning of the strings, which requires a forceful twisting action that quickly leads to painful injury.

Erect posture is as important for the musician as for any worker. This posture provides the best body alignment for breath control in playing brass and woodwinds, and it minimizes stress to muscles of the low back and upper extremities. Chairs used by musicians tend to be uniform in nature, and adjustments for shorter legs and low back support are left to the individual. Use of an

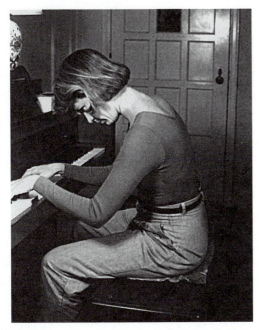

FIGURE 13.7 Pianist striking chord with total upper body tension.

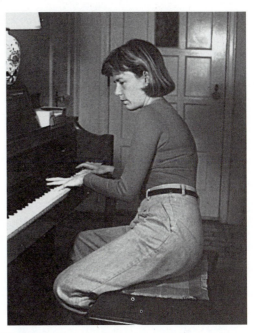

FIGURE 13.8 Pianist leaning body toward upper register.

adjustable piano bench seems to be the only recognition of individual differences. Those who play multiple keyboards must constantly rotate to reach other keyboards; lone drummers must rotate to reach other percussive devices.

■ Erect posture facilitates breath control of wind instruments and minimizes muscle fatigue from an unbalanced spine.

Since most individuals rotate only the shoulders, back problems quickly develop. Considerable effort has been directed toward improving posture of double-bass players as well as to their facility for manipulating a large implement by varying chair height and music stand placement. Guitarists also have problems related to imbalanced positioning of their instrument during play (Silverstolpe 1983).

Control of the instrument itself or of the arms in moving to produce sound frequently leads to problems of the upper extremities and/or low back. Silverstolpe (1983), Fry (1986), and Elbaum (1986) note that musicians suffer from upper limb overuse syndromes. Flute,

double bass, guitar, violin, and cello are particularly problematic instruments for musicians ages 17–24, who have the highest incidence of back pain. Sex differences exist only in relation to those instruments that are predominantly played by males, e.g., double bass (Silverstolpe 1983).

Note the pianist in Figure 13.7 whose upper body is totally tense in playing a cord. If it is not the final chord that ends the musical selection, it would be impossible to reposition the hands on the keys in the upper register. This is similar to the fencer who commits totally to the thrust, without considering the possibility of being parried. Playing from an erect posture allows the pianist to use a slight body lean to play notes in the upper register (Figure 13.8) while remaining prepared to move to another keyboard position. If only the arms are moved to play high octave chords (Figure 13.9), the pianist would quickly fatigue the muscles of the back and shoulder. Sitting erect at the piano (Figure 13.10) and using a bench height that maintains the lower arm parallel to the keyboard is the posture that produces the least tension in the shoulders

Biomechanics in the Arts   **269**

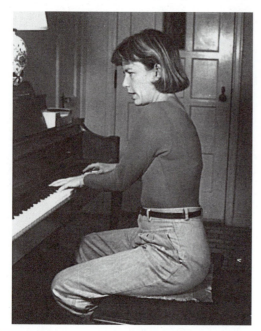

FIGURE 13.9 Pianist moving only the arms toward upper register.

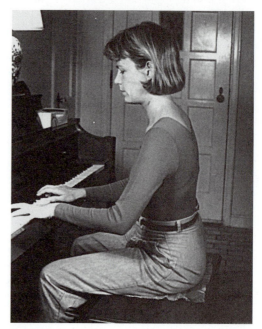

FIGURE 13.10 Correct erect playing posture.

and upper back. The pianist in Figure 13.11 collapses the spine, which produces fatigue in the back and shoulder muscles. To alleviate this discomfort, the pianist retracts the shoulders, allows the pelvis to tilt forward, and sits (Figure 13.12) with a hyperextended lumbar spine to relieve tensions—a position conducive to producing low back pain.

Posture appears to be affected by the demands of the instrument for some musicians (Bejjani and Halpern 1989). Among virtuosi male trumpeters, producing music is clearly a total body effort. Higher notes require higher expiratory air pressure when respiration exceeds 40 l min^{-1}, which is true in trumpet playing (Basmajian and DeLuca 1985). To play these higher notes, especially when sustained, the musician lowers the horn position and tilts the pelvis posteriorly. Constrained by the length of hip flexors and hamstrings, a concurrent knee flexion occurs. Stretching exercises for these muscle groups may effectively increase the ability to hit and sustain high notes.

In singers and wind instrumentalists, abdominal control of breathing is critical. In novices, serious back problems are related to lack of abdominal strength and the inability to control the pelvis during standing and seated playing. It is important that, even during practice, these musicians maintain a balanced, erect posture to facilitate their breathing and performance. Although a relatively lightweight instrument, the flute forces an imbalanced posture because the performer must sit or stand with arms directed to the right side of the body, away from the body center. This posture leads to back difficulties; therefore, flutists are encouraged to execute movements toward the opposite side of the body or to perform relaxation exercises during resting passages (see Figure 13.13).

Injuries

Pianists and drummers are especially susceptible to overuse injuries of the hands. Fry (1986) noted that among injured pianists, the problem was not a simple

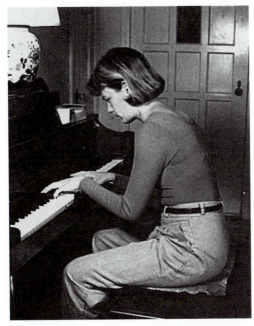

FIGURE 13.11 Playing keys with a collapsed spine posture.

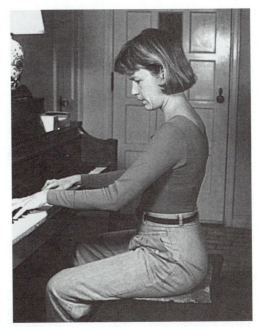

FIGURE 13.12 Pianist compensating for tired upper back muscles.

acute attack of pain. Nearly half had experienced symptoms for a period of one to five years, and one-fifth had suffered longer. As might be expected, the site of pain was predominantly the hand/wrist and all levels of the spine. Leading with a flexed hand in a fast upward run of the piano (Figure 13.14) is more damaging than leading with the elbow and maintaining the wrist as an extension of the forearm (Figure 13.15). Drummers, because they use the sticks almost as if they were weapons, suffer not only from chronic hand problems but may also develop calluses around the nerve that require surgical removal (Lubell 1987; Van Horn 1987).

Efficiency and Control

Instrumental and vocal musicians search for efficiency in the control of airflow as well as the neuromuscular control of the facial muscles and lips, the arm, and the fingers. Several researchers have approached technique improvement by contrasting professional musicians with a student or novice group. Ortmann (1962), an early pioneer in applying science to music performance, focused on the movement patterns of pianists in coordinating the fingers and arms for weight transfer, vertical and lateral

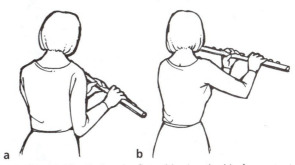

FIGURE 13.13 Playing the flute: (a) using the hip for support; (b) holding the flute correctly.

arm movements, and finger stroking required to play staccato, legato, portamento, octave tremelos, arpeggios, cadenzas, etc. He demonstrated clearly that greater vertical arm motion was required in playing fortissimo than pianissimo, that volume increased relative to the number of body segments (finger, hand, forearm, arm, and trunk) used, and that faster passages were played with less vertical action and increased use of the elbow in pulling the hand away from middle C.

Biomechanics in the Arts   **271**

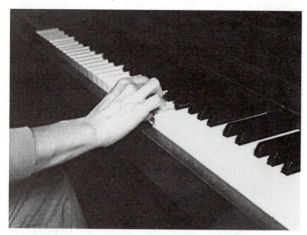

FIGURE 13.14   Scale run with wrist leading a radially flexed hand.

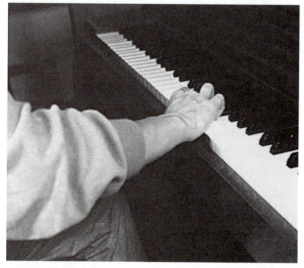

FIGURE 13.15
Run played with elbow leading and the hand and wrist aligned.

Sieber (1969); Polnaur and Marks (1964); Morasky, Reynolds and Clarke (1981) used electromyography to identify bow and finger control in string players. Lammers (1983) focused on the neuromuscular control of the slide in all seven positions of the slide trombone. Henderson (1942), White (1972), and White and Basmajian

(1973) clarified the muscular pattern of the lips in controlling trumpet embouchure. Although White (1972) was also interested in mouthpiece pressure, it was Froelich (1987) who refined the instrumentation and protocol to effectively identify direct (normal) and shear forces applied to the trombone mouthpiece. He found direct pressures higher in trombonists playing in the high registers or playing fortissimo. A high note played loudly used three times the force of a low note played softly (571 vs. 1875 grams). As the first researcher to consider mouthpiece shear force, Froelich suggested greater shear force was used to perform fortissimo and at higher pitches; however, he also noted more force was used to perform low pitches than to perform the middle pitches. He also suggested that less shear force seemed to identify a better quality of sound.

Contrasts between differing levels of instrumental musicians have indicated that professionals generally play more efficiently (with less muscular activity) and control the mouthpiece and bow with less force. In the bowing arm, Sieber (1969) found greater muscular activity among the student violinists compared with professionals.

■ **Keep body parts in anatomical alignment when controlling slides, bows, and sticks and use larger muscle groups to move the implement.**

Lammers (1983) identified professional trombonists as moving the slide more quickly to position with less muscular activity, thus allowing greater time for controlling tonal qualities. Froelich (1987) described professional trombonists as using less direct pressure as well as shear force against the mouthpiece than novices. White (1972) identified that muscular activity in the lips of trumpet players was equally divided between the top and bottom lips in professionals, but more weighted toward the top lip in beginners. Froelich (1987) supported this finding in trombonists suggesting that shear force was detrimental to the quality of the tone produced. Barbenel, Kenny, and Davies (1988) found that more prolific trumpeters tolerated greater maximal mouthpiece force than less-skilled players.

The Dramatic Artist

The dramatic artist is often required to manipulate heavy implements, remain in distorted positions to rehearse, and perform for long hours. Consider the role of Albin in *La Cage aux Folles.* Eight shows a week for more than a year, Walter Charles maneuvered in high-heel shoes, which caused his calf muscles to knot up, resulting in a painful Achilles tendon. The pain was in addition to the risk of falling downstairs due to the unaccustomed footwear. After an ankle fracture, Katharine Hepburn was forced to play her role in *A Matter of Gravity* from a wheelchair. Because of the complex make-up for *Elephant Man,* the actor was trapped for long hours behind the heavy debris configured to resemble the physical change in the man he portrayed. In *Creeps,* actors produced the effect of moving as if they had cerebral palsy. The role gave rise to aches and pains and reactivated old injuries, until physicians and physical therapists, serving as medical choreographers, identified problematic repeated movements and worked with the actors to find a safer way to produce the same effect (Rowes 1986).

Historically, people maneuvered flags, banners, and heavy weapons. Film and theatrical performances require that these implements be handled safely and efficiently in a confined space. Stage fights of all types must be carefully choreographed to prevent injury to the adversaries or the surrounding cast. Movements of flags and banners must be carefully practiced to minimize the low back pain associated with balancing a long, weighty lever. (Tree trimmers who use a saw blade attached to the end of a long pole have similar problems with low back pain.)

■ Weight at the distal end of a long lever may require a hand position near the weighted end to facilitate control of that larger force.

Because of hazardous actions executed in movies and television, stunt men and women have become important performers. In the early stages of a career, an actor or actress may be asked to perform all stunts without a stand-in. Barbara Stanwyck was an excellent horsewoman who made directors very nervous because she insisted on doing her own riding stunts even in the later years of her career. When his or her economic value to the movie or show changes, the star is usually replaced in any dangerous action. The replacement is a stunt athlete, who is an expert at absorbing force in a very short time, with the aid of various shock-absorbing materials such as mats and pits. When the hero is thrown from the second-story window, the stunt man takes the fall, landing on shock-absorbing materials not seen by the audience. In sports we see similar force absorption in the flexing of legs and trunk or the use of a special landing pit. A beginning judo lesson includes practice of various techniques for landing safely.

The Visual Artist

Visual artists manipulate various tools that they grasp and move rapidly for long periods of time. A survey of self-employed artists in New York City revealed that 80% had to work very fast using repetitive motions and in awkward positions. Tomie dePaola, famed children's illustrator/author, was seriously incapacitated by wrist and forearm pain. After seeking medical guidance he was able to work again (and sign autographs for his young fans).

Arts medicine clinics report high incidence of low back, neck, and shoulder complaints in professional artists. A fifteen-minute video of randomly selected senior drawing students at the School of Visual Arts in New York City provided insight into these problems (Chang, Bejjani, and Chyan 1987). Students were engaged in either a small detailed work (15 × 15 cm) or a large piece (60 × 80 cm). Detailed small work led to greater flexion and more stress to the back and neck. Significant sex differences were noted in shoulder angular velocities, with males demonstrating higher values. Calculated muscle tensions were several times greater than those of the neutral body position. When painting for long hours, the artist's arm might well feel as fatigued as that of a baseball pitcher (Rowes 1986).

■ Using large brush strokes controlled by large muscle groups minimizes fatigue for visual artists.

Every visual artist should have a well-lighted, ergonomically designed work station to support creative endeavors. Breaks should be frequent and provide the artist with a different type of motion, preferably total body movement such as walking to another room. Stretching exercises to relieve tensions in the upper back, i.e., the upper trapezius, rhomboids and deltoids that support arm use, and for the lower back are also useful. A video of the artist at work could easily document deterioration of posture and movements due to fatigue.

Trends and Guidelines

Sophisticated technological tools have been used for more stringent scientific analysis of artists' movement patterns. When used by a team of concerned individuals from several professional groups, these tools can reduce the risks to performance and enhance movement efficiency. A three-year program of biyearly screening of dancers at the University of California, Irvine has resulted in reducing the number of alignment problems. More dancers are visiting the trainer or kinesiologist as soon as a problem develops, and the number of debilitating injuries has been reduced. The medical team at Irvine included an athletic trainer, an orthopedic surgeon, an expert in evaluating feet for pointe work, and a kinesiologist, who works closely in monitoring and advising dancers (Plastino 1987). Similar teams have reported positive results with artists at the Miller Health Care Institute for the Performing Arts in New York (Rowes 1986; Van Horn 1987). Early screening to identify functional anatomical or postural alignment problems also plays a role in the development of technique in children. Because of their skeletal immaturity, elementary-age children might be encouraged to play trumpet rather than tuba, and ballet dancers encouraged to wait until they are older to begin pointe work.

Because artists need a healthy body to perform, they are encouraged to use a conditioning and warm-up routine similar to that of an elite athlete. All artists are encouraged to warm up their bodies and the active body parts, their hands, arms and shoulder area, before engaging in their art form. Strength development of important muscle groups is encouraged even to the extent of suggesting that dancers might train with external weights (Plastino 1987). Dancers also need to stretch the agonist and antagonist muscles to facilitate greater range of motion in all planes. To meet the needs for long periods of technique practice, artists should begin work very gradually

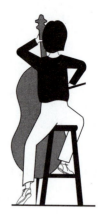

FIGURE 13.16 Posture and compensations for size and height of stool and string bass with respect to anthropometric characteristics of the performer.

after a prolonged layoff. With a better understanding of the anatomical, biomechanical, and physiological aspects of controlling the fingers or bowing arm, and of the limitations of the body, artists can expect to be more successful in preventing injuries that result from overuse or faulty technique. They will also be able to pace their work, cope with fatigue, and perform more effectively.

MINI-LABORATORY LEARNING EXPERIENCE

1. Sit at a piano striking a key or chord. Use the weight of the finger, then add additional segments until finger, hand, forearm, arm, and trunk are involved. What action produces the loudest sound? the best staccato? the fastest tremelo? How is production of a loud tone similar to throwing a ball for distance?
2. While at the keyboard play four notes of a scale with the fingers of one hand. Play first with fingers outstretched, then curve the fingers so that you cannot see the nails as you play. Try each method playing the scale of four notes faster and faster and faster. Which method works better for a fast passage? Why are pianists amazed at Horowitz's flat finger style in very fast passages?
3. String bass players often sit on a high stool to play (Figure 13.16). Sometimes one foot is on the ground

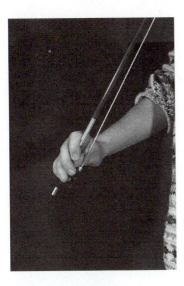

FIGURE 13.17 Bow hand and position of minor radial deviation of the hand. Optimum position for long durations of playing the violin or viola.

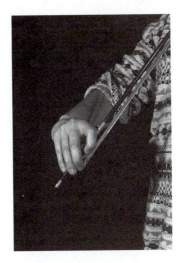

FIGURE 13.18 Potentially traumatic stress levels occur when playing the violin or viola with the bow hand in this flexed, radially deviated position.

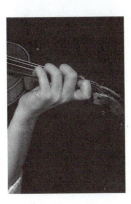

FIGURE 13.19 Hyperextended hand during playing the violin.

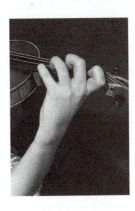

FIGURE 13.20 Hand in alignment with forearm while playing the violin. Note the differences in flexion at the metacarpal joints in this figure and Figure 13.19.

and the other on the low rung of the stool. How does this affect posture? Try sitting with a small paperback book under one hip. How long can you remain in this position without discomfort? How is that alignment of the spine similar to that of the string bass player?

4. Look at the photographs of the violin player (Figures 13.17–13.20). Which bow hand position allows for the best anatomical alignment? Look at the string fingers and select the alignment that is best for that task? How does curving the fingers help the violinist?

5. Hold a canoe paddle as if it were a flag in a parade. Experiment with different angles from vertical to horizontal. Try different placements of the hands: close together at the end of the pole (paddle), separated, close together 18 inches from the end, or separated at least 12 inches from the end. Which is easiest and which is hardest to control? How is this similar to using a lacrosse stick or other sport implement?

6. If you were a harpist in the symphony, what could you do to facilitate moving the harp from one site to another and performing the many repetitions of tuning the strings. *Hint:* Piano tuners demonstrate a longer tool for tuning piano strings to reduce forearm stress.

7. Observe a musician in performance on stage, videotape, or television. Identify correct biomechanical posture, limb positions, and use of hands. Do you note any actions that might lead to fatigue or overuse when performed for several hours?

References

Ames, J., and Seigelman, J. 1977. *The book of tap.* New York: David McKay.

Badler, N. I. 1989. A computational alternative to effort notation. In *Dance technology: Current applications and future trends,* ed. J. A. Gray. Reston, VA: AAHPERD.

Barbenel, J. C., Kenny, P., and Davies, J. B. 1988. Mouthpiece force produced while playing the trumpet. *Journal of Biomechanics* 21(5):417–24.

Basmajian, J. V., and DeLuca, C. J. 1985. *Muscles alive,* 5th ed. Baltimore: Williams and Wilkins.

Beal, R., Scearce, C., and Moore, D. 1976. Electromyographical studies in ballet. Unpublished paper.

Bejjani, F. J., and Halpern, N. 1989. Postural kinematics of trumpet playing. *Journal of Biomechanics* 22(5):439–49.

Bejjani, F. J., Halpern, N., Pio, A., Dominguez, R., Voloshin, A., and Frankel, H. 1988. Musculoskeletal demands on Flamenco dancers: A clinical and biomechanical study. *Ankle & Foot* 8(5):254–63.

Brink, C. 1987: Cinematographic analysis of the sissonne ouverte in female dancers. Ph.D. dissertation, University of Minnesota.

Calvert, T. W. 1989. Toward a language for human movement. In *Dance technology: Current applications and future trends,* ed. J. A. Gray. Reston, VA: AAHPERD.

Chang, W., Bejjani, F. J., and Chyan, D. 1986. Biomechanical basis of musculoskeletal disorders among visual artits. In Bejjani, F. J., ed., *Proceedings of North American congress on biomechanics.*

Clarkson, P. M., Freedson, P. S., Skrinar, M., Keller, B., and Carney, D. 1989. Anthropometric measurements of adolescent and professional classical ballet dancers. *Journal of Sports Medicine and Physical Fitness* 29(2): 157–62.

Dunning, J. 1985. *But first a school: The first fifty years of the school of American Ballet.* New York: Viking Press.

Elbaum, L. 1986. Muscularskeletal problems of instrumental musicians. *Journal of Orthopaedic and Sport Physical Therapy* 8(6):285–87.

Fitt, S. S. 1987. Corrective exercises for two muscular imbalances: Tight hip flexors and pectoralis minor syndrome. *JOHPERD* 58(5):45–48.

Fitt, S. S. 1988. *Dance kinesiology.* New York: Shirmer Books.

Froelich, J. P. 1987. Mouthpiece forces during trombone performances. Ph.D. dissertation, University of Minnesota.

Fry, H. J. H. 1986. Overuse syndrome of the upper limb in musicians. *The Medical Journal of Australia* 144: 182–83, 185.

Gaffney, S. D. 1977. A cinematographic analysis of the straight leg leap (grand jete). Master's thesis, Texas Woman's University.

Gans, A. 1985. The relationship of heel contact in ascent and descent from jumps to the incidence of shin splints in ballet dancers. *Physical Therapy* 65(8):1192–96.

Hagist, F. M., and Politis, G. 1989. A computer program for the entry of Benesh movement notation. In *Dance technology: Current applications and future trends,* ed. J. A. Gray. Reston, VA: AAHPERD.

Hamilton, L. H., and Hamilton, W. G. 1991. Classical ballet: Balancing the cost of artistry and athleticism. *Medical Problems of Performing Artists,* June: 39–44.

Henderson, H. W. 1942. An experimental study of trumpet embouchure. *Journal of the Acoustical Society of America* 13:58–64.

Hinson, M., Buckman, S., Tate, J., and Sherrill, C. 1977. The grand jete en tournant entrelace (tour jete): An analysis through motion photography. *Dance Research Journal CORD* 10(1):9–13.

Howard, P. L. (1982). Gamba leg. *New England Journal of Medicine* 306(18):1115.

Huddleston, C. B., and Pratt, S. M. 1983. Cymbal player's shoulder. *New England Journal of Medicine* 309(23): 1462.

Irvine, J. K., and LeVine, W. R. 1981. The use of biofeedback to reduce left hand tension for string players. *American String Teacher* 31:10–32.

Kelly, E. 1987. The dancer's back. *JOHPERD* 58(5): 41–44.

Kirkendall, D. T., Bergfeld, J. A., Calabrese, L., Lombardo, J. A., Street, G., and Weiker, G. G. 1984. Isokinetic characteristics of ballet dancers and the response to a season of ballet training. *Journal of Orthopedic and Sports Physical Therapy* 5(4):207–11.

Koller, B. A. 1973. A cinematographical analysis of the dance leap. Master's thesis, Southern Illinois University.

Kraines, M. G., and Kan, E. 1990. *Jump into jazz.* Mountain View, CA: Mayfield Publishing Co.

Kravitz, S. R. 1987. Basic concepts of biomechanics relating the foot and ankle to overuse injuries. *JOHPERD* 58(5): 31–33.

Kushner, S., Saboe, L., Reid, D., Penrose, R., and Grace, M. 1990. Relationship of turnout to hip abduction in professional ballet dancers. *Journal of Sports Medicine* 18(3):286–91.

Lammers, M. E. 1983. An electromyographic examination of selected muscles in the right arm during trombone performance. Ph.D. dissertation, University of Minnesota.

LaPointe-Crump, J. D. 1985. *In balance: The fundamentals of ballet*. Dubuque, IA: Wm. C. Brown.

Laws, K. 1984. *The physics of dance*. New York: Shirmer Books.

Levee, J. R., Cohen, M. J., and Rickles, W. H. 1976. Electromyographic biofeedback for relief of tension in the facial and throat muscles of a woodwind musician. *Biofeedback and Self-Regulation* 1(1):113–30.

Levine, W. R., and Irvine, J. K. 1984. In vivo EMG biofeedback in violin and violin pedagogy. *Biofeedback and Self-Regulation* 9(2):161–68.

Lubell, A. 1987. Physicians get in tune with performing artists. *Physician and Sportsmedicine* 15(6):246–56.

MacDuff, N. 1972. Effects of music and rhythm on the biomechanics of a specific dance movement. Master's thesis, Pennsylvania State University.

Micheli, L. J. 1984. Physiologic profiles of female professional ballerinas. *Clinics in Sports Medicine* 3(1):199–209.

Minton, S. 1984. *Modern dance: Body and mind*. Englewood, CO: Morton Publishing Co.

Morasky, R. L., Reynolds, C., and Clarke, G. 1981. Using biofeedback to reduce left arm extension EMG of string players during musical performance. *Biofeedback Self-Regulation* 6(4):565–72.

Norman, D. O., and Grodin, M. A. 1984. Injuries from break dancing. *American Family Physician* 30(4):109–12.

Ortmann, O. 1962. *The physiological mechanics of piano technique*. New York: Dutton.

Piagenhoef, S. 1977. *Patterns of human motion, a cinematographic analysis*. Englewood Cliffs, NJ: Prentice-Hall.

Plastino, J. G. 1987. The university dancer physical screening. *JOHPERD* 58(5):49–50.

Polnauer, F., and Marks, M. 1964. *Senso-motor study and its application to violin playing*. Urbana, IL: American String Teachers Association.

Robertson, K., Hutton, R., Miller, D., and Nichols, T. 1989. Mechanical and anatomical factors relating to the incidence and etiology of patellofemoral pain in dancers. In *The dancer as athlete: The 1984 Olympic scientific congress proceedings,* vol. 8.

Rowes, B. 1986. To deal with their special needs, painters and performers can turn to a new speciality! Arts medicine. *People Magazine* 26(21):101.

Ryman, R. S. 1978. A kinematic analysis of selected grand allegro jumps. In *Essays in dance research: Dance research annual IX*, ed. D. L. Woodruff. New York: Congress on Research in Dance.

Ryman, R. S., and Ranney, D. A. 1978. A preliminary investigation of two variations of the grand battement devant. *Dance Research Journal CORD* 11(1):2–11.

Sataloff, R. T., Brandfonbrener, A. G., and Lederman, R. J. 1991. *Textbook of performing arts medicine*. New York: Raven Press Ltd.

Schafie, M. D. 1990. The child dancer: Medical considerations. *Pediatric Clinics of North America* 37(5):1211–20.

Sieber, R. E. 1969. Contraction-movement patterns of violin performers. Ph.D. dissertation, Indiana University.

Silverstolpe, L. 1983. Ergonomic problems amongst musicians. Lecture Fimm-Congress, Zurich.

Teitz, C. C. 1983. Sports medicine concerns in dance and gymnastics. *Clinics Sports Medicine* 2:571.

Teitz, C. C. 1987. Patellofemoral pain in dancers. *JOHPERD* 58(5):34–36.

Teitz, C. C., Harrington, R. M., and Wiley, H. 1985. Pressures on the foot in pointe shoes. *Foot and Ankle* 5(5):216–21.

Van Horn, R. 1987. Music medicine: The Miller Health Care Institute. *Modern Drummer*: 28–31, 100–105.

Warren, M. P., Brooks-Gunn, J., Hamilton, L. H., et al. (1986). Scoliosis and fractures in young ballet dancers: Relation to delayed menarche and secondary amenorrhea. *New England Journal of Medicine* 314:1348–53.

White, E. R. (1972). Electromyographic potentials of selected facial muscles and labial mouthpiece pressure measurement in the embouchure of trumpet players. Ph.D. dissertation, Columbia University.

White, E. R., and Basmajian, J. V. 1973. Electromyography of lip muscles and their role in trumpet playing. *Journal of Applied Physiology* 35(6):892–97.

14 Collisions and Impacts

Performers in certain sports or work environments learn to catch objects. Falling and landing effectively with a minimum of injury are also necessary skills to attain longevity in sports, industry, and daily living. Special protective equipment, including helmets and footwear, reduces risk of injury due to striking, hitting, falling, and colliding with other objects.

A collision (or impact) is the interaction (contacting) of two or more objects, with at least one being in motion prior to contact. Thus, the momentum of the moving object can be transferred, in part, to the other object. The collisions of greatest interest to biomechanists are those involving two or more human bodies or one human body and an inanimate object, such as the ground.

■ During every collision or impact involving a human body, there is a risk of trauma from the kinetic energy of the colliding bodies.

Understanding and Measuring the Forces of a Collision

As described in Chapter 6, each collision transfers the forces at impact, redistributes them, increases the forces acting on one body and decreases the forces acting on the second body and/or absorbs, dampens, or attenuates the forces of the system. What happens to the forces during an impact can be measured and recorded with dynamometers and accelerometers. Such instrumentation and applications were presented in Chapters 7 and 8. The underlying problem in collisions, commonly occurring in the sports world but also in daily living and work situations, is for the biomechanist to determine the magnitude of the forces and to estimate the expected trauma, since the kinetic energies may be greater than those the human tissues can tolerate. The design of protective equipment to protect against specific collisions in sports has become more important in the reduction of injury.

Mechanics of Stopping Moving Objects

Among the motor skills that human beings perform is stopping a moving object. The object may be external, such as a ball, or it may be the performer's own body, as in landing from a height. The pattern of joint action varies with the situation, but the mechanical principles are the same in all situations.

If a stopping action is skillfully done, the momentum of the moving object is decreased gradually by joint actions. The object is permitted to continue its motion as its velocity is gradually decreased. If the object is contacted with the hands and the arms extended to meet it, the joint actions are those of a pulling pattern, usually extension of the upper arm and flexion of the forearm. Although the joint actions in pulling and stopping are the same, the source of energy differs. The momentum of the oncoming object moves the segments in the direction in which the object was moving; at the same time, muscular effort resists that motion. As the upper arm is extended by the force of the object, the shoulder flexors resist; as the forearm is flexed, the elbow extensors resist. In pulling, the object to be moved resists, while shoulder extensors and elbow flexors contract. Thus, the muscular tension is greater during pulling than catching. Likewise, when the body lands from a height, the momentum of the center of gravity tends to cause flexion at the ankle, knee, and hip joints. These actions are resisted by the extensor muscles at the joints.

The basic mechanical principles involved in stopping a moving object or one's own moving body in action are based on the effective and efficient manner of dissipating the kinetic energy of the moving body without injury to the performer. The kinetic energy ($\frac{1}{2} mV^2$) of an object can be reduced to zero or to other safe limits by the following methods:

1. Using as great a surface area as possible in catching or landing.
2. Using as great a distance as possible. This may be accomplished through movement of body parts, deformation of body parts, or moving the entire body.
3. Using as great a mass as possible in catching or landing.
4. Regulating the position of one's center of gravity for dynamic control. For example, in falling, a person is able to continue movement of the body into a controlled rolling action that terminates in a stance rather than lose equilibrium, which causes the body to tumble several revolutions in uncontrolled directions, terminating in an upside-down position.
5. Using materials other than the human body to perform steps 1 to 4.

Catching

Catching is the act of reducing the momentum of an object in flight to the point of zero or near-zero velocity and retaining possession of it at least momentarily. This is accomplished by using the hands, body, feet, and auxiliary pieces of equipment. The momentum of the object is transferred to the receiving mechanism. When an object is light in weight and traveling slowly, a human being can easily stop it. However, if the object is heavy, traveling at great speed, or both, the transfer of momentum must be gradual to prevent injury to the hands or other parts of the body and to allow the receiver to control the object once in possession of it.

When one part or parts of the body, such as the hands, are held rigid at the moment that a fast-moving object comes in contact with it, they must absorb the full force of the impact. In sports, the momentum of an object being caught is decreased by increasing the distance at which it is caught. This process is known as giving, or recoiling, with the object until it is traveling slowly enough to be controlled accurately.

If the object to be caught is heavy, such as a large medicine ball, or is traveling unusually fast, such as a fastball thrown by a baseball pitcher, to dissipate its momentum over a long distance may be difficult and take more time than can be allotted during the process of playing the particular game. The more practical procedure is to increase the mass (inertia) of the stopping mechanism and decrease the distance over which it travels. For example, the baseball catcher dissipates the momentum of the ball thrown by the pitcher by placing the body directly in front of the path of the oncoming ball. He assumes a stance in which the feet are placed in a stride position with the legs flexed and the center of gravity low. This is the best posture in which to recoil from the force (momentum of the ball) and at the same time offer as much of the body to absorb the momentum of the ball as possible.

The receiver of an object must be careful not to make unnecessary body motions when running to receive it. Unnecessary up-and-down movements, such as raising and lowering the center of gravity and moving the head and eyes up and down through a vertical plane, may cause the receiver to lose track of the flight path of the object. Outstretching the arms while running may cause receivers to reduce their speed because they are not using the arms properly in the run and are also projecting the center of gravity too far forward. It also may tense the arms and cause them to drop the ball.

A ball is not caught with the fingers. Rather, it is received first against the middle of the palm of the hand (which is made into the form of a cup), and then the fingers close around it, preventing it from escaping. If it is caught against the rigid heel of the hand, it is likely to rebound too quickly from the hand and may also cause injury.

TABLE 14.1 Fielding mechanics analysis.

Mechanics (Progressive)	Rating	Comments
Preparation/Ready Position		
Relaxed and comfortable position	_____	_____
Feet shoulder-width apart, parallel/square stance	_____	_____
Base of support includes entire foot, heels down	_____	_____
Hips, knees, and ankles flexed	_____	_____
Trunk straight, slightly inclined forward	_____	_____
Head comfortable, bat level	_____	_____
Shoulders slightly forward; 90 degree angle at elbows	_____	_____
Arms slightly away from body, relaxed	_____	_____
Positioning Phase		
First move, shift of weight in direction of ball	_____	_____
Pivot on foot closest to ball, step forward or backward	_____	_____
Head moves in direction of ball off bat	_____	_____
Rapid run to fielding location	_____	_____
Forward/backward foot position, slightly apart	_____	_____
Body directly behind oncoming ball	_____	_____
Reduction of Force Phase		
Catch is on throwing side	_____	_____
Fingers appropriately upward or downward	_____	_____
Upon ball contact, hands are pulled into body	_____	_____
Weight shift onto flexed back leg, leg on catching side	_____	_____
Trunk rotates to catching side	_____	_____
Transfer of momentum from catch to throw	_____	_____

Rating scale: 4-very good, 3-good, 2-fair, 1-insufficient (Klatt 1990). Reprinted by permission of Lois Klatt, Concordia University, River Forest, IL.

The effective catcher (receiver in any sport or endeavor) has loose, flexible hands to catch the object and to dissipate its momentum gradually. Correct body posture is also essential. Placing the hands in the best possible position is another requirement for success. For example, a ball traveling at a height below the waist is caught with the fingers pointing downward. In all instances, the hands are placed so that they have a basket-like quality. Seldom does a skilled performer not make use of two hands, even though the actual catch is made with one hand. The object (such as a ball) may rebound out of one hand if the momentum is not properly dissipated. The use of both hands aids in trapping the object.

MINI-LABORATORY LEARNING EXPERIENCE

1. Apply the checklist for fielding a softball (Table 14.1) to performance of skilled and unskilled players.
2. Qualitatively determine the risk of injury due to repeated trauma from lack of dissipation of the kinetic energy.
3. Identify and suggest changes to be made in the fielding technique.

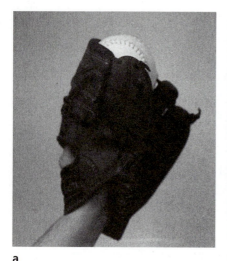 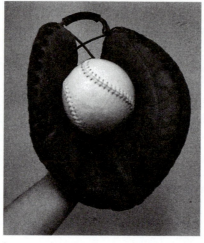 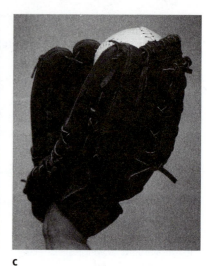

a   b   c

FIGURE 14.1 Catching a softball with three different mitts. Note the differences in moment arms (ball to wrist) among the three ball-mitt systems. **Which one has the greatest extension of the hand?** (a) Represents the system with the longest moment arm; therefore, this mitt absorbs the energy of the ball through a greater distance than the other two mitts. **Which mitt appears to have the greatest amount of material to absorb the energy of the ball through material deformation?**

Large objects thrown with great speed, such as a football (which is also thrown with a spin), are caught and then quickly cradled. That is, the receiver pins the football against the body as soon as possible to prevent its escape because of the reaction. If the arms do not have to be extended fully for the catch, the receiver should not do so in this instance. In the flexed position, the arm muscles can withstand the force of the impact with no chance for injury, since the impact will elicit further flexion.

Protective Equipment for Catching

Baseball and Softball

When gloves or mitts are used to catch fast-moving objects, two principles can be considered. The first principle is to allow some part other than the human body to absorb the force of impact, which can be considered as having a certain amount of either kinetic energy or momentum. The second principle is that of dissipating the force through a distance. The use of catcher's, fielder's, and first-base mitts is based on these principles (Figure 14.1).

The material comprising the mitt usually deforms. The ball embeds in the mitt and dissipates its force (energy), both through a large surface area and increased distance. The first-base mitt functions more on the principle of increasing the distance through which the mitt moves, thus dissipating the kinetic energy of the ball. The distal end of the mitt, and with it the ball, moves approximately 15 cm after initial contact and then, because of its movement of force, causes the hand to move. Then the elbow, shoulder, and other joint angles of the body change. The fielder's glove incorporates certain features of a catcher's and first-base mitt.

New gloves and balls have been designed for greater shock absorption of forces. This is especially true for balls for children and balls for baseball batting practice.

Lacrosse

The quantification of what actually happens during catching may be described by the example of cradling a lacrosse ball in a lacrosse stick (Figure 14.2). When the ball strikes the lacrosse basket, the materials of ball and basket deform, but only the deformation of the basket can be seen. These deformations are not sufficient to prevent rebounding of the ball. Catchers have to move the stick and arms in the direction of the ball flight.

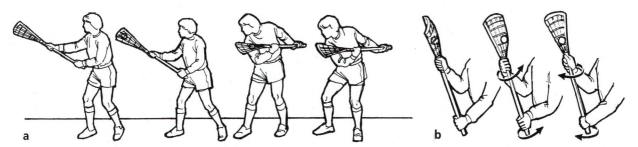

FIGURE 14.2 Catching (a), and cradling (b) techniques used in lacrosse to dissipate kinetic energy of the ball. In a, the player reaches forward toward the ball and during the catch moves the stick in the direction of the ball flight. In b, the ball is caught with a rotational movement of the stick, thereby assuming the momentum of the ball. The ball is then oscillated between the sides of the basket until it comes to rest or is thrown.

If the flight velocity of the ball had been 20 m/sec before impact, its kinetic energy would be $\frac{1}{2}mV^2$, or 48 NM, or joules (based on a ball weight of 2.4 N, which is 0.5 lb). Both deformation of the basket and the reactive forces caused by the lengthening and narrowing of the basket opening reduce the kinetic energy of the ball as much as 90%. Thus, the ball velocity for rebounding may be no more than 5 m/sec. Movement of the arms and stick adds mass to the moving ball system and reduces the ball velocity to 0.2 m/sec, based on the conservation-of-momentum principle. Observation of the performance indicates that a distance of 0.6 m is required to reduce the velocity of the ball and arms to zero.

During the game of lacrosse a catching distance of 0.6 m requires too much time and places the ball and stick in an unsatisfactory position. An alternate method of catching involves the cradling, or rotation, of the stick about its longitudinal axis, which causes the ball to rebound from one side of the basket to the other. Linear displacement is replaced by rotational displacement for the dissipation of the kinetic energy of the ball.

■ In most sports situations, the momentum gained during the catch may be used in starting the next movement. If the next action is to be a throw, the ball is drawn back during the catch in preparation for throwing. Whenever possible, the receiver should move the body into position for the next action as the catch is made, to reduce still further the time required for the complete movement. In addition, the momentum of the ball (since it seldom comes to a complete rest but usually continues in a small angular path as the arm is moved to throw) may be used in moving the ball in the new direction.

Biomechanics of Head Injuries and Protection

Look in your history books and you will note that head protection, for prevention of injuries, has been deemed important for thousands of years. We have progressed remarkably far since the heavy metal helmets of the Middle Ages. Now the helmets consist of lightweight, effective impact-resistant outer shells, resilient energy-absorbing liners, ventilation systems, fire-resistant and shatter-proof shields, and neck protection attachments. Because the brain is inside the skull and the head is a collision site from accidental and deliberate collisions in sports such as football, boxing, ice hockey, motorcycle and auto racing, bicycling, equitation, skiing, and baseball, it has become necessary to design and manufacture helmets for sports participants. In order to design each helmet effectively, the following process is required:

1. Determine the frequency and type of head impact in the sport.
2. Determine the magnitude of the impact force.
3. Develop a test method to evaluate proposed helmet designs and prototypes.

■ Head protection is required in many sports since we cannot prevent the unprotected head from impacting, colliding with, or being accelerated by another object.

Impacts to the head caused by translational forces, rotational forces, and combinations of the two produce accelerations to the head, crushing and fracturing at the impact site, and stresses at the neck, which is the axis of rotation. Thus, we identify flexion and extension bending moments, torsion moments, and pure axial loadings to the head (and neck) as a unit. In addition, however, two other types of effects on the head can occur that are difficult to analyze. These are *stress wave propagation,* waves that transmit throughout the head, producing varying amounts of strain and disturbances and *contact phenomena,* stress that causes physical disturbances at and near the impact site. These occur because the head is comprised of living tissue, mainly fluid, which deforms and can be accelerated. Such accelerations and deformations create reflective forces.

Using videography, cinematograpy, dynamography, accelerometry, electrogoniometry, and electromyography, researchers have estimated forces produced by or acting on the human body and its tissues. For example, accelerometers placed inside football helmets enable us to record the forces of impacts to the head and high accelerations due to the sudden stopping, starting, or trunk impacts that create a "whiplash" condition.

Experimental data are obtained not only from volunteers or unsuspecting participants of a collision, but through the use of human cadavers, living experimental animals, anthropomorphic replications (or simplifications) of the human head or head-neck-torso system, and through mathematical/computer modeling. Mathematical modeling simulates experimental and other conditions in order to predict potential forces, determine safe limits of impacts, and design protective headgear. The use of CAD/CAM to design a helmet is shown in Figure 14.3.

After the protective headgear is designed, testing methods evaluate the effectiveness of the headgear to withstand forces (not break) and to attenuate the acceleration forces. The maximum allowable peak force appears to be 300 Gs (300 multiplied by the acceleration of gravity). More recently, however, there is speculation that 175–200 Gs might be the limit of safety, especially for children. Common test methods are shown in Figure 14.4.

■ An alternative to protective headgear is protective landing surfaces, such as playgrounds, pole-vaulting pits, ice hockey arenas, walls, etc.

Falling

Correctly performed falling involves a gradual reduction in the momentum of the body when it comes in contact with the floor, ground, or other surface. Four general principles and techniques of protection in all types of falling are:

1. In the sit-down-and-roll technique, the center of gravity is lowered. The action in falling is such that the weight of the body is distributed over a large area. If the fall is vertical, the momentum should be transferred from vertical to horizontal as soon as possible to reduce the force of the fall, e.g., in a gymnast's accidental fall.
2. The projections of the body must be protected by using the fleshy parts as striking surfaces as in football.
3. Extended levers offer a greater potential range of motion than do flexed ones. Therefore, when the legs or arms strike the surface in falling, they should be prepared for the contact by being placed in near-extension. Care must be taken to avoid hyperextension, which causes the joint to be rigid and resist flexion of the limb. With the joint at an angle slightly less than 180°, the force of the fall can then be taken by a gradual flexion of the legs or arms, (e.g., in tumbling back handsprings).
4. If during a fall the landing is made on the feet, the person must bring the center of body weight to a position above the feet in order to use the shock-absorbing action of the ankles, knees, and hips, as in a gymnast's controlled fall.

How Severe Is a Fall?

We can estimate the kinetic energy of the body at the instant of impact from a fall by incorporating the law of falling bodies:

A body falls at the rate of 9.8 m/sec^2 (32.2 ft/sec^2), the effect of gravity

The body begins with a zero vertical velocity at the beginning of the fall. Its final vertical velocity will be equal to the square root of twice the acceleration of gravity multiplied by the distance of the fall (or $V^2 = 2as$).

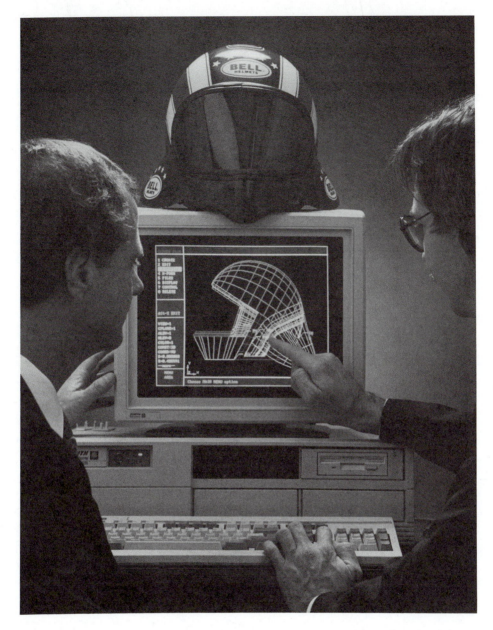

FIGURE 14.3 The use of CAD/CAM (computer assisted design and computer assisted modeling software) to design a sports helmet. (Courtesy of U.S. Pep.)

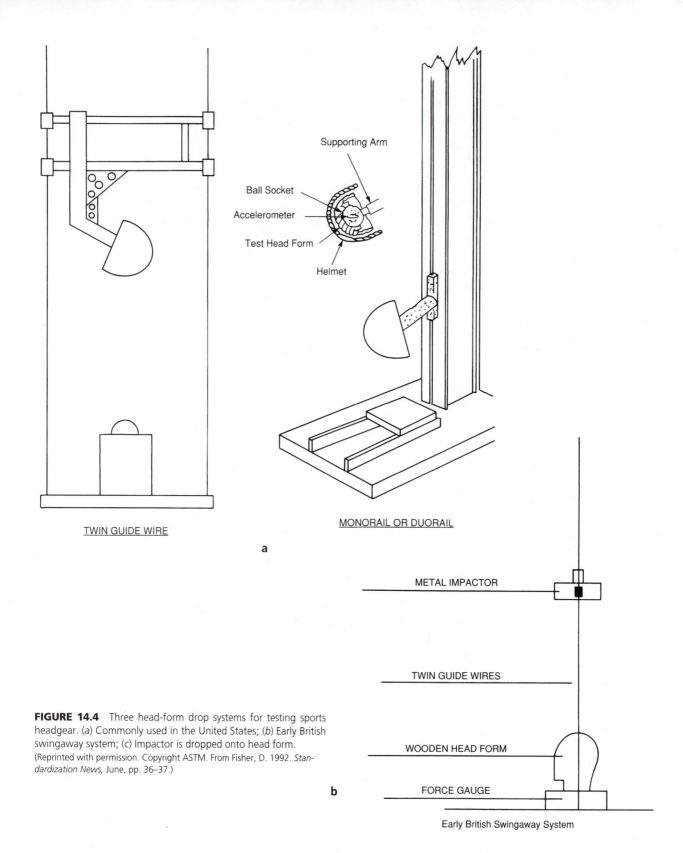

Supporting Arm

Ball Socket

Accelerometer

Test Head Form

Helmet

TWIN GUIDE WIRE

MONORAIL OR DUORAIL

a

METAL IMPACTOR

TWIN GUIDE WIRES

WOODEN HEAD FORM

FORCE GAUGE

b

Early British Swingaway System

FIGURE 14.4 Three head-form drop systems for testing sports headgear. (a) Commonly used in the United States; (b) Early British swingaway system; (c) Impactor is dropped onto head form. (Reprinted with permission. Copyright ASTM. From Fisher, D. 1992. *Standardization News,* June, pp. 36–37.)

FIGURE 14.4 Cont.

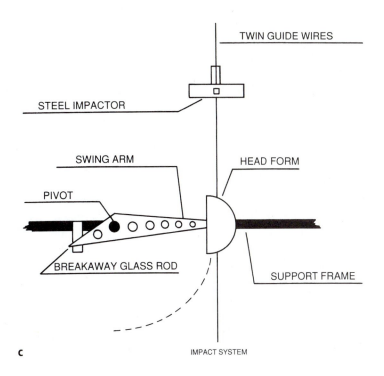

TWIN GUIDE WIRES

STEEL IMPACTOR

SWING ARM

HEAD FORM

PIVOT

BREAKAWAY GLASS ROD

SUPPORT FRAME

c

IMPACT SYSTEM

Knowing the mass of the falling body as weight divided by gravitational force, we can calculate kinetic energy $\frac{1}{2}mV^2$. We cannot, however, know the rate of dissipation of this energy unless we know the strain (deformable or elastic) characteristics of the system. (Refer to Chapter 3 for a review of mechanics of materials.)

Fat and muscle deform more than bone, dissipating the kinetic energy before extensive damage can be done. We can estimate the dissipation by measuring the amount of deformation of body parts and surfaces or measuring the rate of deceleration using an accelerometer.

The recovery from a stumble is mainly reflexive. Both the righting reflex and equilibrium reactions (which are instinctive) are activated. As the toe trips over an obstacle and the body starts to fall forward, reflex and equilibrium reactions are initiated. Normally the head and trunk are extended to counteract the forward momentum. The arms are often abducted to assist in regaining balance.

A person who starts to fall to the right side, for example, usually elevates and abducts the arms and extends the forearms (with arms out to the sides). The body is shifted to the left to help check the momentum

to the right. The side of the buttocks is offered as the landing surface. The legs are flexed to decrease the force of the blow and to lower the center of gravity so that the distance of the fall is reduced. A rotation of the trunk may take place so that the momentum of the fall is dissipated in two directions—opposite and to the rear. Protective extension of the arms is often used to help dissipate the momentum of the fall. This action, however, has proved dangerous when the forearm has gone into hyperextension. Gymnasts, dancers, and others must be cautioned not to use the rigidly extended arm to attempt to stop a fall.

Landing

Landing is a type of fall that is often both controlled and expected and that enables the performer to strike a surface, possibly avoiding injury to the body parts. Landings occur in many activities of life, from the mild ones of foot landings during walking to the landings of ski jumpers, skydivers, and pole-vaulters. When a body falls, its vertical force, kinetic energy, and momentum are directly related to the distance through which it falls. Since the rate of falling is 9.8 m/sec², the velocity of the body increases exponentially, not linearly, as the height of fall increases. Therefore, landing on a rigid, rather nondeformable material is dangerous from heights of 3 m or more. If the landing is headfirst, the result is often death, except for the very young. In the sports arena, specialized landing surfaces are required for high jumping, pole-vaulting, long jumping, and certain gymnastics events. When a landing cannot be made with the feet, the fleshy part of the thighs, hips, and shoulders are preferred landing areas. These parts are the primary landing sites in judo. For ectomorphic persons, however, no area of the body may have sufficient "padding" for a safe landing, even with landing mats. In such instances, the landing should be with the feet unless protective equipment is worn.

Numerous studies have been conducted on landings in gymnastics, volleyball, and track and field events. Biomechanists use ground reaction data to deduce relative impacts to the human body. (See Chapters 6, 8, and 9.)

Protective Equipment Used During Landings

Kneepads are common in volleyball, basketball, football, skateboarding, and soccer. Shin guards are recommended for field hockey and soccer. Thigh pads are used in softball, baseball, and football. It is recommended that hip or thigh protection be used for gymnasts performing on the uneven parallel bars. In this case padding the bars may be an alternative to padding the human body. The higher the skill level, the greater the forces are apt to be. However, the lower the skill level, the more likely it is that there will be uncontrolled landings.

In activities in which the landing is the terminal point in the movement pattern, such as in high jumping and pole-vaulting, the landing surface is padded, rather than the performer. Both the pole-vaulting and landing pits are above ground to decrease the falling height and, therefore, the final velocity of the performer at landing.

MINI-LABORATORY LEARNING EXPERIENCE

1. Investigate the landing forces using one of the following methods: force platform, digital or needle-type weighing scale, or a perceived-shock rating scale. This perceived-shock rating scale is a 7-point scale that the person uses to rate intolerable-to-minimum shock to the body.
2. Use four or more landing conditions from a box approximately two inches high:
   a. land rigidly
   b. land with deep flexion
   c. land on a soft mat placed on the landing surface
   d. land with a double mat placed on the landing surface
3. Note the kinematic chain of the legs and arms during the landings.
4. Record the maximum vertical forces observed or the perceived magnitude of the forces for each condition.
5. Apply the results to sports situations.

The pits are made so that the penetration by the performer into the landing pit is approximately half the depth of the landing pit at the time the performer reaches zero velocity. This distance allows a safe, low rebound from the pit.

Since the vertical drop in long jumping is much less than in pole-vaulting or high jumping, and since the landing is on the feet, an elevated landing pit is not needed. A sand pit in which the body can penetrate from 10 to 30 cm into the sand is adequate for safety. The sand also allows measurement of the jump. In fact, the long jump pit is slightly below the level of the takeoff board.

During recent years, the public has shown a concern for reducing the injury rate in sports. Manufacturers have produced more and better protective devices to be worn by the performer or on which the performance takes place. Sometimes there are conflicting problems in the manufacturing of a product that must be designed not only to improve safety but also to improve performance. Often an improvement in safety alters the performance capabilities or prevents the attainment of a satisfactory performance. For example, shoulder pads restrict the ability of football line players to raise the arms above shoulder height. Original tumbling mat design and construction allowed the impact forces to be absorbed at landing but prevented the execution of a second tumbling movement directly after landing. As new materials were developed, mats with an elastic component were constructed. These mats not only attenuated the energy of landing but gave a "spring" to the performer. As skill levels in tumbling improve and more complex stunts at greater heights are executed, the mats may no longer be safe. It is also possible that the safe mats of today may limit the acquisition of certain skills, especially for Olympic-caliber performers.

A similar inadequacy of sports equipment has been noted in jogging. Millions of people jog several miles on concrete sidewalks and paved streets and compete in long-distance races on similar terrain. Jogging shoes were not originally designed with the shock attenuation qualities necessary for such conditions. Research that identifies the impact forces and the sites of impact is now helping manufacturers to design safe shoes for jogging.

Teachers and coaches must understand the biomechanics of clothing and impacts to avoid the risk of litigation and save students from unnecessary injuries.

■ Excess forces or repetitive forces create trauma.

Is Protective Equipment Required?

To answer this important question, movement analysts must ask:

1. Does the force of the collision approach or exceed human tolerances?
2. Does collision occur frequently?
3. Is there a high rate of injury for this collision?

If the answer is yes to any of these questions, protective equipment should be considered.

Base the selection of adequate protective equipment on the following criteria:

1. Protective equipment must fit the anatomy of all performers. Quite often, protective equipment is designed for the average person and is unsatisfactory for persons at the extremes of anthropometric distribution.
2. Protective equipment must allow freedom of movement. For example, shoulder pads used in football sometimes restrict players' movement to the detriment of performance.
3. Protective equipment must attenuate the "excess" force. Protective equipment must be checked after hours or seasons of use to ensure that attenuation characteristics have not degraded.

Figure 14.5 shows examples of protective equipment. Evaluate each with respect to the above criteria.

People with physical impairments and those with muscular weaknesses may need some type of protective equipment for activities of daily living. The tolerances of their body tissues may be much lower than those of the athletic population. In particular, frictional forces may cause hand injuries to persons with these impairments but may have no effect on the hands of athletes. Anatomic considerations, again, are of vital concern to the movement analyst in identifying the forces and level of safety of movement patterns.

The Committee on Sport Facilities and Equipment of the American Society for Testing and Materials (ASTM) is a standards-setting body in the United States. ASTM studies the safety and performance of sports equipment and facilities. Teachers and coaches can help the committee to identify problems by providing the following information:

1. What types of injuries occur in a specific activity?
2. What landing surfaces and protective devices are in use when injuries occur?
3. Which products are unsatisfactory?
4. What is the nature of the performance in which injuries occur, for example, falling from a height, rotary movements, or absorbing forces?

Contact ASTM at 1916 Race Street, Philadelphia, PA 19103, phone (215) 299–5400

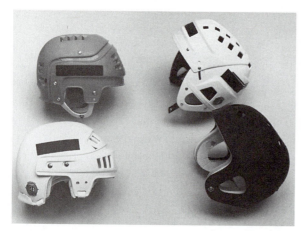

a

MINI-LABORATORY LEARNING EXPERIENCE

1. Rank the kinetic energy (KE) of the following falling bodies (vertical direction) and the approaching objects (horizontal direction), using the formula $KE = \frac{1}{2} mV^2$.
   a. adult, 588 N, jumping from a bus step, 1 m above ground
   b. diver, 490 N, diving from a 3-m board
   c. ball, 19.6 N, traveling 10 m/sec
   d. ball, 9.8 N, traveling 30 m/sec
   e. long jumper, 588 N, with center of gravity 2 m above ground
   f. pole-vaulter, 534 N, clearing a 5-m bar with a 1.5-m landing pit
   List one (or more) factors or methods useful in dissipating the kinetic energy of these moving parts.
2. Observe people catching two medicine balls of different weights. Describe the effectiveness of the action in response to both a moderate speed of flight and a fast speed of flight.
3. Catch a softball in the following manners:
   a. with "board hands," remaining stiff and letting the ball rebound
   b. with hands
   c. with forearms and abdomen
   d. with hands and under conditions of increasing speed of flight until the ball "stings" at impact
   e. with a mitt and at increasing speeds (greater than those used in step d)

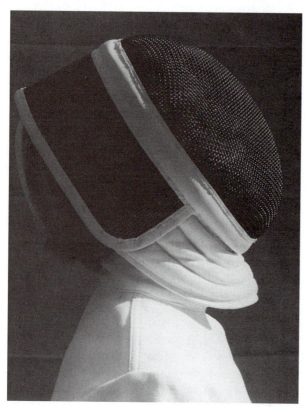

b

FIGURE 14.5 (a) Four protective helmets worn during sports. (b) Fencing mask to protect neck and head.
(a. Photo courtesy of ASTM.)

References

Adams, S., Adrian, M., and Bayless, M. A., eds. 1987. *Catastrophic injuries in sports: Avoidance strategies.* Indianapolis: Benchmark Press.

American Society for Testing and Materials 1994. *Annual book of standards:* Sec. 15, vol. 15.07, End use products. Philadelphia: ASTM.

Coleman, J., Adrian, M., and Yamamoto, H. 1984. The teaching of mechanics of jump landings. In *Second national symposium on teaching kinesiology and biomechanics in sports,* ed. R. Shapiro. Dekalb, IL: NIV.

Della-Giustina, D. E. 1992. Impact of eyeguards on eye injury reduction in the racquet sports. *ASTM Standardization News,* June 1992, pp. 50–53.

Doherty, J. K. 1964. *Modern track and field.* Englewood Cliffs, NJ: Prentice-Hall.

Fisher, D. 1992. History, helmets, and standards: 40 years of advancement in head protection. *ASTM Standardization News,* June 1992.

Frederick, E. C., ed. 1985. Sport shoes and playing surfaces: Biomechanical properties. Champaign, IL: Human Kinetics Publishers, Inc.

Goldsmith, W. 1982. Biomechanics of head injury: Part 1. *Trauma* 24, 3:21–73.

Goldsmith, W. 1982. Biomechanics of head injury: Part 2. *Trauma* 24, 4:5–65.

Goldsmith, W. 1983. Biomechanics of head injury: Part 3. *Trauma* 24, 5:73–101.

Hodgson, V. R., and Thomas, L. M. 1973. Biomechanical study of football head impacts using a human head model, final report. Detroit: National Operating Committee on Standards for Athletic Equipment.

Ireland, D. R. 1992. The shocking truth about athletic footwear: ASTM subcommittee F08.54 develops test method. *ASTM Standardization News,* June 1992.

Morehouse, A., and Morrison, W. E. 1975. The artificial turf story: A research review. Penn State HPER Series No. 9. State College: The Pennsylvania State University.

Nigg, B., and Kerr, B., eds. 1983. Biomechanical aspects of sport shoes and playing surfaces. Calgary, Canada: University Printing.

Roberts, C. C., Jr. 1992. Skiing injuries are going downhill. *ASTM Standardization News,* June 1992.

Too, D., and Adrian, M. 1987. Relationship of lumbar curvature and landing surface to ground reaction forces during gymnastic landing. In *Biomechanics in sports* III, IV, ed. J. Terauds, B. Gowitzke, and L. Holt. Del Mar, CA: Academic Publishers.

Vinger, P. 1985. The eye and sports medicine. In *Clinical ophthalmology,* ed. T. Duane. Philadelphia: Harper & Row.

Vinger, P., and Hoerner, E., eds. 1986. Sports injuries: The unthwarted epidemic, Section IV: Protective devices and rules, pp. 375–400. Littleton, MA: PSG Publishing Company.

PART

IV

Sports Movements on Land

15 Biomechanics of Running*

Running is a form of locomotion. Most children and adults have had the experience of participating in this cyclic repetitive action. In this chapter we will investigate environmental and other influences on running biomechanics.

Running is a modification of walking and differs from it in significant aspects. First, during one phase in running, neither foot is in contact with the ground; second, at no phase are both feet in contact with the ground. Although these distinctions necessitate differences in joint action, the same joints and segments are used in running as in walking. Differences in joint degrees and timing of actions can be anticipated. Since only one foot is on the ground at one time, and both feet are off the ground at one time, it is possible to run relatively smoothly with one leg shorter than the other; in walking, this condition would cause a limp. In addition, once speed in running has been developed, the force of the forward momentum is greater and contributes more to forward movement of the body than during walking. The action of the swinging leg in running is greater in amplitude and velocity and is likely to contribute the most to the forward movement of the body.

*consultant: Phillip Henson, Ph.D.
Assistant Track Coach, Indiana University and Olympic Facilities Manager for the 1996 Olympics

Running is a bipedal, three-dimensional action, just as is walking. (See Figure 9.8.) All the determinants of walking are prominent in running: pelvic rotation, pelvic tilt, lateral motion of the pelvis, flexion at the knee, foot and ankle motion, and knee motion all are present to a greater degree in running than in walking. In addition, there are greater flexion and extension of the legs and arms, resulting in a wider range of motion. Thus, running requires greater lengthening of muscles and greater flexibility at the joints than does walking. The faster the run, the greater the change in movement range. A major difference is that in walking there is an overlapping of the stance phases, while in running there is an overlapping of the swing phase.

Often the factors that are important in speed running are less important in distance running. Proper mechanical positions and speed are essential to a sprinter, while physiological endurance, efficiency, and pace are all important to a distance runner. In races involving both speed *and* endurance, the abilities to use proper mechanics and have sufficient endurance are paramount. The sprinter and the distance runner use both factors. Some element of endurance is necessary in a longer sprint race, and at the end of a distance race, the distance runner may need to become a sprinter and use correct sprinting mechanics.

The distance of a competitive race usually varies from 55 meters to 44+ km; consequently, different factors are necessary for success in each separate distance. Short races are accomplished primarily anaerobically (without much breathing) and long races aerobically (constant breathing).

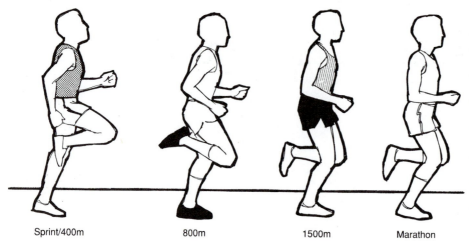

FIGURE 15.1 Four runners are shown, each in the midsupport position: a sprinter and 400 m runner; a 800 m runner; a 1500 m runner; a marathon runner. The runners have certain postural similarities and differences. The trunk angle is nearly perpendicular in all runners. The knee angle of the lead leg is highest with the sprinter and lowest with the marathon runner. The arms are more vigorous and move with more amplitude the shorter the distance, if the runner is running at regular speed.
(Similar to data reported by Slocum D., and Bowerman, W. 1962. The biomechanics of running. *Clinic. orthop.* 23:29.)

Sprint/400m   800m   1500m   Marathon

Researchers have identified minor differences in postures and movement patterns in runners competing in races of varying lengths. For example, four runners are shown in Figure 15.1 at the midsupport position. Number 1 is a sprinter and 400m runner, number 2 an 800m runner, number 3, a 1500m runner, and number 4, a marathon runner. The runners have certain postural similarities and differences. The trunk angle is nearly perpendicular in all runners. The thigh angle and flexed knee of the lead leg are higher with the sprinter and lowest with the marathon runner. The arms are moved vigorously and with more amplitude during the shorter distance when the runner is running at regular speeds. This information is similar to that reported by Slocum and James (1968).

Researchers believe that the mechanics of running have an effect on efficiency of performance. One measure of energy cost in running relates to the rise and fall of the center of gravity (CG). A sprinter produces a pronounced rise and fall, while a distance runner exhibits a more even CG path. A distance runner may delay the onset of fatigue by maintaining a smooth, even, compact stride. Momentum is more constant, since fluctuation of force causes a change in momentum. In turn, more energy is required. It may be possible to delay the onset of fatigue by maintaining effective mechanical positions such as a proper knee lift and an upright trunk.

Excessive height could be detrimental because of wind resistance, and most distance runners are at or below the population mean for height. Extremely short

(several inches below the mean) individuals would have difficulty when a long stride is needed. A light body weight (with low body fat) would be advantageous in distance running. In speed running, fast-twitch muscle fibers are essential.

Step and Stride

Since there is disagreement among some scholars in defining step and stride, a definition of each will be given here. A "step" is that part of the running action that commences at the moment when either foot terminates contact with the ground and continues until the opposite foot contacts the surface. A "stride" consists of two steps, during which there is a period of support and a period of flight. A stride is identified by the termination of contact of a foot with the ground through the next contact of this same foot—it involves two steps.

General Mechanics of Running

Stride Length

Many authors, such as Hoffman (1971), Teeple (1968), and Sparks (1974), have shown that there is a positive relationship between step or stride length and running velocity. Keep in mind that speed of the run equals stride length times stride frequency. A short-legged runner who desires a fast pace will have to take more strides per unit of time than a longer-legged runner, whose stride should be longer. Mathematically, it may be stated as:

$$\frac{DV}{DT} = F - KV$$

F = highest propulsive force

T = time

V = velocity

K = constant

A combination of long stride and high frequency is an indication of a fast runner, all other things being equal. Explosive push off and flexibility help determine stride length. On the other hand, a runner desiring to run a long distance will run with a short stride, depending on pace and low stride frequency to conserve energy.

In most instances, leg length is associated with body height. The taller person usually has longer legs and should be able to take a longer stride than a shorter person. In addition, a positive relationship exists between the force exhibited by the legs at pushoff and length of stride. Furthermore, if there is only a minimum amount of braking force at the foot-down position, the runner can move faster in a forward direction.

Speed runners use the longest stride of all the runners. The stride length is approximately 4.87 m (16 ft) for men and 3.65 to 4.26 m (12 to 14 ft) for women. The top female sprinters have a step frequency of 4.48 steps per second, and the male sprinters, 5 steps per second. (Use half these values for stride frequency.)

It has been reported that initial increases in speed by an experienced runner is a result of increased stride length (SL). After a stride of optimum length has been attained, further increase in speed becomes a matter of increasing stride frequency (SF). A formula for evaluating running is speed = SL × SF. Remember, though, that excessive increase in SL may bring about a decrease in SF. Mechanically, overstriding in speed races shows the heel striking firmly first with evidence of some backward movement of the center of gravity.

Arm Action

The main purpose of the arm action in running is to counterbalance the off-center thrust of the legs. The arms of the fast runner move in opposition to the legs and are 180° out of phase with the adjacent leg, as in walking. However, as the speed increases, the arms move more rapidly in a flexed to partially extended position. The arms move toward the midline of the body in the forward position and then to the rear, with the hands seldom going beyond the hips. (See Figure 15.1.)

Aristotle (384–322 B.C.), who has been called the father of kinesiology, observed arm action and its contribution to the running motion. He wrote:

> The animal that moves makes its change of position by pressing against that which is beneath it. Hence, athletes jump farther if they have the weights in their hands than if they have not, and runners run faster if they swing their arms, for in extension of the arms there is a kind of leaning upon the hands and wrists. (p. 41)

Center of Gravity

Beck (1965) studied the path of the center of the body during the running stride. The subjects, twelve boys ages 6 through 12 and representing the first six grades, were selected from their classmates as having the better time scores in a 27.4 m (30 yd) run. Beck found that, regardless of the runner's age, all paths were wavelike, reaching the high point shortly after the body became airborne. After the high point the center of gravity moved downward through the next foot contact and for a short time afterward. The next rise began while the foot was in contact with the ground and continued through the takeoff, and the cycle was then repeated. With increased age, there was an increase in the horizontal and vertical distances traveled by the center of gravity during each stride, and the stride also became longer. With age, the percentage of the total stride time represented by foot contact decreased, and, of course, that of flight time increased. The horizontal velocity of the center of gravity also increased with age. For the flight phase, however, the percentage of the horizontal velocity decreased, and for the support phase it increased. The rise and fall of the center of gravity is greater in running than in walking (5 to 6.3 cm [2 to 2.5 in.]), but not as great in marathon running.

Speed/Tension

To prevent tension from occurring in the arms and neck, the runner must learn to run explosively but in a semi-relaxed manner. A runner should try to run as fast as possible without unduly contracting the arm and neck muscles or other muscles extraneous to the action. This is termed *differential relaxation*. Runners use the following strategies to reduce tension:

Relax the hands by closing the fingers without clinching the fist. During distance running, the hands are held very loosely.

Relax the jaw by keeping the mouth open and the jaw loose.

Tension usually begins in the neck, jaw, and arms, proceeds to the torso, and finally to the legs. As a result of extraneous tension, the legs may rotate so much externally that the stride of the sprint runner is decreased considerably and the speed is reduced.

Foot Position

The contact of the runner's foot with the ground at foot strike is slightly different from that of the walker's foot, the degree of difference depending on the velocity of the run. At high speed, the contact is first made on the lateral edge of the ball of the foot. The heel is lowered, but a controversy exists as to whether it actually touches the ground. In middle-distance running, the first contact is made with the rear part of the foot. In the case of slower-speed or distance running, the heel does come down so that the foot is flat on the ground at contact. In very slow running, the heel strikes the ground first. The body weight moves forward after foot contact, as in walking. However, the contact time of the foot in running is much shorter than in walking, being slightly less than 0.01 second for speed runners and greater for other runners, depending on their body velocity. In walking, it is about a second, depending on speed.

In reviewing research on the direction of foot movement immediately before contact, Fortney (1963) found that authors did not agree on the direction. In most cases, they also did not make clear whether they referred to movement with reference to a fixed point in space or to a fixed point in the body. In studying film of eight elementary school boys whose runs were photographed when they were in the second grade and again in each of the three following years, Fortney found that the heel moved forward with reference to a fixed point in space and that there was no apparent difference between runners classified as good and those classified as poor. However, she found that the heel moved backward with reference to a point within the body (the knee). Since the forward movement of the total body was greater than the backward movement caused by flexion at the knee and extension at the hip, the foot moved forward immediately before contact.

Other findings by Fortney point out differences between the skilled and the unskilled runners:

1. At the beginning of the flight phase, the skilled runners had greater flexion in the leading limb at the knee and the hip, the latter bringing the thigh closer to the front horizontal.
2. At the beginning of the contact phase, the skilled runners had greater flexion at the knee of the rear limb, bringing the heel closer to the buttock.

Elite Sprinter Characteristics (Dillman 1971)

1. slight vertical displacement of the body
2. long length of stride
3. small amount of time on the ground
4. greater flexion at the knee during recovery of the leg
5. backward rotations of leg segment just before foot contact
6. strong and complete extension during thrust phase of support

---

Knee Action

During speed running, the knee lift (thigh flexion) should reach nearly the level of the hip, and the rear "kickup" of the foot (flexion of leg during swing phase) should again be nearing the horizontal. Knee lift and rear kickup are not as pronounced in the distance runs.

The position in which the heel is moved high and just to the edge of the buttocks during the running cycle is an advantage. The radius of rotation is decreased as the heel moves high and closer to the edge of the buttocks, a position characteristic of a fast runner.

Flexion at the knee occurs at foot-down, and extension occurs as the toe-off movement takes place. There is some disagreement regarding the amount of extension present as the foot leaves the ground. Apparently, with the world's top sprinters, complete extension does not occur because of the short time the foot is in contact with the ground (support time). Some researchers have found an increase in flexion at foot-down concomitant with an increase in running velocity.

Braking Force

Some have hypothesized that if the foot of a runner is moving backward as it strikes the ground with a negative velocity equal to the positive velocity of the center of gravity moving forward, the **braking force** would be zero. It is known that faster runners show a greater negative foot velocity than do slower runners. It appears that this diminution of the braking force aids in speed running. Most researchers agree that if the foot at foot strike is directly under the center of gravity, the braking force is reduced to a minimum.

■ There is a power flow for the lower limbs of a sprinter. The hip joint musculature is the main power source.

Hip Action

Considerable rotation occurs at the hip during the sprint action, while much less occurs during long-distance running. The former motion results in a long stride and facilitates the development of greater stride frequencies. The reverse is desired in long-distance running.

Support and Nonsupport Time

The writers of this text have found (unpublished research) that as the speed of running increases, the nonsupport time increases and the support time decreases. Most researchers have found that the respective times may be close to 50% for each. With distance runners, the ratio may be reversed. World-class sprinters show an increased nonsupport time (52% nonsupport and 48% support). It is just the opposite in the fatigue situation; the more fatigued the runner, the more time spent in support.

Trunk Angle

The trunk angle, or upper body lean, during running has been a subject of debate for some time. Body lean is intertwined with acceleration, forward lean occurring during acceleration, backward lean occurring during deceleration. There is some agreement that after the initial starting distance, which is 13.71 to 28.28 m (15 to 20 yd) in sprinting, there need be very little lean or inclination. Many coaches are now advocating an almost upright position after an optimum running posture is attained.

Sprinters do not accelerate after running 54.8 to 64.0 m (60 to 70 yd, 6 seconds) from the start; they just try to maintain a constant velocity as long as possible. On the other hand, distance runners set a pace and may accelerate at times to obtain a better position among the other runners or to relieve monotony or tension. In the latter instance, they may lean forward to increase velocity, and then, as they assume a more even pace, become more upright.

There is a trunk lean of 5 to 7° forward during sprint running. Some sprinters have a trunk lean a few degrees to the rear. In distance running, the trunk lean is about the same as in sprinting. Depending on the wind or air resistance, the lean may be greater or less than upright. The important factors are that muscle effort should not be used to maintain body lean and the respiratory muscles must be free to function.

Body Lean of a Sprinter Compared to a Distance Runner

We have found that the sprinter inclines the trunk (which is synonymous with body lean) more than does the long-distance runner. Slocum and James (1968) question whether any skilled runner, regardless of the distance of the run, inclines the trunk forward beyond the vertical after the acceleration of the start. They also maintain that there is a backward tilting of the pelvis, accompanied by flexion of the spine, and that this "flat-backed" position increases the ability to rotate the thigh laterally. (Lateral

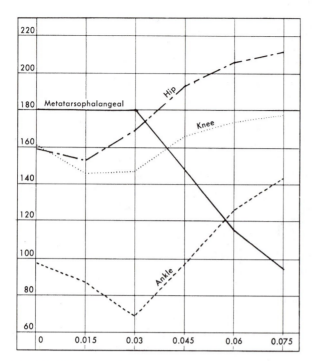

FIGURE 15.2 Joint actions of supporting limb of male Olympic contestant during foot contact in running. Time in seconds is shown at bottom; angles between body segments are shown in degrees at left. Kinematic analysis of leg action.

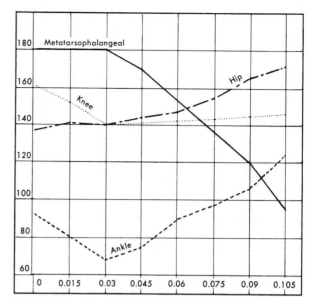

FIGURE 15.3 Joint actions of supporting limb of college woman (with no special training in running) during foot contact in running.

rotation of the thigh is needed to place the foot in the desired direction as the pelvis is rotated forward over the supporting hip.) The lower-limb actions of a sprinter and distance runner are the same in general appearance, but there are differences in detail. The sprinter has greater thigh flexion in the swinging limb, raising the flexed knee higher. The stride is also longer, there are more strides per second, and a smaller area of the foot contacts the ground. Other investigators (e.g., Sparks 1974) found trunk inclination to be 2 or 4 ° forward of the vertical.

Joint Actions of Supporting Limb

Figure 15.2 shows the angle of the lower limb measured on film of a male Olympic competitor as he neared the finish line in the 1500m race. The time per frame for this film is based on the speed, which is assumed to be approximately 64 frames/second. The support phase was therefore approximately 0.075 second. The runner

landed with full foot contact, and the foot flexed immediately and continued to do so for 0.03 second. This action is caused by the forward momentum of the body and consequent rotation at the ankle joint. At 0.03 second, extension at the ankle begins, the forward momentum cannot now rotate the body around the ankle joint, and its force must act at the metatarsal joints. This action continues to the takeoff. Extension at the ankle, as the foot (except for the toes) is lifted, moves the leg backward and upward from the positions to which it would be carried solely by the metatarsophalangeal action.

The leg flexes at contact, easing the force of impact as the foot touches the ground. During the final 0.045 second, there is extension at the knee, carrying forward the entire body except the supporting leg and foot. This action is due to contraction of the knee extensors and the forward momentum of the body. Flexion at the hip joint occurs at impact, followed by extension to maintain the angle of inclination of the trunk.

It is interesting to compare the joint actions of the skilled runner with those of a college woman who had no special training in running. The joint actions of the woman as she ran at her top speed are shown in Figure 15.3. The pattern of action is the same for the two

TABLE 15.1 Comparison of joint actions of trained and untrained adults.

Joint Action	Trained			Untrained		
	Range	Time	Velocity (degrees/sec)	Range	Time	Velocity (degrees/sec)
Metatarsophalangeal extension	86	0.045	1911	85	0.075	1133
Ankle extension	73	0.045	1622	56	0.075	746
Knee extension	32	0.045	711	6	0.075	80
Hip extension	59	0.06	983	32	0.075	426

Note the lesser angular velocity in support phase.

runners; that is, the direction of joint angle change is the same. The differences are in speed of action and range and are shown in Table 15.1. Compare the information in Figures 15.2 and 15.3. Except for the metatarsophalangeal joints, the range of movement for the man is greater, especially at the knee and hip joints. The speed of the man's actions is also greater at all joints; in particular, at the knee, it is more than 8.8 times as great. Further comparisons can be made of the angles of inclination.

Joint Actions of Swinging Limb

The joint actions of the swinging limb can be seen in Figures 15.4 and 15.5, which show the differences in segmental inclinations of both supporting and swinging limbs. This description is of the runner in Figure 15.6. In the takeoff, the rear limb is about to leave the ground, and the swing will begin with the hip and knee at 180°. During the period of no contact, this limb will reach the position of the rear limb shown at contact. During this time, which for the 1500m male runner equals the support phase, the runner has not yet brought the thigh in line with the trunk. But the lower leg has flexed through almost 120°, bringing the heel to hip level. At contact, the runner flexes rapidly at the hip, bringing the thigh in line with the trunk and then up toward the front horizontal at takeoff. During the first two-thirds of support, the swinging lower leg flexes, bringing it closer to the thigh. This moves the center of gravity of the limb toward the fulcrum (the hip) and facilitates its flexion. The speed with which the thigh and lower leg are swung forward and upward (closer to the front horizontal) during contact

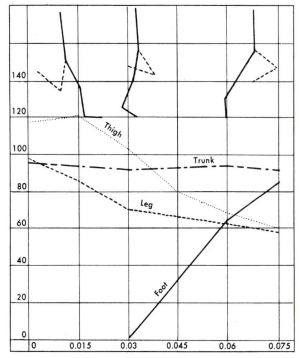

FIGURE 15.4 Segmental inclinations of supporting limb of male Olympic contestant during foot contact in running. Time is in seconds at bottom. Angles between body segments are shown in degrees at left.

Biomechanics of Running **301**

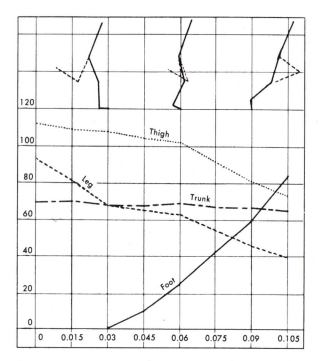

FIGURE 15.5 Segmental inclinations of supporting limb of college woman with no special training in running. Time in seconds and angles between body segments are shown on left.

since this action rotates the distal end of the leg backward. As foot contact is made, flexion at the ankle rotates the proximal end of the leg forward. Thus the direction of leg rotation before contact is continued after the foot is placed on the ground.

Angles of Inclination of Supporting Limb

The graphs in Figures 15.4 and 15.5 show that to understand movement in running, one must consider both angles at the joint and inclination angles of body segments. The inclinations of the trunks of both runners remain at an almost constant angle during foot contact, yet the angle at the hip joint (which moves the trunk) increased 59° in the man and 32° in the woman (Table 15.1). In both runners, thigh inclination has equalled hip action. Foot inclination is the same for both runners, approximately 85°; leg inclinations differ, indicating a difference in ankle action. During foot rise, the man's leg inclines 12° and the woman's more than twice that amount. If the man is using better running mechanics, the primary cause of the woman's lesser performance may be the small range of extension at the ankle. Do her extensor muscles lack strength, or does the reflex for foot flexion fail to respond with sufficient strength? Leg inclination could explain the difference in thigh inclination. That of the woman is less. Greater thigh inclination combined with her leg inclination could be too much for balance. These possible causes of lesser performance have been suggested; they require further testing. This example demonstrates both the values and limitations of film analysis.

Additional Joint Actions

In reviewing the film (Figure 15.6) of the male sprint-runner, we noticed that the pelvis rotates to a greater degree in running than it does in walking. When the thighs are separated, the pelvis is rotated on the supporting femur. As one thigh is swung forward, the pelvis rotates forward on the same side, adding length to the step. Thus, part of the male's greater speed in running is due to an increase in stride length.

adds to the projecting force. Observation of a vigorous kick shows that the swinging limb can move the whole body forward. (One film of an expert football punter shows that the body is moved forward more than 0.6 m (2 ft) with no observable action in the supporting limb.) According to Fenn and Fortney, better runners bring the thigh closer to the horizontal at takeoff.

From the position at takeoff, the leading limb during flight prepares for contact by extension at the hip, lowering the entire limb, and the lower leg is extended, increasing the length of the stride. In other film observations, some runners have been seen to flex at the knees just before contact. This action moves the foot back under the body and may decrease the possible backward push on contact, but it does decrease braking force and enables the runner to move the leg rapidly forward. In many cases, the forward movement of the total body is greater than the backward movement of the foot because of flexion at the knee. This seems to be advantageous,

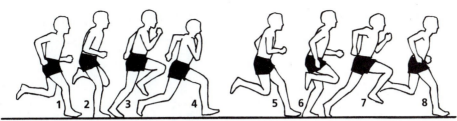

FIGURE 15.6 Sprinter in action. Reading from left to right the sequence is as follows: (1) foot strike on outside border of foot near ball; (2) foot-down position with foot completely flat (some sprinters show heel not touching surface); (3) toes almost ready to leave surface (7's supporting foot's toes just touching surface); (4) both feet are off ground (non-support); (5) rear foot lift (also see 1 and 8); (6) knee lift in front, almost complete; (7) high knee lift and long stride potential; (8) foot strike as seen in 1.

Notice that the arms swing in opposition to the legs. They aid in maintaining a forward position of the upper trunk, which would otherwise tend to face in the same direction as does the pelvis. The arm swing also affects the center of gravity of the whole body. At takeoff, one arm is raised to the front and the other to the back. These positions raise the center of gravity of the total body, which reaches its highest point at takeoff. Shortly after contact, when the thighs are parallel, the arms are at the side of the body, with the forearms approaching extension. The arms now tend to lower the center of gravity of the entire body, which reaches its lowest point at this time. Modern sprinters are de-emphasizing the backward extended movements of the forearms for a more rapid arm movement forward. This seems to be associated with increased leg action.

Types of Terrain

Curve Running

Running a curve is relatively easy at a slow pace. As velocity is increased, the runner must make certain accommodations to negotiate the curved path effectively. For example, the center of gravity is moved laterally to the inside of the track oval (body lean toward curb), and a wider base of support is achieved with the feet spaced somewhat apart to give better balance. The runner may accelerate part of the way on the straightways, but must run under control at the initial entrance onto the curve; then the runner may accelerate on the curve. These accommodations are necessary because of centrifugal force. To overcome this force, the runner initially pushes outward with the feet and leans the body toward the inside to reduce the radius of rotation and increase the lateral ground reaction forces. Otherwise the runner would be forced toward the outside and would not be able to run the curve effectively.

■ The greater the velocity of the runner, the greater the lean on a curve.

Grade Running

Henson (1976) studied six male cross-country runners while they were running on a treadmill at fifteen combinations of speed and grade. He found that when increasing speed on a downhill slope, the runner should do so primarily by increasing the length of stride. This results in a more bounding type of movement but makes greater use of the pull of gravity as the runner moves farther down the hill with each stride, increasing the flight phase. The muscle contractions are primarily eccentric opposing the pull of gravity, which do not require the same amount of energy as concentric contractions, which dominate when running on the level or uphill. The least mechanical energy is expended running downhill, next least running on the level, and the most running uphill. Also, because fewer strides per minute are required in this bounding type of movement, the limbs are not required to oscillate as rapidly or as frequently. Additional energy is saved in accelerating and decelerating the limbs. When running up a long incline, the runner should shorten each stride and lean into the hill slightly, slowing the pace to avoid producing excessive oxygen debt. These techniques should aid the novice runner in making the most efficient adjustment to a hilly cross-country run and result in maximum improvement of performance (Henson 1976).

Track Starts and Initial Sprinting Phase

In most running races, it is desirable to move the body forward as rapidly as possible from the start. This is especially important in sprints, and most investigators have found that the start is faster when executed from a crouching position than a standing position. A crouch start places the sprinter in a position to move the center of gravity rapidly well ahead of the feet. The runner must then accelerate very rapidly or fall. In longer races, the runner usually uses a standing start because rapid acceleration at the start is not necessary.

It has been found through experience that the start is faster if blocks are provided for the backward push; they too increase the amount of push that can be directed horizontally. (Some recent starting blocks are shown in Figure 15.7.) One track coach has increased the height of the front block in order to decrease the amount of backward movement of the front foot and thus decrease the time that the front foot pushes against the block.

As the runner takes the crouching position, hands, feet, and rear knee are in contact with the supporting surface, with the rear foot supporting little of the body weight. The distance between the hands and the forward foot is short enough to force the spine to flex (arch). The value of this flexion will be shown later.

The latest starting techniques involve having the hands apart as much as 30 inches or more. Also, the sprinter tries to reach an upright position as soon as possible to be in full running stride much sooner than was previously advocated.

In the "get set" position, which precedes the actual start, the rear knee is raised from the surface until the rear leg is inclined some 25 to 30° as measured from the front. (Some runners, however, completely extend the rear leg.) Both thighs are moved upward and forward by extension at the knee, which moves the trunk and the center of gravity farther forward. At the same time, the spine flexes more; the head is held at the same height as in the first position.

As the trunk is raised, the rear foot pushes by sudden knee extensor action, which moves the thigh forward.

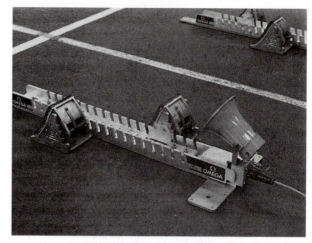

a

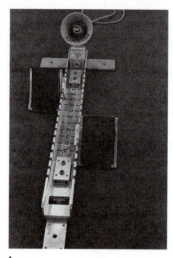

b

FIGURE 15.7 Two views of contemporary starting blocks. The light on the rear flashes if a runner starts too soon (false start). Also, there is an electronic sound device so that all runners hear the starter's commands and the gun signal at the same time.

As viewed on film, the feet are moved slightly backward preceding the push. This push is of short duration because the limb must be moved forward quickly for the first step. Before the rear foot has left the block, leg extension at the front knee begins, moving the front thigh forward. Both knee actions are examples of reversed muscle action and are the primary sources of power for putting the body into motion. The leg of the front foot keeps a fairly constant inclination, adjusting its position to the movement of the foot. The trunk, which has been inclined slightly above the horizontal during the push of the rear foot, is raised somewhat as the rear foot is moved forward for the first step. Since the center of gravity is ahead of the supporting front foot, gravity will rotate the foot about the metatarsophalangeal joints. In general, the action is that described in the discussion on mechanics of the stepping pattern.

The first five or six steps after the push differ from the steps of the run. There is only a short period in which both feet are off the surface. Because the center of gravity is so far ahead of the takeoff foot, little upward projection is given to it, and the succeeding step must be taken quickly to prevent it from falling below the desired line of flight. After the first step (contact with ground 0.015 sec), the trunk is gradually raised, increasing the amount of upward direction given to the center of gravity. With this change, the steps can be gradually lengthened to equal those used in the sprint stride.

During the striding action of the lower limbs, the arms move in opposition to them. The upper arms are moved by shoulder joint muscles, and the forearms are held in approximately 90° of flexion to shorten the moment arm of the shoulder levers.

At the starting signal, the contacting segments leave the surface in sequence. According to Bresnahan (1934), who observed twenty-eight trained sprinters, all right-handed, the order of breaking contact in all subjects was left hand, right hand, right foot, left foot. The average time between the signal and the left-hand break was 0.172 second and between the signal and the left-foot break 0.443 second. Bresnahan also observed one left-handed sprinter whose breaking order was reversed—right hand first and right foot last.

As the hands are raised, the spine extends, counteracting the pull of gravity on the upper trunk while the lower trunk is supported by the feet. As the spine extends, it moves the head and the center of gravity forward. In looking at film of this action, we are reminded of Gray's statement: "By arching and extending its back, a galloping dog greatly increases the power and length of its stride" (1960, p. 15).

The forces made against starting blocks by runners using the crouching starts are shown in Figure 15.8. In the crouching start, note that the front foot in most instances exerts force over a longer time but for less maximum force than does the back foot. (The impulse is greater for the front foot since impulse force is integrated over the time.)

Siegerseth and Grinaker (1962) studied the effect of foot-spacing on velocity in sprints. The subjects were twenty-eight male college physical education majors. In the crouching start, the feet were separated 10, 19, or 28 inches, and times were checked at 10, 20, 30, 40, and 50 yards. At every distance, the time for the 19-inch start was the lowest, but the records were statistically significant only when the means for the 19- and 28-inch starts were compared for the 10, 20, 30, and 50 yards.

Sprint Starting Mechanics

The following are certain starting mechanics agreed on by investigators Barlow and Cooper (1972):

1. Block spacings vary from 27.9 to 38.1 cm (11 to 15 in.), partially according to leg length. This arrangement enables the sprinter to attain a fast start.
2. In the set position, the front knee joint angle should be near 90°, since the sprinter remains longest over this leg before leaving the blocks.
3. The rear leg is near extension (varying from 140 to 170°) to react to the gun signal as soon as possible and to apply nearly maximum thrust.
4. The head of the sprinter is relaxed. It is the first body part to move the body in the desired direction.
5. A sprinter usually takes about 0.11 second to react to the gun.
6. The time of exit of the rear foot from the rear block (mean time, 0.270 second) was less than Morris (1971) found for untrained sprinters (mean time, 0.343 second).
7. The mean time spent in the blocks by the front foot was 0.446 second.
8. The greatest horizontal force against the blocks was exerted by the rear foot. However, the front foot generates slightly less force over a longer time, producing greater impulse.
9. The first step by the best sprinter off the blocks was longer and closer to the ground than for the other sprinters.

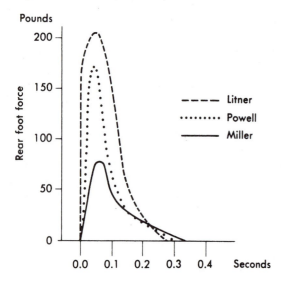

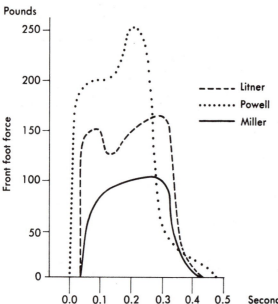

FIGURE 15.8 Starting block force-time curves for three runners using the crouching start. Note similarity in the rear foot impulse. Note differences in the front foot impulse.

Overstriding and Understriding

Studies have looked at overstriding and understriding. In overstriding, "a 10% increase in stride length resulted in an increased peak shank deceleration (leg shock) upon landing," (Messier, Franke, and Rejaski 1986, p. 176). Overstriding results in increased cardiorespiratory demands (Cavanagh and Williams 1982). It would appear that overstriding mechanically causes increased tension and some malfunction of the rhythmic contraction of leg and even arm muscles. If the stride is decreased, there is less peak shank deceleration. Deshon and Nelson (1964) found that, in sprint overstriding, there was a decreased angle at touchdown. This, in turn, results in greater braking force. There is deceleration at foot, forefoot, or heel. If the foot decelerates, the only way the runner can maintain constant velocity is to increase the forces at toe-off. This, coupled with increased braking force, would call for the expenditure of increased energy. The runner who runs correctly from a biomechanical standpoint should not be required to overcome inertia at every step.

Atwater (1979) reports that overstriding may cause increased tension stress on both pubic and femoral attachment of the adductor muscles. Her subjects were female runners and military recruits.

Understriding results in the lead foot being placed almost under the runner's center of gravity. Thus, the center of gravity of the runner is not elevated vertically as much and the flight time is reduced. Advantageously, there is a decrease in braking force at heel strike when understriding. Cavanagh and Williams (1982) found that understriding was more efficient than overstriding. However, Messier, Franke, and Rejaski (1986) found that a small decrease in stride length did not adversely affect a runner's performance. On the other hand, they discovered that a large reduction in stride length did.

Running Economy

Style, technique, training, and age affect the amount of energy expended in running. Obviously, the longer the distance of the run, the more important the conservation of energy becomes. Extraneous movements also add to the cost; even the excess use of the arms in a long-distance run may exact a toll. There is argument as to optimum stride length and frequency. If 148 cm is the stride length of a given runner, a shift of −5 to +10 cm will change the energy output. Pugh's data (as reported by Best and Bartlett) on comparing track and treadmill running in relation to energy are:

1. There was a marathon-pace difference of 7–8% at the middle-distance pace.
2. There was 20% decrease in energy cost during drafting. Also, they reported one runner got a decrease in energy cost due to clothing changes and a haircut.

Optimum stride length and frequency changed slightly (4%) when the arms were held across the chest. When the trunk movement was overemphasized, there was 16% change. Also, there were changes when the legs were lifted higher than in normal running.

No difference was found in VO_2 max (the maximum amount of oxygen that can be consumed by the body) between running on the ball of the foot and having the heel planted first.

Length of stride in speed running is dependent on several factors:

1. It is positively correlated with the ratio of leg length to body height.
2. It is directly proportional to the amount of force extended to propel the body into the air during push off.
3. It is inversely proportional to the amount of braking force at touchdown.

Fatigue Effects

In middle-distance running, Sparks (1974) found the following:

1. The best runners depend on their ability to consume and use oxygen efficiently. These same top runners supply more energy by the aerobic system and therefore produce less oxygen debt.
2. The better runners are more airborne during the race; that is, they are in the air slightly longer than on the ground. The reverse often happens as they become fatigued.

3. As the stress of the run becomes greater toward the end of the race, the stride often is shortened, and to keep up the pace the runner increases the stride frequency. The center of gravity is lowered, and the knee lift (leg flexion) is decreased as fatigue sets in.

In distance running the same mechanical effects from fatigue often occur. Stress tolerance and ability to consume and use oxygen efficiently may delay or even prevent the occurrence of mechanical faults.

It is known that experienced runners tend to use running strides that are near to their optimum stride. From a mechanical viewpoint, after years of experience these runners have found through trial and error, the most relaxing stride without reducing their momentum. Their measuring stick is in the preconceived cost in energy output and their times in races. We advocate experimenting with a measured length of stride.

Kaneko has stated that, in running, the muscles acting internally on the body and externally against the ground (by each foot) move the body's center of mass forward. He stated that the mechanical work may be found by calculating the net energy consumed. Segmental analysis is another method used to determine mechanical work. Cavagna and Kaneko (1977) found that efficiency increased with running speed from 45–70% with elastic energy recoil helping. This increase was found without calculating oxygen debt in the cost. Also, they found that efficiency of distance runners is higher than sprinters under normal circumstances. They also found an economical step rate at any given constant running speed.

Characteristics of a fatigued runner:

1. lower center of gravity of the body during air phase
2. greater forward body lean
3. lateral extension of the arms
4. decreased leg lift
5. shorter strides
6. decreased step frequency
7. wider base of support, with the legs rotated laterally (externally)

Speed and Efficiency

In sprinting, the runner attains maximum velocity at 60–70 meters from the starting position. The fastest reaction time in leaving the blocks is an asset, provided the sprinter has fast leg speed.

Short sprinters tend to start fast and reach maximum acceleration first. But they usually have difficulty maintaining top speed in a race. In a recent 20.46 second 200-meter dash, the top sprinter had a speed of nine strides the last 20 meters. The less time it takes for each stride, the faster the runner. However, the very best runners are able to maintain a fast speed longer. Sprinters pump their arms but use very little shoulder movement, while distance runners use less arm action and more shoulder twist.

In walking, the energy absorption period in which one second elapses is from heel strike to heel strike. In running, the runner decreases the time the foot is on the ground up to 0.2 seconds (200 m/s). The events occurring during the stance phase in running happen three times or more faster during sprint running. This points out the necessity of a runner being mechanically correct and efficiently sound to run at top speed.

Dillman (1975) discusses the mechanical aspects of running that affect the efficient use of human resources in distance running. Since it is impossible to run at top speed for any great length of time or distance, the distance runner must conserve energy. The velocity of a competent distance runner ranges from 4.5–6.5 meters per second (m/s), which is from 10–14.6 miles per hour. Contrast this with the velocity of a sprinter, which is 21–23 miles per hour.

The average horizontal velocity of a skilled runner is 5.2 m/s. A runner at this speed in a six-mile race would have an elapsed time of 30 minutes.

■ Dillman (1975) calls running "a series of projections that results in translation of the body over the running surface," and adds "Running speed can be varied by manipulating both the impulse of the thrust force and the frequency of application." (p. 40)

To conserve energy, the distance runner must run at a relatively constant pace (stride frequencies) through most of the race. Most top runners do vary their stride lengths, which, in turn, affects their speed. They also have less knee lift and less arm action than sprinters.

Forces and Anatomical Adjustments

Mann (1982) has stated that in running, as regards the vertical force curve, the initial contact of the running foot on the ground is approximately 150–200% of body weight, forward shear force is about 50% of body weight, and medial shear force is about 10% of body weight. At contact of the foot with the ground, there is rapid extension at the hip and knee and further dorsiflexion at the ankle. There is also pronation of the foot and internal rotation that occurs throughout the lower limb. This, in turn, causes eversion of the calcaneus, which unlocks the transverse tarsal joint bringing about flexibility with the entire foot. Adduction at the hip also occurs. It is easy to see this is a coordinated effort, as the muscles that cross the hip, knee, and ankle joints help maintain stability at those joints.

■ The jarring effect of jogging can be reduced by using rubberized or foam insoles, which reduce the friction and vertical force to the body. They have a cushioning effect of up to 20 to 30% more than a regular shoe and can help many who jog, including elderly persons.

The swing leg is flexed during the rapid extension of the stance leg—a coordinated and related occurrence. The absorption of force at impact lasts for 50% of the stance phase with continuous dorsiflexion at the ankle joint and flexion at the knee joint. On passing the stance leg (the supporting mechanism), the swinging leg causes the center of gravity to move again in front of the stance foot. Then, external rotation occurs in the pelvis. This rotation is caused by the swinging leg, which rotates the stance leg pelvis by activation of the adductor muscles. The center of gravity is lowest during the stance phase just before the extension at the knee joint and plantar flexion at the ankle joint take place. At this time, the leg is also being adducted. The vertical force at the time of midstance is 250%–300% of body weight, with the aft shear force approximately 60% of body weight. Most of the muscles cease to fire during the last third of the stance phase. This is probably because the center of gravity has gone beyond the stance leg foot. Therefore, the forward propulsion of the body is caused by the swinging leg and arm motion. The force vectors during the support phase of running are shown in Figure 15.9.

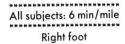
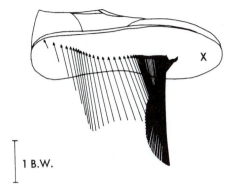

****
All subjects: 6 min/mile
****
Right foot

1 B.W.

FIGURE 15.9 Computer graphics of magnitude and direction of force vectors acting on shoe during running.
(Courtesy Pennsylvania State University Biomechanics Laboratory.)

Active peak flexion at the hip occurs during the latter part of the swing phase. No forces are active against the foot after it leaves the ground. During the last fourth of the swing phase, many of the muscles become more active, namely the hip extensors and hamstrings, the quadriceps about the knee, and the posterior calf muscles, in preparation for the initial contact with the ground.

Pronation of the foot at initial contact is one way the body (part) helps in decreasing the force. Also, the whole foot and ankle enter into the action. There is eversion of the subtalar joint as pronation of the foot takes place. The eversion brings rotation of the tibia—the greater the eversion, the more rotation. In walking, it is normally 6 to 9°; runners usually exhibit greater than 9°.

Gender Differences

Atwater (1989) noted that researchers have found very few differences between female and male distance runners in such elements as percent of body fat, absolute pelvic width, even relative pelvic to height and shoulder width. These measures show no real differences, and neither do kinematic values expressed in relative terms such as stride length and stride frequency. Comparing times for various distances, women are improving more rapidly than men.

Racewalking

Racewalking is a specialized walking technique, usually found in a competitive situation in which the walker comes very close to running. The speed of the movement is faster than that of brisk walking. (The heart-rate attainment is often the same as in running at average speeds.) The distances raced are usually 20 and 50 kilometers. Racewalkers try to keep their walking action as continuous as possible.

The interaction of the ground and the push off, including the reaction of the walker to these forces, is a factor in executing the walking technique. The knee moves first, then the ankle follows in the action. The knee joint has a velocity of more than 7 m per second. To be classified as a legal walking action, "the forward foot of the walker must make contact before the rear foot leaves the ground, and the supporting leg must be straight in the vertically upright position" (Cairns 1987). (See Figure 15.10.)

TABLE 15.2 Running mechanics analyses.*

Mechanics	Rating	Comments
Side View (Frontal Plane):		
Foot strike (heel, mid, toe)		
Slightly bent hip, knee, and ankle		
Knee angle approximately 170° at contact		
Center of gravity over base of support, braking force		
Midsupport phase-lowest center of gravity, knee approximately 145° (diff. approx. 25°)		
Takeoff (following, highest center of gravity, diff. 4 in.)		
Extension of driving hip, knee, and foot		
Rear leg kick-up		
Stride length (longer increasing speed–shorter decreasing speed; consistency; individual optimum)		
Length ground contact relative to nonsupport phase (less–greater speed)		
Pelvis and shoulder posture (square)		
Trunk-straight line (back flat) throughout stride; body lean		
Head erect, no strain anterior/posterior		
Rhythmic leg movement (consistency)		
Arm action; elbow at approximately 90° angle, relaxed; arms working in opposition-balance factor		
Relaxed run; jaw easy; all body parts effortless		
Front or Rear View (Sagittal Plane):		
Foot plant relative to midline—foot forces: inside to outside border, head of metatarsals at time of push off		
Ankle: pronation in, supination out (right/left)		
Knee bows in/out (right/left)		
Hip inward/outward rotation, pelvis alignment		
Direction of forces, forward/backward		
Head and trunk/spine control fixed position; arms and legs working together, independent of trunk		

* Prepared by Lois Klatt, Concordia University

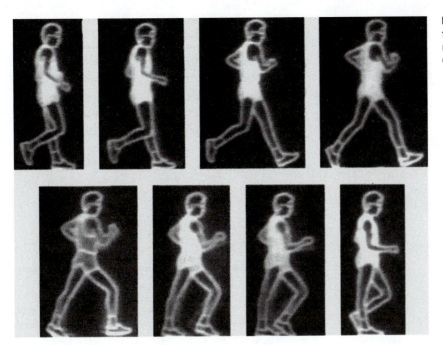

FIGURE 15.10 Racewalking sequences taken from videotapes produced from biomechanics research at the 1985 European Championships.

Analysis of Racewalking

Racewalking is a heel and foot action with the outside edge of the heel contacting the ground first. As the body weight moves forward, it is slightly on the outside edge of the foot. Then the toes of the rear foot push the foot off the ground, and the body continues forward.

The walk should be direct, or as straight as possible, to conserve energy. The center of mass should move vertically as little as possible. After the heel contacts the surface, the forward leg is straightened immediately. It remains so until the pushoff from the back leg commences. The straightened leg and the hip rotation help to keep the center of mass from rising too drastically.

Overstriding expends unnecessary energy. A beginner should start with short strides. As the speed of the walk increases, the length of stride will increase. The forward leg moves the pelvic area on that side forward. The forward and backward movement is accomplished without too much twisting so as not to interfere with the rapid and lengthening action of the legs.

The trunk is held upright with the head kept vertical. Any large degree of head-forward inclination affects the stride length. The upper body is erect and some forward lean occurs, putting the center of mass ahead of the push off foot. A backward lean will cause shortening of the stride and may cause back problems to develop.

The racewalker reaches maximum velocity sooner than in running. The faster the striding rate, the faster the walker will move. As the support phase decreases, the recovery phase increases. At landing or striking of the lead foot and in transversion or conversion, the center of mass remains higher and doesn't go up and down as much as in running.

The arms remain flexed and are moved in synchronization with the leg action, moving just across the midline of the body at sternum level. The arms remain near the body, not laterally away from it, as they are pumped vigorously. On the backswing of the arms, the elbow may be raised vertically near shoulder level. The hands are relaxed, passing back and forth near the pelvic region.

As the speed of the walk increases, the arms move faster to counterbalance the action of the lower body. This vigorous action of the arms is similar to the arm action in running, but of lesser amplitude.

Biomechanics of Running **311**

MINI-LABORATORY LEARNING EXPERIENCE

Compare racewalking and walking using films, EMG, dynamography, and other instrumentation.

Murray et al. (1983) compared racewalkers from a temporal and angular perspective, and racewalkers and fast walkers using a conventional or normal style. The racewalkers had longer strides than the walkers and faster rates, with the stance and swing times approximately equal. Other comparisons were:

1. The racewalkers had increased dorsiflexion at heel strike.
2. The racewalkers had increased hyperextension at the knee in midstance.
3. Racewalkers had increased flexion at the knee and hip during the leg swing.
4. Racewalkers had increased pelvic rotation.

Cairns et al. (1986) found similar results in comparing gaits of walkers and racewalkers in stride lengths, cadence, stance time, swing time, peak ankle dorsiflexion, knee extension at midstance, peak hip flexion, peak pelvic displacement in all three planes, and peak vertical, anterior, and medial components of the ground reaction force. They found considerable difference in these values between the racewalkers and fast walkers

Cairns et al. also stated:

The seemingly exaggerated angular motions of racewalking are necessary to attain increased velocities within the rules of racewalking and to modulate the excursions of the center of mass. The increased vertical and anterior components of the ground reaction forces are related to the increased propulsive forces associated with increased stride length and velocity in racewalking. The increased medial component of the ground reaction force seems to be a compensatory force related to lateral pelvic shifting. There is a support and recovery phase, as is present in conventional walking. (p. 447)

In reviewing the film of the 1983 European Track and Field Championships, researchers found that the racewalker's center of gravity is shifted 3–6 cm as the pelvis is rotated. This is a minimum shift and considered to be

TABLE 15.3   Racewalking data.

Horizontal velocity of arms	2–6 meters per second
Vertical velocity of arms	.5–2 meters per second
Angular velocity of upper arms	8 radians per second
Angular velocity of forearm	9 radians per second
Angular velocity of thigh	12–13 radians per second
Angular velocity of lower leg	15 radians per second
Linear velocity center of gravity	4.1–4.3 m/sec., 20K race
	3.7–3.8 m/sec., 50K race
Stride length	220–260 cm, 20K race
	220–240 cm, 50K race
Linear velocity of knee	7 meters per second
Linear velocity of ankle	9 meters per second

the newest trend in racewalking technique. Previously, the pelvic rotation, and consequently the center of gravity shift, was more exaggerated to produce a long stride. The minimum shift has been found to permit the walker to increase the leg velocity and yet attain a long stride.

The arm actions are an integral part of the walking technique. They are moved very vigorously in synchronization with the leg movements. Kinematic data are listed in Table 15.3. Note the high vertical velocities of the arms and the ratio of ankle speed to speed of the racewalker (center of gravity data).

The decrease in pelvic turn enables the walker to increase leg velocity. The emphasis is on economy of effort and relaxation during certain phases. Fast leg action should be executed with a minimum elevation of the center of gravity.

Cairns (1987), using the best performers, found the following mean values: velocity, 4.07 m/sec; stride length, 2.56 meters; stance time, .40 sec; stance and swing time, .89 sec. (See Table 15.4.) She summarized the results of her study: "It is evident from this investigation that increased stride length, an increased anterior component of the ground reaction force, and a stance time/swing time ratio which approaches 1.00 are characteristic of increased velocity and better performance times in racewalking." (p. 56)

TABLE 15.4 Means of selected variables that differentiate between two performances of racewalkers.

Variable	Performance Group 1	Performance Group 2
Velocity (m/s)	3.13	4.07
Stance time (sec)	.40	.40
Stance time/Swing time ratio	1.14	.89
Anterior GRF (× *bw*)	.29	.39
Stride length (m)	2.17	2.56
Leg length (m)	80.06	83.82
Max. knee extension (deg)	184.00	190.00

References

Abbot, R. R. 1985. Cinematographic analysis of the techniques of hurdling. In *Encyclopedia of physical education, fitness and sports,* ed. T. Cureton. Reston, VA: AAHPERD.

Adrian, M. 1972. Sex differences in biomechanics. In D. V. Harris (Ed.), *Women in sport: A national research conference,* vol. 2, ed. D. V. Harris. University Park, PA: The Pennsylvania State University.

Al-Kurdi, Z. 1991. The angular pattern of the leg during sprinting event. Paper presented at the Asian seminar, Yarmonk University, Irbid, Jordan.

Anderson, R. et al. 1982. A comparison of stride length and stride time using radio telemetry recording techniques. Unpublished report, Dept. of Human Kinetics and Leisure studies, George Washington University, Washington, D.C.

Aristotle. 1945. Parts of animals and Progression of animals. Loeb Classical Library, Cambridge, MA: Harvard University Press.

Atwater, A. E. 1979. Kinematic analysis of striding during the sprint start and mid-race sprint. *Medicine and Science in Sports* 11(1):85.

Atwater, A. E. 1980. Kinematic analysis of sprinting. In *Proceedings of the Biomechanics Symposium,* Indiana University. Oct. 26–28, 1980, ed. J. M. Cooper and B. Haven. Bloomington, IN: The Indiana State Board of Health.

Atwater, A. E. 1989. Gender differences in distance running. *Journal of Sport.*

Bale, P., Rowell, S., and Colley, E. 1985. Anthropometric and training characteristics of female marathon runners as determinants of distance running performance. *Journal of Sports Sc.* 3:115–126.

Barlow, D. A., and Cooper, J. M. 1972. Mechanical considerations in sprint start. *Athletic Asia* 2:27.

Beck, M. C. 1965. The path of the center of gravity during running in boys grades one to six. Ph.D. dissertation, University of Wisconsin–Madison.

Berg, K., and Bell, C. W. 1980. Physiological and anthropometric determinants of mile run time. *Journal of Sports Medicine and Physical Fitness* 20:390–96.

Cairns, M. 1987. Contribution of kinematic variables to racewalking velocity. *Proceedings of ISBS biomechanics in sports,* III & IV, eds. J. Terands, B. Gowitzke and L. Holt. Del Mar, CA: Academic Publishers.

Carter, J. E. L. 1984. Age and body size of Olympic athletes. In *Medicine and sport science,* vol. 18, pp. 53–79, ed. J. Carter. Basel, Switzerland: S. Karger.

Cavagna, G. A., and Kaneko, M. 1977. Mechanical work and efficiency in level walking and running. *J. Physical.* 268:467–81.

Cavanagh, P. 1990. *The mechanics of distance running: A historical perspective: Biomechanics of distance running.* Champaign, IL: Human Kinetics.

Cavanagh, P., and Kram, R. 1990. Stride length in distance running: Velocity, body dimensions and added mass effects. Champaign, IL: Human Kinetics.

Costill, D. L., Bowers, R., and Kammer, W. F. 1970. Skinfold estimates of body fat among marathon runners. *Medicine and Sc. in Spts.* 2 (2):93–95.

Cox, J. S., and Lenz, H. W. 1979. Women in sports: The naval academy experience. *American Journal of Sports Medicine* 7:355–57.

Dillman, C. J. 1971. A kinetic analysis of the recovery leg during sprint running. In *Selected topics on biomechanics,* ed. J. M. Cooper. Chicago: Athletic Institute.

Dillman, C. J. 1975. Kinematic analyses of running. In *Exercise and sport sciences reviews,* vol. 3, eds. J. H. Wilmore and J. F. Keogh. New York: Academic Press.

Dintiman, G. B. 1974. Research tells the coach about sprinting (pamphlet). Washington, DC, AAHPERD.

Drinkwater, B. L. 1984. Women and exercise: Physiological aspects. In R. L. Terjung (Ed.), *Exercise and sport sciences reviews,* vol. 12, pp. 21–51. Lexington, MA: Collamore.

Fleck, S. J. 1983. Body composition of elite American athletes. *American Journal of Sports Medicine* 11(6):398–403.

Fortney, V. 1963. Trends and traits in the action of the swinging leg in running. Ph.D. dissertation, University of Wisconsin–Madison.

Gregor, R. J., and Kirkendall, D. 1978. Performance efficiency of world class female marathon runners. In *Biomechanics, VI-B ed.* E. Asmussen and K. Jorgensen. Baltimore: University Park Press.

Henson, P. L. 1976. Pace and grade related to the oxygen and energy requirements and the mechanics of treadmill running. Ph.D. dissertation, Indiana University.

Hoffman, K. 1971. Stature, leg length, and stride frequency. *Track Technique* 46:1463–69.

Hult, J. S. 1986. The female American runner: A modern quest for visibility. In *Female endurance athletes,* ed. B. L. Drinkwater. Champaign, IL: Human Kinetics.

James, S. L., Bates, B. T., and Osternig, L. R. 1978. Injuries to runners. *American Journal of Spts. Medicine* 6(2):40–50.

Kaneko, M. 1990. Mechanics and energetics in running with special reference to efficiency. *Journal of Biomechanics,* vol. 23, Supp 1:57–63. Pergamon Press, Great Britain.

McBryde, A. M. 1985. Stress fractures in runners: Clinics in sports medicine. *Symposium on Running,* 4(4):737–52.

McMahon, T. A., and Chang, B. C. 1990. The Mechanics of running: How does stiffness couple with speed? *Proceedings of the XII International Society of Biomechanics,* Pergamon Press, New York.

Miller, D. I., Enoka, R. M., and McCulloch, R. G. 1980. Influence of speed on thigh and knee kinematics of female distance runners. Unpublished manuscript.

Murray, M. P., et al. 1983. Kinematics and electromyographic patterns of olympic racewalkers. *American Journal of Sports Medicine* 11(2):68–74.

Ozburn, M. S., and Nichols, J. W. 1981. Pubic ramus and adductor insertion stress fractures in female basic trainees. *Military Medicine* 146 (5):332–34.

Slocum, D. B., and Bowerman, W. 1962. The biomechanics of running. *Clin. Orthop.* 23:39.

Sparks, K. E. 1974. Physiological and mechanical alternations due to fatigue while performing a four-minute mile. Unpublished paper.

Tanaka, K., and Matsuura, Y. 1982. A multivariate analysis of the role of certain anthropometric and physiological attributes in distance running. *Annals of Human Biology* 9:473–82.

Teeple, J. B. 1968. A biomechanical analysis of running patterns of college women. Master's thesis, Pennsylvania State University.

16 Biomechanics of Jumping

Jumping is one of the fundamental movements of children after they learn to walk and run. Many children practice it to some degree at least until the teenage years, and it is a highly specialized activity of a few adults, such as Olympic competitors.

There are many similarities among the different kinds of jumps: standing long jump, standing vertical jump, long jump, high jump, pole vault, and hurdling, as well as certain specialized jumps made in games and contests.

Jumping is a projection of the body into the air by means of a force made by the feet or hands against a surface. Often the jump is made after a run, and the takeoff may be made from either one or two feet. The ability to project the body at an optimum angle at the takeoff is one of the factors determining the distance or height of the jump. Takeoff speed is another factor involved in the quality of jumps. Usually, the force multiplied by the time of application ($F \times t =$ Impulse) determines the longest or highest jump, with the best jumpers having the greatest impulse. In addition, they apply the force in the shortest time and have greater vertical force than the poorer jumpers.

Whenever a run precedes the jump, there is a problem of redirecting some of the horizontal velocity into vertical velocity. Inevitably, there is some sacrifice of one in an attempt to optimize the other.

The path of the jumper who is in the air is that of a parabola, except in a purely vertical jump. The crossing of a bar or a landing for distance involves manipulating the center of gravity to gain advantages in its placement in the body or outside the body.

There is a rotational component connected with the takeoff in jumping. Most researchers consider the rotational component to be in a forward direction (e.g., Bedi 1975). Either using this force or counteracting it may aid the jumper.

A one-foot takeoff provides the greatest forward momentum at takeoff, but is the hardest to control in relation to timing a hit while the jumper is in the air, such as in a block in basketball. For distance, such as in the long jump, or height, such as in the high jump, the one-foot takeoff after a run is preferred.

Movement of the center of gravity within the body or outside of it can be accomplished by moving the body parts. However, moving the arms and legs while the jumper is in flight (airborne) does not add to the distance covered or to the height of the center of gravity of the body. Many of the leg, trunk, and arm movements are made for balance purposes or to project the center of gravity vertically or horizontally within the path prescribed.

If the airborne jumper moves a part of the body in one direction, another part will move in the opposite direction. For example, movement of the head and torso forward and downward (clockwise) cause the feet and lower body to move downward and forward (counterclockwise). This action-reaction principle may be an asset or a liability, depending on its use. In addition, the timing of one movement to cause reaction in another is crucial to performance. One arm moving clockwise too soon may cause the performer's other arm to move counterclockwise, striking a crossbar and nullifying an otherwise effective action.

The basic jumps of track and field events are found in appropriate sections, as are some specialized jumps.

Standing Jumps (Pushing Off with Both Feet)

Standing Broad Jump

The standing broad jump is most frequently used in schools and colleges as one measure of motor ability and physical or motor fitness. It is a modification of the walking step—a modification that low-level performers frequently do not achieve effectively. These performers take off from one foot when they attempt to take off from both. This is a reflex, or inherent, reaction to maintain balance.

Joint Actions in Takeoff Phase. The following analysis of the mechanics of the jump is based on a film of a 12-year-old girl whose score ranks above the ninety-fifth percentile in a nationwide sampling of girls 12 to 17 years of age. The discussion is based on graphs of joint angles and segmental inclinations shown in Figures 16.1 and 16.2. The lines in the illustrations begin at the time that the heels leave the ground and show that the propelling actions occur in slightly more than 0.25 second from raising of the heel until the final thrust is made. For the first 0.18 second, as the foot is raised from the floor, no action (or very little) occurs at the ankle joint, except for the slight flexion and immediate recovery at 0.09 seconds. This lack of extension at the ankle is noteworthy, since many authors attribute raising

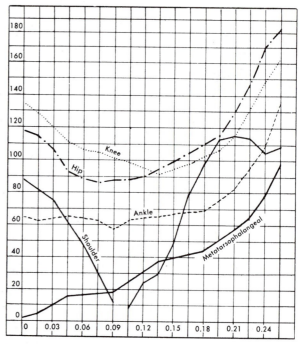

FIGURE 16.1 Kinematics of jumping. Joint actions during the propulsive phase of the standing long jump of a highly skilled 12-year-old girl. Time in seconds is shown at bottom; 0.24 sec is the instant of takeoff. Angles between body segments are shown in degrees at left. For all angles, the downward direction of lines represents flexion and upward slopes represent extension. Note nearly constant angle at the ankle during the majority of the jump. During the last 0.18 sec prior to takeoff, the extension at most joints increases rapidly.

on the toes to extension at the ankle. These graphs, like many others, show that as the center of gravity of the body is moved downward by gravitational force, the foot rotating at the metatarsophalangeal joint is moved in an upward direction. This occurs only when the ankle extensors prevent flexion at the ankle. This apparent paradox—movement in an upward direction because of gravitational force—was also noted in connection with teeterboard action.

Once the leg has reached the desired angle of inclination, extension at the ankle parallels extension at the metatarsophalangeal joint from 0.135 to 0.21 second (Figure 16.1), and by this means the inclination of the leg is kept almost constant (Figure 16.2). In the final

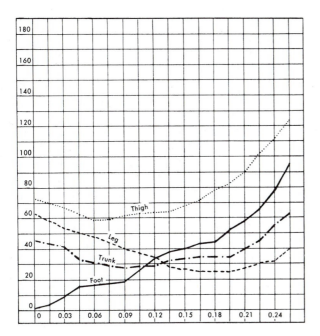

FIGURE 16.2 Kinematics of jumping. Angles of inclination of body segments during the propulsive phase of the standing long jump of the same highly skilled 12-year-old girl as in Figure 16.1. The propulsive phase begins at time zero and takeoff occurs at 0.24 sec. The angles are in degrees. Note the foot consistently changes its angle of inclination starting with a zero position (horizontal) and moving to the vertical position prior to takeoff.

0.03 second, extension at the ankle exceeds action at the metatarsophalangeal joint, and the leg is raised 10°, adding to the upward thrust.

The lower leg flexes for the first 0.135 second, carrying the thigh downward and backward in reference to the knee. However, from 0.06 to 0.135 second, the thigh is not inclined backward with reference to the horizontal because the forward inclination of the leg at this time exceeds flexion at the knee. At 0.21 second, the thigh reaches the vertical, and after this point all limb actions increase in speed. Up to 0.21 second, thigh extension has lifted the thigh and the torso against gravitational pull. After that time, both thigh extension and gravity are applying force in a downward direction. All joints (metatarsophalangeal, ankle, knee, and hip) react to this change in gravitational pull; all rotations at these joints increase in speed. Here is an example of the marvelous capacity of a living organism to adjust to a situation;

these adjustments are not voluntarily controlled. The nervous system reacts to balance and to the speed of the thigh. Guided by the intended action, it provides the necessary movements at the joints.

The shoulder measures shown in Figure 16.1 are those of the angle formed by lines drawn though the upper arms and the trunk. As the heels leave the ground, the arms are back of the trunk at an angle of 88°. They are moved downward by flexion at the shoulder, pass the trunk between 0.09 and 0.105 second, and reach the height of their swing just before the thighs reach the vertical. In this swing, the arm movement affects the position of the center of gravity of the entire body, tending to move it forward and downward until the arms pass the trunk, and then forward and upward.

In studying the standing broad jump of 20 boys (five each at ages 7, 10, 13, and 16 years) who were selected as average jumpers, Roy (1971) found that the peak angular velocities at the knee, ankle, and metatarsophalangeal joints reached maximum values at takeoff, except for one 10-year-old boy whose maximal velocity at the knee occurred 0.07 second before takeoff.

■ Using measures derived from film and a force platform, Roy (1971) concluded, "Kinematics of jumping are well established by the beginning of school age and remain essentially constant through mid-adolescence for average performers." (p. 35)

Factors Affecting the Distance of the Jump. The standing broad jump is customarily measured from the toes at takeoff to where the heels touch the ground in landing. This distance is determined by four factors: (1) the distance to which the center of gravity of the body is carried forward by the lean at takeoff; (2) the horizontal distance through which the center of gravity is projected during flight; (3) the distance beyond the center of gravity that the heels reach on landing; and (4) the time spent on the takeoff surface. Felton (1960) compared these factors in the performances of five high-scoring college women, whose jumps averaged 2.19 m (86.22 in.), and five low-scoring ones, whose jumps averaged 1.08 m (42.78 in.). At the time of takeoff, the centers of gravity of the high-scoring group averaged 78 cm (30.62 in.) in front of their toes; for the low-scoring group the average distance was 45.9 cm (18.74 in.). The heels of the high scorers landed 14.1 cm (5.56 in.) ahead of the center of gravity, and the heels of the low scorers 9.14 cm (3.6 in.) ahead.

The degree to which the center of gravity is in front of the toes at takeoff is affected mainly by the degree of extension at the knee. The 12-year-old girl whose angular kinematics were shown in Figure 16.1 reached an extension at the knee of 164°. In Felton's comparison of high-scoring and low-scoring women, the average extensions at the knee were 165.7° and 141°, respectively. The degree of extension may be due to the balance mechanism. The strength of the ankle extensors could also influence the amount of lean, for the tension in these muscles must move or hold all parts of the body above the ankle joint.

Thigh Position. The position of the thigh at landing is the determining factor in the length of the reach with the heel. The more closely the thigh approaches the horizontal, the longer the reach. When the thigh is nearly horizontal on landing, the legs are almost vertical. This landing position enables the body momentum to carry the center of gravity over the stationary feet. In a running long jump, the horizontal velocity during flight is greater, and the legs can reach farther without the likelihood of the body's falling back of the contact point. The horizontal position of the thighs changes the position of the center of gravity and permits the point to approach closer to the ground before the landing contact is made. This increases the time of flight, adds to the horizontal distance gained during flight, and facilitates forward rotation of the body at the ankle, thus decreasing the possibility of falling backward. Glasgow and Kruse's (1960) observation of hundreds of films of children has shown that the position of the thighs at landing is a distinguishing feature between high-scoring and low-scoring broad jumpers.

The flight adds the greatest proportion to the distance of the jump. The range of flight is determined by the angle and speed of the projection (velocity).

Measures of Velocity and Distance. We rarely measure the velocity of the center of gravity; yet this is the most valid evaluation of the force developed in the takeoff. Halverson (1958) found an average velocity in

the jump of kindergarten children to be between 1.8 and 2.1 m/sec (6 and 7 ft/sec), and the highest was 2.52 m/sec (8.28 ft/sec). Felton (1960) calculated the mean velocity of the five high-scoring women to be 2.47 m/sec (8.11 ft/sec) and that of the low-scoring women to be 1.72 m/sec (5.66 ft/sec). The highest velocity was 2.81 m/sec (9.22 ft/sec) and the lowest 1.53 m/sec (5.02 ft/sec). The increase from age to age was due to greater horizontal velocity, while vertical velocity changed little, indicating that with age the center of gravity is lowered at takeoff.

Different scores for various age groups are fairly common. For example, in unpublished scores for elementary-school boys found in studies at the University of Wisconsin, the first-grade boys averaged 1.16 m (46 in.), and the eighth-grade boys averaged 1.93 m (76 in.). The scores for intervening grades fell between these; the score for each grade was higher than that for the grade below it. The shorter time spent on the takeoff surface, exhibited by the best performers, varied from 0.24 to 0.29 second.

Standing Jump for Vertical Height

The standing jump for height is widely used as a test item, and its successful performance adds to playing ability in many sports. Sargent (1921) was the first to propose the jump for height as a measure of motor ability. He said, "I want to share what seems to me the simplest and most effective of all tests of physical ability with the other fools who are looking for one." Since that time many investigators have found the Sargent jump test, or the "jump and reach," a valuable item in a test battery. For games in which an attempt is made to catch or to strike a high ball, the ability to jump is an asset. Receivers of a forward pass in football, infielders and outfielders in baseball, spikers in volleyball, and basketball players who attempt to tip a ball toward the basket or to a teammate will play more effectively if they can add to their reach by a jump for height.

Henson, Turner, and Lacourse (1986) have developed a predictive test of explosive power for track and field athletes. Those with the highest scores are considered potentially outstanding prospects for sprints, hurdles, and field events. Success is predicted for women who jump more than two feet vertically and almost nine feet

TABLE 16.1 Test for determining potential for track and field athletes: sprinters, hurdlers, throwers, and jumpers.

File Name: Variables:	Brown VJ* SLJ** Age	N = 98	Men	
Variable: Low		High	Mean (in inches)	STD Dev
5. VJ 14.00		(N = 97): 34.00	26.0928	3.3004
6. SLJ 80.00		(N = 97): 127.00	106.6804	8.8881
13. AGE 18.00		(N = 97): 23.00	19.4536	1.3151
File Name: Variables:	Smith VJ SLJ Age	N = 37	Women	
Variable: Low		High	Mean (in inches)	STD Dev
5. VJ 15.00		(N = 37): 26.00	20.2973	2.8271
6. SLJ 70.50		(N = 37): 104.00	90.1554	8.5591
13. AGE 18.00		(N = 37): 22.00	19.3243	1.3345

*VJ Vertical Jump
**SLJ Standing Broad Jump
From Philip Henson, Paul Turner, and Mike Lacourse. Paper presented to Tac Olympic Development Committee, 1986.

horizontally. Similarly, men who can jump almost three feet vertically and more than eleven feet horizontally probably will score well in sprints, hurdles, and field events. (See Table 16.1.)

Hudson (1987) found the following interesting information as a result of studying the vertical jump:

1. In the crouch or preparatory position, the muscle-connective tissue system is "stretched" in eccentric tension, or more specifically, elastic energy is stored. She stated that if the eccentric contraction is followed immediately by concentric contraction, some of the stored elastic energy is reused during the concentric contraction. This seems to imply that the crouch should be followed as soon as possible by the jump.

2. The two groups (male and female) used as subjects jumped approximately 23% of their height and crouched 17% of their height.

3. The mean angle at the knee for the two groups was slightly less than 90° at maximum crouch and the start of the movement upward in the propulsive phase.

4. The angle at maximum flexion at the knee, but not hip or ankle, was related to the use of stored energy.

5. Those subjects having faster extension time used more stored energy.

6. The ability to integrate the downward movement of the legs and to integrate the movement of the arms were related to use of stored elastic energy.

7. The more-skilled performers were able to execute the upward propulsion in 100 ms less than the less-skilled performers.

8. The more-skilled performers crouched to a 96° angle at the knee, while the less-skilled performers flexed 12° beyond 90°.

9. The center of gravity descended 25 cm for the more-skilled performers and 34 cm for the less-skilled ones.

10. The takeoff velocity of the more-skilled performers was higher than that of the less-skilled subjects. Coordination and integration of the body segments, coupled with rapid contraction and a smaller range of motion, seemed to characterize the more-skilled performers.

11. She stated, "The skilled jumpers had very brief timing lags between adjacent segments at both the start and the end of the propulsive phase of the jump."

12. Hudson said it was more important to time the pattern of movement correctly than it was to have the action move from proximal to distal.

13. She also found it was more important to have a "synchronization between the trunk and thigh" than "between the thigh and shank."

14. If the purpose of the vertical jump is to gain greater height, the range of motion in the preparatory position should be slightly more than 90° and full extension of the body.

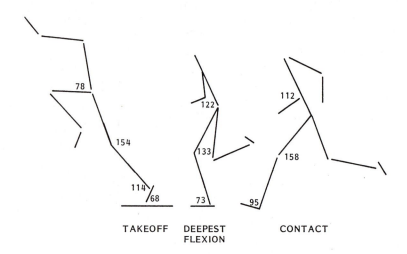

FIGURE 16.3 The final step and takeoff of the running long jump. The numbers represent the angles (in degrees) at the joints during contact, deepest flexion at the knee and takeoff.

TAKEOFF   DEEPEST   CONTACT
           FLEXION

MINI-LABORATORY LEARNING EXPERIENCE

Compare height of jump using the following measures and techniques:

1. Start with legs flexed 90° and jump upward with no prebounce.
2. Start with legs flexed 30° and jump with no prebounce.
3. Use a shallow prebounce (30°).
4. Use a deep prebounce (90°).
5. Use a depth jump (drop from a height and immediately jump at landing).

Discuss principles involved in achieving high/low performance.

Comparison of the Standing Broad Jump and Vertical Jump. Since the inclination of any segment affects the inclination of all segments above it, in spite of the similarities of proximal joint actions in the two jumps the difference in foot inclinations results in differences in inclination of the remaining segments. In the observed actions, the inclinations (measured from the horizontal counterclockwise and with those in the jump for height given first) were as follows: leg, 91° and 44°; thigh, 102° and 60°; and trunk, 80° and 37°. In the standing broad jump, gravitational force adds to the final push; in the high jump, it adds little or nothing. Without the aid of gravity, the velocity in the jump for height is slower than that for the standing broad jump.

Running Jumps (Single-Foot Push)

Running Broad Jump

The running broad jump involves an approach run and a jump that is a modification of the running step. At foot plant in the jump, the center of gravity is farther back than during the run. (See Figure 16.3.) After contact the jumper relies on the momentum of the run to carry the body mass forward with flexion at the ankle joint of the takeoff foot.

Adjustments to bring the center of gravity of segments closer to the fulcrum (the contact point) are made by flexion at the knee and hip in the supporting limb and by flexion at the hip in the swinging limb. As the supporting limb reaches the point of deepest leg flexion, ankle extensors prevent further flexion at the joint, and the pattern described for walking, running, and the standing long jump follows; that is, the heel is raised from the ground.

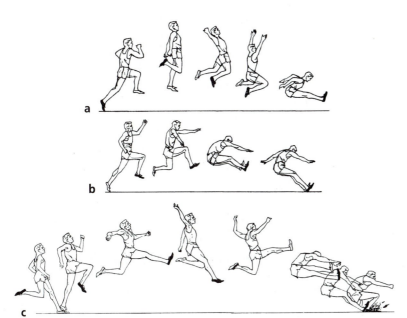

FIGURE 16.4 Three commonly used styles of flight during the long jump. (a) The hang is a held, upright posture requiring rapid flexion at the hip at the appropriate time for a reach at landing. (b) The sail is a held position requiring strong flexor muscles crossing the hip. (c) The hitch kick is a dynamic movement simulating running more nearly than the other styles.

At deepest leg flexion, the center of gravity is almost over the foot and will be moved forward rapidly by extension at the knee of the supporting leg, flexion of the swinging limb, and flexion of both arms.

No action occurs at the ankle joint as the foot begins to rise. Extension at the ankle begins as the center of gravity passes the metatarsophalangeal joints, but the range of this extension is approximately slightly more than half of that at the metatarsophalangeal joint. Therefore, the leg is inclined downward by foot action.

As shown in Figure 16.3, the force of the joint actions at takeoff are directed upward more than forward. This force has been found to be 3.6 Gs (3.6 times the performer's weight). If the jumper has not lost the momentum of the run, there will be a forward component acting on the body mass, and the resulting angle of projection will be between the horizontal and that suggested by the takeoff position. In the depicted jumper, it was calculated to be 33°. Bunn (1955) reported that Jesse Owens' angle of projection was between 25 and 26°. Findings from recent studies show the takeoff angle to be even less, around 17° for world-class jumpers. This low angle is indicative of the inability to transfer the horizontal velocity into vertical thrust and reliance, to a great degree, on horizontal velocity.

Angles of much less than 45° are essential for maximal distance, since the center of gravity at landing is lower than at the beginning of flight and increased vertical projection greatly reduces the horizontal speed. Minimization of the angular momentum is one of the reasons for the world-record broad jump of more than 29 feet by Bob Beamon in 1968. Recently, an even longer jump of 29 feet 4½ inches was recorded by Mike Powell.

The movement in the air of the arms and legs is for balance and to counteract the forward rotation produced at the time of takeoff. (Three styles are shown in Figure 16.4.) The arms and legs each produce a secondary axis of rotation, which causes the body as a whole to rotate backward around the center of gravity. This places the body in a better landing position by extending the lower limbs ahead of the path of the center of gravity to increase the measured distance of the jump.

The reach on landing can be longer than in the standing long jump. A horizontal position of the thighs and a greater degree of extension at the knee add to the measured distance. The trunk is hyperextended at midpoint in the flight and then flexed to prepare for projection of the center of gravity forward past the feet. Flexion at the hip, to raise the thighs before landing, will also incline the trunk, bringing the center of gravity forward. By

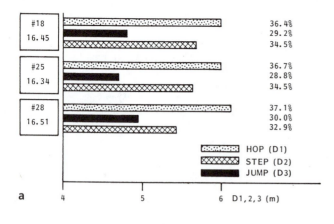

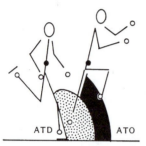

ATD- TAKEOFF ANGLE
b   ATO- TOUCHDOWN ANGLE

FIGURE 16.5 (a) Percent of contribution to distance jumped by three athletes jumping approximately 16.5 meters at the 1987 European Cup. (b) Angle of touchdown and takeoff for each of three propulsion phases. The angle was measured as the angle through the estimated center of gravity of the body with respect to the horizontal in the triple jump.
(Courtesy of Petr Susanka.)

swinging forward, the arms can assist in carrying the body over the landing contact. The legs are flexed to absorb the shock.

Bedi (1975), investigating the broad jumps of medium-skilled performers, concluded:

1. The jumpers in their run up to the board averaged 8.1 m/sec (26.6 ft/sec), with the best performers running the fastest.
2. The vertical force averaged 4133.64 N (930 lb), with the best jumpers exceeding the amount by more than 441 N (100 lb) of force.
3. The braking force was 3036.04 N (683 lb) on the average.

4. The largest impulses (force multiplied by time) were recorded by the best jumpers.
5. The best long jumper spent 0.11 to 0.12 second on the board, while the poorest jumper spent 0.13 to 0.14 second.
6. The jumpers all had a forward rotation at the takeoff, with a large horizontal braking force contributing to this rotational component.

Bedi believes that to jump farther, the performers need to reduce the horizontal braking force at takeoff. This would minimize the forward rotation and maintain horizontal velocity. To achieve this, jumpers adjust their last six to eight steps of the approach. They visually perceive the best step placement for an effective and legal takeoff.

■ The flight of the center of gravity cannot be altered after the takeoff. The path is determined by the angle and speed of projection and by gravitational force once the body is in the air. The only aids to distance possible during flight are positioning of the thighs and legs for the reach and of the trunk and arms for carrying the center of gravity forward on landing.

Triple Jump

The actions of a triple jumper are also those of a long jumper (Bedi 1975), especially at the instant of the final takeoff. The triple jump involves more than a true jump. Once the triple jump was called the hop, step, and jump, which is more descriptive because it encompasses these three movements. The approach, aside from the run-up, used in the modern period might be described as a hop, a bound, and a jump.

While in the long jump there is one flight period, in the triple jump there are three flight periods. Couple these with not one, but three, takeoffs and three landings, and this event is an intriguing one to study. Figure 16.5 contains data from a European Cup meet in 1987.

The ratio of the distance of the three movements (jumps) might become nearly even in the immediate future, as triple jump athletes improve. In 1970, Yoon found the ratio to be 7:6:7 for the hop, step, and jump, respectively. Today, many coaches are proposing a 36:30:34 ratio.

The triple jump is a beautiful motion when executed by an outstanding competitor. The performer's rhythmic sounds could be recorded and used by the beginner to facilitate improvement.

Here are some observations on performance in this event.

1. The initial takeoff in the triple jump is at a lower angle than in the long jump. Descriptive terms might be low, higher, and highest for the three phases, in that order. The takeoff angle at each stage is 8–12°.
2. There is a continuous compromise made between horizontal speed and vertical lift, and the angle of takeoff is considerably lower than in the long jump.
3. The movements must be executed so that the movement is as nearly continuous as possible. The momentum of the jumper must not be decreased too much at each takeoff position; that is, he or she must minimize the braking forces.
4. There is a forceful downward extension at the hip, knee, and ankle joints of the takeoff leg at each position.
5. The center of gravity is maintained in front of the takeoff foot at each takeoff position.
6. The torso of the jumper is essentially an erect one so that the landing leg can be extended and the force of the foot against the ground can be exerted somewhat vertically.
7. The arms move laterally, backward and then forward together to provide a transfer of momentum from one movement to another and to help in maintaining horizontal momentum.
8. The landing foot first moves forward and then backward to ensure that the foot is moving backward faster than the body's center of gravity is moving forward. This enables the jumper to move to the next phase.
9. The landing shock is attenuated by the flexion at the hip, knees, and ankles. The arms move forward in extension, and the torso's forward lean (flexion) enables the jumper to fall forward at landing.

A Brazilian study of the triple jump (Amadio 1989) shows the transfer of mechanical energy that takes place from the hop, step and jump phases. (See Figure 16.6.)

Larkins and Ramey (1991) theoretically deduced that a triple jumper having a velocity at takeoff of 17.2 m/sec could not attain equal distances for the hop, step, and jump phases. To attain this equality and jump farther is not possible because the step phase would exceed velocity beyond human capability.

Running High Jump

The takeoff for the running high jump is in some ways similar to that of the running broad jump. However, most world-class high jumpers use the flop style, which is not similar to the broad jump. The principal difference is that the CG is projected at a much greater angle at takeoff in the high jump. This is accomplished by taking a longer penultimate step, which lowers the CG just before takeoff. The takeoff foot is then planted in front of the CG, which helps to convert the horizontal momentum into vertical lift. Much as in the long jump, the high jumper should strive to take a quick last step, although the step will still be considerably in front of the CG. As shown in the description of the standing jump for height, the inclination of the foot affects the inclinations of all other segments. As in the standing jump for height, actions at the ankle and hip serve to maintain the desired direction. The final force is derived from running momentum, from extension at the knee, and from the forceful swing of the free lower limb and the arms. Segmental inclinations of the foot, leg, thigh, and trunk are closer to the vertical and takeoff than in the long jump.

The flop style high jump uses a curved approach, which allows centrifugal force to be exerted at the instant of takeoff. This centrifugal force helps in (1) providing a lifting component at the time of takeoff; (2) providing a horizontal component to carry the jumper into the pit; and (3) providing rotation to help the athlete rotate around the crossbar for optimum bar clearance.

The height of the center of gravity at takeoff is important. If a jumper is 1.82 m (6 ft) tall, the center of gravity in the normal standing position, according to Palmer's formula, would be 1.036 m (40.65 in.) above the soles of the feet. In rising to the tip of the toes at takeoff, the jumper could raise the CG 17.78 cm (7 in.). The position for the elevated arms and the swinging leg could add another 20.32 cm (8 in.), bringing the position of the CG 1.41 m (55.65 in.) above the ground at takeoff. How high would and could the velocity of the jump carry the center of gravity to enable the jumper to

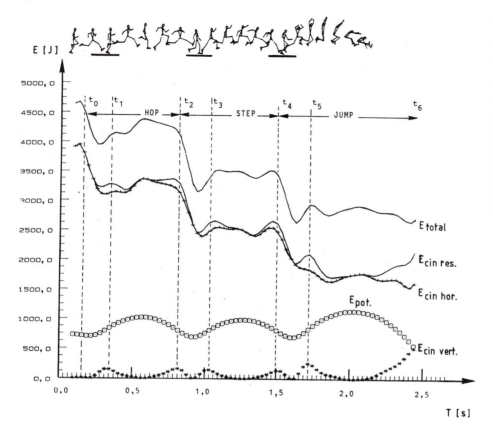

E [J]

FIGURE 16.6 External characteristics of mechanical energy for the triple jump as a function of time and stick figures of each movement phase. Example: for one subject with a performance of 17.33 m, that means: Hop (first jump), step (second jump), jump (third jump): $t_0 - t_1$; support phase hop; $t_2 - t_3$, support phase step; and $t_4 - t_5$, support phase jump.
(Translated from Portuguese.) Reprinted by permission of Alberto Carlos Amadio, Ciencia e Cultura 41(8) 811–817 Agesto, Brazil, 1989.

clear the bar at 2.28 m (7.5 ft)? If a superior jumper could raise the CG another 0.76 m (30 in.), the attained height would be slightly over 2.13 m (7 ft). Additional height is gained by manipulation of the body segments, which allows the CG to pass almost under the bar.

One researcher (Cooper 1968) has listed these requirements for world-record high jumping in order of importance:

1. enough speed and strength at takeoff to give an upward thrust of considerable magnitude
2. long legs and high center of gravity

The Fosbury flop style is shown in Figure 16.7. The ease of execution and high lift of the hips (center of gravity) may make this style mechanically best. The flop style performer usually develops and uses greater horizontal velocity than do practitioners of other jumping styles. Consequently, it is the style now used by almost all elite high jumpers.

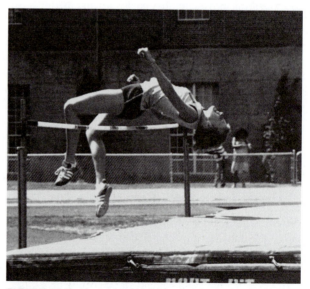

FIGURE 16.7 Flop style of high jumping.
(Courtesy of Sports Information, Washington State University.)

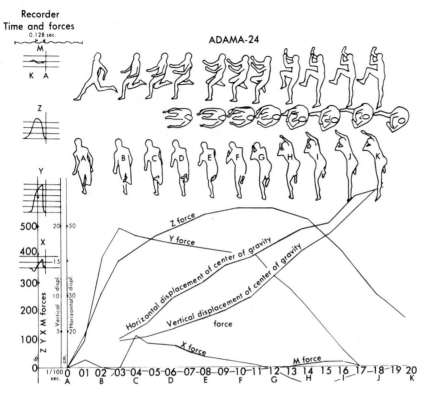

Recorder
Time and forces
0.128 sec.

ADAMA-24

FIGURE 16.8 Force-action-time relationships during propulsive extension of takeoff leg for straddle roll-type high jumper. Contourograms of three planar views are synchronized in time with force platform recordings and calculated displacement plots of the center of gravity.
(From Ward, R. D. 1971. An investigation into the use of computer integration of kinematics, kinetics, and cinematography data in motion analysis. Ph.D. Dissertation, Indiana University.)

Ward (1971) has shown that force, action, and time aspects of high jumping can be synchronized as illustrated in Figure 16.8. Such a study involves using a force plate, three cameras, and an oscillograph recording device. The jumper shown here is a straddle roller. The shortest time on the ground at takeoff (0.15 sec) and the most vertical thrust (4 G) have been recorded for the best jumper.

Research on High Jumping. Dapena and Bahamonde (1991) have used elite high jumpers as subjects, plotting their actual takeoff angle and bar clearance with film analysis. They then used simulation to increase the speed and height of the CG at takeoff. They also changed the body position in the air slightly. By this means, they were able to increase the height of the jump

without having the performers actually jump. One or more of these changes accounted for the simulated increase (see Figures 16.9a, b, and c).

Pole Vault

In the running high and broad jumps, the momentum of the run rotates the body over the supporting foot. The foot and lower limb serve much the same function as the pole does in the vault. During the run, the pole is carried by the front arm in medial rotation, and the shoulder is adducted with some flexion. The forearm is flexed and pronated. In the rear arm, there is some extension at the shoulder and the forearm is also flexed (Figure 16.10). Horizontal velocity is imparted to the pole by the run, and since the pole is raised upward and pointed downward in the final step, it will be rotated upward and forward, after contact with the box, by the horizontal velocity.

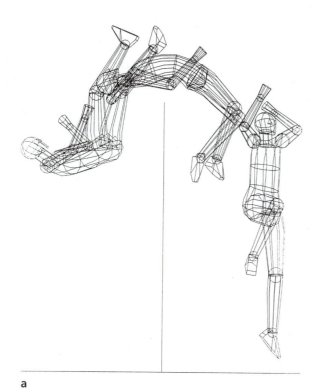

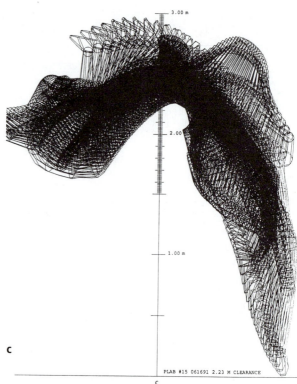

FIGURE 16.9 High jump computer simulation.
(Courtesy of Dapena and R. Bahamonde.)

a

c

PLAB #15 061691 2.23 M CLEARANCE

c

SIDE VIEW

BACK VIEW

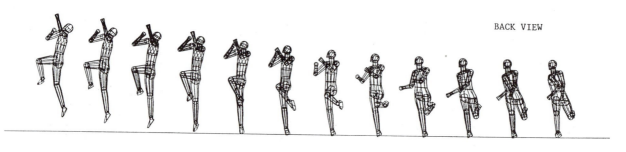

10.22   10.20   10.18   10.16   10.14   10.12   10.10   10.08   10.06   10.04   10.02   10.00

b

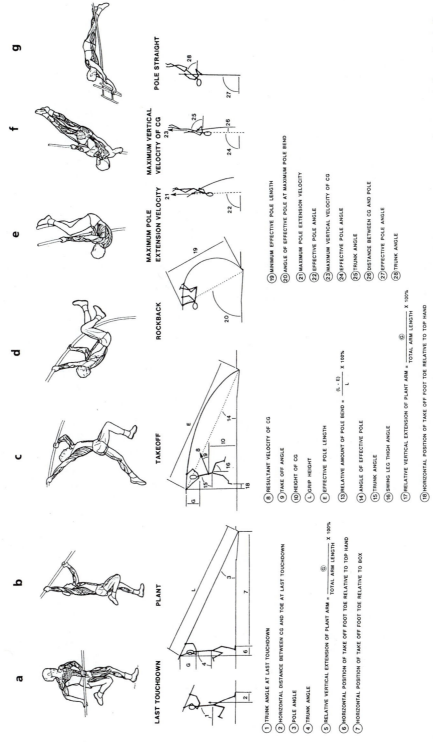

a   b   c   d   e   f   g

LAST TOUCHDOWN   PLANT   TAKEOFF   ROCKBACK   MAXIMUM POLE EXTENSION VELOCITY   MAXIMUM VERTICAL VELOCITY OF CG   POLE STRAIGHT

(1) TRUNK ANGLE AT LAST TOUCHDOWN
(2) HORIZONTAL DISTANCE BETWEEN CG AND TOE AT LAST TOUCHDOWN
(3) POLE ANGLE
(4) TRUNK ANGLE
(5) RELATIVE VERTICAL EXTENSION OF PLANT ARM = $\dfrac{G}{\text{TOTAL ARM LENGTH}} \times 100\%$
(6) HORIZONTAL POSITION OF TAKE OFF FOOT TOE RELATIVE TO TOP HAND
(7) HORIZONTAL POSITION OF TAKE OFF FOOT TOE RELATIVE TO BOX

(8) RESULTANT VELOCITY OF CG
(9) TAKE OFF ANGLE
(10) HEIGHT OF CG
(L) GRIP HEIGHT
(E) EFFECTIVE POLE LENGTH
(13) RELATIVE AMOUNT OF POLE BEND = $\dfrac{(L - E)}{L} \times 100\%$
(14) ANGLE OF EFFECTIVE POLE
(15) TRUNK ANGLE
(16) SWING LEG THIGH ANGLE
(17) RELATIVE VERTICAL EXTENSION OF PLANT ARM = $\dfrac{G}{\text{TOTAL ARM LENGTH}} \times 100\%$
(18) HORIZONTAL POSITION OF TAKE OFF FOOT TOE RELATIVE TO TOP HAND

(19) MINIMUM EFFECTIVE POLE LENGTH
(20) ANGLE OF EFFECTIVE POLE AT MAXIMUM POLE BEND
(21) MAXIMUM POLE EXTENSION VELOCITY
(22) EFFECTIVE POLE ANGLE
(23) MAXIMUM VERTICAL VELOCITY OF CG
(24) EFFECTIVE POLE ANGLE
(25) TRUNK ANGLE
(26) DISTANCE BETWEEN CG AND POLE
(27) EFFECTIVE POLE ANGLE
(28) TRUNK ANGLE

FIGURE 16.10 Sequential contourogram and muscle tracings of pole-vaulter during approach, pole plant, takeoff, rockback, pullup, inverted pushup, and release. **List the primary muscles acting at each of these phases as shown. Estimate the position of the center of gravity of the body and determine its distance to the pole. How do the movements of the arms and legs and the position of the center of gravity influence muscle contraction?**

(Reprinted with permission from Railsback, D. 1987. The pole vault. *National Strength and Conditioning Association Journal* 9(2), April/May, pp. 5–8, 78–80. Illustrations by M. L. Eitel.)

Plant. At the plant of the pole in the box, the right hand is placed as high above the head as possible and should be directly over the left foot. The horizontal velocity at plant and the height of the right hand are the two single most important preparations for a successful vault. The right arm is laterally rotated and flexed at the shoulder. There is extension at the elbow. The left arm has flexion at the shoulder and some at the elbow (stage *c* of Figure 16.10). The left hand is open and then closed, momentarily releasing the pole and then regrasping it. The tracings in Figure 16.10 were taken from a film in which the performer used a glass pole.

As the pole is placed on the ground and the final thrust is made by extension of the thigh and plantar flexion of the foot of the supporting limb, the left forearm is extended and the arm is flexed at the shoulder. The right forearm extends to retain the grasp on the pole as it rebounds from its compressed position. Note that the hands are spaced well apart. Assisting the thrust of the lower limb is the rapid upward movement of the pole and of the swinging right lower limb.

Takeoff. According to Ganslen (1970), at takeoff the supporting leg is inclined 78° since the trunk remains vertical, the thrust of the supporting joints can be assumed to be close to the vertical. As the pole rotates upward around its ground contact, the body rotates around the hand contact on the pole. The body rotation will be faster than that of the pole, and as the extended body passes the pole, its speed of rotation will be increased by flexion at the hips and knees.

For elevation of the lower part of the body above the hands, first there is flexion at the hips and the knees (Figure 16.10), then the knee position decreases the amount of force needed to flex the legs by moving the center of gravity of the lower limbs closer to the fulcrum (the hip joints). As the thighs approach the vertical, extension at the knees occurs to bring the legs in line with the thighs. The body's center of gravity is now close to the pole so that the vaulter is able to take greater advantage of the pole action. In *f*, the trunk has begun to rotate to the left; pelvic rotation will follow, and the right leg will scissor over the left. As the jumper's center of gravity passes the pole, the pulling is converted into a pushing movement, which is achieved by flexion at the shoulder and extension

at the elbow. This action is completed in one continuous movement, and the left hand is released from the pole first. The forearms are pronated as the release of each is accomplished. To project the legs as high as possible, the vaulter should keep the chin down toward the chest in preparing to go over the bar. The movement of the lower limbs downward after crossing the bar raises the trunk and arms. Elevating the arms still higher helps keep them from striking the bar as they go over. The vaulter must be sure to wait until the pole has almost reached the vertical position before executing the pull-up.

Hand Placement. The higher the vaulter places the hands on the pole at the start, the faster the run, the steeper the parabola of the path of the center of gravity in flight, and the higher the vault. Using rather elaborate electronic equipment, including force plates, special slow-motion camera, force transducers, recording oscillograph, and necessary accessories, Barlow (1983) was able to secure kinematic and kinetic parameters of the pole-vaulting of top performers. Barlow analyzed these data with a computer and digitizing system. Some of his findings are:

Kinematic Factors

1. The last stride of all vaulters was shorter than the preceding stride.
2. The second-to-last stride was longer than either the third-to-last or the last stride.
3. The best vaulter (who was of world class) took longer strides throughout than did any of the other subjects and shortened his last stride the least.
4. All pole plants of those who vaulted 4.87 m (16 ft) or higher were initiated in 0.423 second (mean time), compared with 0.408 second for the pole plants of those who vaulted less than 4.87 m.
5. Considerable deceleration over the final three strides occurred for those who vaulted less than 4.87 m.
6. The best vaulter accelerated longer in the run and decelerated less during the final strides.
7. Those who vaulted over 4.87 m attained a maximal velocity of 8.83 m/sec (28.97 ft/sec) during the second-to-last stride, while those who vaulted less than 4.87 m attained a maximal velocity of 8.30 m/sec (27.26 ft/sec) under the same conditions.

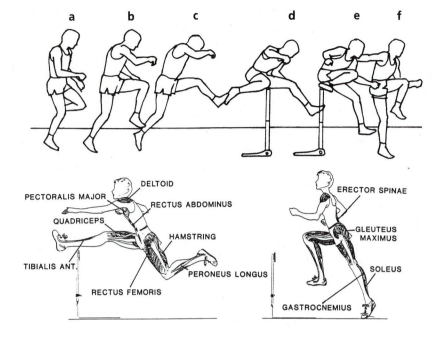

FIGURE 16.11 Sequence of contouro-grams of hurdler and takeoff and flight phase of one hurdler, with muscles high-lighted. **What are the major differences in kinematics of the two hurdlers? Which muscles contract for takeoff, but not flight action, and which muscles contract at both times?**
(From McFarlane, B. 1986. High Performance Hurdling—The Women's 100m Hurdles. *National Strength and Conditioning Association Journal* 8(6) pp. 4–13. Illustrations by Patricia Rowan Hays.)

8. The average takeoff angle for the center-of-gravity projection of all vaulters was 21.9°.
9. The angle of takeoff tended to increase as the height of the crossbar was elevated.
10. When the pole was perpendicular, the top vaulters had no vertical acceleration, and the poorer ones had negative vertical velocity.

Kinetic Factors

1. The average time on the force plate (of the takeoff foot) was 0.122 second.
2. The fastest time was 0.116 second for the top vaulter.
3. The peak vertical striking force at takeoff was an average magnitude of 3635.8 N (819 lb).
4. The top performers attained greater vertical force at takeoff than did those who were poorer vaulters.
5. The top vaulters supplied greater braking impulse at takeoff.
6. The vertical extension force tended to increase with the increased height of the crossbar.

What meaning can be derived from these data? We now know that the pole-vaulter, in fact, does jump at the takeoff, attempts to generate considerable vertical force,

and runs at close to top sprinting speed. Finally, by studying such data, we may find distinguishing factors characteristic of the better vaulters. McGinnis (1986) has done this; his analysis is discussed in Chapter 8.

Hurdling

The high hurdler is a runner who vaults a series of hurdles. The run must be slightly modified on the approach to each hurdle. There is flexion and abduction at the shoulders and the scapulae are elevated (Figure 16.11). As the body's center of gravity is moved forward by the momentum of the run, the heel is raised (*b* to *d*). At the same time, the shank of the supporting limb extends. Considerable flexion at the hip of the lead limb takes place as the limb is swung forward with the leg extended. (Most hurdlers attempt to prevent the leg from extending into a locked knee position.) The skilled hurdler flexes the neck as well as the trunk so that the center of gravity will not go too high over the hurdle and contact with the ground will be made sooner.

The high point of the parabola should occur in front of the hurdle. The athlete is actually on the way down when crossing the hurdle. This helps in spending as short a time as possible off the ground and prevents

Biomechanics of Jumping   **329**

"floating" the hurdle. Note that the hurdler starts flexion of the trunk and neck before leaving the ground (*c*). The rear leg (*d*) is brought forward by flexion at the hip. As the thigh is moved forward, it is abducted and rotated medially, bringing the flexed leg close to the horizontal (*d* and *e*). At the same time that the trail leg is being brought forward, the arm on the same side is driven forcefully to the rear. This creates an action-reaction situation and assists in bringing the trail leg through quickly and back down into a sprinting position.

After the hurdle is cleared, the lead thigh extends to lower the foot and the leg flexes, moving the foot backward with reference to the knee (*e* and *f*) and decreasing the possibility of backward push, at contact. After the hurdle is cleared, the rear thigh adducts and rotates laterally (*f*) to bring the foot in line for the next step. After contact, body momentum helps to extend the supporting limb.

■ The hurdler attempts to raise the center of gravity only high enough to clear the hurdle.

The hurdler tries to get the lead leg down as soon as possible so that the feet are in contact with the ground and he or she is able to run rapidly to the next hurdle. This involves an action-reaction phenomenon in that as the hip flexes, it aids in balance when the thigh is extended. The reason is that the extension of the thigh creates the action-reaction and brings about an extension of the trunk.

Kinematic Analysis. McDonald and Dapena (1991) used three-dimensional filming techniques to secure linear kinematic data on men in 110m and women running in 100m hurdle race. They found an increase in vertical velocity and a decrease in forward horizontal velocity during the takeoff of the hurdle step. The hurdlers recovered most of the velocity lost during the second support phase after clearing the hurdle. The CG downward motion was not stopped until the second support phase after hurdle clearance. The peak height of the parabola path was directly over the hurdle in men and 0.30m before the hurdle in women. They believe it would be a mistake to have a lower parabola for women because this would shorten the hurdle step and lengthen the three between-hurdle steps. It would also make the airborne phase of

the race too short. The women would not give their legs time enough to prepare for landing after clearing the hurdle if they used a lower parabola.

Steeplechase

The **steeplechase** is a type of endurance run coupled with a hurdling and jumping action. The mechanics used in running 3000 meters are similar to those used in any run of that distance. However, scaling five hurdles or obstacles over each 400 meters, with one located just before the water barrier, puts considerable emphasis on the endurance factor. Many performers in the past have jumped on top of the barrier and then attempted to clear the water area. Steeplechasers jump the other four hurdles or leap on top of the barrier and then jump into a running stride. We discuss the water jump here.

MINI-LABORATORY LEARNING EXPERIENCE

1. Use the Sargent (vertical) jump to determine the best vertical jumpers in class. Then list the reasons why some individuals jump higher than others.
2. Do a standing long jump. Observe and analyze each jump.
3. From a standing position, do a sail, a hitch kick, and a hang as represented in the long jump. These three positions are depicted in Figure 16.5. Discuss how these movements influence the distance of the jump.
4. Using a three-step approach, perform the coordinated pattern of the triple jump: hop, step, and jump. Note which foot is used for the hop. Discuss the perceived force of impact for the three landings. Next, use the other foot to initiate the hop and repeat the triple jump. Discuss differences in speed, distance, coordination, balance, and perceived impact force.

Many authors contend that a fast approach and rapid mount (if this is used), followed by a smooth takeoff, are the ingredients for success in this event. Formerly, the steeplechaser usually tried to maximize the horizontal displacement and minimize vertical displacement. The jumper usually landed in the water about 0.60 m (2 ft) from the forward edge of the water area in a stride position and accelerated from a flexed front leg (which reduces the body's moment of inertia) out of the water as rapidly as possible. A runner from the University of Wisconsin introduced a new technique: he jumped the water hurdle (rather than mount the barrier and then jump into the water) and landed just beyond the middle of the water hazard. He landed sooner and was out of the water sooner than his opponents. His technique is now commonly used, possibly because athletes are stronger, taller, and have improved technique.

Plyometrics (Depth Jumping)

Plyometrics is a form of training used to condition athletes for various jumps. It involves dropping from a small or sometimes high height, followed by a countermovement of jumping upward to another starting position. This has proved to be an asset to some performers. (See Chapter 10, "Biomechanics of Exercise," for more details.)

References

Alexander, R. 1989. Sequential joint extension in jumping. *Journal of Human Movement Science* 8(4):339–45.

Barlow, D. A. 1983. Kinematic and kinetic factors involved in pole vaulting. Ph.D. dissertation, Indiana University.

Bedi, J. F. 1975. Angular momentum in the long jump. Ph.D. dissertation, Indiana University.

Bedi, J. F., Cresswell, G. A., Engle, J. T., and Nicol, M. S. 1987. Increase in jumping height associated with maximal effort vertical depths jump. *Research Quarterly for Exercise and Sport* 58:11–15.

Bobbert, M. D., Mackay, M., Schinkelshoek, D. P. A., Huijing, P. A., and Van Ingen Schenau, G. J. 1986. Biomechanics analysis of drop and countermovement jumps. *European Journal of Applied Physiology* 54:566–73.

Bunn, J. W. 1955. *Scientific principles of coaching.* Englewood Cliffs, NJ: Prentice-Hall.

Cooper, J. M. 1968. Kinesiology of the high jump. In *Proceedings of the first international seminar on biomechanics,* eds. J. Wartenweiler, E. Jokl, and M. Hebbelincks.

Dapena, J., and Bahamonde, R. 1991. Report for scientific services project, (The Athletic Congress): Biomechanics analysis of men's high jump, Biomechanics Laboratory, Indiana University.

Doherty, K. 1984. *Track and field.* Swarthmore, PA: TAFMOP Publishers.

Dowell, L. J., and Lee, B. 1991. A comparison of the effect of transferring momentum from the part to the whole in the vertical jump and the standing long jump. *Biomechanics in Sports IX.* College Station, TX: Texas A & M University.

Felton, E. 1960. A kinesiological comparison of good and poor performers in the standing broad jump. Ph.D. thesis, University of Wisconsin–Madison.

Ganslen, R. V. 1970. *Mechanics of pole vault,* 7th ed. Denton, TX: R. V. Ganslen.

Ganslen, R. V. 1985. Triple jump. In *Encyclopedia of physical education, fitness and sports,* ed. T. Cureton. Reston, VA: AAHPERD.

Glassow, R., and Kruse, P. 1960. Motor performance of girls 6 to 14 years. *Research Quart* 37:3.

Gros, H. J. 1984. Computerized analysis of the pole vault utilizing biomechanics, cinematography and direct force measurements. Ph.D. dissertation, University of Alberta, Canada.

Halverson, L. 1958. A comparison of the performance of kindergarten children in the takeoff phase of the standing broad jump. Ph.D. dissertation, University of Wisconsin–Madison.

Henson, P., Turner, P., and Lacourse, M. 1986. Test for determining potential for track and field athletes. Paper presented to Tac Olympic Development Committee.

Hudson, J. L. 1987. What goes up. Paper presented to AAHPERD National Convention.

Hul, He. 1990. Study of characteristics of female triple jump technique and training: Changsha, China: Human Research Institute of Sports Science.

Jensen, J., and Phillips, S. 1991. Variations on the vertical jump: Individual adaptations to changing task demands. *Journal of Motor Behavior* 23(1):63–74.

Larkins, C., and Ramey, M. R. 1991. Can triple jumpers really use an even ratio strategy? University of Michigan, Ann Arbor and University of California, Davis. *Biomechanics in Sports IX.*

McDonald, C., and Dapena, J. 1991. Linear kinematics of the men's 110m and women's 100m hurdles races. *Medicine and Science in Sports and Exercise* 23.

McGinnis, P. 1986. Pole vault reports. USOC/TAC Sports Science Project.

Oddsson, L. I. E., and Westing, S. H. 1991. Measurements of muscle strength and biomechanical parameters. Karolinska Institute, Stockholm, Sweden. *Biomechanics in Sports IX*.

Roy, B. 1971. Kinematics and kinetics of the standing long jump in seven, ten, thirteen and sixteen year old boys. Ph.D. dissertation, University of Wisconsin–Madison.

Sargent, D. 1921. Physical test of a man. *Am. Phys. Educ. Rev.* 26:188.

Ward, R. D. 1971. An investigation into the use of computer integration of kinematics, kinetics, and cinematography data in motion analysis. Ph.D. dissertation, Indiana University.

Yajun, Lu. 1990. Dynamic research of the pole vault. Tangshan, China: North China Coal Mining Medical College.

Yoon, P. T. E. 1970. The triple jump. In *International track and field coaching encyclopedia,* eds., F. Wilt and T. Ecker, West Nyack, NY: Parker Publishing Co.

17 Biomechanics of Throwing

Throwing is the act of propelling an object through the air by means of the action of the body, climaxed by the arm and hand. The release is through extension or by a whirling motion of the upper limb and parts of the body assisting in the action. Researchers can measure the percent of contribution of each lever to ball velocity.

Throwing includes a rapid acceleration of the trunk and arm segments, usually after a step and just before release of an object. Sometimes it involves a summation of the velocities of the body parts, all adding up to a crescendo at the time of release. At other times, some body parts are moved for positional purposes to allow for the freedom of the body parts engaged in the primary action. In addition, an axis (pivotal point, fulcrum) around which the body rotates as the throwing action takes place is established so that the movement is effective.

Factors Affecting Flight of Objects

General concepts of aerodynamics are described in Chapters 6 and 21 and are also applicable to throwing. Specific factors, however, relate to the effects of flight of thrown objects. For example, most objects are thrown (released) with a backspin. A human being can release an object with the greatest velocity (because of the final position of the fingers) if the object is spinning. However, a spinning ball travels slower in the air than one that is not spinning. If the object is light in weight, there is lateral deflection as it progresses toward its destination. Watts (1985) explains this curve phenomenon, with respect to pitching, by stating that it involves a boundary layer of thin fluid (air) very near the object. The air moves around the front half of the object, in this case a ball. This involves creation of a downstream separation point, called the wake, that occurs away from the front of a ball. The flow of air over the ball is equal in speed to the velocity of the ball. The pressure in the wake region (drag) is lower than the pressure on the front of the ball. This tends to slow the object. If the wake is not symmetrical, the flow of air is redirected off the rear of the ball, causing deflection.

A baseball can be made to curve or fall more slowly or more rapidly in regard to its normal parabolic path. However, this is only possible if the force generated to spin the ball is large enough. Watts (1985) reports that an investigator (Briggs) found that baseball pitchers rotated the ball seven to sixteen times (revolutions) on the throw to home plate. This rotation creates high and low pressure areas (drag and lift forces) that produce the change in flight.

Because of their greater weight and spherical shape, smooth surface, and coincident geometric center of mass, the flights of the shot and hammer are not observably affected by spin, lift, or drag.

Putting a substance on the baseball, such as petroleum jelly, saliva, and sweat drops, reduces the spin. The knuckle ball, thrown with the first knuckle of the throwing fingers, has a similar effect. The effect of scuffing up the ball causes the ball to spin toward the roughened area. This is an illegal pitch, but it has been used.

MINI-LABORATORY LEARNING EXPERIENCE

1. Throw a football, rugby ball, baseball and/or other balls, differing in size, weight, and shape. Identify the types of spin easily imparted to each ball and the type of throwing pattern naturally used.
2. View videos of each of the above to determine the similarities and differences in the actions.

High-Velocity Throwing Concepts

Throwing a lightweight object such as a ball usually consists of accumulated accelerations of successive segments, especially of the upper extremity. This movement can be labeled concurrent motion; that is, all successive limbs move in the same direction. The result is much greater contraction of the large muscles, such as the pectoralis major and the latissimus dorsi (which are actually arm muscles, in terms of action, even though they are located on the thorax and back), that attach to the humerus in the bicipital groove.

This type of high-velocity throwing calls for greater contractile length of the muscles of the throwing arm than of some of the lower-extremity muscles. The reason is that many of the arm muscles are biarticular in nature; that is, they usually move two joints in the same direction at the same time. This factor calls for proper timing of the action so that the thrower is able to be consistent. A slight error in any part of the movement is accentuated at the time of release. If accuracy rather than velocity is the objective, the thrower uses the least number of segments possible. The pattern in such a case may be quite different because only a few segments are involved.

The movements involved in a high-velocity throw are:*

1. The center of gravity shifts backward and then is displaced forward.
2. The performer steps forward with the leg opposite the throwing arm.
3. The upper portion of the body is flexed after being extended (first acceleration).
4. The trunk rotates about its longitudinal axis to pull the throwing arm forward (second acceleration).
5. The scapula moves forward over the back (torso), as much as 15.24 cm (6 in.) or more. This is one key to the ability to throw efficiently. A large scapula is considered an asset in high-velocity throwing.
6. The humerus acts in conjunction with the scapula as the former flexes on the latter over a range of 90°.
7. The humerus rotates internally around its long axis up to 90° (another major acceleration). Just as the throw of an object is near the release point, there is some retraction of recoil in the shoulder area.
8. The extension at the wrist at the end of the backward motion of the arm and the flexion at release together add another acceleration. (There is some controversy regarding this statement. Some researchers contend that there is no acceleration involved in the extension at the wrist and that the situation is only positional. Also, to speak of the "cocking," or flexing, and then extending at the wrist is misleading. It is the hand that does most of the movement, not the wrist.)
9. The fingers are extended first and then flexed to add a final acceleration.

Axes of Rotation

Four axes (fulcrums or pivotal points) of rotation are often involved in high-velocity throws. They are the planted foot on the opposite side of the throwing arm, the hip opposite the throwing arm, the spine, and the shoulder of the throwing arm. The body as a whole rotates about one axis—the foot—while the other body parts rotate about various axes, such as a joint or joints.

---

*Adapted from Gaul, 1968

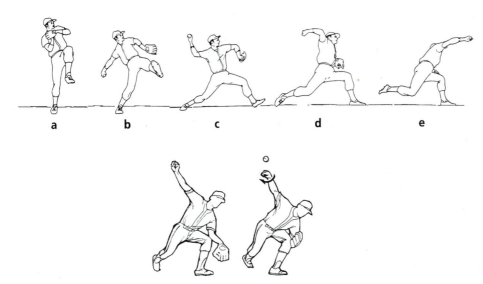

FIGURE 17.1 A high-velocity throw is characterized by a step forward, counter rotation and forward rotation of the trunk, and lateral and medial rotation of the arm. Note at the termination of the throw there is pronounced lateral body lean and pronation of the forearm.

In the so-called overhand throw, the throwing arm begins the action from an extended-arm position with the hand pointing downward. The arm moves in an angular path to the rear and upward. From this rearward, fully extended position, the arm translates upward and backward. Then the arm flexes and moves forward at the elbow to increase the angular motion, after which it extends laterally before release takes place. This latter action gives the opportunity to apply centrifugal force. The lateral body lean in the opposite direction enables the arm to be extended upward (Figure 17.1). The non-throwing hand moves backward, assisting in the torso rotation and arm motion. Almost all throwing action has some or all of these segmental movements. Small, light objects are released in a plane lying parallel to the body and tangential to the movement. Heavy objects such as a shot put are released in front of the body; otherwise, injury to the elbow would occur frequently. These objects are linked to the length of the moment arms.

The function of the arm in a throwing situation is to position the hand for the throwing action and to help develop efficient velocity of the hand. (The object is released with that velocity that the hand has accumulated.) For a better understanding of the upper limb complex and the amazing action that occurs during the throwing action, let's look at some anatomic and bio-medical aspects.

Shoulder Girdle Complex

A total of 28 bones in the arm-shoulder area are used in the whip-rack, flail-like action occurring during throwing. The scapula, humerus, radius, ulna, proximal row of carpals, distal row of carpals, metacarpals, and finally the phalanges are involved. In addition, the clavicle serves as a strut supporting the whole arm during the act of throwing.

The astounding thing about the shoulder girdle complex is its lack of stability, which results in great freedom of motion. In the upper swing of the arm, the great range of movement is further enhanced by the broken hook structure involving the clavicle, acromion process, top of glenoid fossa, and coracoid process. Furthermore, the scapula moves on the clavicle, and the clavicle moves on the sternum. The shallow depth of the glenoid fossa pushes the humerus farther away from the center of the joint, promoting still more freedom of motion. The joint then has to rely on the rotator cuff muscles—the subscapularis, supraspinatus, infraspinatus, and teres major—as well as on other shoulder girdle muscles to preserve its integrity. Many pitchers in baseball, as well as those involved in other throwing activities involving high velocity action of the arm, may have rotator cuff muscle injury. These small muscles sometimes have difficulty withstanding the strain forced on them in such a stressful situation.

The spins and swings of the arm about its long axis, in which acceleration is produced from a small radius of gyration, enable the arm to have great spinning motion. Its motion has been compared to that of a jackhammer in the overhand motion.

Muscles Involved

The main muscles of the arm and adjacent region involved in throwing, as determined by electromyography, are the pectoralis major, latissimus dorsi, deltoid, trapezius, serratus anterior (magnus), rhomboids, and levator scapulae. The muscles acting on the scapula function as a force couple: One group produces an upward rotation, and another causes a downward rotation. This is similar to the action of a revolving door. The longer in length the scapula, the farther down the muscles attach, creating the possibility of a large force. This is one of the reasons tall people can throw at the rate of 160.9 kmph (100 mph), while smaller people throw at slower speeds.

■ There is usually a proximal-to-distal action of the segments during throwing. This means that the heavier parts initiate the movement, and the distal, lighter segments benefit by transfer of momentum and also are easier to move at the crucial point of release.

Action of the Hand

The grasping aspect of the hand is used in throwing. For example, there is opposition of the thumb, which is used only during the early stages of the throwing motion but is not evident at the release of lightweight objects. The skin of the hand on the palmar side is tight for grasping and flexibility, but on the back the skin is loose. The skin creases of the fingers are not located only over the joints, but are on either side, allowing for greater flexibility. A natural pocket is formed by the thenar and hypothenar muscles and the metacarpals, and there is an increased angle of application of the profundus and superficilis when they are lifted upward to produce more effort.

All forceful throws from almost any position are characterized by medial rotation of the humerus and pronation of the forearm and hand (Figure 17.2). The radius of movement of the forearm ranges from long to short to long, which gives the arm the longest moment

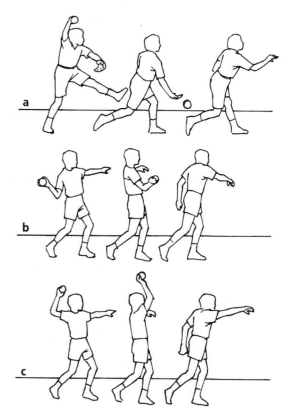

FIGURE 17.2 Evidence of pronation of the forearm during the underarm (a), sidearm (b), and overarm (c) throwing patterns.

arm and raises the possibility that the radius and the moment arm will be the same length. A throw of high velocity is likely to be the result.

Thrower Airborne

In certain situations, such as shot putting and discus throwing, it is possible for the thrower to have lost contact with the ground and to be airborne before releasing the object. The object has by this time accumulated its own momentum and will continue unimpeded on its course, even though a foot of the thrower is not anchored to the ground.

Throwing Patterns

Mechanics of Underarm Pattern

The underarm pattern is most frequently seen in skills that project an object by a throw. Its outstanding characteristic is movement of the arm, usually with extension at the elbow, by action at the shoulder. At the height of the backswing, the arm is approximately at shoulder height. During the force-producing phase the arm is moved rapidly downward, and at release or impact it reaches a position that is usually parallel with or slightly beyond the line of the trunk.

Arm Lever. The lever of this arm action includes the bones of the upper arm and forearm, the wrist and hand, and, in the throw, the portion of the phalanges up to the center of gravity of the projectile. If an implement is used, all the phalanges will be included, in addition to the length of the implement from grasp to point of impact. The resistance arm includes the same rigid masses as does the entire lever; the fulcrum is in the shoulder joint. The length of the moment arm at the time that the object is started on its flight will be the distance from the proximal end of the humerus to the point of impact or the center of gravity of the projectile. This line will be perpendicular to the axis and to the line of the applied force (known as the principle of perpendicularity).

Other Levers. Various levers can be added to this primary action to increase the amount of applied force. Among the most common is that which moves the pelvis by rotation at the hip joint. This lever includes the pelvis, the spine, the throwing arm side of the shoulder girdle, and the rigid masses included in the shoulder-action lever. (The following description refers to a right-handed performer.)

The resistance arm includes the same masses as does the entire lever. At release or impact the length of the moment arm is the distance from the axis (a line passing through the hip joint about which the trunk is rotating) to the point of release or impact. This line, perpendicular to the axis and to the direction of applied force, can be changed in length by the positions of the trunk and the arm. If the trunk is flexed to the right, the moment arm will be lengthened; if the trunk is flexed to the left, the

moment will be shortened. If the arm is abducted, the moment arm will be lengthened. In some underarm patterns, although pelvic rotation occurred during the force-producing phase, studies did not find it to occur at the time of application of force. Thus, if the linear velocities of moment arms acting at release or impact are determined, and if the velocity of pelvic rotation is not one of them, pelvic rotation makes no direct contribution to the force at that time. Most likely its contribution, made before the final phase, is reflected in the actions at the other joints.

Rotation of Pelvis. Pelvic rotation is facilitated by a transfer of weight of the total body. In the preparatory phase the weight is transferred to the right foot, and the pelvis is rotated to the right. Rotation can be more than 90° from the intended direction of flight of the projectile. This range of rotation is not possible unless the weight is taken from the left foot. Pelvic rotation facilitates arm action. As the pelvis turns, it carries the torso with it until it too is at right angles to the intended line of flight. As the arm is raised upward and backward, it is abducting instead of extending, as it would be if the torso were facing forward. This action increases the range of motion and speed of the segment.

Length of Step. While the weight is on the right foot, the left foot can be lifted in preparation for a forward step. No evidence is available to indicate the most advantageous length of this step. Researchers do show that more skilled performers take longer steps than those who are less skilled and that the length of the step is a feature that distinguishes between these two categories of performers. As the forward step is taken, some forward movement of the whole body occurs. This adds to the force that can be imparted to the projectile, but, compared to that developed by trunk, spine, and arm action, this force is small. The step alone is not an important factor in increasing force; it does, however, facilitate increased range of trunk and arm action. It is important for this reason.

Rotation of the spine can add another lever to the pattern. Compared to other levers that may be a part of the pattern, the spine makes a small contribution. Although the action occurs in many vertebral joints, the fulcrum can be considered to be located at the level of the sternoclavicular joint. The lever includes the right clavicle and the masses included in the shoulder lever; the resistance arm includes the masses of the entire lever. The length of the moment arm is the perpendicular distance from the axis, and it will pass through the upper spine to the point of release or impact. The length of the moment arm can be altered by changes of trunk or arm position, as described for the moment arm of pelvic rotation.

Wrist Action. An important lever acts at the wrist joint, because the wrist can be the fastest of the acting joints and because the length of the moment arm can be greatly increased by an implement. For the throw, the lever arm and the resistance arm include the bones of the hand and fingers to the center of gravity of the projectile. For the strike, they include the bones of the hand and fingers and the implement, if one is used, to the point of impact. In a throw, depending on the size of the hand, the moment arm from the wrist to the center of gravity of the projectile could be 7.6 to 10.1 cm (3 to 4 in.) in a child and 20.3 and 22.8 cm (8 to 9 in.) in an adult.

The levers described in the preceding paragraphs, acting at shoulder hip, spine, and wrist, are those most commonly used in a variety of underarm patterns. Whether more than one is used in the pattern depends on the demands of the situation. Movements from the shoulder axis will always be used, since it is the basis for the underarm classification. It is possible that in some situations movements about other joints can be used efficiently, but such additions will not change the classification. (See Figure 17.2.)

Mechanics of Overarm Pattern

The overarm pattern, like the underarm, is commonly used in throws and strikes. Its distinguishing feature is action that rotates the humerus laterally during the preparatory phase and medially during the force-producing phase. To help you visualize these actions, try going through the following movements: Hold the upper arm at the side in such a position that, when the forearm is flexed 90°, the forearm will be horizontal and pointing directly forward. (If necessary review Chapters 3 and 4 on anatomical terminology.) Keeping the upper arm at the side, move the forearm to the right 90° in the transverse plane; the forearm will now point directly to the side. The

joint action that brought about this change in the position of the forearm was lateral rotation of the humerus. If the forearm is now moved back to the original position, the action involved is medial rotation of the humerus.

These rotations at the shoulder can be made while the upper arm is in many positions. One position frequently used is as follows: With forearm extended, abduct the entire arm 90° to the horizontal. Adjust the position of the upper arm so that when the arm is flexed 90° at the elbow, the forearm will point directly forward. Move the forearm until it points directly upward. You do this by 90° of lateral rotation of the humerus. Lower the forearm until it again points forward; you have moved it to this position by 90° of medial rotation at the shoulder joint. This rotation of the humerus is the outstanding characteristic of the overarm pattern; this bone is usually abducted in the force-producing phase.

Feltner and Dapena (1986) calculated the resultant joint forces and torques at the shoulder and elbow joints in baseball pitching throughout the entire motion. They found that as the forward step came in contact with the ground, there was a horizontal adduction torque at the shoulder joint and the shoulder was externally rotated at the same time. As the upper arm began to rotate internally, (they stated this was 30 ms before release of the ball), it was still in a state of external rotation at the time of release of the ball.

It is probable that, next to hand flexion, medial rotation of the humerus is the fastest action of the upper limb. Apparently there is a limit to the speed with which each body segment can be rotated. Because the moment arm of humeral medial rotation can be longer than that acting at the wrist joint, its linear velocity, and therefore its contribution to the force imparted to a projectile, can be greater than those contributed by action at the wrist (hand movement). (See Figures 17.1 and 17.2.)

Lateral and Medial Rotation. In lateral and medial rotation of the humerus, the axis passes through both the shoulder and elbow joints and the length of the humerus. In the other actions at the shoulder, the axis passes through only the shoulder joint, humerus. The length of the moment arm in the rotating actions (lateral and medial) is the distance from the axis to the point of release or of impact. The line representing this distance must be perpendicular to the axis and also to the line of applied force. The moment arm is longest when the forearm is perpendicular to the humerus; when the forearm is flexed either more or less than 90°, the moment arm is shorter.

With the forearm extended (but not locked), medial and lateral rotation can be used effectively when an implement is held in the hand. If the arm is held at the side, with the elbow extended, and a tennis racket held in the hand so that it is at right angles to the arm, the racket can be moved through 180° in the transverse plane. In this action, pronation and supination of the forearm add to the range and the speed as the humerus is rotated.

Other levers commonly combined with arm action in the overarm pattern are the same as those described for the underarm pattern. They are brought into action by pelvic and spinal rotation and hand flexion, and their resistance arms are those described for the underarm pattern. The lengths of the moment arms for pelvic and spinal rotation are likely to be longer in the overarm than in the underarm pattern because the humerus is usually abducted.

According to Tarbell (1971), the variety of types of the overarm pattern that the upper limb can perform is characteristic of the versatility of this section of the body. This limb can apply great force and also act with extreme precision. In part, this versatility is due to the structure of the connection with the trunk. The humerus is connected to the freely movable scapula. The humeral head, which is almost half a sphere, fits into a cup of cartilage attached to the inner surface of the fossa on the upper distal section of the scapula. This attachment permits flexion, extension, and abduction of the humerus and the antagonistic actions. Variations are increased by movements of the scapula, which has no direct connection with the trunk. The scapula and clavicle are functioning parts of the upper limb and take part in practically all movements of the humerus, not adding to strength of action but, rather, increasing range and versatility.

Mechanics of Sidearm Pattern

The sidearm pattern, like the underarm and overarm ones, is generally used in throws and strikes.

■ Unlike the underarm and overarm patterns, the distinguishing feature of the sidearm pattern is not the type of shoulder action but the lack or limitation of action at this joint.

The main action in the sidearm pattern is pelvic rotation, with the arm held fairly stable in an abducted position. The lever and the resistance arm for this action include the segments described for it for the underarm pattern. The moment arm for the pelvic lever can be one of the longest found in common throwing activities. It extends from the axis passing through the left hip (for right-handed performers) to the line of applied force and includes the width of the pelvis, often the length of the whole arm, and part of the hand. The length of the moment arm is increased by the length of any implement used. With a tennis racket or baseball bat, the length of the moment arm could be 1.828 m (6 ft) or more in an adult. Other actions commonly combined with pelvic rotation in this pattern are spinal rotation, hand flexion, and often a small range of arm adduction.

Another outstanding feature of the sidearm pattern is the plane in which the movements are made—the transverse. Many movements of the underarm and overarm patterns are made in the sagittal or diagonal plane.

The basic sidearm pattern, in which the shoulder and elbow joints are fixed, is rarely used in throwing light objects. Only when heavy objects are projected and in young, inexperienced children is the basic pattern likely to be observed. In a study of the sidearm and overarm throwing patterns of a highly skilled man and woman, the preliminary parts of the movements were found to be much alike. The differences were in the position of the arm and the degree and timing of extension at the elbow. The arm in the sidearm pattern was close to the horizontal as rotation at the hip began, and the forearm was more fully extended at release. These arm positions lengthened the moment arms at pelvic and spinal levels and shortened the moment arm for shoulder rotation. The pelvic action in both subjects contributed a greater proportion of the velocity in the sidearm throw than it did in the overarm pattern. The ball velocity for the man's sidearm throw was 3.657 m/sec (120 ft/sec) and for the woman's 2.73 m/sec (89 ft/sec).

Continued study of the so-called sidearm throws of skilled performers has shown so much similarity with the overarm throw, especially those in which medial rotation of the humerus is followed by forearm extension, that some researchers have questioned classifying them as different patterns. Other observers believe that a distinguishing feature in the sidearm throw is a circular arm movement preceding release and that this is never seen in the overarm throw. These observers say that the throw with the circular pattern should not be classified with the overarm throw. The overarm and sidearm patterns may be primarily diagonal patterns with different directions of trunk lateral flexion. The sidearm includes a lean of the trunk toward the throwing arm; an opposite lean occurs during overarm throwing. (See the discussion on the discus throw.)

MINI-LABORATORY LEARNING EXPERIENCE

1. Put up a target and have class members throw at it, using underarm, overarm, and sidearm patterns, and using only the arm segment. Record the differences in accuracy.
2. Bring to the laboratory pictures of all types of throwing actions, preferably in sequence. Note segmental action.
3. Have a skilled performer demonstrate and explain his or her throwing action. Compare the statements to what the performer demonstrated.
4. Contrast unskilled and skilled performances in a throwing action.

Biomechanics of Selected Throwing Skills

Analyses of selected throwing skills involving sidearm, underarm, and overarm patterns are presented here. We have not attempted to include all the movements; only a representative sample is discussed. In the sidearm example, we present only the discus throw. However, many striking patterns use sidearm actions and we will describe some of them in the next chapter.

Sidearm Throw: Discus

The discus throw is a type of sidearm throwing action. Throwers use this throwing movement because it enables them to attain the greatest possible distance. Factors influencing the flight pattern are height, velocity at release, and angle at release. In addition, the discus in flight is subject to aerodynamic factors and angle of attack (air resistance), which influence the distance traveled.

Velocity. The velocity of the released spinning discus accomplished by top performers is 24.38 m/sec (80 ft/sec) or more, and the angle of release is approximately 35°. The angle of attack, about 15°, is the angle of the plane of the discus and the relative wind. The discus is thrown with a slight tilt so that the lift factor is greater than the drag factor. (See Chapters 6, 21 and the javelin section in this chapter for more information on lift and drag.) A headwind coming toward the performer at an angle of 45° from the right (with a right-handed competitor) is the most advantageous wind, in terms of direction, for top performers.

If the radius of the throwing arm is long (externally extended) and coincides with the moment arm, great velocity is generated at release. Furthermore, the throwing arm is extended downward at the start of the spin and then extended laterally and upward, taking advantage of centrifugal force at release.

Action of Discus Thrower. The discus throw is an excellent example of the basic sidearm pattern, to which has been added a preparatory movement of the entire body. In the area, a ring with a diameter of 2.5 m (8 ft 2.5 in.), within which the body is permitted to move, the progression includes total rotation of the body one and one-half times, as well as movement from the back to the front of the space. Some of the world's best performers use all of the ring, starting well to the back and ending with the final step at the front of the ring. Some performers are now using two full turns.

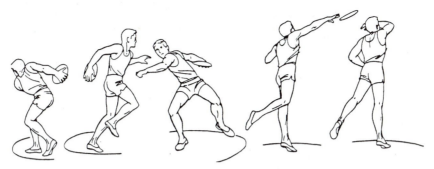

FIGURE 17.3 The discus throw is characterized primarily by rotary movements. The discus is kept close to the body during the initial turn, then the arm is abducted and the forearm extended prior to release. Often, release velocity is limited by the angular momentum that can be developed and controlled during the body spins.

TABLE 17.1 Kinematic data for Olympic discus throwers.

	Speed of Discus	Height of Release	Distance between Feet	Trunk Angle at Release	Release Angle from Ground	Distance of Throw
males Ht = 1.73 m	24.8 m/s	1.73 m	.80 m	97.4°/sec	35.6°	65.6 m
females Ht = 1.48 m	25.0 m/s	1.48 m	.85 m	97.5°/sec	34.7°	63.5 m

The first step is taken with the left foot, which is moved toward the front of the ring and placed in line with the right foot. As the steps continue, they resemble those of a sprinter more than do those shown in Figure 17.3. As the turns are made, the legs are flexed, and the right arm is held fairly close to the side, with the discus dragging behind.

These actions lower the center of gravity of the body and aid in balance. The arm position also moves the center of gravity of the rotating body closer to its axis and enables it to turn with greater speed. The speed of rotation during the stepping should accelerate; it should be as fast as possible and still allow the performer to maintain balance. The general concept is that the thrower moves slowly during the first turn, accelerates during the step phase, and explodes into the throwing action.

On the final step, the right arm is abducted, lengthening the moment arm of the pelvic lever, which can also be increased if the discus is held as close to the end of the fingers as possible and is still controlled. Adduction of the arm at release will start the flight well beyond the front of the ring. Hand action in the final phase can be added to impart more velocity. The discus is released by rolling it off the index finger with the thumb providing the control.

Study of Discus Throw. Gregor et al. (1985), studying the 1984 Olympic male and female winners and placers of the discus throw, found some very interesting results. Height, angle, and velocity of the discus and the thrower's trunk angle were measured using film data. They found little difference between men and women (women throw a smaller discus) in regard to the kinematics of the throw. There were, however, anthropometric differences that influenced the kinematics. The higher standing height of the men meant that the release of the discus was at a higher arm position than that of the women. Table 17.1 compares these performances.

Gregor et al. (1985) stated that the release velocity and the release height are the two most important variables in determining distance of throw. Many other investigators support these comments.

Underarm Patterns: Softball Pitching, Hammer Throw, Bowling, and Curling

Pitching Underarm (Softball)

In the basic underhand pattern, the joints about which levers rotate in the direction of the throw normally occur in the following sequence: pelvis (rotation), spine (rotation), arm (adduction and flexion), and hand (flexion). As the trunk is rotated backward, the arm is raised to the rear in a combined abduction and extending action. As the arm is moved forward, it is kept in the sagittal plane by a combination of adduction and flexion at the shoulder. The underarm throw and pitch (see Figure 17.2) are very similar in joint and lever actions. We described the moment arm lengths for this form of throwing previously. However, observers will find many individual modifications of the basic joint actions.

Normally, the first forward movement is a step with the left foot (right-handed pitcher). This necessitates first putting the weight on the right foot, facilitates pelvic rotation over the support, carries the left side of the pelvis forward, and increases the length of the step. As the left foot contacts the ground, the right arm usually reaches a horizontal position and is ready to begin its forward swing. For most effective action the upper torso should at this time be facing to the right with the shoulders in line with the direction of the throw. Unskilled performers often fail to take advantage of this position. Instead, they tend to keep the upper torso facing the direction of the throw, which decreases both hip and spinal actions, sometimes with complete loss of the latter. The major forward movement of the body is made as the left foot moves forward; the left foot rarely slides, as in bowling. At the time of release, forward movement of the body contributes little to the force of the throw. A 3-D representation of a skilled woman's fast-pitch underarm throw is shown in Figure 17.4.

The lead foot moves directly forward toward the batter. At release, the contributing joint actions are left hip (rotation), right shoulder and wrist (flexion), and left ankle (flexion). Medial rotation of the humerus and supination of the forearm impart rotation to the ball. Based on film observations, men frequently flex at the elbow and use either lateral or medial rotation of the humerus to develop speed. In doing so, they decrease

the amount of flexion at the shoulder. Present information does not indicate whether rotation of the humerus develops more speed than does greater flexion at the shoulder with the forearm extended.

Contribution of Each Lever. Measurements of the basic pattern provide insight into the potential contributions of each lever. The authors of this text observed the film of a skilled college woman pitcher. The measurements were made for two frames, including one showing the release; the time for all limb actions except the hands was 0.03 second. The action at the wrist occurred in less than the time of one frame, and the time of this action was calculated to be 0.008 second. In the measurements in Table 17.2, the range is expressed in degrees, the angular velocity in degrees per second, the moment arm length in centimeters (feet), and the linear velocity in meters (feet) per second.

The sum of the velocities in Table 17.2 is 21.5 m/sec (70.59 ft/sec); the ball velocity in the film was measured at 21.4 m/sec (70.26 ft/sec). Using the sum of the linear velocities as the total, the contributions of limb segments rotation about the following joint (expressed in percentages), are as follows: hip, 14.3; spine, 7.9; shoulder, 45.3;

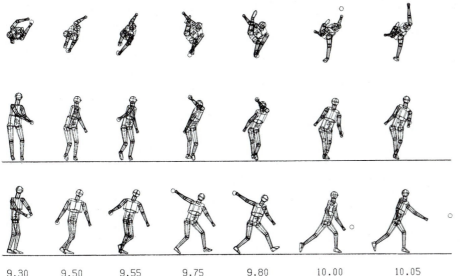

FIGURE 17.4 The action of the slingshot style of fast-pitch softball is displayed as 3-D computer-generated contourograms. Note the nonplanar path of the arm at the height of the swing and the speed at the lowest part of the arc. Note the differences in action of the lead leg between this particular pitcher and that of the overarm pitcher in Figure 17.1.

9.30   9.50   9.55   9.75   9.80   10.00   10.05

TABLE 17.2 Lever contributions to ball velocity in underarm throw (pitch).

	Range (degrees)	Angular Velocity (degrees/sec)	Moment Arm Length		Linear Velocity	
			cm	ft	m/sec	ft/sec
Hip rotation	12	400	44.7	1.45	3.08	10.12
Spinal rotation	6	200	48.7	1.60	1.70	5.59
Shoulder flexion	22	733	76.2	2.50	9.74	31.98
Wrist flexion	30	3750	10.6	0.35	6.97	22.90

and wrist, 32.4. Arm flexion at the shoulder is the major contributor. Hand flexion about the wrist in the throw with the lighter ball is more forceful than in bowling.

■ Velocity measures of ball projections are a more valid measure of the force imparted by body levers than is a measure of distance.

Glassow (1932) found that two male pitchers on softball teams had velocities of 32.91 and 33.22 m/sec (108 and 109 ft/sec). Two women majors in physical education threw balls at 19.81 and 19.50 m/sec (65 and 64 ft/sec). A teenage girl and outstanding pitcher in a city softball league delivered a ball at 24.68 m/sec (81 ft/sec). In addition, Joan Joyce, once the outstanding women's fast-pitch softball pitcher, is reported to have thrown a ball at approximately 193 kmph (120 mph).

MINI-LABORATORY LEARNING EXPERIENCE

Time the speed of a pitched softball in the following situations:

1. Legal slow-pitch softball (ball must have an upward arch).
2. Legal fast-pitch fastball.
   a. Windmill style
   b. Sling-shot style
   c. Figure-8 style

Compare results. State the mechanical principles as you explain the results.

Hammer Throw

The hammer throw is an underarm, two-handed throw unique in that a weight of 7.25 kg (16 lb) is attached to a wire string 117 to 121 cm in length. This increases greatly the moment arm length of the thrower. This sport is one of few activities in which centrifugal force is exceptionally high. A relatively lightweight object such as a hammer can be propelled into the air rather easily by using this force.

There are two or three twisting actions of the hammer around the body prior to the actual true turns about the circle. These preliminary moves are done so the thrower gets a feel of the hammer in relation to the body. Then the hammer thrower executes the three or four turns about the circle, advancing slightly from rear to the front each turn.

Two factors stand out as important in gaining velocity at release and, consequently, greater distance in the throw: a long turning radius and an increased turning speed. Black (1980) stated:

> In an analysis of the Munich competition, we found that the top throw by A. Bondarchuk of the USSR of 247'8''(75.48 m) was achieved with a turning interval of 1.51 seconds. A further breakdown shows the increased body speed from one turn to the next.

The hammer is released at more than 26 m/sec by the top throwers. Thus, a decrease in turning time increases the final distance, provided that all other factors are held constant.

The thrower must keep in balance and control, gradually accelerating the hammer during the turns. There is torque between the upper and lower portions of the body. In a sense, the hammer thrower hangs onto, or some say against, the hammer as velocity increases.

The thrower establishes an orbit, or path, turning about the circle and a high and a low point of the hammer's path. A right-handed thrower flexes the right arm and then extends it to regain a tighter hold on the handle. The left arm is kept straight (extended) throughout the movement. During this acceleration phase, the plane of the hammer is relatively level. Any additional force, such as a pull inward, will decrease the radius and also prevent pelvic rotation (causing the hip to lead the movement).

As the thrower winds the hammer about the body, the center of rotation being the right shoulder, the degrees of rotation change from a low point of 280–290° to a maximum of 320–325°. These windups, or sweeps, have to be done with no loss of balance and with increased velocity of the hammer.

A "sit-and-stretch" action helps the shoulders relax and increase the radius. Doherty (1976) has stated that for every inch gained in radius, there is a possibility for a six-foot gain in distance. The flexing at the knees helps increase the length of the radius and also aids in maintaining balance by lowering the center of gravity.

The period of maximum acceleration is during the hammer's descent. The thrower at this time "sits" vigorously, increasing the centrifugal pull. The "sit" is necessary to keep the center of gravity over the feet, especially the left heel (for a right-handed thrower). Usually the left foot stays in contact with the circle area throughout the turns.

As the thrower moves about the hammer ring, he or she attempts to increase the time of double support of the feet and to decrease that of single support. It has been shown that the hammer acceleration occurs only during the double-support period. Double support is referred to as the "power" aspect and single support as the "gliding" phase.

The thrower must turn fast enough to stay ahead of the rotating hammer on the turn. Failure to do so causes a decline in acceleration, especially during the second and third turns.

To increase the torque in the body (a twist between the upper and lower portions), the thrower rotates the hips ahead of the shoulders during the turns. The hip lead with respect to the hammer is anywhere from 45–90°.

The height of release is governed by the physique of the thrower and the position of the hammer. The angle of release is considered to have the greatest influence on the distance of the throw. It is a result of the application of the horizontal and vertical forces at the moment of release. The best release angle for distance is between 42 and 44°, since the hammer is released at shoulder height.

Force Couples. Two force couples act in the hammer throw. The first one is the outward, centrifugal pull of the hammer, which is countered by the inward, centripetal force exerted by the thrower. The latter involves the pulling of the thrower's weight through the center of mass downward. This force is opposed by the pushing of the ground upward against the thrower's feet. More centripetal force is needed to counteract the centrifugal pull as the speed of the turns increases. Russian researchers have measured the strain on the handle of the hammer during the throwing action, as have Hwang and Adrian (1986).

Within each wind and turn, the force increases and decreases, but it consistently increases from the first wind to the last turn. The maximum force at release was measured to be 1400–2000 N and was positively related to the distance of the throw.

Model Approach. Using Schultz's mathematical model, the muscle forces and compression on the lumbar spine were estimated. The basic theory underlying this modeling approach was that only the muscles that are necessary to contract would do so; the other muscles would relax. Each contraction composite would produce precisely the required force to produce or oppose the force measured on the hammer. This means that each muscle contributes according to its estimated line of pull and estimated cross-sectional area. These concepts are based upon the Optimization theory: Every force is optimum.

The authors calculated estimated stress to the lumbar spine (L3) and found it to be greater than forces occurring during lifting tasks as used in various occupations. The latter also were estimated through modeling using *Optimization theory*. Such modeling has value in predicting risk of injury or levels of physical conditioning to prepare for high-level sports competition.

Relaxation of the shoulders helps increase the radius. There is an optimum position of the central axis of rotation within the hammer-athlete-lever system. To keep the system stabilized, the athlete must center the base of the axis over the left heel, thus increasing the smoothness of execution. The left heel is not only the center of rotation, but also the axis of the lever system.

Dapena (1986) has made a technical study, including calculations of center of mass of the thrower, the hammer, and a hammer-thrower system. He found that the up-and-down motions of the center of mass of the thrower was ahead of the hammer by about a third of a cycle, and this made it possible for the upward "vertical acceleration of hammer-thrower system to almost coincide with the double-support phases." In the horizontal direction, the center of mass of the hammer and the thrower in their rotations were out of harmony by about half a spin.

Hwang and Adrian (1986) also reported on the kinematics of the hammer. Regarding the displacement of the hammer head, they found the pattern to be neither symmetrical nor purely circular. There was a continuous changing of the shape and slope of the elliptical pattern as the turns occurred. (See Figure 17.5.)

Bowling

Among the least complex of the underarm patterns is the bowling delivery. Obviously, the major contribution to the velocity of the ball is the force derived from arm action. It is also apparent that rotation at the hip and spine about the vertical axis is limited, since the bowler tends to keep the upper torso facing the lane, and the weight of the ball limits hand action.

Although each bowler's performance differs in detail from that of others, the following analysis gives a general idea of the contribution of each acting lever. Film of the delivery of a male physical education major disclosed that at the time of release, spinal rotation and flexion at the shoulder occurred, but there was no rotation at the hip or flexion at the wrist. An unexpected action was flexion at the elbow.

To determine the contribution of each acting joint, the authors made the following measurements for the two frames preceding release: (1) the range of action of each joint (Table 17.3A), and (2) the time during which this action occurred. The time per frame was 0.0158 second, and for 2 frames was 0.0316 second, or approximately 64 frames/sec. The length of each moment arm at the time of release was measured from a side view. These moment arms were (1) from shoulder to center of the ball; (2) for the elbow (from each elbow to center of the ball); and (3) for the spine (a horizontal line from the upper spine to a vertical line passing through the center of the ball).

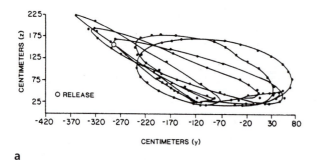

a

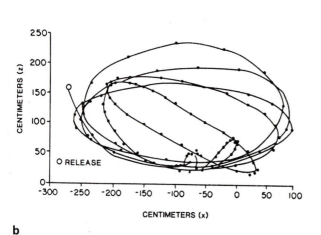

b

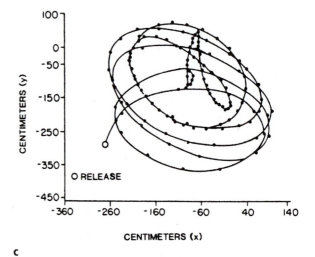

c

FIGURE 17.5 Three planar views of the path of the hammer during the hammer throw event. (*a*) Sagittal views (side viewing orothogonal to throw); (*b*) frontal view (viewing from in front of thrower); (*c*) transverse view (viewing from above the thrower). Note especially the change in the slope of the path as seen in the sagittal view. The open circle denotes the release point.

(Reprinted from Hwang, I., and Adrian, M. 1986. In proceedings of the 1984 Olympic scientific congress, eds. Adrian, M., and Deutsch, H. Microfilm Publications.)

The sum of the linear velocities of the three levers is 7.8 m/sec (25.60 ft/sec). The velocity of the ball as it moved away from the hand was measured and calculated at 8.8 m/sec (29.11 ft/sec). The difference may be attributed to a contributing factor not included in the analysis or errors made in measurement. The former was found to be true, based on further study of the films. The torso moved forward during the two frames because of sliding on the left foot and flexion at the left ankle. The distance that the shoulder moved forward was measured as 44 mm (0.144 ft). The linear velocity of this movement was 1.4 m/sec (4.56 ft/sec). The summed velocities were now 1.4 m/sec (30.16 ft/sec), or 0.32 m (1.05 ft) more than the measured velocity of the ball. The discrepancy is less than the 1.07 m (3.51 ft) before the forward movement of the body was observed. However, better techniques are needed to provide greater accuracy.

Anhalts (1966) studied the film of a highly skilled woman bowler, whose season's average score in three leagues was 182. Results are shown in Table 17.3B. The measurements were made from a side view.

Levers at Release. As shown, the moving levers at release were the shoulder-arm, elbow-forearm, and wrist-hand. The sum of their linear velocities is 6.64 m/sec (21.81 ft/sec). The body was moving forward at the same time at a rate of 1.4 m/sec (4.72 ft/sec). This, added to the lever velocities, totals 8.08 m/sec (26.53 ft/sec). The measured velocity of the ball in the film was 8.15 m/sec (26.74 ft/sec) after release. The degree to which the summed velocities agree with the ball velocity indicates the accuracy of the measurements.

TABLE 17.3A Lever contributions to ball velocity in bowling.*

	Range (degrees)	Angular Velocity (degrees/sec)	Moment Arm Length cm	ft	Linear Velocity m/sec	ft/sec
Shoulder	14	443	74.67	2.45	5.770	18.94
Spine	6	190	31.69	1.04	1.050	3.45
Elbow	4	127	44.20	1.45	0.978	3.21

*Skilled man bowler.

TABLE 17.3B Lever contributions to ball velocity in bowling.*

	Range (degrees)	Angular Velocity (degrees/sec)	Moment Arm Length cm	ft	Linear Velocity m/sec	ft/sec
Shoulder	12	400.00	75.59	2.480	5.27	17.31
Elbow	2	66.66	46.63	1.530	0.54	1.78
Wrist	11	366.66	12.95	0.425	0.83	2.72

*Skilled woman bowler.

■ No definitive research has been conducted regarding hooking and finger-thumb release of the bowling ball.

Optimum Velocity of Ball. Increased velocity of the ball should be a goal for beginning bowlers but observations have not been extensive enough to set such goals with confidence. Casady and Liba (1968) recommend that women bowlers should impart a velocity to the ball that would send it from the foul line to the head pin in 2.50 to 2.75 seconds (7.31 to 6.67 m/sec [24 to 21.9 ft/sec]), and men bowlers in 2.0 to 2.5 seconds (9.14 to 7.31 m/sec [30 to 24 ft/sec]). How much speed must a bowler impart to the bowling ball? Review Table 17.4, which lists data from randomly selected league bowlers. Since the expert does not deliver the ball with the greatest possible velocity, but only with enough to make effective impact with the pins, the velocity of the highly skilled performer is one that the beginner can attain.

Action of Bowler. Both the man and the woman whose bowling delivery was studied derived over 60% of their velocity from the lever acting at the shoulder joint. Bowlers should strive to use this action effectively. It is

TABLE 17.4 Ball velocities and time to travel the length of bowling alley (60 feet) of league bowlers.

	Ball Velocity (average)	Time of Ball (sec) (average)
Men (+190)	8.65 m/sec (28.38 ft/sec)	2.11
Women (+180)	8.61 (18.26)	2.12
Men (150–160)	8.8 (29.12)	2.06
Women (120–130)	7.29 (23.94)	2.50

frequently said that the arm should reach the horizontal at the height of the backswing. Shoulder hyperextension, when the body is erect, will not carry the arm to this height. By flexing at the hips, therefore, the bowler inclines the trunk forward. In this position, although the range of shoulder hyperextension is not increased, the arm, depending on the degree of trunk inclination, can approach, reach, or pass the horizontal. Widule (1966)

Biomechanics of Throwing **347**

found in the groups that she observed that the upper arms reached the following positions: skilled men, 185°; average men, 180°; skilled women, 199°; average women, 163°. (The horizontal is represented by 180°; more than that means higher than the horizontal.) Inclination measured from the horizontal of the trunk for these groups were 35° for skilled men; 51° for average men; 41° for skilled women; and 54° for average women. (If the trunk were erect, the inclination from the horizontal would be 90°; the greater the forward inclination of the trunk, the smaller the inclination measure.)

■ The height of the arm on the bowling backswing depends on the degree of trunk inclination and the degree of hyperextension at the shoulder joint.

At the height of the backswing, Widule (1966) found the following hyperextension measures: skilled men, 40°; average men, 52°; skilled women, 59°; and average women 37°. (The greater the measure, the greater the degree of hyperextension.)

Length of Bowler's Arm. The length of the bowler's arm also affects the linear velocity of that lever. In the measurements shown in Table 17.3, had the moment arm for arm flexion been 0.67 m (2.2 ft) instead of 0.74 m (2.45 ft), and had the angular velocity been the same (443°/sec), the linear velocity would have been 5.18 m/sec (17.01 ft/sec). A difference of 7.62 cm (3 in.) in length decreased the velocity almost 0.60 m/sec (2 ft/sec).

Curtis and Sabol have shown the strength of grip to be related to the speed of the swing. The difference in grip strength enables men to use a heavier ball than women usually use.

The contribution of the approach steps is not entirely shown in the forward movement of the torso at the time of release. As the ball is moved backward past the right leg by the arm, the approach steps are moving it forward. In the film study (Curtis and Sabol 1962) the ball was observed to move forward faster than it moved backward, so that during the backswing the ball was moving forward. Visualize this by thinking of a person walking toward the rear of a railway car as the train moves forward. The person is walking backward but

moving forward. As the bowling swing begins its downward, forward action, the ball already has a forward velocity, and the body levers add to this, rather than beginning from a zero velocity. The velocity of the approach increases with each step. The frequency of the steps is usually kept constant, but the length of each increases over that of the preceding one.

If the velocity derived from the body levers is to be fully used, there should be no downward direction in the ball's movement as it touches the floor. The arm should be a degree or two past the perpendicular at release, even if this means that the ball is released a few centimeters above the alley. The impact with the floor from this height will be slight and will be decreased by the roll given to the ball at release. Widule (1966) found that the upper arm had passed the perpendicular at release and also that the arm was flexing at the ball release. This action not only raises the ball slightly but adds to the velocity. (See Table 17.4.)

Speed Factors. The analysis of the swing so far has dealt with factors affecting the **speed** of the ball. The *direction* given to the ball is an important factor in the number of pins knocked down. In the distance that the ball travels from release to the pins, approximately 18 m (60 ft), a slight deviation from the exact line to the point of aim can result in marked deviation as pin contact is made. For every 0.25° deviation, the ball will miss the point of aim by approximately 7.62 cm (3 in.). A variation of 1° in direction would miss the point of aim by 30 cm (12 in.). A ball started at the midpoint of the alley, if it deviated by 2° from a perpendicular to the foul line, would end up in the gutter. Since slight deviations in direction have this marked effect on point of contact, the bowler must give careful attention to factors affecting accuracy.

Among these factors is the point at which the ball crosses the foul line. The starting position should be carefully determined with reference to this line, and the approach should be consistently straightforward. From the point on the foul line, the ball should be directed along the selected line of direction. The bowler should clearly visualize that line, and the arm should swing along this line even after the ball is released.

1. Time the speeds of balls rolled by bowlers of different skill levels. Explain reasons for differences.
2. Compare speeds of balls bowled from a stationary position, one-step approach, three-step approach, and five-step approach. Explain the results.

The Curling Delivery*

Many skills are required to successfully make shots and score points in the game of curling. Of particular importance is the delivery of the curling rock. The performance objectives of the delivery action are target accuracy (hitting the broom) and weight control (imparting the required momentum to the rock). Bothwell-Myers (1982) identified the importance and specific roles that each of the seven phases of the delivery action has in propelling the rock and curler forward toward a target. (See Figure 17.6.)

Stance.   This is the stationary positioning of the curler in the hack (foot hold) prior to the delivery. The functions of the stance phase are target viewing, alignment of the body and rock with target, and positioning of the hack foot (right foot for right-handed curlers) for balance and leg drive leverage. (See Figure 17.6.)

Backswing.   Backswing is the delivery motion, backward, from the point the rock loses contact with the ice to the maximum vertical displacement of the rock (top of the swing). The functions of the backswing are positioning of the body, body levers, and rock for the production of forward motion and controlling the weight of the shot. The height of the backswing serves only to position the rock and body for the generation of momentum (predominately rock momentum). Thus, the height of the backswing reflects the amount of rock momentum that the curler can control and comfortably integrate into the delivery, rather than the called-for weight of the shot. Actions in the backswing include a slight forward motion of the rock and body to help overcome the inertia of the stone, elevation of the body from the stance position, backward pull or swing of the rock, and counterbalancing movement of the broom and sliding foot (Figure 17.6b and c).

Downswing.   The downswing, or forward swing, begins at the top of the backswing and ends when the rock contacts the ice surface. The function of this phase is the production of rock and center of mass momentum, but predominately rock momentum. Actions in the downswing include forward swing of the throwing arm and rock, body fall forward, and placement of the sliding foot forward to receive the body's weight (Figure 17.6d).

Transition.   This phase relates to the actions occurring between rock touchdown (end of the downswing) and the beginning of leg drive—i.e., extension of the hack knee. The function of this phase is the conversion of angular rock momentum to linear rock momentum. Actions include rock touchdown (initial contact of the rock with the ice surface), rock soled (entire running edge of rock contacts the ice surface), and hack knee flexion. Flexion at the hack knee appears to coincide with the soling of the rock and occurs after initial rock-ice contact. These specific events require more study to further understand the relationship between the downswing and leg drive and the conversion of angular motion to straight line motion (Figure 17.6e).

Fall Forward.   This consists of the forward displacement of the curler's center of mass or forward lean of the curler, which occurs as the rock touches the ice and before hack leg extension begins. The functions of this phase are acceleration of the curler toward the target and positioning of the curler's center of mass for the acceptance of force from the leg drive action. This serves to

*Contributed by Connie Bothwell-Myers

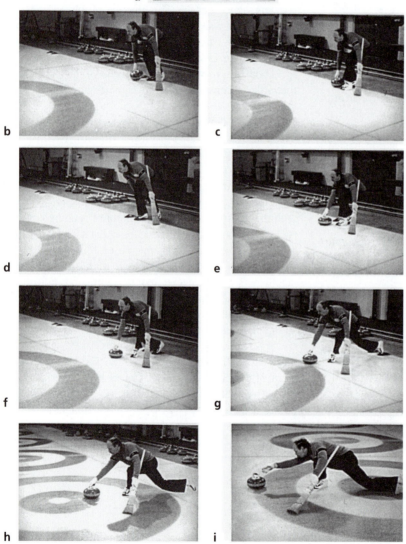

FIGURE 17.6 The sequence of a curling delivery. (*a*) Stance; (*b*) start of; (*c*) backswing; (*d*) downswing; (*e*) transition; (*f, g*) leg drive; (*h*) glide; (*i*) release.

propel the curler forward and upward, but primarily forward. The body, as a unit, falling forward or pivoting from the hack is the observable action.

Leg Drive. Extension at the hack knee, after the forward fall, that results in the forward propulsion of the curler from the hack is the leg drive. Functions of this phase include propulsion of the curler and rock closer to the target, acceleration of the curler to the speed of the rock, regulation of the release velocity of the rock either in conjunction with the backswing or alone, and provision of forward (horizontal) momentum to the rock and curler. Observable actions are extension at the hack knee and at the hip and plantar flexion of the ankle (Figure 17.6*f* and *g*).

Glide or Slide. If the curler is propelled forward from the hack with sufficient momentum, a gliding phase is observed. The functions of this phase are to bring the rock and curler closer to the target and to correct for the weight of the rock by adjusting the length of the slide and, therefore, the release point. The body is extended behind the rock during this phase and is sliding along the line of delivery toward the target. A number of important weight and accuracy control mechanisms are active during this phase (Figure 17.6*h*).

Release. The function of the release is to impart a clockwise or counterclockwise rotation to the rock (Figure 17.6*i*).

Determinants of Success. Identifying the primary function of a specific action is an essential step in movement analysis. Grouping actions by function can further assist the coach with fault identification and correction. The actions observed in the delivery motion can be categorized into three functional groups:

1. *Actions that generate momentum.* That is, those actions that propel the rock and curler out of the hack toward the target. Key actions that serve this function are (a) angular acceleration of the rock during the downswing, which contributes to rock momentum; (b) the smooth soling of the rock during the transition phase, which contributes to the maintenance of rock momentum; (c) angular acceleration of the curler during the forward fall; (d) hip, knee, and ankle flexion during leg drive, which contribute to rock and curler momentum; and (e) trunk flexion, shoulder and elbow extension during the glide phase, which contribute to rock momentum.

2. *Actions that correct or adjust the amount of rock momentum (weight control mechanisms).* Examples of observed weight control actions that result in braking are (a) lengthening the slide, causing deceleration of the rock and curler; (b) lifting the trunk during the slide, which shifts the curler's weight backwards, producing a drag; (c) shifting body weight to the broom or rock during the slide; and (d) flexing the throwing elbow during the slide to pull back on the rock, decelerating it. Actions that may result in enhancing momentum are (a) increasing the height of the backswing; (b) increasing the angular acceleration of the rock and throwing arm during the downswing; (c) falling forward faster by flexing the hack knee; and (d) increasing leg drive propulsion by more complete and forceful extension of the hack leg.

3. *Actions that contribute to target accuracy.* These actions include (a) body alignment in the stance; (b) "straight back" displacement of the rock during the backswing; (c) balancing and counterbalancing actions of the throwing arm, broom arm, and sliding foot; (d) flat-footed sliding position; (e) elongated position of the body behind the rock during the sliding phase; and (f) lengthening the slide, bringing the rock closer to the target before release.

The pattern of acquisition of momentum (i.e., horizontal velocity) for the delivery of the rock and the forward propulsion of the curler is as follows: (a) at the end of the downswing phase, approximately 90% of the final release velocity of the rock has been acquired, compared to approximately 35% of the final release velocity of the center of mass (curler); (b) at the end of the forward fall phase, the rock center of mass velocity has been increased by approximately 20%; (c) at the end of the leg drive phase, the rock velocity has been augmented again by approximately 20%; the center of mass velocity has been increased by 55% or more; and (d) at the end of the glide phase (slide), the rock velocity has been diminished by between 12% and 26%. The rock decelerated more than the curler during the slide for a given type of shot.

Based on these results, the downswing (forward swing) phase contributes most to the acquisition of rock momentum. The forward fall phase contributes equally to the rock and curler momentum. The leg drive phase contributes most to the acquisition of curler momentum and the slide phase contributes to deceleration of the rock and center of mass for both draw shots and takeout shots. That is, the rock is decelerated more than the curler during the slide. Also, the rock is decelerated more for draws than for takeouts during the slide.

There appears to be a close association between curler and rock during the downswing phase that is not present during the other phases of the delivery. In fact, during the leg drive and slide, the rock and curler are essentially acting independently or in a more complex manner not yet identified.

Weight control mechanisms in curling were investigated by Bothwell-Meyers (1982) by looking at force production during the delivery. For comparative purposes, the total force required to produce the known release velocity of the rock and curler was estimated and then compared to the force actually generated for the shot. For takeouts, approximately seven times more rock force was generated than required; for draws, approximately ten times more rock force was generated than required. Why such inefficiency? Possibly, excessive momentum is generated to overcome the retarding effect of sliding friction during the slide phase. In a practical sense, it is possible that the curler makes a "rough" assessment of the momentum that must be generated during the downswing, forward fall, and leg drive phases, (i.e., weight) and then fine tunes or corrects the momentum during the slide.

Overarm Patterns: Football Passing, Baseball Pitching, Shot Put, and Javelin Throws

When great speed and control are desired in a throw, the overarm pattern is often used. (See Figures 17.1 and 17.4 for baseball pitching; Figure 17.7 for football passing;

Figure 17.11 for shot put; and Figure 17.12 for javelin throws.) This throw uses the two joint actions that appear to have the highest speeds: flexion at the wrist and medial rotation at the shoulder. The sequence of joint actions can be seen in the football pass (Figure 17.7) and the baseball pitch (Figure 17.1). Both show the step forward with the left foot, pelvic and spinal rotation, and medial rotation of the humerus. Apparently, less hand action occurs with the football throw than with the baseball pitch, which partly explains (ignoring air resistance) the greater velocity obtained with the smaller ball. Note in both series of pictures that, as the torso is rotated forward by pelvic and spinal actions, the humerus is rotated laterally. This timing is an important feature of complex movement patterns. The slower joints begin their forward movement as the faster, more distal joints complete their backswings. No appreciable pause between the backswing and forward swing of these faster-moving joints is necessary. The muscles responsible for the forward swing can begin contraction to stop the backswing. The combination of backward movement and beginning contraction stretches the tendons and connective tissue in the muscles, allowing the forward movement to be more forceful.

Linear Velocity

Note that in both throws the forearm extends somewhat before the ball is released, shortening the moment arm for shoulder medial rotation. Apparently, then, this action develops its greatest **linear velocity** before release, and this velocity must be used by the joints acting at release. However, forearm extension lengthens the moment arms for the pelvic and spinal levers and adds to the linear speeds of these levers at release. In both performances the right foot, as it supports the body weight during the backswing, is placed at right angles to the direction of the ball flight, which permits a greater range of pelvic rotation at the right hip.

Figure 17.8 shows the path of the wrist in two throwing actions. The release of the ball by the pitcher is at the height of the movement at the wrist. But the football passer, because of the spin that must be imparted to the ball, releases it when the hand is moving downward.

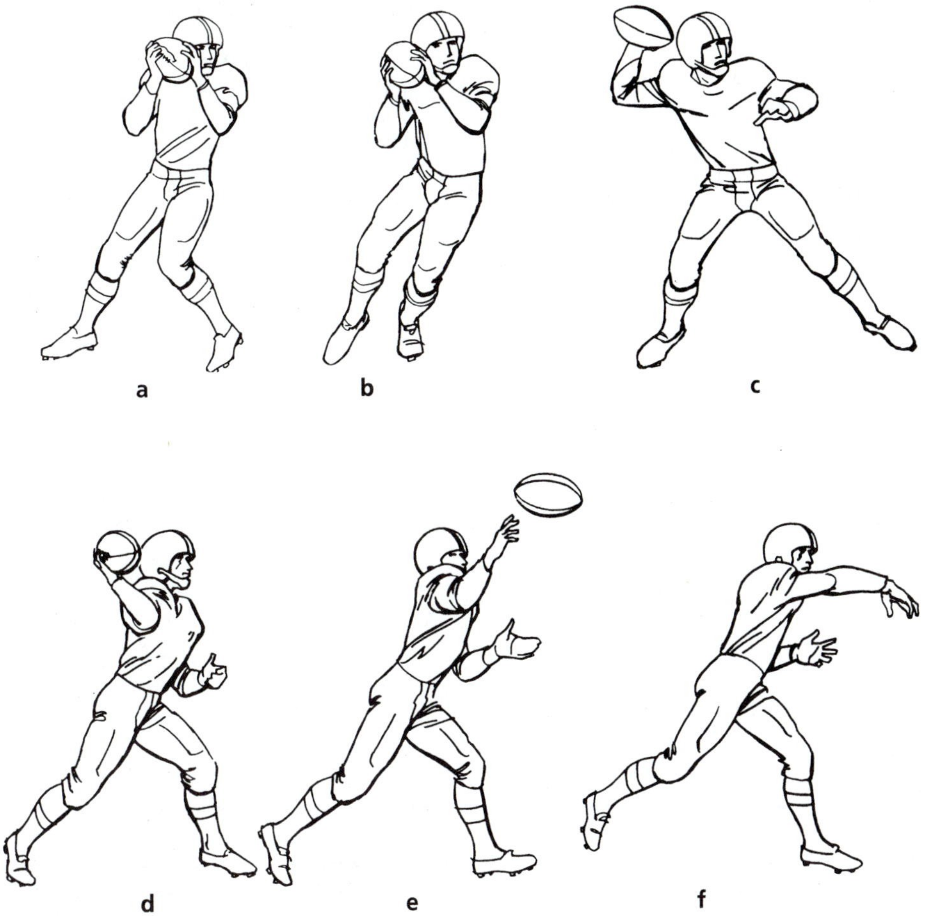

FIGURE 17.7 The football pass uses the typical lever systems of the overarm throwing pattern. Note the lateral and medial rotation of the humerus. Note the differences in step length compared to a baseball pitch (depicted in Figure 17.1). **What other differences are there between a baseball pitch and football pass?**

a   b   c

d   e   f

A physical education major, in analyzing his own football passes, measured the ball velocity as 18 m/sec (60 ft/sec) immediately before release. Humeral medial rotation contributed 62%, spinal rotation 35%, and hand flexion 3%. He had no rotation at the hip during the release phase.

Baseball Throw

A film study by Casady and Liba (1968) of the overarm baseball throw of a skilled man (a major league player) and a highly skilled woman was useful in determining contributions of the four levers of the pattern and in studying individual adjustments in it. (See Table 17.5.)

The time in which the limbs moved through the given range was 0.025 second for the man, except for the hand, for which the time was 0.007 second. For the woman, the time was 0.028 second except for the hand, for which the time was 0.008 second. The high linear velocity for hand flexion shown in Table 17.4 has been questioned by later research, and the way it was determined may be of interest to those who study film. Note that in the table the time for the measured range for the hand is less than for the other joints. In the frame before

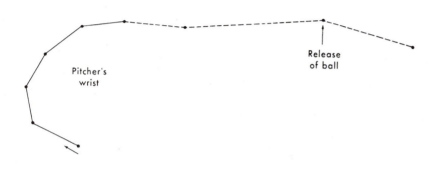

Football passer's wrist

Release of ball

Pitcher's wrist

Release of ball

TABLE 17.5 Lever contributions to ball velocity in overarm throw.

	Range (degrees)	Angular Velocity (degrees/sec)	Moment Arm		Linear Velocity	
			cm	ft	m/sec	ft/sec
Man						
Hip rotation	20.6	824	64.6	2.12	9.29	30.5
Spinal rotation	9.6	384	83.8	2.75	5.60	18.4
Shoulder rotation	38.5	1540	8.2	0.27	2.22	7.3
Wrist-hand flexion	60.0	8571	14.9	0.49	22.34	73.3
Woman						
Hip rotation	20.6	735	70.7	2.32	9.08	29.8
Spinal rotation	20.9	746	67.7	2.21	8.77	28.8
Shoulder rotation	29.0	1036	10.6	0.35	1.92	6.3
Wrist-hand flexion	42.0	5250	11.2	0.37	10.33	33.9

Prepared by Adrian. 1982. Unpublished material. Champagne-Urbana, IL: University of Illinois.

release, the angle at the wrist-hand was measured; in the next frame, the ball had been released and the wrist angle had changed. The change was assumed to have occurred during the time that the camera shutter was closed, and time, rather than the frames per second, was used to determine the velocity at the wrist-hand joint. If this procedure is acceptable, the time cannot be longer than shutter time, and it could be less. In that case the angular velocity would be even greater than reported.

The sum of the linear velocities for the man is 39.50 m/sec (129.6 ft/sec); the ball velocity measured on the film was 39.90 m/sec (130.9 ft/sec). For the woman, the sum of the linear velocities is 30.11 m/sec (98.8 ft/sec); the measured film velocity was 29.24 m/sec (95.93 ft/sec) (Adrian 1982).

Hand Velocity

The hand action in both performers is the greatest contributor to the linear velocity; the trunk ranks second and arm (shoulder) last. Both performers extend at the elbow just before release, shortening the length of the moment arm of the shoulder lever.

A study of the moment arm lengths in the overarm throws of high school girls found that the highest velocities were developed by the girls who had the longest moment arms for the hip rotation levers and consequently the shortest moment arms for the shoulder medial rotation levers (Glasson 1962).

The tabulation of moment arm lengths shows that, for the man, the moment arm for the hip is shorter than that for the spine. This is due to a leaning to the left so far that the upper spine is to the left of the hip joint at release. The lateral flexion may be the cause of the small range of movement in the spine.

■ Keep in mind certain limitations about these reported contributions of limb actions to the velocity of an overarm projected ball. In each case, the measurements were made for one or two subjects and were taken during the release phase, so that they do not indicate contributions made in earlier phases.

Joint Action of Overhand Throw

The earliest, most detailed and extensive study of joint actions in the overarm throw was reported by Atwater (1970), who observed action in three planes, using side, overhead, and rear camera views. She included fifteen subjects to provide opportunity for comparison: five skilled college men and women, and five average college women. Her observations include not only the release phase but also the 400 m/sec preceding the release. For the skilled groups, that time period encompassed almost all the overarm pattern, including the backswing. For the average women, only the later stages of the backswing occurred in the selected time. She measured displacement of the ball in three planes, and combined the three velocities determined algebraically into one "resultant velocity." She related the measured joint actions to ball displacement on the basis of observation and logic; she did not study moment arms and linear contributions of joint actions.

In observing displacement of the ball before its release from the hand, Atwater (1970) found that although the movement is primarily forward, vertical and lateral movements also occur. None of the subjects accelerated the ball continually, but all accelerated rapidly shortly before release: the men as much as 457.20 to 609.60 m/sec (1000 ft/sec); skilled women, 304.80 m/sec (2000 ft/sec); and average women, 121.92 m/sec (400 ft/sec). (See Figure 17.9.)

Comparing limb actions, Atwater found that all skilled subjects used essentially the same actions but that the range and speed were generally greater for the subjects who had the fastest ball velocities at release. Some of these differences can be seen in Figure 17.9, which represents positions at times of approximately 0.070 and 0.025 second before release of the ball and 0.005 second after release. Note that in the lowest tracing for each subject the ball is behind the hand and that this distance is greatest for the skilled man and least for the average woman. Differences in ball position at this time can be attributed largely to trunk position; the trunk of the

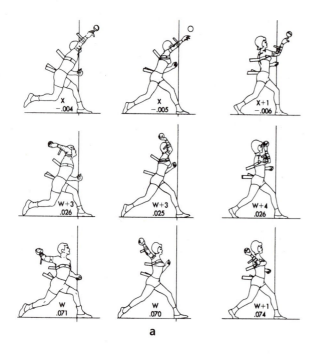

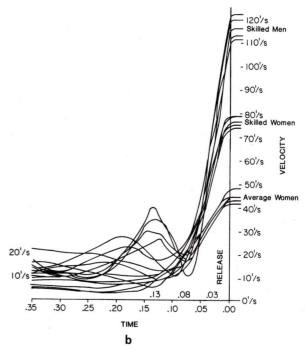

a

b

FIGURE 17.9 (a) Tracings (contourograms) from movie film of skilled man (left column); skilled woman (middle column); and woman with average skill (right column) at the end of backswing, 25 ms prior to release, and immediately after release. Qualitatively assess the differences in step length, counter-rotation, lateral rotation of the humerus, and extension to the arm. (b) Resultant velocities, calculated from displacements measured from displacement data merged from analysis of side, rear, and overhead views. (From Atwater, A. E. 1970. Movement characteristics of the overarm throw. Ph.D. dissertation, University of Wisconsin.)

skilled man is not yet facing slightly beyond that direction. To reach the positions shown in the top tracings, the man's trunk moves through a greater range than does that of the woman, and its rotation must therefore be at a faster angular velocity. Note also that the forearm of the average woman is flexed 50–60° at release, while those of the skilled performers are almost completely extended.

The differences in length of stride are not as clearly seen. Atwater reports considerable differences in the average stride length for the three groups: that of the skilled men was 1.18 m (3.87 ft); that of the skilled women was 15.8 cm (0.52 ft) shorter, and that of the average women 47.8 cm (1.57 ft) shorter than that of the men. A similar finding related to stride is reported by Ekern (1969), who studied the overarm throw of boys and girls selected as the better throwers from second, fourth, and sixth grades. Within that group, she found that the better throwers, whose projected balls were fastest, took longer steps.

Fisk (1976), in a review of the data in his study "The Dynamic Function of Selected Muscles of the Forearm: An Electromyographical and Cinematographical Investigation" made the following comments:

EMG Analysis was made of electromyographical data obtained from 12 subjects in the study. A great deal of individual variety in the function of the four muscles (identified in Figure 17.10) during the performance of the overhand straight throw and the overhand curved throw was found. Conclusions drawn from the study indicate that the electrical response generated in the muscles took place during the final movements of the "laying back of the arm," just prior to when the elbow begins its forward movement and the hand assumes its "cocked position." Once the forward movement of the arm begins, the flexors diminish electrical activity. All four muscles were more active during the throws with spin than during the straight throws: therefore, it is assumed that greater muscular effort was required to perform the throws with spin. The onset of the maximal action potential response occurred earlier and endured

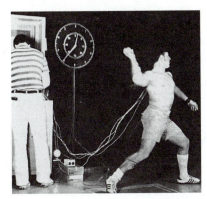

FIGURE 17.10 Electromyographic instrumentation used to study muscular involvement during overarm throwing. In-dwelling fine wire electrodes were located in the lateral head of the triceps brachii, in the flexors carpi ulnaris and radialis, and pronator teres muscles. Dynamographic instrumentation records ground reaction forces simultaneously. The step has been taken and the rear foot has exerted force against a force plate embedded in the floor.

longer for the throws with spin, and occurred earlier and endured longer among the experienced performers. The contribution of the pronator teres muscles still remains partially unsettled; however, this muscle contributed to the spin imparted to the ball at release when the throws with spin were performed.

■ Throwing a curve ball frequently and with high intensity commonly results in permanent damage to the shoulder and elbow because of the torquing action.

Shot Put

Shot putting is a modification of the throwing action. It is a combination of overarm throwing and pushing because the shot cannot be thrown as in many high-velocity throws (Figure 17.11), since the rules state that the put must be initiated from in front of the neck and above the shoulder. This results in a push put instead of a true throw.

Dessureault (1976) found the following in his kinematic and kinetic study of unskilled and world-class shot putters:

1. The entire action lasted 2.16 mean seconds.
2. The best shot putters extended their bodies farther outside the rear of the circle and flexed at the right knee more before beginning the move across the circle.
3. The shot putters' mean displacement of the center of gravity was 1.52+ m (5+ ft) during the action.
4. The path of the shot followed a linear and slightly upward direction by the best performers and dropped nearly vertically during part of the movement by the poorer performers.
5. The angle of release for the best performers was 38–41° and was as low as 27° for the poorer performers.
6. The majority of shot putters lost contact with the ground and became airborne at release.
7. All performers had greater horizontal than vertical velocity at release.
8. The shot was released at a linear velocity of 13.52 m/sec (44.36 ft/sec) for the best performer; other velocities were less, the slowest being 9.14 m/sec (30 ft/sec).
9. The superior performers were in contact with the ground for a shorter time after the glide. (Mean time for all subjects was 0.296 second in the vertical plane and 0.287 second in the horizontal plane.)
10. There was a mean value of 2781.4 kg (613.2 lb) of peak vertical thrust by the supporting foot, and a mean value of 1337.9 N (301 lb) by the front foot.

The shot putter faces to the rear, as seen in Figure 17.11a, in preparation for moving across the ring. The weight is on the right foot. From position a, the performer hops on the right foot to place it in the position shown in c. This action gives a forward movement to the shot, which should be used by adding to it the final lever actions (c to e). Flexion at the knee (c) is important for development of force. As the left foot makes ground contact (d to e), the torso can be moved rapidly upward by extension of the rear (right) thigh, and as the left foot takes the weight, the pelvis can rotate on the left limb. These two actions can accelerate the movement of the shot. Note that the upper arm is abducted to the horizontal in d; this position lengthens the moment arm for the lever moving at the left hip.

In the last phase of trunk rotation, adduction, and flexion at the shoulder, the upper arm moves forward and upward. At the same time, the forearm extends, moving the forearm forward and counteracting the upward movement of the upper arm. Final impetus is given by hand flexion. Although all these levers contribute to

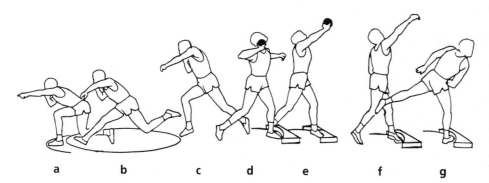

FIGURE 17.11 Performance of shot putter. Observe the height of the shot put at the start, at final step, and at release. In this performance the initial position is half as high as the release position. Measure it for yourself. The athlete should utilize the complete diameter of the circle. **Does he?** Note in the final two figures that the momentum of the body has been dissipated by changing the supporting foot.

a b c d e f g

the force developed, as does the initial glide, the major contributor is the pelvic lever. The actions occurring from *e* to *g* are made to maintain balance.

Because the velocity of the shot is much slower than that of many objects that people project, and because its release point is higher than the landing point, the projection angle should be less than 45°, above the horizontal, as indicated by Dessureault's findings (1976).

Instead of a glide across the ring, many of the world's best shot putters are now using a spinning action similar to that used by discus throwers to attain higher velocity rates at release. A kinematic and kinetic study of this new method should be made to determine its potential and actual advantages and disadvantages.

■ The flight of the shot is not observably influenced by spin, lift, or drag.

Javelin Throw

The javelin throw is similar to other types of overarm throwing actions in which the throwing objective is distance; the extreme stretching of the arm-throwing muscles facilitates the throwing motion. The various axes of rotation—namely, the opposite hip, the spine, and the shoulder—increase the radius and moment arm at release (Figure 17.12). The shape of the javelin, however, is unique as a throwing implement in that it is long and relatively light in weight.

MINI-LABORATORY LEARNING EXPERIENCE

1. View videotapes to analyze the shot-put action.
2. Observe two shot putters attaining greatly different throwing distances to ascertain the reasons for the disparity in performance.
3. Obtain a film of the new spinning action throw and analyze it for possible differences in velocity and distance.
4. Construct two physiques for an ideal shot putter. Do so first within the limits of the body as we know it now, and then construct a physique that transcends our current physical/anatomical structure.

The 1991 NCAA rule book includes the following standards for the javelin:

| | Length | | |
	Minimum	Maximum	Weight
Women	2.20 m (7ft 2.78 in.)	2.30 m (7 ft 5.459 in.)	600 GM (1 lb 5.16 oz)
Men	2.60 m (8 ft 6.375 in.)	2.70 m (8 ft 10.250 in.)	800 GM (1 lb 12.25 oz)

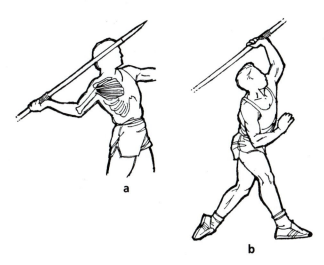

FIGURE 17.12 (a) Final position of the preparatory phase of the javelin throw showing the pectoralis major as the primary muscle for initiating the arm action in the delivery phase. (b) Illustration of Detlef Michel of East Germany, winner of the first I.A.A.F. World Championship in Helsinki, Finland, 1983. First left-handed thrower to win a major international meet. Note the position of the non-throwing foot and throwing leg.

a

b

There are certain rules to follow, such as the thrower must stay within the lane markers in the run-up, must stay behind the scratch line in the follow-through, the point of the thrown javelin must land first, and the discus-type spin of the body is prohibited. In addition, the javelin must meet the standards set by the governing bodies relative to its shape, and particularly in reference to the location of its center of gravity.

The angle of projection of the javelin is determined by the height of release above the ground, air resistance, the direction of the wind, and the velocity of the javelin at release. The javelin has aerodynamic qualities and is released at a lower angle than might be anticipated. Although some javelin throwers release the javelin at an angle of 42–50°, the best throwers in the world release at about 30°.

Best and Bartlett (1987) investigated the characteristics of the javelin used by women and reported smaller lift, drag, and pitch coefficients than for the men's javelin. Lift/drag ratio was also smaller for the women's javelin in comparison with the men's javelin. The center of pressure of the women's javelin was behind the center of gravity. The men's had a constant site for the center of pressure and the women's did not. They predicted the ballistic range of the women's javelin to be 3–4% shorter than the men's. They also stated that the release speed is the greater determinant of range than is the run-up or delivery angle.

The transverse moment of inertia is such that wind effect is negligible in flight, though tail wind is the best

wind direction for performance. Gyration of the javelin reduces the total amount of pitch. Optimum conditions to produce greatest distance for the women were: 78 m/sec, 35° angle of release, 0.8 angle of attack and −20°/sec pitch rate. The men's optimum conditions for a javelin thrown at the same speed and same release angle are −.28 angle of attack and −8.3°/sec pitch rate. The javelin, however, will not have reduced range until a wide variation from the optimum occurs.

The javelin thrower attempts to release the javelin with as much velocity as possible (27.43 to 30.48 m/sec [90 to 100 ft/sec]). The thrower often goes into the air one step before release. Horizontal momentum is created during the run, and a braking force occurs at release, causing the momentum of the run to be transferred to the arm and to the javelin.

The Run Up. The run is executed at a controlled speed and involves an acceleration in its last stages. Before the last step is taken, the body weight is on the right foot; with the penultimate step, the pelvis rotates at the right hip, adding to the length of the step. As the weight is shifted to the left foot, the humerus is rotated medially and the forearm is flexed. The final force, added to the forward movement of the body, is derived from pelvic and spinal rotation, medial rotation and slight adduction of the humerus, and flexion of the hand.

Note the position of the pectoralis major in Figure 17.12. This muscle is well suited for medial rotation of the humerus. In addition, the action of the latissimus dorsi should be visualized here, since it too is a medial rotator and its contraction would lower the humerus and pull it backward. The latter two actions are prevented from occurring by the pectoralis major. Acting together, these two muscles are excellent rotators of the arm. Note that in the javelin throw the forearm is not fully extended during the final thrust, and the moment arm for medial rotation at the shoulder is almost a maximal length. In this skill, medial rotation of the humerus is a greater contributor than is hand flexion.

The release of the throw is crucial, not only because of its length and low weight, but because of the effect the wind may have on its flight. Injury to the shoulder and arm muscles often occurs because of the position of each during or prior to release. There is a large torque at the humerus.

■ There is no pure parabolic flight in javelin throwing.

Javelin Flight. Certain factors stand out in regard to javelin performance. There are lift and drag components while the javelin is airborne. Lift is the component of the total air force on the javelin perpendicular (normal) to the direction of the air flow. Drag is the component of the total air force on the javelin parallel to the direction of the air flow.

The lift on the javelin in flight is not as influential as the angle of attack, which is the acute angle between the long axis of the javelin and the direction of the air flow. The angle of attack is in the vertical aspects; the positive angle is with the tip up and the negative angle with the tip down. When the angle of attack during the flight is small, the lift of the javelin is not optimum. Conversely if the angle of attack is too great, the javelin stalls in the air and lands short of the obtainable distance. New javelins have a larger diameter in the rear position. This contour of the javelin is called planform and enhances flight.

The attitude angle is the acute angle between the long axis of the javelin and the horizontal. When the javelin's front point is above the horizontal, as at the release, the attitude angle is positive; if the point is below the horizontal, it is negative. In order to have a fair throw, the javelin must land with a negative attitude angle (Terauds

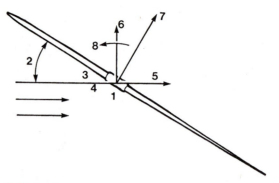

FIGURE 17.13 The javelin in flight is subjected to environmental forces and motion forces that negate the usual parabolic flight of balls. The javelin is revolving about its long axis during flight and the javelin flight will be affected by the following: (1) axial force; (2) angle of attack; (3) center of gravity; (4) center of pressure; (5) drag; (6) lift; (7) normal force; and (8) pitching moment.

1985). If there is headwind, the attitude angle at release should be reduced; if there is a tailwind, the angle should be increased.

The center of pressure on the javelin is the point at which it is in balance. This varies with the angle of attack and the amount of rotation along its long axis. Terauds (1985) has stated that there are 16–24 revolutions per second for top performers. This helps stabilize the javelin in flight.

The magnus effect is present when a javelin is airborne. This is the force produced that is perpendicular to the motion of its long axis in flight (Figure 17.13).

The moment of inertia of the javelin is the sum of the mass of the javelin times the distance between the mass and the javelin's axis of rotation squared. An understanding of the magnus effect and moment of inertia is important for predicting stalling of the javelin.

The grip is important to the execution of the throw. The thumb and middle finger grip just behind the cord or binding appears to be the best for most throwers. The thrower can get rotation on the javelin (its long axis) by pushing against the cord as the javelin is released. Some javelin throwers also obtain rotation about the short axis of the javelin.

The javelin thrower usually takes ten to twelve strides prior to release. A cross-over step is used to enable the

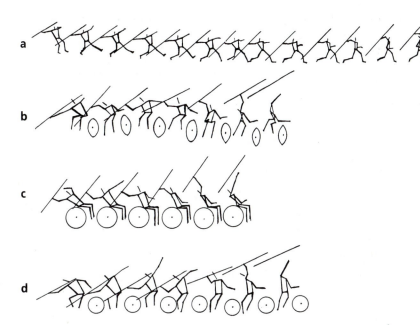

FIGURE 17.14 Line-segment tracings of performances of throwing a javelin with a runup (a) and from stationary wheelchairs (b, c, d). **Compare the performances.**

performer to have the feet in front of the upper part of the body. This enables the thrower to land on the front foot, so the throw can be executed effectively. About five strides from the scratch line, the javelin is started back toward a throwing position. The runner-thrower moves the legs rapidly just prior to the release at about six feet in height. It takes a javelin thrower about six steps to recover and not go over the restraining line.

Importance of Release Velocity. In the final analysis, the most important aspect in throwing the javelin is the release velocity. All other aspects have their influence, but only in contributing to the final action. Most throwers have strong, but short levers (especially arms). Strength is essential. The acceleration of the throwing arm and hand is crucial to high release values.

Komi and Mero (1985) conducted a study of performances of both men and women finalists in the javelin throw at the 1984 Los Angeles Olympic Games. They found that the men had the higher release velocity, 29.12 m/sec, and that there was a strong positive relationship between the release velocity and the distance attained. However, with the women, the release velocity—in spite of a wide range in distance attained (55 m+ to 69 m+)—was relatively close. Both the men and women had high

impact loading with the last foot to contact the ground, which was of short duration (0.0325). They also had high velocity of flexion at the knee.

MINI-LABORATORY LEARNING EXPERIENCE

Compare (from Figure 17.14) the mechanics of throwing the javelin from a wheelchair and from a running approach.

Injuries

Throwing injuries often occur because of using incorrect mechanics, as well as repetitive overuse syndrome conditions. This latter may happen even if the performer is using correct throwing mechanics, especially in high-velocity throws. The olecranon process, part of the elbow joint structure, may chip, or the shoulder girdle may be stressed. Often the rotator cuff muscles are injured. Refer to Table 17.6 and analyze a throwing action with respect to injury potential.

TABLE 17.6 Throwing mechanics checklist.

Mechanics (Progressive)	Rating	Comments
Preparation Phase:		
Relaxed standing position	_____	_____
Pitching arm extends down and back	_____	_____
Weight on bent back leg (hip, knee, ankle)	_____	_____
Front leg up and bent at knee	_____	_____
Trunk lean back on pivot foot	_____	_____
Pivot foot, hips, and shoulders 90° to flight line	_____	_____
Back leg and hip coiled on inside	_____	_____
Force Phase, Release:		
Weight shift forward	_____	_____
Stride leg swings forward (knee bent)	_____	_____
Nonpitching arm swings back and across body (elbow bent)	_____	_____
Shoulders outward (lateral) rotation	_____	_____
Shoulder/humerus at 90° angle to trunk	_____	_____
Back hip and leg drive body forward, inwardly rotate, extend	_____	_____
Stride forward, counterforce maintained	_____	_____
Consistent stride length and direction (left of flight line)	_____	_____
Trunk rotation, flexion, lateral flexion	_____	_____
Shoulder outward to inward rotation, elbow lead	_____	_____
Trunk lean away from throwing arm	_____	_____
Elbow extension, 110–160° angle maintained	_____	_____
Release of ball slightly above head	_____	_____
Follow-Through Phase:		
Balance after ball release, front leg planted	_____	_____
Direction of arm: across body and down toward front foot	_____	_____
Direction of trunk: flexed and rotated around	_____	_____
Weight shift slightly forward	_____	_____
Back leg and foot automatically move to ready position	_____	_____

Rating Scale: 4-very good, 3-good, 2-fair, 1-insufficient
Prepared by Lois Klatt, Concordia University, 1990.

References

Adrian, M., and Enberg, M. L. 1971. Sequential timing of three overhand patterns. *Kinesiology review,* ed. C. Widule. Reston, VA: AAHPERD.

Al-Kurdi, Z. 1990. The release parameters of shot-putting. Irbid-Jordan: Yarmouk University.

Ariel, B. C. 1973. Computerized biomechanics analysis of the world's best shot putters. *Track and Field Quarterly Rev.* December.

Atwater, A. E. 1970. Movement characteristics of the overarm throw: A kinematic analysis of men and women performers. Ph.D. thesis, University of Wisconsin–Madison.

Bartlett, R. M. 1983. A cinematographic analysis of an international javelin thrower. *Athletic Coach,* September.

Bothwell-Myers, C. 1982. Kinematic characteristics of the curling delivery. Dissertation Abstracts International, 43,3840A. (University Microfilms NO. DA 8308845.)

Canadian Curling Association 1991. Discover curling. Ontario, Canadian Curling Association Publishers.

Casady, D., and Liba, M. 1968. *Beginning bowling.* Belmont, CA: Wadsworth.

Changjian, Zhang, et al. 1990. Some main factors involved in shot put: An analysis based on the elite national female shot putters. Beijing, China: Beijing Normal University.

Curtis, E. 1950. The relationship of strength of selected muscle groups to performance in bowling. Ph.D. thesis, University of Wisconsin–Madison.

Dapena, J. 1986. A kinematic study of center of mass motions in the hammer. *J. Biomechanics* 19(2):147–58.

Dessureault, J. 1976. Selected kinetics and kinematic factors involved in shot putting. Ph.D. dissertation, Indiana University.

Doherty, J. 1976. *Track and field omnibus,* 2nd ed. Los Altos, CA: Tofnews.

Ekern, S. 1969. Analysis of selected measures of the overarm throwing patterns of elementary school boys and girls. Ph.D. dissertation, University of Wisconsin–Madison.

Feltner, M., and Dapena, J. 1986. Dynamics of the shoulder and elbow joints of the throwing arm during a baseball pitch. *Jnl. of Biomechanics* 19(2):147–58.

Fisk, C. 1976. The dynamic function of selected muscles of the forearm: An electromyographical and cinematographical investigation. Ph.D. dissertation, Indiana University.

Glassow, R. 1932. *Fundamentals of physical education.* Philadelphia: Lea and Febiger.

Glassow, R. 1962. Unpublished student studies. University of Wisconsin–Madison.

Gregor, R. J., and Pink, M. 1985. Biomechanical analysis of a world record javelin throw. *International Journal of Sport Biomechanics* 1:73–77.

Gregor, R. J., Whiting, W. C., and McCoy, R. W. 1985. Kinematic analysis of Olympic discus throwers. *International Journal of Sport Biomechanics* 1:131–38.

Hwang, I., and Adrian, M. 1986. Biomechanics of hammer throwing. In *Proceedings of the 1984 Olympic scientific congress,* ed. M. Adrian, and H. Deutsch. University of Oregon: Microfilm Publications.

Komi, P., and Mero, A. 1985. Biomechanical analysis of Olympic javelin throwers. *Int'l. Jnl. of Sport Biomechanics* 1(2).

Lize, Kang. 1990. A study of important technique links of the top hammer throwers in China. Xi'an, China: Xi'an Institute of Phys. Ed.

Sabol, B. 1962. A study of relationships among anthropometric strength and performance measures of college women bowlers. Ph.D. dissertation, University of Wisconsin–Madison.

Schwartz, G. 1983. Two major obstacles to effective discus throwing. *Track and Field Quarterly Review* 83(1):25.

Tarbell, J. 1971. Some mechanical aspects of the overarm throw. In *Proceedings of the committee on institutional cooperation symposium on biomechanics,* ed. J. Cooper. Chicago: The Athletic Institute.

Terauds, J. 1985. Biomechanics of the javelin throw. Del Mar, CA: Academic Publishers.

Uebel, R. 1986. *The effects of varied weighted implements on the kinematics of the shot put.* Eugene, OR: University of Oregon, Microform Publications.

Watts, R. C. 1985. The kinematics of baseball. In *Yearbook of science and the future.* Chicago: Encyclopaedia Britannica.

Widule, C. 1966. A study of anthropometric strength and performance characteristics of men and women league bowlers. Ph.D. dissertation, University of Wisconsin–Madison.

Widule, C., ed. 1971. *Kinesiology review.* Reston, VA: AAHPERD.

Zollinger, R. L. 1973. Mechanical analysis of windmill fast pitch in women's softball. *Research Quarterly* 44: 290–300.

18 Biomechanics of Striking and Kicking Skills

Striking action involves the fundamental patterns common to throwing. Differences lie in the momentums and the characteristics of the colliding objects. These differences create slightly different kinematics, especially where only one foot or hand is used. Striking often involves unique trajectories, which, while not always predictable, are interesting to analyze.

Striking is the act of one object hitting another (kicking is a striking activity). For example, it may involve moving the hand or foot (in soccer, sometimes the head) in the striking action, as in throwing, or an extension of the arm, such as a bat or a racquet, may be used. This latter type of implement increases the radius of motion. The run or step made before an object is contacted increases the momentum of the foot or hand at contact because of transfer of momentum from a part to the whole.

Striking an object at rest, such as a golf ball or a stationary soccer ball, is somewhat different from striking a moving object, such as a baseball. Counteracting the momentum of a ball traveling at 144.81 kmph (90 mph) means that the mass times velocity of the bat must be greater than the velocity of the ball times its mass.

The stationary object must be struck with a force of sufficient magnitude to overcome its inertia. This involves the application of Newton's first law of motion. In addition, performers can attain the maximum distance or velocity in the flight of the struck object if the striking implement contacts the object at a point tangential to the swing and through the center of gravity of the object. The takeoff angle of the struck object must be high enough to achieve maximum distance of flight if distance is the objective. Some of the struck objects have aerodynamic qualities, and the resistance to flight or form drag is increased. The dimples in a golf ball help a golfer attain a greater distance in a drive. Both the number and depth of the dimples influence the distance of the flight. Why is this so? Use the information in Chapters 5 and 21 to answer this question.

The spinning ball traveling through the air exhibits the so-called **magnus effect.** For example, catchers in baseball know that a pop fly struck into the air behind home plate will curve toward the stands on the way up and toward the infield on the way down. Consequently, to avoid missing the catch on the ball's return to the ground, they station themselves with their backs toward the infield. In this position, a catcher who slightly misjudges the flight path can block the ball with the body and then catch it. Likewise, a spinning baseball, hit to the outfield along or near the foul line on either side of the field, will curve toward the outside. Outfielders know this and play the ball accordingly.

Velocity of the Striking Instrument

Based on cinematographic research, the velocities of a badminton racquet, tennis racquet, baseball bat, and other striking implements were found to decrease slightly at contact. In addition, there is a short period when the object struck is compressed, sometimes to as much as half its normal shape, before it rebounds. Furthermore, there is a period when the object struck adheres to the striking implement's surface before rebounding from it. The type of surface, the velocity of the implement, the type of object, and the material of the object determine the degree of compression.

There are other considerations that relate to the striking action. For example, vibration of a compound pendulum occurs in various striking actions. If a bat is suspended from one end, its parts will vibrate at different rates. In a sense, pendulums of different lengths are involved, since the weight is distributed along the length of the bat.

Particles of the bat vibrate more slowly near one end than elsewhere. A particle that vibrates at the same rate as the undivided bat is located at the center of oscillation. The real length of the bat swinging as a pendulum is thought of as the distance between the center of suspension and the center of oscillation, comparable to center of gravity.

If the bat is struck at its center of oscillation with a sledge as it is suspended, it will swing evenly without shocking or jarring the hands. If the bat is struck at any other point along its length, it will not vibrate smoothly and will sting the hands of the striker. This center of oscillation is identical with the center of percussion, which is that point along a suspended object where a blow to it produces the least detrimental effect. A ball can be hit with more velocity if it is struck at the center of percussion, called the "sweet spot" by performers. The location of the center of percussion varies according to the length and composition of the bat. The same is true of tennis racquets and other striking implements.

It has been found that a baseball hit with a metal bat rebounds at a faster velocity than one hit with a wooden bat. This is due to the flexibility of the metal bat.

Baseball and Softball Batting

The objective in baseball/softball batting is to use a bat to strike a ball thrown with varying velocities by a pitcher. The softball batter has a smaller range of motion in the swing than the baseball batter. The softball pitcher is closer to the batter and often throws with greater velocity.

The bat is cylindrical in shape, and the ball is small and usually spinning as it is struck, making an effective striking action difficult. The magnus effect has influence, through air resistance, on the thrown and struck ball's flight. The stance of the batter and subsequent mechanical actions of the batter determine the ability to hit the ball in a consistent manner.

Unskilled Batter

The path of the center of gravity of an unskilled batter may show a drop of as much as 15.2 to 20.3 cm (6 to 8 in.) during the swing. None of the skilled batters shows a drop of more than 7.62 cm (3 in.). The skilled batters also turn their heads more to face toward the pitcher, to enable them to see the ball longer. The long radius and long moment arm aid the batter in achieving high bat velocity. Unskilled batters often pull the handle of the bat toward their bodies as they swing, reducing the length of the radius; skilled batters extend their arms.

There is some "hitch," or backward movement, of the batter's arms before they move slightly downward and forward. Depending on the height of the thrown ball, the path of the bat may follow the body's center of gravity or move downward and upward.

The rapid extension of the arms just before or as the step toward the pitcher is taken increases the speed of the end of the bat. Not only are the radius of swing increased and the moment arm lengthened, but centrifugal force comes into play to aid in bat velocity. Breen (1985) has calculated the bat swing time to take 0.19 to 0.23 second for the top hitters and 0.28 second for the poorer hitters, as calculated from the time the bat started movement toward the ball until it made contact with the ball.

Swing of the Bat

During the swing, the body weight of the above-average batter shifts forward, moving the center of gravity forward. The shoulder turn causes the batter to be facing the pitcher as the ball is contacted. The rear foot is in plantar flexion, with only the toes touching the ground. Approximately 75% of the body weight is forward at the time of contact.

The head is held relatively stationary during the action. The eyes follow the ball until it is within 0.914 to 1.52 m (3 to 5 ft) of the plate. This is called "looking the ball into the catcher's glove," but in reality the eyes do not quite accomplish this task.

Start of Striking Action

Hubbard and Seng (1954) found that batters reacted to the initial flight of the ball in 0.24 to 0.28 seconds. Breen (1985) found that the skilled batters started their swing when the ball reached half the distance of the plate, and that unskilled batters started their swing sooner, or before the ball reached half the distance to the plate.

The action used in batting normally starts from a position in which the performer has assumed a relatively wide base of support. Usually the feet are approximately 43.2 cm (17 in.) apart. The step is 25.4 cm (10 in.) as the ball approaches the plate (Figure 18.1). The weight is mainly on the right foot (for right-handed batters), which is at right angles to the intended flight of the ball to permit freedom of pelvic rotation at the right hip. As the weight is transferred to the left foot, the pelvis is rotated at the left hip, turning through 90°. The bat is moved forward in the transverse plane, first by the turning of the torso and finally by action at the wrists. A slight movement at the shoulder joints takes the upper arms forward and away from the trunk. The main contributing levers are those acting at the hip and wrist joints; the lengths of the moment arms for these levers have been greatly lengthened by the bat. Strong muscles acting at the wrist are important because they must hold the bat in the horizontal position, resisting gravitational pull, and move it with great speed in the final force-producing phase.

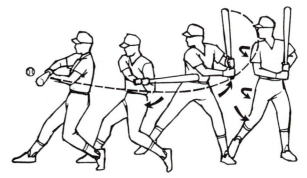

FIGURE 18.1 Body rotation and hip action during batting. The sequence is leg step with rotation of the femur to open the hips, pelvic rotation, which provides the momentum for the upper spine rotation, and the arm swing.

Note that the head is turned to the left to focus on the approaching ball. As the torso turns to the left, the head does not turn with it but remains facing toward the ball. Many coaches believe that if the batter's head moves to the left as the bat is swung, the left shoulder will be elevated, thus changing the path of the bat and reducing the possibility of contacting the ball. A tonic neck reflex may also interfere with the swing.

After studying film, Breen concluded the following:

1. The center of gravity of the body follows a relatively level plane, thus indicating a level swinging of the bat.
2. Hitters are able to adjust their heads to a position from which they can obtain a better look at the flight of the ball for any given pitch.
3. The leading forearm tends to straighten immediately as the bat is swung toward the ball, immediately moving the end of the bat and resulting in faster bat speed.
4. The length of the stride is the same for all pitches for any single skilled hitter.
5. The body is flexed in the direction of the flight of the ball after contact has been made, thus putting the weight on the front foot.

TABLE 18.1   Batting mechanics analyses checklist.

Mechanics (Progressive)	Rating	Comments
Preparation/Stance Phase:		
Upright, relaxed stance	_____	_____
Back foot, hips, and shoulders at 90° angle to flight line	_____	_____
Body weight over bent back leg (hip, knee, and ankle)	_____	_____
Front foot light-weighted approximately shoulder-width	_____	_____
Front arm and elbow at top of strike zone	_____	_____
Hands at top of rear shoulder	_____	_____
Bat between horizontal and vertical	_____	_____
Back leg and hip coiled on inside	_____	_____
Force/Swing Phase:		
Stride forward 8–12 inches	_____	_____
Consistency of stride	_____	_____
Center of gravity or body weight shifts forward	_____	_____
Pelvic rotation (belt buckle toward pitcher)	_____	_____
Trunk rotation	_____	_____
Immediate straight front arm (elbow)	_____	_____
Back arm "throws" from inside out	_____	_____
Horizontal-level swing	_____	_____
Head remains stationary with slight adjustment to see ball	_____	_____
Follow-Through Phase:		
Balanced body position ground up	_____	_____
Upper body in direction of ball flight	_____	_____
Arm and wrist roll	_____	_____
Full level follow-through; around to opposite side	_____	_____

Rating scale: 4-very good, 3-good, 2-fair, 1-insufficient
Prepared by Lois Klatt, Concordia University 1990.

Contact Point

Contact of the ball with the bat is most effective if made at the center of percussion. If the baseball batter undercuts the ball slightly (if too much of the ball is undercut, it will pop up), the distance the ball will carry will be increased significantly by as much as 50 feet (15 m). Additionally, by undercutting, the number of revolutions of the ball may increase by 1,000–2,000 rpms. Undercutting and getting backspin results in a lifting force. Backspin without undercutting is almost impossible since the coefficient of friction between a wood bat and a baseball is low. A sticky substance, such as pine tar, placed on the bat would increase the coefficient of friction. However, there are rules restricting the amount of the surface of the bat that can be covered with friction-enhancing substances (Watts 1985).

■ Klatt (1977) has constructed a rating scale on batting to determine the mechanical performance of the batter. (See Table 18.1.)

Racquet Sports

Tennis, badminton, racquetball, and squash involve the use of an implement that has strings to "catch the ball" and propel it back in the relative direction from which it came. This catching, of course, cannot be seen because the ball or shuttlecock are in contact with the strings for only a few milliseconds. Through the analysis of high-speed film, however, researchers have been able to identify the amount of depression of the ball and the deflection of the strings as well as deflection of the racquet frame itself during the contact of tennis balls. A novice experimenter will be able to see this depression if the strings are loose and the racquet frame is very weak and fatigued. The speed of the ball and the shuttlecock leaving the racquet strings are influenced by string tension, the size of the racquet head, the shape of the racquet head, the materials from which the racquet head has been made, and the type of material used for the strings, as well as the site of ball/racquet contact. In the non-racquet sport table tennis, the surface of the paddle also has a significant influence on the flight of the ball. Sandpaper paddles, rubber-covered paddles, cork paddles, and other materials have been used to influence the ball rebound and ball spin.

MINI-LABORATORY LEARNING EXPERIENCE

Weigh a shuttlecock, tennis ball, racquetball, and squash ball. Next weigh the four racquets. Assume the racquetball is traveling 140 feet per second, the squash ball is traveling 180 feet per second, the tennis ball is traveling 125 feet per second, and the badminton shuttlecock is traveling 180 feet per second. Calculate the momentum of each ball. Calculate the momentum of the racquet, assuming the racquet is traveling half the speed of the shuttlecock before impact.

Discuss the law of conservation of momentum during a collision. Discuss the effect of the strings on the object's velocity after rebound.

Racquet Characteristics

The weight of the racquet, length of racquet, and the size of the grip with respect to the hand size and muscular strength of the player all influence the development of speed. The badminton racquet is lightest and can be swung fastest of the four racquets; a tennis racquet is heaviest and is swung at the slowest speed. The difference in momentum, however, may be negligible. Linear momentum is necessary to provide the force to impact the ball or shuttlecock. Since the shuttlecock is very light in weight, the momentum that is necessary to counteract the momentum of the shuttlecock is not great and need not be great.

Stroke Mechanics in Racquet Sports

It is evident that the same general principles used for throwing are also used in the stroking skills of racquet sports. The objects are hit in a rather horizontal stroking pattern, a high-to-low stroking pattern, a low-to-high stroking pattern, and backhand and forehand stroking patterns. The player uses the legs either to take a step, obtain rotation at the trunk, or push from the ground. The step creates linear momentum to facilitate the angular momentum of the torso. Pelvic or lower trunk rotation usually occurs prior to an upper body rotation. The armstroke then lags behind and begins with an upper arm movement, then a forearm movement, and lastly a hand movement. Independent action of the hand and the forearm are more common in badminton and racquetball than in tennis and squash; however, the action at the hand is very common in squash as well. In all cases, the action is a sequential kinematic link system, in which each body part develops a force and helps form a kinetic chain, in which the forces are summated. This summation provides the linear velocity to the head of the racquet, allowing the ball or shuttlecock to be hit with a high velocity.

The following section describes selected strokes in the various racquet sports, as well as table tennis. Since information from one sport can easily be transferred with slight or no modifications to the other racquet sports, we will list basic principles applicable to all racquet sports.

Principle 1. To create maximum force, a follow-through is necessary. The follow-through assures that maximum velocity occurs at the time of impact. The deceleration of the racquet then will not occur until well after the ball or shuttlecock has left the strings. The follow-through also is a protective mechanism to prevent too rapid reduction of momentum to zero.

Principle 2. The player has very little control on how long the ball or shuttlecock remains on the strings. The duration of impact is governed by the type and tension of strings and compressibility of the ball and shuttlecock head.

Principle 3. String tension is parabolically related to control and ball velocity. Loose tension in the strings will decrease velocity up to an optimum point; ball velocity will increase with increase in string tension. With further increased tension on the strings, the ball velocity decreases. The greater the string tension, the shorter the racquet/ball contact time. A probable explanation for this phenomenon is that when the strings and the ball deform, energy is absorbed and then given back to the ball in instances where string tension is lower. To impart spin, the ball is hit outward and upward for topspin, forward and downward for backspin. Topspin is rarely used in squash, but is common in tennis.

Principle 4. Acceleration rates of the hand, forearm, and upperarm create stress and possible trauma to the wrist, elbow, and shoulder in racquet sports. Strength training of supporting structures is required to protect against these acceleration forces.

Tennis

With respect to technique, there are several general concepts of value to players. These concepts are based on Groppel (1986).

The fewer the body segments used, the less chance for error. Therefore, players should use a minimum number of segments during the toss of the ball for the service. When lobbing or merely meeting the ball at the net for a volley, a minimum of body movement will also achieve greater effectiveness and more accurate ball placement. A player should not jump into ground strokes but, rather, remain on the ground to create a ground reaction force to be transferred to the angular momentum of the racquet. If there is a jump, it should occur near the instant of contact. This means that the push is used in the stroke. The belief that one should always turn with the side to the net when hitting ground strokes is not true. In many cases, there may be inadequate time to take the turn with the body; the ball may be coming so fast that there is no necessity to add to the momentum of the ball in the return stroke. A player might also want to use another movement pattern in order to return the ball very quickly. This pattern is the open-stance forehand. A sidestep is taken to create the angular rotation at the hip. This trunk rotation can be extremely effective for forehand drives. A two-hand backhand drive is as effective, with respect to reach, as is the one-hand drive. It is fairly common practice now to teach the two-hand backhand, since it is a simple segmental link in keeping with the principles identified in gymnastics. The two-hand backhand creates a two-link system composed of 1 the trunk rotation and 2 the arm swing. With the one-hand backhand, the trunk is rotating, one arm is swinging, and the second arm is a third link in a three-link system. Greater speed and control and less fatigue probably are advantages of the two-hand backhand drive over the one-hand backhand drive. Young tennis players who consistently use two-hand backhand and two-hand forehand strokes frequently experience back pain due to high torsional forces.

MINI-LABORATORY LEARNING EXPERIENCE

Identify the active muscles in Figure 18.2. Contrast this stroke to the batting stroke.

Tennis Serve. The tennis serve is an overarm-type of striking movement. At the beginning, the trunk is rotated to the right (in a right-handed player) with the weight shifted to the rear foot. Note in Figure 18.3, as in football passing and overarm pitching, that the right foot is placed at a right angle to the intended flight of the ball. This

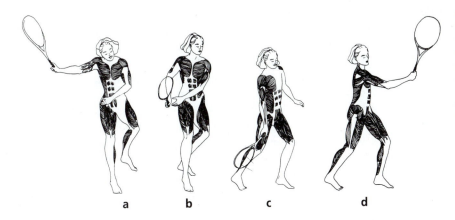

FIGURE 18.2 The muscles involved in the forehand drive in tennis. **Identify the role each group of muscles has during the respective phases of this stroke.**

(Groppel, J. L., Conroy, B., and Hubb, E. 1986. Sports Performance Series: The Tennis Forehand Drive. *The National Strength and Conditioning Association Journal* 8(5):5–79. Illustrations by Patricia Rowan Hays.)

a b c d

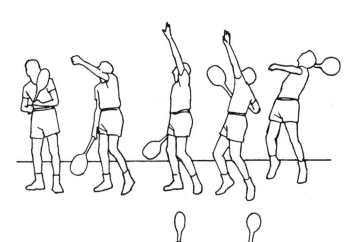

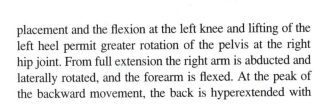

FIGURE 18.3 The tennis service as viewed by the receiver. Note trunk lean and rotation, lateral and medial rotation of the humerus, and other similarities with the basic overarm pattern of throwing. **What major differences exist between the tennis service and the overarm pitch?** (See Figure 17.1.)

placement and the flexion at the left knee and lifting of the left heel permit greater rotation of the pelvis at the right hip joint. From full extension the right arm is abducted and laterally rotated, and the forearm is flexed. At the peak of the backward movement, the back is hyperextended with the hand extended. Note the continuation of the head of the racquet downward as the player's body moves forward. As the player moves the racquet toward the ball, the right arm is medially rotated and the forearm is extended. The trunk and pelvis are rotated to the left.

Biomechanics of Striking and Kicking Skills

The tilting at the torso to the left, which is due to abduction at the left hip, is frequently seen when height of reach is desired. This raises the right shoulder girdle and increases the length of the moment arm for spinal rotation.

Major Contributor. In the tennis serve, medial rotation of the humerus is a major contributor to the speed of the racquet. However, as in the overhand throw, this action makes its major contribution before the impact phase. The humerus is laterally rotated, close to 90°. Here medial rotation imparts speed to the racquet. Next the forearm extends to achieve height. Also during this time the hand makes its contribution by flexing. Except for the position of the upper arm, the tennis serve and the overhand pitch are much alike. The moment arm for hand action is lengthened by the racquet, and here, as in the golf swing, hand action is of major importance. Plagenhoef (1971) stated that racquet speed is no more important than firmness of grip.

The velocity of the ball and the height of impact determine the angle at which it should be directed to clear the net and to land in the service court. Pancho Gonzales, whose serve was measured electrically at 50 m/sec (164 ft/sec), was reported to have the fastest measured serves of his era. Jack Kramer's serve was measured as 46.6 m/sec (153 ft/sec). These velocities permit the ball to be directed below the horizontal and still clear the net. Stan Smith's serve has been reported to travel at the rate of approximately 60.6 m/sec (199 ft/sec). Some of the younger current international players exceed this speed by the rate of 2 m/sec.

A beginning player, before attempting to direct the ball downward, should develop enough velocity in the serve that when the ball is projected horizontally, it will clear the net and land in the service court. If the impact is 2.4 m (8 ft) above the ground and the projection is horizontal, gravitational force will bring the ball to the ground in 0.704 seconds (solved using $d = \frac{1}{2}gt$).

In this time, the horizontally directed ball must travel approximately 17.6 m (58 ft); its velocity would be 0.704 $V = 17.6$ m or $V = 25$ m/sec (82.4 ft/sec). If the impact were 12.2 m (41 ft) from the net, the ball would clear the net in 0.485 second, and gravity will have moved it downward 1.15 m (3.79 ft). Thus, the net is

cleared by 37 cm (1.21 ft). It is evident that a beginning player should develop a velocity of at least 24.4 m/sec (80 ft/sec) before attempting to direct the ball downward, unless the height of impact is considerably more than 2.4 m. The average tennis player can develop this velocity.

A velocity of 30.5 m/sec (100 ft/sec) has been measured in the better tennis players among college women. If impacted at a height of 2.4 m and directed downward at an angle 3° below the horizontal, the ball will clear the net by 10.6 cm (4.2 in.). That angle allows little margin for error and shows the importance of the height of impact. These calculations were made without consideration of air and wind resistance and ball spin.

Ball Velocity. If players are able to develop a ball velocity well over 30.5 m/sec, they should impart spin to the ball. Plagenhoef (1971) reported that five men whose serves he studied had ball velocities of approximately 44.5 m/sec (146 ft/sec), or 160 kmph (100 mph). For these projections, the racquets were moving at approximately 36.5 to 37.8 m/sec (120 to 124 ft/sec), showing that, as reported for golf, the ball can move with greater speed than does the striking implement. This phenomenon is a result of the duration of force application (Impulse = Ft), or the work (Fd) on the ball while the ball and the racquet strings are in contact with each other.

Smith (1979) did a comparative study of the kinematic and kinetic parameters of the flat and slice serves in tennis and found the following:

1. The mean backswing time in the serve was 1.62 seconds and composed 92% of the serving time.
2. The temporal analysis revealed that the mean total serving time was approximately 1.74 seconds.
3. The center of gravity of the racquet reached a mean linear velocity of 33.6 m/sec (84+ ft/sec), with the flat serve being slightly faster.
4. The mean ball velocity for the flat serve was 43.8 m/sec (143.9 ft/sec) and for the slice serve 40.5 m/sec (133 ft/sec).
5. The mean angle of projection was different for each serve: 6.67° for the flat serve and 8.00° for the slice serve.

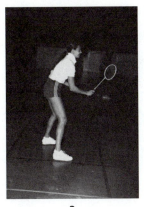 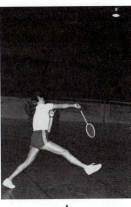

a   b

FIGURE 18.4 (a) This basic defensive position (ready or preparatory position) for badminton is typical of many sports. The anti-
gravity muscles are contracting to support the trunk and thighs in
their semiflexed positions. (b) Attack movements can require large
ranges of motion that could result in unbalanced terminal positions. Note the extreme inward rotation of the striking arm and
large movement of the ipsilateral leg. From such a position the
badminton player must quickly return to a.
(Original photos by Bob Clay.)

6. The ball was tossed approximately 0.76 m (2.5 ft)
   before contact was made with the racquet.
7. In the kinetic analysis, the vertical peak force,
   corrected for body weight, was 480 N (108.2 lb) for
   the flat serve (2.79 N per kilogram of body weight)
   and 521.8 N (117.4 lb) for the slice serve (3.05 N
   per kilogram of body weight).
8. The peak force of the swing before racquet contact
   with the ball occurred at 0.046 second for the flat
   serve and 0.051 second for the slice serve.

Much research has been conducted on the design of
tennis racquets, including the following:

1. There is a lower incidence of "tennis elbow"
   occurring from midsized racquet heads than for
   oversized racquets. Nirschl (1974) collected clinical
   research data to substantiate this.
2. Graphite baron and special dampeners dampen the
   vibration impact more than wood and metal.
3. Changing the center of percussion in racquet design
   and identifying power spots have led to more
   effective tennis racquets and less trauma from off-
   center contacts.

Badminton*

■ Badminton is a game that challenges the player's
reflexes and demands the most precise timing. This is
true because of the uniqueness of the flight of the
shuttlecock.

The shuttlecock's weight and shape is affected by air
resistance, which reduces the velocity rapidly. This necessitates timing that is quite different from striking a
ball because the shuttle's flight does not follow a true
parabolic curve.

Since the shuttle can travel faster (214.8 mph) or slower
(almost zero mph) than almost any struck object and can
be played with a variety of spins and slices, the possible
flight trajectories outnumber those in other racquet sports.
Badminton is also the only racquet sport in which the
struck object is not allowed to bounce; therefore, an opponent has only a short time to prepare for the return.

The player must develop footwork (Figure 18.4) that
allows him or her to recover immediately and return to a
center court position in a minimum amount of time.
Many strokes are executed while the player is airborne.

The racquet and the shuttlecock are both very lightweight; therefore, players can produce great force by increasing racquet acceleration. Because the shuttlecock is
so light, there is a minimum deceleration of the racquet
at contact. The key to a powerful smash, as stated by
Gowitzke and Waddel (1980), is to increase "optimum
ranges of movement coupled with precise timing with a
series of purposeful joint actions" in order to achieve
maximum racquet acceleration. (Remember Newton's
second law: $F = ma$.)

Similarities to Throwing. Badminton strokes are similar in some ways to fundamental throwing motions.
Some underhand strokes (see Figure 18.5a) include:
serves, redrops at the net, underhand clears, and defensive blocking actions. The deep singles serve best follows the mechanical principles of a basic underhand pattern. The stroke that best fits the mechanical principles of
a sidearm pattern is the forehand or backhand drive
(Figure 18.5b). The overhead strokes include drops,

---

* Contributed by Dawn Patel

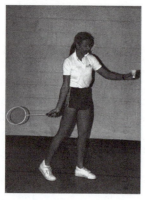
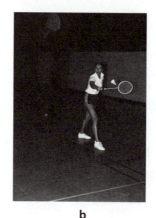
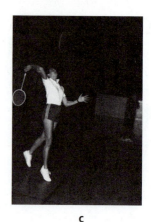

a **b** **c**

FIGURE 18.5 The three fundamental throwing patterns are prevalent in badminton. (a) The underhand serve in badminton has similarities to the underhand throw. However, the distance between the feet is shorter and the trunk remains more erect. Because of the aerodynamic characteristics of the shuttlecock, the height of the badminton net, and the distance to be served, other differences also can be noted between the two skills.

(b) The backhand stroke (sidearm pattern) in badminton is similar to the drive in tennis. (c) The smash, drop, and clear are basic overarm patterns with the characteristic lateral rotation of the humerus that occurs in the baseball pitch. Badminton players attempt to initiate all the overarm patterns from this basic position to deceive the opponent.

(Original photos by Bob Clay.)

clears, and smashes hit from forehand, backhand, and round-the-head positions. The most powerful badminton stroke is the overhead forehand smash (see Figure 18.5c).

■ There are many similarities between the baseball and javelin throws or the volleyball and tennis serves and the overhead badminton smash. All follow the basic mechanics of a high-velocity overarm pattern.

Since the smash is the most powerful technique of all the strokes, we will describe it in more detail. You can analyze other strokes using information found in other literature, including chapters in this book.

Elements That Assist in Power Development.

Summation of Forces. Following Newton's first law, the larger muscles contract first to overcome the inertia of the body. The principle of summation of forces dictates that the larger, more proximal body segment leads the movement pattern, followed by the smaller, more distal segments. (Refer to Table 18.2, time-phase relationships chart.) The main contributing levers are medial rotation of the upper arm and pronation of the forearm. Lateral flexion of the trunk aids in this lever action. The radius of movement of the forearm should be

long-short-long. More than 50% of the force comes from this lever's action while airborne. Since 1980, almost all the skilled players, even the very tall, jump to hit smashes, clears, and drops. They come out of the back-court and jump in the air with a scissors-kick action as they play the stroke. Short players tend to use a "cheerleaders arched" action. All the top-level players also jump to strike the shuttle early at the net. The resultant speeds attained during the badminton smash have been reported by numerous researchers, some of which are tabulated in Table 18.3.

Continuous Loop. There is no hesitation at the end of the backswing. The movement should continue to follow as each joint action continues the kinetic chain. When the objective is power, the backswing should be timed to loop into the forward swing. The acceleration of the racquet reaches its maximum velocity at or near the reversal of direction enabling a greater velocity at the forward swing. Gowitzke and Waddell (1980) suggest that "techniques of getting the racquet back early and waiting for the shuttle should be discouraged for the advanced player." Although successful as a timing technique, it will not produce speed effectively. Players would have to relearn the smash to improve beyond a mediocre smash level.

374   Sports Movements on Land

TABLE 18.2 Time-phase relationships of the badminton overhead forehand smash. Gowitzke and Waddell (1980) have shown that the characteristic features of a badminton stroke, from backswing to follow-through, take place in less than 0.1 second and can only be revealed when data are sampled at frequencies of 0.01 second or less. Note the nonsignificant action at the wrist and the significant radio-ulnar pronation, humeral medial rotation, and flexion at the elbow all being initiated at less than 0.02 second prior to shuttlecock contact.

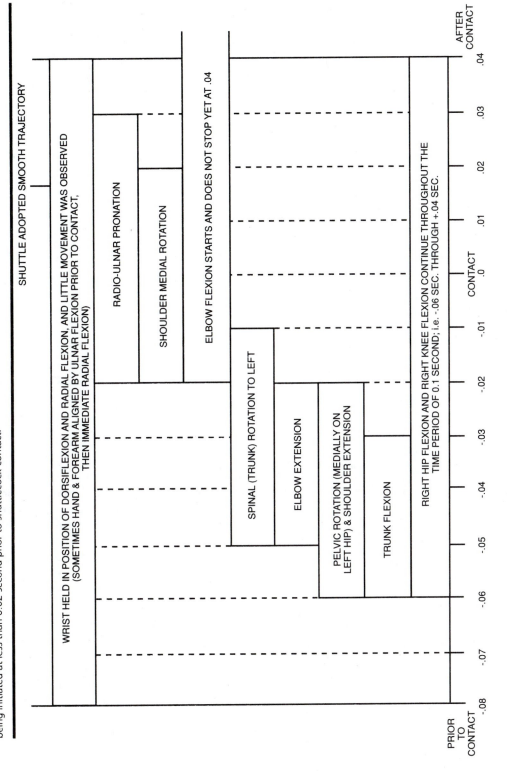

TABLE 18.3 Comparison of forehand badminton smash velocities as reported by researchers. These speeds can shatter nonsafety eyeglasses and cause bruises, as well as prevent the opponent from being able to respond quickly enough to execute a successful stroke.

Study Identified by Author	m/s	ft/sec	km/hr	mi/hr
Adrian-Enberg (1973) (reported in ft/sec)	56.0	183.6	201.6	125.2
Poole (1970) (reported in ft/sec) *				
Subject A	42.1	138.2	151.6	94.2
B	30.1	98.8	108.4	67.4
C	21.1	69.2	76.0	47.2
D	26.6	87.2	95.8	59.5
Gowitzke-Waddell (1979)				
Subject 1	80.0	262.5	288.0	179.0
2	55.7	182.7	200.5	124.6
3	65.4	214.6	235.4	146.3
4	72.7	238.5	261.7	162.6
5	83.1	272.6	299.2	185.9
6	71.0	232.9	255.6	158.8
7	76.7	251.6	276.1	171.5
8	96.0	315.0	345.6	214.8
Mean of 8 subjects	74.9	245.7	269.6	167.5

Abbreviations:　meters per second: m/s
feet per second: ft/sec
kilometers per hour: km/hr
miles per hour: mi/hr

*Poole totaled the velocities of elbow, wrist, and racket head to attain a "final velocity."

Sequential Actions With Increased ROM. Figure 18.6 shows a four-sequence portrayal of the badminton smash propulsive phase.

Preparatory Phase. Basic biomechanical principles:

1. Place muscles on stretch.
2. Position for largest range of motion.
3. The "ready" position for a forehand overhead smash should be a semisquat balanced position with the racquet held waist-to-shoulder height in front of the body. The hand in radial flexion is ready to whip up and back at the appropriate time.
4. The knee and hip angles of both lower extremities should show some degree of flexion as the racquet is drawn backward.

5. The shoulder of the hitting arm should be drawn backward by a combination of lateral rotation at the hip joint of the non-racquet side and rotation of the trunk and intervertebral joints.
6. The non-hitting arm should be raised and the hand pointed at the shuttle to aid in trunk rotation (force couple), shoulder leverage, and better body balance.
7. The trunk should show some degree of hyperextension at the conclusion of the backswing.
8. The elbow should be drawn back initially by a combination of lateral rotation at the hip joint of the non-racquet side and rotation of the trunk and intervertebral joints. Horizontal abduction at the shoulder joint also brings the elbow into proper position.

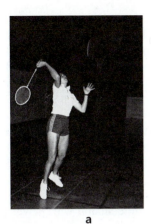 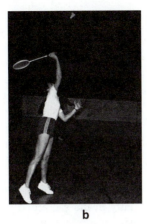 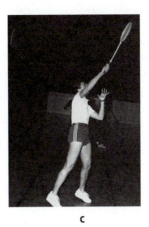 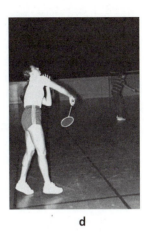

| a | b | c | d |

FIGURE 18.6 The propulsive phase of the badminton smash. Note the extreme rotation of the upper arm and the pronation of the forearm. It is no wonder that badminton players hypertrophy the forearm muscles. (Original photos by Bob Clay.)

9. The racquet face should be seen from a side view and the edge should be seen from a back view. The racquet head is well below the wrist and hand.

10. The racquet head should circle backward and then downward by a combination of previously described movements and by lateral flexion at the shoulder joint, supination of the forearm, and dorsiflexion and radial flexion at the wrist joint.

11. Gowitzke and Waddell (1977) observed that "the hand stayed in one place as though it were the center of rotation for these movements."

Because the badminton player uses a continuous motion to move from the backswing to the forward swing, it is extremely difficult to depict a precise point in time when the backswing ends and the forward swing begins. Gowitzke and Waddell (1977) stated that "the lower extremities have started to move forward while the racquet head is still being drawn backward." The force-producing phase is considered to be when all joint actions are moving in the "hitting direction."

Propulsive Phase. Basic biomechanical principles:

1. The feet should be well balanced over the base of support and relatively close together prior to the airborne takeoff.

2. The position of the lower extremities varies according to court position and ability. The more skilled the player and the deeper the position on the court, the more pronounced the forward leg split should be. This extreme forward stride position aids in achieving better body balance while the player is airborne and recovering to the midcourt position.

3. The trunk should medially rotate over the forward leg at the hip joint as the intervertebral joints are still counter-rotating backwards.

4. The spinal rotation should reverse to a forward motion and the trunk should rotate toward the forward leg while the elbow is still moving backwards.

5. Spinal rotation should continue as the joints of the upper extremity reach the limits of their range so that it gives the impression of the body "moving out from under the arm" with the hand staying almost motionless in space behind the head, according to Gowitzke and Waddell (1977).

6. The upper arm should be extremely abducted with the elbow held high.

7. The racquet should be thrown forward and upward as the player stretches the body up to make contact with the shuttle in front of the body.

8. The hitting arm should be slightly flexed, but near 180° just prior to contact.

9. Medial rotation at the shoulder and forearm pronation are the major force-producing components. The hand should roll through the shuttle in a position of radial flexion. (The frying pan grip is discouraged because it forces one to play "patminton" instead of badminton.)

Biomechanics of Striking and Kicking Skills   **377**

Follow-Through Phase. Basic biomechanical principles:

1. The racquet head should continue to move forward and downward until the racquet shaft is in a vertical position below the hand level and in front of the body. The edge of the racquet should point toward the body.
2. After contacting the shuttle, the racquet reaches the above position by continuing forearm flexion, maximum pronation of the forearm, and radial flexion of the hand.
3. Spinal rotation and arm adduction pull the hitting arm down and across the body to complete the follow-through.

Backhand Overhead Smash. The mechanics of the backhand smash are a reversal of the forehand smash. The forearm is markedly flexed, the force-producing motions are lateral rotation at the shoulder and supination of the forearm. Each body segment moves through its full range of motion. The racquet face should be seen in full from a side view after the follow-through.

Round-the-Head-Smash. The mechanics of the round-the-head smash are similar to the forehand smash; however, there is a considerable amount of lateral flexion of the trunk. The trunk should remain parallel to the diagonal of the court in a position to throw (hit) as opposed to squaring off to the net before the forward swing. This will help reduce the errors of hitting the shuttle wide of the sideline. There is a side split of the legs instead of the forward split to return to the ready position.

Many players tend to feel off balance when learning this shot because often the body has been placed in an awkward alignment in trying to hit the shuttle. This occurs due to the lateral flexion of the upper body toward the sideline, and at the same time taking a scissor-kick split step toward the center of the court. A beginner must learn to place the foot of the non-hitting side parallel to the net with the toes directed toward the center of the court. One would almost be in the same position as in a forehand smash except the shuttle would be farther toward the non-racquet side of the body. Laterally flexing and horizontally rotating the trunk are the keys to executing a proper round-the-head smash. The initial foot placement greatly affects the ability to make a powerful stroke and an effective recovery.

Trunk Flexibility. Trunk flexibility is crucial to permit the player to reach more shuttles and to execute a quick stroke with deception and power. Players with good trunk flexibility reach more shots with fewer steps and keep their body close to the center of the court. This gives the players quick recovery as the trunk flexes laterally toward the shuttle.

The trunk muscles, especially the intercostals, can be injured if a player takes a stance that is square (parallel) to the net prior to contact with the shuttle. This position causes extreme lateral flexion to take place and delay in horizontal rotation of the trunk. Lumbar injuries, especially in the sacroiliac joint, are common with players using incorrect mechanics.

There is a lack of speed (shuttle rebound or racquet velocity) if a player is off-balance at the moment of impact. Another fault is poor footwork—not assuming a stable stance.

The use of the round-the-head smash allows the player to have fewer backhand shots, which tends to be the weakest shot for most players. The player using the forehand shot is in a better position to watch the opponent's readiness prior to contact and during the follow-through. It also permits the performer to return more quickly to the ready position than when using the backhand.

Coaching Principle	*Biomechanical Principle*
Sit to hit. Be as erect as a fencer.	Dynamic balance is established if hips are positioned on the same vertical line as the shoulders.
Play badminton, not "patminton."	Acceleration of racquet head forward of the wrist will produce required momentum at contact of strings with shuttlecock.

Golf Stroke

Golf is a game in which the golfer uses a variety of clubs, depending on the distance from the target (green). The clubs have different lofts of striking area. The golf

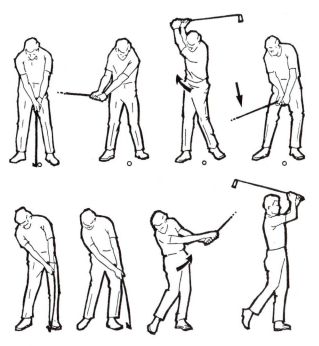

FIGURE 18.7 The golf swing is a two-arm underarm pattern in which the arms move primarily in the frontal plane and the trunk rotates in the transverse plane. Differences in position of the club at the height of the backswing are influenced by strength and anthropometric characteristics of the golfer. Note the characteristic counter-rotation and caudal-cephalic summation of forces.

stroke is an underarm striking pattern similar to throwing, with modifications in the arm action. It might be called a reversed underarm pattern, since for the right-handed performer, the left arm is the guiding force, and in the downward swing the left arm action is in abduction rather than adduction. The skill also differs from the usual underarm pattern in that both arms are active. (See Figure 18.7.) Although the right arm does contribute to the force, it is used mainly to support the club, except for the hand action. Broer and Houtz (1967) have classified this skill as a sidearm pattern. However, we justify its classification as an underarm pattern on the basis of the movement of the left arm from a horizontal position above or at shoulder level at the height of the backswing downward to a position parallel with the trunk axis at impact. Broer and Houtz observe that there is greater activity in the muscles of the left arm, supporting their statements that this arm action contributes more force than the right. This concept is subject to debate. The sequence of joint involvement is the usual hip, spine, and shoulder, with the wrist being last. No step is taken, since the feet do not move from the starting position.

But the weight shifts to the right foot on the backswing and back to the left foot on the forward swing. This shifting of weight increases the range of hip rotation.

Back Swing

At the height of the backswing, pelvic action is seen to have rotated the pelvis almost 90° and spinal rotation to have turned the upper torso more. As the weight is transferred to the left foot, medial rotation at the left hip turns the pelvis toward the line of ball flight. In the skilled performer, rotation at the hip begins before the shoulder and wrist have completed the backward movements. As the pelvis rotates forward, it carries the arms downward. Action at the shoulder begins approximately at the time that the arm has reached the horizontal; action at the wrists is delayed until the arm approaches the vertical.

Moment Arm

The moment arm lengths of hip and spinal levers must be measured from pictures taken with a camera placed in line with the flight of the ball. The moment arms are

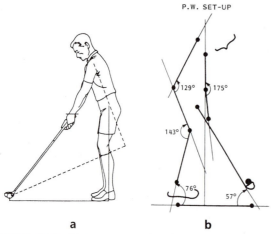

P.W. SET-UP

DRIVER SET-UP

5-IRON SET-UP

a   b   c   d

FIGURE 18.8 (a) Moment arm lengths in the golf stance are measured as the perpendicular distance from the spinal rotation axis (passing through the forward hip) to the center of the ball. Note how the stance changes for a given golfer when using a pitching wedge (b), driver (c), and 5-iron (d). Construct the moment arms of b, c, d as shown in a and relate their lengths, ranking them from longest to shortest. Determine percentage of difference based on the longest moment arm (100%).

(b, c, and d courtesy of Brian Magerkuth.)

illustrated in Figure 18.8. Depending on the length of the club and the performer's arms and on the amount of spinal flexion, the moment arm length for hip action is 0.9 to 1.2 m (3 to 4 ft). These factors also affect the length of the moment arm for spinal action, which is greater than that for the hip. The angular velocity at the hip and spine is considerably less than that at the shoulder. A rough approximation of the linear contributions at the acting joints is 70% at the wrist, 20% at the shoulder, and 5% each at the hip and spine.

Because extreme accuracy is necessary in golf, Cochran and Stobbs (1968) recommend that the movement pattern be as simple as possible. They believe that the important levers are those acting at the shoulder and wrist joints, and state that the difference between skilled and unskilled golfers may lie in the simplicity of action and the ability to generate power in the acting muscles.

Different Clubs—Same Lever Actions

Full swings of the various clubs have the same lever actions and the same proportion of linear contribution to the speed of the club head at the time of impact. In comparing full swings with the driver and with the 7-iron as made by five women golfers (handicaps 4, 5, 7, 9, and 12), Brennan (1968) found that the same body segment actions were used in the two swings. In the degree of body segment action in the forward swing and backswing, she found only one significant difference in the mean measures. Although the degree of pelvic rotation in the backswing did not differ, with the driver the pelvis had rotated 7.2° farther at contact than with the iron. The length of the club affects the length of all moment arms and also the path of the club head. As the club is shortened, the path becomes shallower and shorter. Photographs of a 2-iron and a wood swung by golfing great Bobby Jones show velocities of 40.23 and 43.28 m/sec (132 and 142 ft/sec), respectively, at the time of impact. The shorter distances obtained with shorter clubs result from the lower linear velocities of the lever, as well as from the higher angles of projection.

Lever action in striking activities cannot be evaluated by comparing the summed linear velocities of acting levers to the velocity of the projectile. In throwing, the distal end of each lever is the center of gravity of the

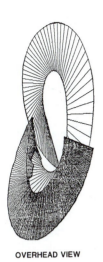
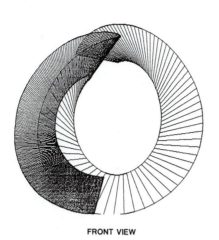
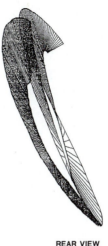

OVERHEAD VIEW

FRONT VIEW

REAR VIEW

FIGURE 18.9 A computer-graphics display of three planar views of the path of the golf club of a golf swing of an experienced golfer.
(Courtesy of James Richards.)

object to be projected. As each lever moves, this center of gravity is moved, and at release its velocity equals that of the contribution of the levers. In striking, the projectile is moved by body levers only during the brief period of contact.

Swing Time

Using film measures of the swings of an average golfer, a college woman, Broer and Houtz (1967) found the average swing time with a 5-iron to be 1.41 seconds and with a 9-iron to be 1.34 seconds. The downswings were three times as fast as the backswings. Drives from the tee made by two highly skilled women golfers as they participated in a tournament were measured with a stopwatch and were found to average 0.64 (Berg) and 0.85 (Suggs) second. Top long hitters among the current women golfers use a somewhat longer swing because of their height and wider range of motion. The swing of a highly skilled college man, measured on film, took 0.77 second; the downswing was twice as fast as the backswing. Films of Bobby Jones show that his backswing was completed in 70 frames and the downswing in 30 frames. His downswing was two-and-one-third times faster than his backswing.

Velocity of Ball

The velocity of the golf ball can be greater than that of the club head at impact. Cochran and Stobbs (1968) reported that a top golfer can have a club velocity of 272.2 m/sec (880 ft/sec). This is equivalent to 160.9 kmph (100 mph). The subsequent ball velocity will be 362 m/sec (1188 ft/sec). The difference between club velocity and ball velocity is due to the smaller mass of the ball, the fact that the ball is flattened on impact, and that during the 0.0005 second of contact the elastic ball pushes away from the club. These authors state that contact time is the same for almost all shots, even for a putt—always less than 1 ms.

Speed of Swing

The swing of a skilled golfer is so fast that detailed movement analysis can be made only with some device to aid vision. In the film of a professional golfer, Cochran and Stobbs (1968) found the time from the start of the swing to impact to be 0.82 second and that from the start of the downswing to impact to be 0.23 second. The downswing was more than two and one-half times as fast as the backswing. Computer graphics, as depicted in Figure 18.9, are valuable aids in pattern recognition, changes in velocity, and spatial orientation.

Dynamics of Ground Reaction Forces

Cooper et al. (1974) used a force platform to study the dynamics of the golf swing. Their major conclusions are:

1. The **line of gravity** was midway between the two feet at the beginning of the downswing. This means that the force for each foot was the same.
2. The weight shift was such that 75% occurred on the front foot and 25% on the rear at impact (mean shift).
3. After impact, there was a continued shift of some weight toward the front foot with most clubs, the greatest being with the high-loft club and the least with the driver.
4. After the impact position was reached, the performers using the highest-numbered club had a force distribution between the feet of approximately 75% on the front foot and 25% on the rear foot. With the driver the weight distribution was approximately equal on each foot.
5. There was some change in the force distribution at the end of the follow-through, in that the shift was almost up to 80% on the front foot with the high-loft club and nearly 70% with the driver.
6. The total vertical force exerted from the downswing to just at or before impact was from 133% of body weight with the high-loft club to 150% with the driver.
7. The total vertical force decreased with all clubs as impact occurred.
8. The total force exerted in the vertical direction was reduced to 80% of the total body weight, indicating that the centrifugal force of the club had pulled the body upward (Figure 18.10).

The Golf Model

Mann (as reported by Carney 1986) used a special computer to electronically chart 32 points on the body and 7 on the golf club during golf swings of 52 leading male professional golfers. Based on these data, he was able to create an ideal or model golfer. Information concerning the golf swing of the model golfer follows.

1. The head remains relatively stationary during the swing and moves no more than two inches in any direction.
2. The backswing and the downswing are not identical. It is not a single swing.
3. The hands and the clubhead move on a "warped" path up and down. The hands tend to move on a flatter path than the club head. This range for the hands is 10° off the vertical with the driver and 18° for the 9-iron.
4. The top right-handed golfers do not have a straight left arm. Mann states that "the left arm flexes more than 30° at the top of the backswing." He believes amateurs, in attempting to have a straight arm, cause tension to develop in that arm.
5. The "butt" of the club does not point toward the ball at the beginning of the downswing. The top players keep the "butt" end from pointing toward the ball by the natural extension of the arms.
6. The outside-to-inside swing concept is generally not true, but the golfer should "feel" as if it were true. The hips prevent this from happening. The downswing is outside the backswing.
7. It is impossible strengthwise for a golfer to control the clubhead at ball contact. The proper positioning of the body, grip, and the position of the clubhead are determined early in the downswing.
8. The change in body weight-shift with each club is not correct. There is almost the same weight shift, regardless of the club used. Mann states that "with the driver, weight-shift is 50% left and 50% right. With the 9-iron, the weight-shift is 55% right and 45% left. The ball is positioned within 2.5 inches for all clubs."
9. The concept of one-piece take away of the club is only true to a point. "From the address until the hands pass the right pocket, it is virtually a one-piece movement. Arms and trunk turn together. The butt end of the club remains the same distance from the body." To try to keep the club and the body together any more would cause the arms to move away from the body. He contends there is only a small amount of hand flexion (cocking).
10. Most top golfers have similar swings. Shorter golfers have flatter swings than taller golfers. Aside from this, their swings are almost identical. The width of the shoulder, length of arms, and standing height are among factors that should influence the club lengths.

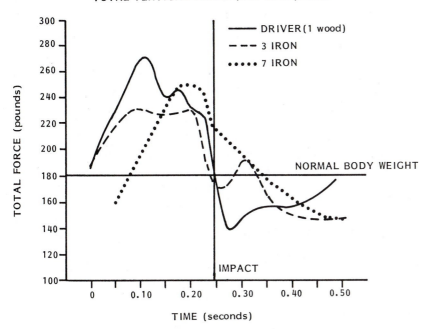

TOTAL VERTICAL FORCE (foot force plates)

- —— DRIVER (1 wood)
- – – – 3 IRON
- •••• 7 IRON

NORMAL BODY WEIGHT

IMPACT

TIME (seconds)

TOTAL FORCE (pounds)

FIGURE 18.10 Total vertical force during three golf swings, measured by foot force plates. Note that the force on the plates varies from approximately 1221.06 N (275 lb) during the downswing of the drive to 621.3 N (140 lb) immediately after impact with the ball. Note the unique force-time patterns for the three clubs used by this golfer. **Although each is unique, two patterns are more similar to each other than to the other pattern. Identify these and speculate why it is so.**

11. There is basically one swing for all clubs. There is a difference in the backswing because of the length of the clubs. Slight changes in the body positions for the various clubs are due to club lengths.

12. The so-called setup at the beginning often dictates what follows in the swing. Mann states that the setup is 100% of an effective swing.

13. Swing errors, or compensating for the swing, include the following: "Stiff-leggedness creates an overly upright swing. Too much leg flexion produces too flat a swing. Weight too far to the left results in a turn centered too far left. Ball position too far to the rear (from driver to 9-iron, only 2.5 inches difference) causes a player to hang back to the right side."

14. Finally, Mann says the legs initiate the downswing, not the arms. As the hands complete the backswing, the hips and legs have started to move toward the ball. The hips and legs have almost returned to the starting position before the hands have made much movement. Upper trunk and lower trunk rotation are the most difficult to measure, but may be the significant factors in long drives. For example, the ratio of shoulder rotation to hip rotation amplitude is 1:0.5 for long hitters, but only 1:0.7 for short hitters.

Putting

Some golfers contend that 50% of their game depends on skill in putting. Certainly to be a low-handicap golfer, one must be able to putt consistently. Most of the people who study the putting action list the following as important for success in putting:

1. Remain stationary over the ball with only the arms, wrists, and hands moving to make the stroke.

2. Keep the head as stationary as possible, since upward head action shifts the center of gravity, causing a change to take place in the arc of movements of the arms.

3. Keep the body weight evenly distributed over the feet in order to have a firm base and to prevent swaying.

4. The backward take-away movement of the putter must be close to the ground and executed smoothly. Any extra movement by the golfer's body or arms may interfere with the stroke action.

5. Maintain a firm left side (right-handed putter) with the left hand and left wrist firm. This action, coupled with the acceleration of the clubface through the ball, is considered effective putting form. The clubface must strike the ball squarely.

The old adage "Never up, never in" should be kept in mind. Many believe that the golf ball must be struck firmly enough to always reach the hole. If it misses, it should travel past the hole approximately 15 to 20 inches. This means that there was enough velocity imparted to the ball to make it go in the hole, provided it was aimed and hit properly.

Other influences must be considered such as the break, grain of the grass of the green, spike marks, footprints, wind, and moisture on the greens.

General Comments

Additional general mechanical comments on optimum performance in golf include:

1. The hands are placed ahead of the ball at address. This enables the club head to contact the ball squarely as the downswing takes place.
2. Too much wrist action is worse than no wrist action. Power hitters use a great deal of wrist action. If too much is used, it results in a duck hook (closed club head before contact) or in a draw (club head closed during impact).
3. The right forearm moves over the left forearm gradually during the follow-through to enable the arms to extend fully.
4. If the grip is too loose at the top of the backswing, the club centrifugal force will turn the club in the performer's hands, resulting in the club head not meeting the ball at the "sweet spot."
5. The key fingers in the grip for right-handed golfers are the ring and middle fingers. However, all the fingers to an extent must have some feel either of the fingers of the opposite hand or the club. The kinesthetic or tactile aspects of the grip are vital in making a rhythmic (smooth) swing with the club.

Kicking

The kicking action is a striking pattern used to apply force with the foot. It is a variation of running and thus is a modification of the walking pattern. The kick differs from the walk and the run in that force is applied with the swinging limb rather than with the supporting one. In the final force-producing phase, the primary action is

MINI-LABORATORY LEARNING EXPERIENCE

1. Have several members of the class demonstrate the golf swing hitting a whiffle ball. Discuss their actions in class. Why do some appear more skilled than others? What parts of the swing can you actually see?
   a. Construct two pendulums of varying weights and radii and then strike a golf ball or table tennis ball with each pendulum. Using the work-energy and impulse-momentum equations, explain the different results.
   b. Construct a large sling shot and release golf balls at varying angles and velocities. Chart the trajectories and ranges of the balls. State conclusions. Relate to the game of golf.
2. Observe the stance (set-up) with different golf clubs as depicted in Figure 18.8. Note the relationship of club length to the given body angles.

extension at the knee. The lever and the resistance arm include the leg and the part of the foot between the ankle and the point of impact. The length of the moment arm is approximately the distance from the knee to the point of impact.

Although little or no action at the hip occurs in the final phase, this joint makes an important contribution in the earlier force-producing phase. As the thigh is swung forward from the hip, it carries the leg and foot with it. During this time the lower leg flexes—an action that moves the foot backward. Based on film tracings, in spite of this lower leg action, the foot moves forward during this phase. Thigh action in this pattern contributes to the forward movement; this action is similar to the contribution of the approach steps in bowling, which move the ball forward as the arm is swinging back. The leg, then, has not only the velocity developed by lower leg extension but also that developed by thigh flexion, even though the latter action does not occur at impact. Immediately after impact, the thigh again flexes and moves the entire limb speedily upward in the follow-through. Unless one has studied this with slow

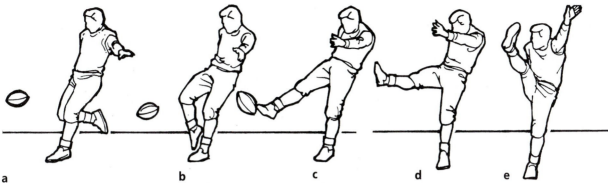

a   **b**   **c**   **d**   **e**

FIGURE 18.11 The football punt. Note backward body inclination to enable the punter to extend further at the hip and knee during the forward swing. The head is relatively stationary through contact with the ball and the supporting leg receives the force of the kicking action.

motion film, the pause in thigh action is not likely to be observed. Thigh action is often thought to be continuous, but cannot be because of the nature of the quadriceps muscle crossing both the hip and the knee.

Another valuable lever can be added to the kick by pelvic rotation, which can be acting at the time of impact. This lever is used most frequently by performers who have had training in soccer and is effective when the ball is approached diagonally. The lever and the resistance arm of this action include the pelvis, the thigh, the leg, and the part of the foot between the ankle and the point of impact. At impact the length of the transverse moment arm, which is perpendicular to the axis passing through the left hip (if the kick is made with the right foot) and to the line of force, is approximately equal to the width of the pelvis.

Punting in Football

Researchers of punting skills used in football have shown that the major contributor at the time of impact is the lever action at the knee joint; the lever at the hip joint makes its major contribution before impact. The pattern is illustrated in Figure 18.11. From *a* to *b* the thigh can be seen to have flexed. From *b* to *c* the inclination of the thigh has changed little if any. After *c*, the thigh flexes rapidly, carrying the entire limb forward and upward.

From 90° of flexion in *a*, the lower leg extends; it has contacted the ball before *c*. Impact is likely to be made before the lower leg is fully extended; this and the rapid flexion at the hip after contact protect the knee joint. Rotation of the pelvis can be seen from *a* to *c*.

Differences in hip action at the time of impact have been observed. Some performers have no hip action; some have slight flexion, and others have slight extension. Thus, it is probable that at impact hip action is an adjustment of the position of the ball relative to the supporting foot. If this is true, studies are needed to determine whether a particular position of the supporting foot relative to a stationary ball will result in greater velocity and accuracy. The drop of the ball with reference to the foot should also be studied. Whether the foot is contacting a stationary or a moving ball, the eyes should be focused on it. Therefore, the performer approaching the ball should flex the head and upper spine.

When a step or a run precedes the kick, forward movement of the body can contribute to the force of impact. The placement of the final step differs from that of the running step. In the latter, the leg flexes just before the foot makes contact with the ground, so that the foot is brought more directly under the body's center of gravity. In the kick, the foot is placed well ahead of the body's center of gravity so that the body can be carried forward by flexion at the ankle, thus adding its forward movement to the force. More important is the greater range of pelvic rotation that this foot placement permits.

Biomechanics of Striking and Kicking Skills   **385**

Similarities in thigh and lower leg actions are reported by Glassow and Mortimer, who studied film of an untrained 9-year-old boy punting a ball and of an experienced male player, executing a placekick. The greatest degree of flexion at the knee was the same for the two performers, slightly more than 90°. The rate of extension at the knee at impact was also the same, approximately 1280° per second (22+ radians). The man, whose leg was longer, had a longer moment arm for the lever acting at the knee and, therefore, greater linear velocity for this lever. Flexion at the hip, moving the thigh forward and slightly upward, occurred in both man and boy while the lower leg was flexing. The lower leg rapidly extended. Both performers extended the thigh a few degrees just before impact. This action has been observed in several studies; it does not add to the force of impact but is probably an adjustment to the ball position.

Much greater lower leg angular velocity is reported by Macmillian (1970) for the kicks of three highly skilled Australian men. These average velocities for each man were 1521.3°, 1788.6°, and 2008.7° per second immediately before contact. During the same time, the average foot velocity was 23.3 and 23.7 m/sec (76.5 and 77.9 ft/sec). The maximum ball velocities were faster than those of the impacting foot: 27.2 and 25.0 m/sec (89.2 and 82 ft/sec). We noted this phenomenon in the discussion of golf and tennis in connection with racquet and ball velocity.

The velocity of the force as it strikes the ball, coupled with the angle of release, determines the distance attained. A high vertical velocity and a high angle (60°) bring about a high-lofted kick. Conversely, a high horizontal velocity and a low angle (40°) may cause the ball to travel a longer distance. A high angle is used with the wind, and a low angle against the wind.

The ball is spinning as it leaves the foot. The reason is that the leg and foot move internally toward the middle of the body on the follow-through. At contact, the foot cuts across the underneath side of the ball, causing the spin. The ball rides on the foot for a few centimeters.

Alexander and Holt (1974) found that before contact the superior punter's kicking foot had a linear velocity of 25.3 m/sec (83 ft/sec). The punters in their study struck the football with the kicking leg flexed at the hip, a maximum of 77°. The ball was dropped so that it struck the foot at an angle of 25° across the forepart of the foot to produce the spinning action or spiral during its flight. The foot contacted the ball at approximately 38 cm (15 in.) above the ground and stayed on the foot for a fraction of a second. The more horizontal the drop, the more effective the punt.

Barr and Abraham (1987) conducted a biomechanical analysis of 22 punts of an outstanding punter using templates with each projected image. They used a Filter-Spline-Filter smoothing scheme for the film data. The punter was described by 21 body points; the ball by 2 points. Their findings were:

1. On a gross basis, the biomechanical patterns were consistent regardless of the distance attained. The action of the punter's kicking leg was described as that "of a simple rotating limb."
2. The motion patterns of punting were found to be very similar to that of a soccer toe kick.
3. The differences between the farthest and shortest kicks appeared to be in the ankle parameters.
4. Using the ankle point (near the point of contact), they found that the peak resultant velocity occurred just prior to contact with the ball. The longest kicks had resultant peak accelerations in the range of 700–800 ft/s².
5. What they called the ankle angle (anterior angle between the foot and the lower leg) moved quickly toward 180°, varied from 158–168°, as the punter contacted the ball, and was largest for the longest kicks. This provided a flat, rigid surface for contact.
6. A shoeless kicker has an advantage. (See discussion on p. 387.)
7. The resultant linear velocities and accelerations were only slightly higher for the longest kicks. They believe that this is due to the fact that there is greater action in the hip flexors in the longest kicks, yet this is tied to the total limb mechanics of the swinging leg.
8. In the case of the knee joint, maximum angular acceleration occurred just prior to contact, followed by maximum angular velocity at contact.
9. Rotation at the hip was similar in pattern to that at the knee with the maximum acceleration coming prior to maximum velocity.
10. The lower leg was not fully extended at contact (130°) regardless of distance of kick.

11. The acceleration at the hip in punting came prior to acceleration at the knee. They suggested that this means there is a "transfer of power from the upper to the lower leg."

12. The resultant ball takeoff velocity after contact was greater than ankle velocity, due to the coefficient of restitution. The ball is compressed when contacted and then regains its original shape. The angle of takeoff of the ball varied from 54–40° with a mean average of 50°.

Flight in the Air

Because of loss of friction, a spiralling ball will go farther into the wind than one punted with an end-over-end turning action. Conversely, an end-over-end punt tends to go farther with the wind than against it. Coaches talk about the ball "turning over" at the height of the flight path. This occurs with a spiralling ball and helps direct the ball less rapidly downward because of lift action of the spinning ball.

A shoeless foot enables the punter to flex the ankle more easily than with a shoe, presents a flatter surface to the ball, and has a peak ankle point velocity just prior to contact. A dominant ankle velocity and a high follow-through results.

Since the kick is initiated after the stepping action by the increase in angular acceleration at the hip and then transferred to the foot, the line from hip to knee and to ankle is extremely critical.

MINI-LABORATORY LEARNING EXPERIENCE

Almost no research exists on the support leg. Observe kickers, placekickers, and punters, and the role of the support leg. Discuss your findings.

Soccer Kicking*

In soccer, kicking is used for passing and shooting the ball. (Other aspects of soccer are found in Chapter 19.) Elements of kicking include distance, accuracy, and speed. The relative importance of these elements in each pass and shot varies with the conditions of play at the time the ball is kicked.

There are several individual techniques for kicking a soccer ball (instep, outside of the foot, inside of the foot, toe poke, and back heel) and many variations of these. Specific information about individual techniques and their variations is beyond the scope of this section. However, we will present four components of the instep kick that are relevant to most kicking techniques. You should understand these before attempting to learn more about other individual techniques and their variations.

Components of Kicking.

Kicking. The movement of a player toward the ball is the approach. A fullspeed run to the ball is not usually desirable because a player will not likely be able to control the kick that follows. There are two types of approaches—*straight* and *angled*. In the straight approach, the path a player takes to the ball is in alignment with the direction of the intended path of the kicked ball. In the angled approach, a right-footed kicker starts from behind and left of the ball and a left-footed kicker starts from behind and right of the ball. The last step of the approach, whether straight or angled, should be a leap. A leap provides time for and aids in the backswing of the kicking leg. During the leap, the shank of the kicking leg should be flexing and the thigh of the kicking leg should be extending. The degree to which these actions occur should be directly related to desired ball velocity. For maximum ball velocity, maximum thigh extension is critical.

Pre-Impact. Pre-impact follows the approach (see Figures 18.12 *a* to *f*). It begins with the placement of the supporting foot on the ground, at the end of the leap, and ends immediately before the instep impacts the ball. Fabian and Whittaker (1950) studied the instep kick and recommended that the support foot be placed alongside of the ball. The support foot should point in the direction of the intended kick. As the support foot contacts the ground, the support leg acts like a strut to block the

---

* Contributed by Eugene W. Brown

Biomechanics of Striking and Kicking Skills

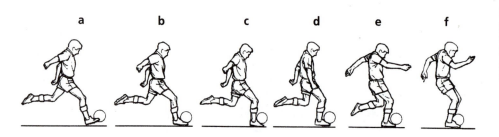

FIGURE 18.12 Saggital plane view of sequential drawings of pre-impact in a soccer kick.
(Used with permission from WCBC.)

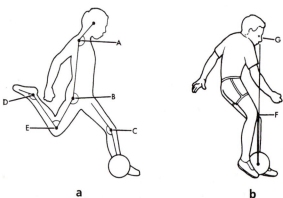

FIGURE 18.13 The critical positions in soccer kicking. (*a*) The planting of the support foot and the extreme backswing of the kicking leg. The pertinent body angles are labeled. (*b*) The position of the eyes, knee, and foot at the time of striking the ball. The vertical line through the center of the ball, the outer edge of the knee, and the eye has been drawn.

forward movement of its hip, start rotation of the opposite hip in a transverse plane toward the ball, and initiate the forward swing of the thigh of the kicking leg. The shank of the kicking leg, however, continues to flex so that the heel is well back. Just before impact, the angular velocity of the thigh of the kicking leg rapidly decreases and the angular velocity of the shank of this leg dramatically increases resulting in an extension at the knee into impact.

It is evident during pre-impact that the angled approach has a greater potential for maximizing ball velocity. The angled approach provides for greater rotation of the pelvis in the transverse plane and permits a fully extended leg (greater lever length) to clear the ground and impact the ball. In contrast, in the straight approach there is relatively little rotation of the pelvis in the

transverse plane and the knee of the kicking leg must maintain some degree of flexion in order for the foot to clear the ground and impact the ball. This conclusion is supported by Plagenhoef (1971), who found the angled approach to produce a ball velocity of 28.9 m/sec (95 ft/sec) and the straight approach to produce a ball velocity of 25 m/sec (82 ft/sec).

The arms are used to counterbalance the forceful forward swing of the kicking leg. They are generally held out to the sides of the body. As the kicking leg is swung forward, the arm of the same side of the body is swung back and the arm on the opposite side is swung forward. The function of the arms is to counterbalance the action of the kicking leg as it continues through impact and follow-through.

Impact. For a low-drive instep kick using the straight approach, the laces of the kicking foot strike the ball through its center at the bottom of the arc of the kicking leg. At this point, the body is over the ball and the eyes, knee of the kicking leg, and ball are in alignment (see Figures 18.13 *a* and *b*). If the objective is an elevated projection of the ball, the support foot is placed 10 to 15 cm (4 to 6 in.) to the rear of the ball, and the body leans backward forming a hip angle of 180° so that contact occurs on the upswing of the arc of the kicking leg. In comparison to kicking with the toes, the instep kick provides greater accuracy because a greater surface area of the foot contacts the ball.

Follow-Through. The movement of the body that occurs immediately after the completion of impact is the **follow-through.** During the follow-through, the speed of the kicking leg is decreased and controlled. It is during this time that the player gains control of body movements in order to proceed to subsequent activity.

388   Sports Movements on Land

TABLE 18.4 Body angles at the shoulder, hip, knee, ankle, and supporting knee of subject during three phases of soccer instep kicking. **Compare the amplitude of the changes at the various joints. Does the soccer kick require extreme ranges of motion at any of these joints? Which one?**

Body Angle*	R shoulder	R ankle	R knee	L knee	R hip
At placement of support foot	137	121	100	140	195
When kicking foot contacted ball	125	125	139	121	160
At highest point of follow-through	112	115	152	117	153

* Body angles are expressed in degrees.
R, right; L, left.
Adapted from Abo-Abdo, H. A cinematographic analysis of the Instep Kick in Soccer. Unpublished report, Indiana University, 1979.

The follow-through does not have any effect on the ball because the kicking foot and ball are no longer in contact. However, the follow-through is the result of the approach, pre-impact, and impact. Thus, from a coaching perspective, it is important to observe and analyze how the body parts move during the follow-through. These movements may provide insight into previous components of the kick.

Contributing Joint Actions. Abo-Abdo (1979) found that the mean linear velocity of the soccer ball was 19.5 m/sec (63.85 ft/sec) and of the kicking ankle 17.6 m/sec (57.86 ft/sec). He supported the concept that the velocity of the ankle and foot depends on the velocity of the thigh and shank and the linear velocity of the body's center of gravity.

Abo-Abdo drew the following conclusions regarding joint actions (see also Table 18.4):

1. From the initial leap through the follow-through, the head-to-trunk angle progressively increased the degree of forward flexion until the kicking foot began descending to the ground. Then the degree of forward flexion decreased. The trunk moved closer to the ball during the kicking action but remained to the rear of the ball.

2. From the initial leap through the follow-through, the right thigh-to-trunk angle was first greater than 180° (thigh was hyperextended behind the trunk) and less than 180° (thigh was flexed in front of the trunk)

as the kicking leg moved forward in the kicking pattern. The forward motion of the kicking leg was started after the leap and before the nonkicking foot touched the ground.

3. As the right foot left the ground on the initial leap, the right thigh-to-shank angle began to decrease in size. This flexion continued until after the nonkicking foot had landed; then the shank (foreleg) began extending forward forefoot contact with the ball and follow-through. As the kicking foot returned to the ground, the degree of flexion increased again.

4. At the time of contact with the ball, the position of the knee of the kicking leg and the focus of the eyes with respect to a vertical line through the center of the ball were as follows: (a) the knee of the kicking leg was in front of the center of the ball; and (b) the eyes were focused on the back of the center of the ball.

5. From the initial leap through the follow-through, the foreleg-to-kicking foot angle was one of extension. The angle decreased at the time of contact with the ball, increased immediately after the ball left the foot, and decreased again at the highest point of the follow-through.

6. The placement of the nonkicking foot in relation to the center of the ball was alongside the ball. The nonkicking foot remained in approximately the same position throughout the kicking pattern. In the follow-through movement the heel of the nonkicking foot was not raised off the ground.

7. From the initial leap through the follow-through, the left thigh-to-foreleg angle progressively increased in the degree of flexion until, at the moment before contact, this angle started to extend from the position of the foot at contact until the highest point of the follow-through. Although the increase in flexion at the knee joint of the supporting leg appears to indicate that the center of gravity was lowered throughout the progression of kicking, the reverse was found to be true. The center of gravity was progressively raised throughout the kicking action and reached its highest point just before impact with the ball. This increase occurred because the body was raised by its rotation over the supporting leg, and increased flexion at the knee joint of the supporting leg was not enough to lower the body's center of gravity before contact. Immediately after contact was made with the ball, the displacement of the center of gravity decreased during the movement from impact to follow-through.

MINI-LABORATORY LEARNING EXPERIENCE

1. Kick a soccer ball and a football at various angles of projection and with spins or end-over-end action. Use moderate force to obtain consistency of kicking effort. Compare results and explain the differences in distances attained and flight patterns.
2. Drop balls from various heights onto different tennis racquets. Note string tension, racquet head size, and other racquet design characteristics. Compare rebound heights and discuss results.
3. Compare flights of indoor, outdoor, and competition shuttlecocks.

References

Adrian, M., and Jack, M., 1980. Characteristics of the badminton smash stroke. In *Proceedings of the national symposium of the racquet sports,* ed. J. Groppel. Champaign–Urbana: University of Illinois.

Alexander, A., and Holt, L. E. 1974. Punting: A cinema-computer analysis. *Scholastic Coach* 43:14.

Al-Kurdi Ziad, D. M. 1991. The linear translation speed on the arm joints in tennis forehand stroke. Special paper presented at Asia Conference.

Barr, R. F., and Abraham, L. D. 1987. The punter's profile — A biomechanical analysis. SOMA (Engineering for the Human Body). Baltimore: Williams and Wilkins.

Breen, J. L. 1985. Baseball batting techniques. In *Encyclopedia of physical education, fitness and sports,* ed. T. Cureton. Reston, VA: AAPHERD.

Brennan, L. J. 1968. A comparative analysis of the golf drive and seven iron with emphasis on pelvic and spinal rotation. Ph.D. dissertation, University of Wisconsin–Madison.

Broer, M., and Houtz, S. 1967. *Patterns of muscular activity in selected sports skills.* Springfield, IL: Charles C. Thomas.

Brown, E. W., and Williamson, G. 1991. Kicking. In *Youth soccer: Complete handbook,* ed. E. Brown. Dubuque, IA: Brown & Benchmark.

Cochran, A., and Stobbs, J. 1968. *The search for the perfect swing.* Philadelphia: Lippincott.

Cooper, J. M., Bates, B. T., Bedi, J., and Scheuchenzuber, J. 1974. Kinematic and kinetic analysis of the golf swing. In *Biomechanica IV,* ed. R. C. Nelson and C. A. Morehouse. Baltimore: University Park Press.

Cunningham, J. E. 1976. A cinematographic analysis of three selected types of football punts. Ph.D. dissertation, Texas A&M University.

Glassow, R., and Mortimer, E. 1966. *Soccer-speedball guide.* Washington, DC: AAHPERD.

Gowitzke, B. A., and Waddell, D. B. 1977. The contributions of biomechanics in solving problems in badminton stroke production. Conference Proceedings, International Coaching Conference, Malmö, Sweden.

Gowitzke, B., and Waddell, D. 1979. Technique of badminton stroke production: Science in badminton. In *Racquet sports,* ed. J. Terauds. Del Mar, CA: Academic Publishers.

Groppel, J. L. (1986): The biomechanics of tennis. In *The encyclopedia of physical education,* ed. T. Cureton, Reston, VA: AAHPERD.

Groppel, J. L., Shin, I. S., Spotts, J., and Hill, B. 1987. Effects of different string tension patterns and racket motion on tennis racket–ball impact. *International Journal of Sports Biomechanics* 3(2): 142–58.

Groppel, J. L., Shin, I. S., and Welk, G. 1987. The effects of string tension on impact in midsized and oversized tennis rackets. *International Journal of Sports Biomechanics* 3(1): 40–46.

Huang, T. C., Roberts, E. M., and Yonn, Y. 1982. Biomechanics of kicking. In *Human body dynamics,* ed. D. Ghista, Oxford: Claredon Press.

Hubbard, A., and Seng, C. 1954. Visual movements of batters. *Res. Q.* 24, March.

Jones, Diana L. 1991. Tennis anyone—Or is bird watching your game? *JOPERD,* Sept.

Klatt, L. A. 1977. Kinematic and temporal characteristics of a successful penalty corner in women's field hockey. Ph.D. dissertation, Indiana University.

Knudson, D., and White, S. 1989. Forces on the hand in the tennis forehand drive: Application of force sensing resistors. *International Journal of Sport Biomechanics* 5:(3).

Macmillian, M. 1970. Unpublished material, Monash University, Victoria, Australia.

Mann, R. (as reported by Robert Carney). 1986. Shattering the swing phase and other teaching myths. *Golf Digest,* July.

Nirschl, R. 1974. Etiology and treatment of tennis elbow. *Jnl. of Sports Medicine* 2:(6).

Olson, J., and Hunter, G., 1985. Anatomic and biomechanics analyses of the soccer style free kicks. Sports performance series. *NSCA Journal* 7, November 6.

Plagenhoef, S. 1971. Patterns of human motion: A cinematographic analysis. Englewood Cliffs, NJ: Prentice-Hall.

Poole, J. 1970. A cinematographic analysis of the upper extremity movements of world class players executing the basic badminton strokes. Ph.D. dissertation, Louisiana State University.

Smith, S. 1979. Comparison of selected kinematic and kinetic parameters associated with flat and slice serves of male intercollegiate tennis players. Ph.D. dissertation, Indiana University.

Terauds, J., ed. 1979. *Science in racquet sports.* Del Mar, CA: Academic Publishers.

Waddell, D. B., and Gowitzke, D. B. 1977. Analysis of overhead badminton power strokes using high speed bi-plane cinematography. Conference Proceedings, International Coaching Conference, Malmö, Sweden.

Watts, R. 1985. The kinematics of baseball. *Yearbook of science and the future.* Chicago: Encyclopeadia Britannica.

Williams, N. 1991. The ten commandments of racquetball. *JOPERD,* February.

Zhifeng, Qin, et al. 1990. Similated training—A study on its scientific principles and its application in the Chinese national table tennis team. National Research Institute of Sports Science.

19

Biomechanics of Selected Team Sports

The team sports analyzed in this chapter use primarily components of running, jumping, throwing, or striking patterns. The basic patterns are modified to fit the strategies, situations, rules, and regulations of each game.

Basketball

Basketball is a multidimensional game in that more than one skill is involved. The environment is constantly changing: positions on the court, the size and speed of opponents, the effect of screens, and the closeness and distance of the crowd are all environmental factors affecting play.

Basketball is similar to other sports because the fundamental locomotor patterns of running and jumping, along with throwing and other related movements, form the major part of the sport. The physical principles and factors that govern movements in other activities also prevail here, for example, ground reaction forces, pull of gravity, acceleration, momentum, braking force, path of the center of mass, friction, and lever principles. (See Chapter 5.)

Since basketball is a hand-ball skill, the size of the hand often determines level of accomplishment. For example, youthful players should have a smaller-than-regulation basketball for learning the skills. Research study findings were the basis for adopting a smaller basketball for women's intercollegiate competition. On the average, women were more proficient in ball-handling skills when using the smaller basketball than with the regular basketball. This is not to say a player with small hands can't be a top performer. Other factors, such as quickness, may offset the lack of big hands.

Dribbling

Dribbling is the act of applying force against the ball by the hand and causing it to move forward and downward. The pull of gravity and the force exerted by the dribbler determine to an extent the velocity of the ball as it leaves the hand and continues to the floor.

The dribbler must be adept in using both hands since the rules prohibit use of both hands simultaneously. The action moves from one hand to the other and often at different heights depending on the position of the defensive player. The ball rests for a fraction of a second against the hand before it is propelled toward the floor. The inflation of the ball, the resistance quality of the floor, and the height of release affect the velocity and the rebound of the dribbled ball.

Dribbling Principles. Dribbling follows several pre-determined principles, including Newton's third law, the law of interaction or the law of action-reaction: There is for every action an equal and opposite reaction. The dribbled ball follows a curved flight path until it comes in contact with the floor. The floor offers resistance to the ball and is compressed, but only insignificantly. The ball flattens a considerable amount and then rebounds at an angle into the air. The height of the rebound is determined by the coefficient of restitution, which is a value derived from the ratio of rebound velocity to inbound velocity. It is dependent on the property of both elastic bodies and their ability to regain their original shapes after compression. Theoretically, the maximum coefficient is 1.00. A basketball dropped from a height of six feet that rebounds 75% of that height, or four-and-one-half feet, is considered a "playable" ball. If it rebounds less than that height, it is a "flat" ball and must be pumped with air. A firmer ball is too lively and must be deflated.

The coefficient of restitution is also involved in a rebound off the backboard or rim. Aside from the inflated condition of the ball, the stiffness or looseness of the rim and backboard affects the rebound.

The dribbler must be moving at approximately the same average horizontal velocity or near to the velocity of the rebounding ball as it returns to the hand. Since the ball rests against the hand for a fraction of a second before being pushed toward the floor, the ball takes on the momentum of the dribbler.

When the dribbler is in a situation where the path toward the basket (goal) is open, several steps may be taken between dribbles and the ball pushed as far forward as deemed appropriate, since running without dribbling is faster than dribbling for 47 feet (half the length of the court). Dean Sempert, basketball coach at Lewis and Clark College, Portland, Oregon, conducted an experiment and reported to the authors that, indeed, running without the ball was faster than dribbling.

Certain dribbling techniques are indicative of a skilled player. They are:

1. The ability to dribble around an opposing player in a curved path (see Figure 19.1). This involves using centripetal force and overcoming centrifugal force.

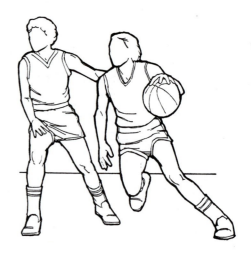

FIGURE 19.1 Dribbling a basketball around an opponent has many of the characteristics of the lean of a skier or surfboard rider described in Chapter 5. Note also the use of the fingers and their size with respect to the ball.

The dribbler must lean into the circle after setting into a curved path. The player pushes with the outside foot toward the outside. This causes the center of gravity to move toward the inside of the curve. The dribbler, on moving into the curve, accelerates, causing the defensive player to be left behind the dribbler.

2. The behind-the-back dribble enables the player to change direction before the opposing player can shift the center of gravity in the new direction. (See Figure 19.2.)

Role of Friction. Friction, which is the resistance to motion due to the contact of two surfaces moving relative to each other, is involved in dribbling. The dribbler creates friction when the shoes contact the floor. A push in one direction enables the offensive player to move quickly in the opposite direction and move past the defender.

The dribbler protects the ball by placing the body between the ball and the defensive player. The dribbler also uses friction in stopping and starting to confuse the opponents.

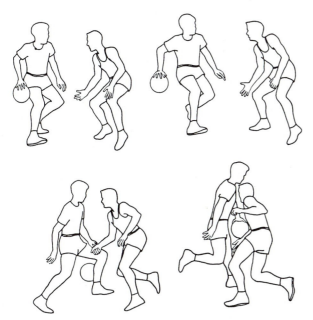

FIGURE 19.2 The behind-the-back dribble is an example of the necessity for kinesthesis and tactile development since vision cannot be used to direct the angle of the bounce. Note the movement to the left of the center of gravity of the guard in response to the position of the ball at the dribbler's right side.

(Reprinted from Cooper, J., and Seidentop, D. 1969. *The theory and science of basketball*. Philadelphia: Lea and Febiger.)

Passing

Passing is the act of throwing the basketball (which includes bouncing it against the floor) from one player to another, usually done in advancing the ball downcourt.

Passing in basketball is often done with the passer not looking directly at a receiving teammate. In other words, the ball is thrown with deception and frequently not as accurately as when the passer looks directly at the target. Some sacrifice of accuracy occurs when precise accuracy is not necessary. There are several types of throws, such as the one-hand bounce pass, the two-hand push or chest pass, and the baseball pass.

The ball thrown into the air assumes a curved flight path. Gravitational pull causes the ball to descend as it traverses through the air. The effect is barely discernible in short passes, but is easily visible in longer ones. In the case of a ball thrown full court, the passer must throw the ball at approximately a 45° angle for it to reach a teammate.

Allsen and Ruffner (1969) studied the types and frequency of passes used in men's basketball games. They found that the two-hand chest pass was the one most often used (38.6%); the one-hand baseball pass was the next most frequently used (18.6%). The two-hand overhand pass was used 16.6% of the time. Other types of passes were less frequently used. These proportions are still valid today, although different levels of physical condition, age, sex, and experience may alter the type of pass used.

An effective passer is one who can pass immediately from the position at which the ball is received. This prevents the opposition from being able to assume a more favorable guarding position in order to intercept the passed ball or prevent it from being passed. Over-the-head and volleyball type passes can be released so quickly the opponents have no opportunity to step into the pathway of the ball in flight. The passer and the guarding opponent wage a constant battle, with the passer having the advantage by being able to determine the direction and the velocity of the ball. In turn, the guard reacts by trying to anticipate and hopes the passer "telegraphs" the direction and speed of the ball. The "look-away" pass is one thrown by a passer looking one way and passing another. The look-away pass is effective because the defensive players are forced to shift the center of gravity toward the direction of the look and are unable to recover quickly into an effective defensive position.

Most effective passers pass the ball to a teammate so that it arrives near waist height, unless a lob pass over an opponent who is fronting a teammate is used. A tall player may want to receive a passed ball out in front and at a high position above the head, since a height advantage may be used.

The ability to pass on the run is a part of the excellent passer's skills. Also, to pass off the dribble just as the ball bounces up from the floor is an added skill that keeps the defensive player from being too aggressive.

Cooper and Siedentop (1969) have listed the following ten principles for skilled passing performance:

1. Successful passers make optimum use of peripheral vision.
2. Except in unusual situations, passes should be executed so the ball is received at waist to chest-high elevation from the floor.
3. Except in unusual situations, passes should be accomplished so the ball is delivered in as nearly a horizontal plane as possible. *Note:* Because of gravity, a horizontal path flight is impossible to attain. However, a pass with too much of an "arched" path is often a dangerous one and subject to interception.
4. The vulnerable places to pass the ball depend on the foot stance and hand positions of the defensive player. Usually the ball is passed through the following areas: over the shoulder of the down arm; under the raised arm; above the head where the arms are both lowered or extended sideward; and between the legs of a wide-feet position.
5. The closer a defensive player is to the passer, the easier it is to pass the ball past the defense. *Note:* This is because the ball can be moved faster than the defensive player can move the hand and arm, since the offensive player moves the hands and arms through a smaller range and knows where the ball will be thrown.
6. A passer must be able to pass the ball as quickly and as forcefully as possible from any receiving position.
7. A definite target spot to pass to should be selected. *Note:* Normally, a pass to the side away from the defensive player should be used. If the teammate is much taller or can jump much higher than the defensive player, then the pass may be thrown to a high target, such as hands extended above the head. The receiving player may often come to meet the ball to get away from the defensive player.
8. Leg extension, medial rotation of the arms, and forearm pronation contribute to the force (velocity) when the ball is thrown.
9. The greater the release velocity the ball attains, the more forearm pronation used.
10. The objective in passing is to get the ball to the desired teammate as quickly as possible without telegraphing the path of the ball to the defensive player.
The following should be added to this list:
11. All two-hand passes are actually one-hand in that the dominant hand comes off the ball last.
12. The index and middle fingers are in contact with the ball the longest. They give the final impetus to the ball. (p. 39)

There are commonalities in the mechanics of the throwing-pushing action in the execution of the four most-used passes: we will analyze the chest pass, the overhead pass, the baseball pass, and the bounce pass.

Chest Pass. Allsen and Ruffner (1969, pp. 94, 105–107) mention that the chest pass is the most common and the least likely to result in turnovers. The passer releases the ball at or near chest level. The ball is gripped with the fingers, spread on the sides of the ball and toward the rear. The thumbs are placed to the rear and parallel to each other. The ball is moved backward so the hands can be extended before being flexed. Some call this action "cocking the wrists," which is not precisely true, since the wrist bones move very little. The thumbs come off the ball as the ball moves forward. (The hands at release are behind the ball to apply impetus to it.) The thumbs do not contribute to the forward propulsion but do aid in gripping the ball prior to release.

Extending the hands puts the muscles that control the hand on stretch and causes them to contract over a longer distance, generating more force. To increase the velocity of the ball at release, the passer takes a step forward, with the body weight being moved in the direction of the throw. When time, however, is a factor, velocity may be sacrificed so that a quick pass can be thrown. Increased velocity may be gained with the arms and hands moving through a wider range of motion. But again this action increases the time needed and also may telegraph to the defensive players the direction of the pass.

The accurate, relatively long passes are ones with a long follow-through, indicating that great force is generated. The backs of the hands often end up within six inches of each other because of the pronating action of the forearms and hands.

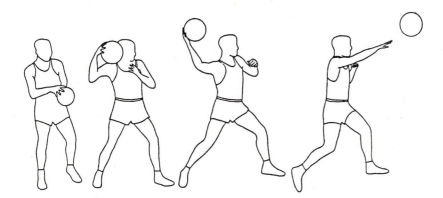

FIGURE 19.3 The baseball pass with a basketball resembles the baseball throw with the classic overarm pattern. Because of the size of the ball with respect to hand size, differences occur with the upper-limb movements. **Can you describe these differences?** (Refer to Figure 17.1 for comparisons.)

The follow-through after a short pass is much shorter than after a longer pass. This indicates a reduced velocity, with a small amount of forearm extension, hand flexion, and pronation. If the ball is passed with high velocity to a teammate in close proximity, the catch is difficult because the attenuation of the force of the ball is nearly impossible. In this case, "a soft pass often turneth away errors." This is not true in a long pass, especially a cross-court pass when the reverse is true. At best, a cross-court pass is a risky pass.

Overhead Pass. The overhead pass is executed similarly to a chest pass in that there is leg extension, medial rotation, and forearm and hand pronation. Often it is not possible to step forward during the throw, so the velocity at release is generated almost without the transfer of momentum from the step. Most offensive guards make use of this pass, especially if they are tall and can see over the defensive players.

The ball is held above the head initially, and, as the pass is being executed, the forearms flex and the hands extend, moving the ball backward before it is moved forward to the release position. Strong forearms and hands permit greater release velocity. The same hand and thumb positions are used as in a chest pass. The follow-through is not as pronounced as in the chest pass since the release velocity is not as great and the flight path is usually forward and more downward, taking advantage of gravity.

Bounce Pass. The bounce pass is used in a situation where the ball strikes the floor before the defensive player can intercept it as it goes under the defensive

players' arms and rebounds into the arms of a teammate. A "look-away" turn of the head makes the pass more effective. The beginning of this pass is identical to the chest pass if delivered with two hands. The ball may be released with a backspin that causes the ball to have a higher angle of reflection and reduces its speed due to friction on impact with the floor. This makes the ball easier to catch.

If topspin is used, the ball bounces off the floor lower, goes a greater distance, and is more difficult to catch. Sidespin passes are used occasionally by some passers.

Because the ball velocity at release in a bounce pass must be sufficient to travel downward, impact the floor, and bounce to a teammate, delivery time is increased. More force from the legs, arms, and trunk muscles is needed than in a regular chest pass. The bounce from the floor is not always as accurate as a common chest pass. For these reasons some coaches prefer to limit the use of the bounce pass.

The one-hand bounce pass has many of the same mechanical aspects, except that the ball is released with one hand. Less spin can be imparted to the ball with a quick one-hand release than in other passes and the ball rebounds from the floor at a higher angle because there is less friction.

Baseball Pass. The baseball pass (Figure 19.3) is the type of throw usually used when the distance to be traversed is equal to or greater than half the court, and the ball must be moved quickly as well. This usually occurs on a fast break following a defensive rebound, an out-of-bounds situation under the basket from a turnover, or after a successful goal by the offensive team. A strong passer can throw the ball the entire length of the floor. (Sometimes a hook pass is used in such situations, but it has sideward spin, curves in the air, and on contact with the floor moves in the direction of the spin.)

The baseball pass is executed with the ball held low (how low depends on the distance the ball is to be thrown) in one extended hand (right for a right-handed thrower), with the hand behind the ball. The other hand helps support the ball. At the initiation of the throwing action, the fingers of the right hand are spread slightly and face upward. The feet are apart with the left foot slightly in advance of the right. The direction the front foot points helps dictate the direction of the throw. The ball is then moved to the rear, and the forearm flexed following this action. Next, the ball is moved farther to the rear and behind the right shoulder. When it is possible, a small step by the left foot may be taken prior to the release. The legs may be flexed. The body action may start with the left side slightly rotated to the rear so that, as the action takes place, the hips may be turned (opened) in the direction of the throw.

The slight step forward with the left foot, the rotation of the hips toward the front, and the wide range of the movement of the arm help to add momentum to the ball as it is released.

The flexion at the elbow occurs prior to the forward movement of the arm with the ball moving above shoulder height. As the arm and hand move forward to begin the release, the forearm extends and moves sideward at shoulder height. The ball is released a slight distance in front of the body. The follow-through will indicate that, as the release takes place, the thumb and left hand are not touching the ball. The legs are extended, the right arm is medially rotated, and the forearm and hand are pronated. The greater the extent of these actions, the greater the possibility for attaining high velocity at release. Immediately after release, the velocity decreases because of the pull of gravity and air resistance.

This type of pass may be thrown while the player is in the air, when less distance is required. The turn to face the court would be initiated before leaving the floor in the jump.

Shooting

One of the most difficult, and perhaps the most important, skills in basketball is shooting. It takes years of practice for the action to become automatic. As in other aspects of the game, the player shouldn't have to think with the higher brain mechanisms while in the act of shooting. Shooting should be intuitive. Changes in shooting style are difficult to perfect for the older player. When players learn a motion as a youngster, even though it may be considered incorrect (and corrected to a degree later), they often revert to it under stress. Bad habits die hard.

Shooting is a type of specialized throwing action in which the ball is usually propelled upward toward an elevated, fixed target. Wooden (1980, p. 71) calls the throw "a pass to the basket." The throw at the basket is released quickly but with much less force than in a throw for distance or high velocity. However, from a mechanical point of view, some of the principles involved in most throwing actions are present in basketball shooting.

Sighting and Aiming. Cousy and Powers (1970) distinguish between sighting and aiming. To many, this would be only a study in semantics. However, in support of Cousy's concept, the shooter first attempts to focus on locating the target, the basket, by sighting, to determine how far and high the opponent guarding will attempt to jump up in the air to block the shot. All such necessary calculations are accomplished before the ball is projected toward the basket. Thus, sighting is an act of locating, focusing, and determining a target out in space. Aiming involves deciding on a specific target, such as the front rim of the basket, a spot on the backboard (glass), or the center of the basket. A type of training procedure involved in this process of aiming is mental imagery. Mental imagery enables a basketball player to prepare for shooting a ball at the goal by just reflecting on the image of the action.

Furthermore, the muscles performing the act of shooting have memory, in a sense. If a shooting action is successful and satisfying, this action is recorded and later fed back to the shooter. At a later moment, the muscles again are called on to contract (flex and extend) and "communicate" to the shooter if they have duplicated the action. The player calls this having a "feel" (kinesthesis) for what was achieved.

A player usually has only a few tenths or hundreths of a second to make decisions on range, angle, and velocity. The path of the ball is parabolic. This means the ball will be elevated gradually in the first part of the parabolic path. A shot blocker must recognize this path.

The word "flip" is used sometimes to describe shots that use fast hand action as well as softness of the throw. A quick release is essential. Brancazio (1984, p. 308) says that in basketball the shooter is launching "the projectile (ball) up an incline."

In modern-day basketball, the dominant hand is the last hand to be in contact with the ball as it is released toward the basket. Additionally, slow-motion film study of shots of the past, such as the underhand shot, two-hand set shot, and the two-hand jump shot, shows that the right hand and fingers of that hand (for right-handed shooters) were the last to give impetus to the ball before it was released. So it is with the one-hand set, the jump shot, the hook shot, the underhand layup, the scoop shot, the push one-hand layup, etc. There is a similar pattern in each, and the relationship to each other, and to the past styles, is remarkable.

Cooper and Siedentop (1969) have formulated certain shooting principles:

1. *Good shooters should always aim at a specific target.* The target area might be the front of the rim of the basket, the back of the rim, the open area within the basket, or a spot on the board (glass). In the past, the good shooter often used the backboard as a target at a distance of 20 feet or more from the basket and to the side of it or at an angle to the basket. There was greater friction of the spinning ball against the wood backboard than against a glass backboard. Accuracy was high at this distance for the wooden backboard; this is not true to the same extent with a glass backboard. Close-to-the-basket shots, such as a layup and close-in hook shots, however, will usually rebound off the glass board into the basket if thrown to the correct spot.

2. *Good shooters should maintain constant eye focus on the target until the ball is released.* Some shooters raise their eyes to observe the flight of the ball toward the basket just prior to releasing the ball. This eye, and consequently head and even torso, movement raises the center of gravity of the player and changes the ball's flight path. This may cause enough of a deviation in the ball's flight path to cause it to miss the basket.

3. *The ball should be wiggled, if possible, just before the release is begun in order to have good touch in shooting.* This action activates the nerve endings in the fingers and the proprioceptors in a joint so an acute awareness of the ball and its position in the hands is communicated to the player. Some call this a "feel" for the ball.

4. *The shooter should not hold the body (especially the arms and hands) in a fixed position for a long time before releasing the ball.* It has been found that to remain in a state of readiness more than 1.7 seconds causes the body to lose some of its fluid, smooth muscular coordination and efficiency of movement.

5. *The ball should be delivered with a reverse spin in most instances.* In order for the ball to rebound effectively away from the glass or other type of backboard as well as from the rim of the basket, shooters should impart reverse spin. The spin creates friction, which causes the ball to lose some of its speed and rebound more softly and relatively higher than if there were no spin. The action of the ball under these conditions makes it easier to rebound defensively and to tip in offensively. In addition, because of the softness and higher bounce, the ball may strike the goal or backboard and still go into the basket.

6. *The better the shooter, the more intense the concentration on the act of shooting.* The successful shooter is one who is prepared to shoot at the basket when within range and partially free from a defender. The skilled shooter-passer is one who is able to change from a shooter to passer or the reverse within fractions of a second. Such a player is rare since the body is being called on to change movement patterns rapidly and as intuitively as possible. If the player has to "cerebrate," that is, think before acting, the opportunity to shoot or pass may be lost.

7. *Shooting is characterized by slight and almost imperceptible medial rotation at the shoulder, by extension at the elbow, by forearm pronation, and by flexion at the wrist.* A clear understanding of the extent of these actions is necessary.

Shooting in modern-day basketball rarely takes place farther than 20 feet from the basket. Therefore, the less pronounced the limbs' actions are, the more accurate the toss and the slower the ball velocity in flight. The legs are slightly flexed and the forearm and hand actions are less pronounced. The release is slightly out in front of the body, so the actions mentioned above are seen to a far lesser extent than those seen in a baseball pitcher. Although the actions are the same, they are not performed to the same extent.

Jump Shot. The most common shot is the jump shot. It began as a two-hand jump, but it was actually a one-hand shot as the dominant hand was the last to touch the ball as it was being released. Many historians of the game, including Stephen Fox, believe that text authors John Cooper and Glenn Roberts were the first to use the jump shot in the late 1920s. The following discussion of the jump shot from Gates and Holt is summarized:

1. More-successful shooters demonstrated a greater angle at the shoulder at the point of releasing the basketball (lateral view).
2. More-successful shooters used a smaller elbow angle at the start of the shot than did the poorer shooters.
3. A greater backspin during flight was associated with the high-performance shooters.
4. The successful shooters demonstrated a closer alignment of the upper arm with the vertical at release than did the lower-percentage shooters.

Cousy and Powers (1970, p. 46) remind the readers that the jump shot can be executed from "a standing position, off a dribble and after a cut is made and the ball is received." While the mechanics of delivery are the same in each instance, the mechanics of preparing for the shot prior to launching the shot are different.

The mechanics used in the three-point shot are similar to the normal jump shot. However, since the distance from the basket is greater, the trajectory of the ball is altered because the angle of release is steeper. The parabolic path is higher than a shot close to the basket, except for one launched within a very few feet of the basket over a taller opponent.

Many authorities believe that a one-step method is the best to use in an approach to executing the jump shot from a dribble, receiving a pass while stationary, or while moving and receiving a pass. The front foot is planted, then the trail foot joins it. The jump is accomplished by flexing the knees and pushing against the floor with the feet (action-reaction). The body position in shooting the jump shot is facing the basket. Students of shooting call this position "squaring up" to the basket with the feet parallel in the air.

Shoulder Position. This "squared-up" position (right shoulder slightly in front of the left shoulder) is the one assumed by all performers in throwing and striking as the object is being thrown or struck. The basketball jump-shooter's position is comparable to the final position of all throwing action. But Gates and Holt found that the most-successful shooters were slightly less "squared" to the basket than the less-successful shooters. The dominant eye focusing on the basket causes the head to be turned toward the basket.

Depending on what the shooter wants to do, the legs may be flexed or extended while in the air. A quick, not very high, jump may be necessary in order to fool the defensive player. Prior to takeoff, the feet should be six to ten inches apart and under the center of gravity.

It is necessary to keep the head, shoulders, and trunk (torso) over the feet. As the push against the floor takes place, the floor pushes back; this force should be through the feet and center of gravity in order for the shooter to be in balance.

Students of the shooting phase of basketball believe that the position of the elbow and hand is the key to successful shooting. The starting position of the elbow is not as important as the release position. Some coaches believe that the elbow of the shooting arm should be pointed toward the basket as the ball is released. Lehmann says that the elbow should be kept within the plane of the body, not lateral to the body.

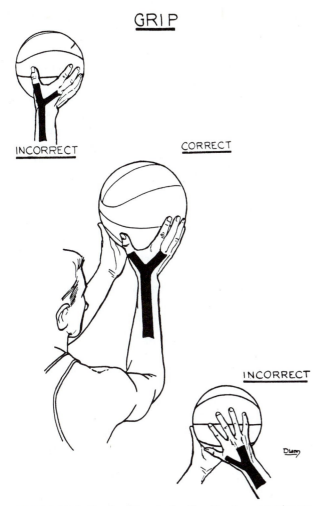

GRIP

INCORRECT

CORRECT

INCORRECT

FIGURE 19.4 Hand positions in shooting. Two incorrect grips are depicted. The correct grip is a Y position such that the ball is well balanced between the thumb and fingers with the distal phalanges holding the ball. The fingers are spread in a comfortable position for maximum control of the ball and subsequent shooting accuracy. (From Sharman, by permission.)

Hand Position. The hand position in gripping the ball for the shot is generally thought to be one in which most of the ball rests on the fingers. Some modern players' hands, however, are so large that the ball, out of necessity, needs to be resting slightly on the palm of the shooting hand. As a rule, however, a true palm shooter is an unsuccessful shooter. Sharman believes the thumb and the index finger of the shooting hand should form a

V and should be in line with the shoulder of the shooting arm. The correct position and two incorrect positions are shown in Figure 19.4. Visualizing the line of force, can you explain why the two incorrect positions are likely to result in an unsuccessful shot at the basket? Do Sharman and Lehmann agree? At what point in the jump shot is the ball released?

■ Strength of the shooter, distance from the basket, and position and size of the defender are among the variables that help determine the release points.

Most writers, such as Brancazio (1984), Hess (1980), Martin (1981), and Macaulay (1970), favor shooting at the peak of the jump.

Release of Ball. Shooting occurs at the peak of the jump because at this position the upward momentum and the force of gravity are neutralized. It is easier to perform an action under these circumstances. It may be necessary to shoot quickly with only a slight jump to outmaneuver a tall defender. To shoot on the way down also confuses a defender. A shooter who is a long distance from the basket (35 feet or more) may release the ball on the way up.

Follow-Through. The follow-through in jump shooting is a continuation of the shooting procedure. It prevents the shooter from stopping the shooting action too soon and having a jerky motion. It makes the shooting rhythm natural and smooth in transference of action from one component part to another.

Many shots are taken at the basket when the offensive player is running, jumping, and shooting on the move. The player tries to shoot before the defense is ready. At release, the shooter must have control over the speed of movement and the angle of projection.

Balance. Students of basketball have discussed balance on the floor and in the air. It is generally believed that the best shooters are balanced when they shoot. It is easy to visualize balance being maintained on the floor. An unbalanced position in the air is often initiated by a push of the feet when they are not under the center of gravity. Misalignment of the head and shoulders with the rest of the body may also cause imbalance.

Other Shots. A variety of other shots, such as the one-hand set, the hook, front scoop, reverse layup, free throw, and even the dunk have some of the same mechanical elements as the jump shot. These include target area selection, pronation of forearm and hand, maintenance of head and shoulder level, eye focus on the target, and follow-through. The fade-away jump shot involves most of the mechanics mentioned in this discussion, with the exception that the center of gravity moves to the rear. The actions in the air, however, are similar to the regular jump shot.

Many students of the game predict that in the future the in-the-air shot will be performed with the ball held above and behind the head, as in a jump shot, while facing the basket. Inside players will combine the hook shot with a jump shot, creating a kind of half-hook. These positions of the ball will prevent defenders from blocking the shot.

Foul Shooting. Foul shooting is similar to one-hand jump shooting and to the set jump shot, in that this 15-foot shot involves a balanced stance, usually with the feet parallel and shoulder width apart. The foul shooter's head remains stationary. There is medial rotation at the shoulder and pronation of the forearm and hand. The elbow faces the basket at release and the body of the shooter is "squared up" to the basket. Hudson (1986) found that women performers were characterized by a high point of release, well-balanced weight distribution, and minimal trunk inclination. Also, the best women players had a higher angle of projection (62°) and greater projection velocity.

The following principles of performance in foul shooting are from Cooper and Siedentop (1969):

1. The player should dry the fingertips.
2. The feet are placed in a stride position close to the foul line, the right foot is in advance of the left (right-handed shooter). The toes of the right foot should be pointing inward and the toes of the left slightly outward. The head is kept down to observe correct foot placement; the ball is kept just overhead or close to the waist to avoid creating tension in the arms.
3. The ball is moved so that the same grip is used as in one-hand set shooting. The ball rests on the fingers, not in the palm of the hand. The ball is loosely placed in the hands to establish the sense of feel; the ball is either shaken with the hands by moving at the wrists or the ball is bounced on the floor once or twice. Such movements release tension.
4. The player now takes a deep breath. This helps relax the shooter and also prevents the chest area from moving while shooting, which would interfere with accuracy. The shooter looks up at the goal, and focuses attention on shooting just over the rim (a target point must be selected). The head is held up and the back kept straight.
5. The legs are slightly flexed, the ball is brought back and down, the hand is flexed, and the ball is released. The hand and finger action is executed as the ball is released and then the follow-through is done rhythmically. There is a dip in the knees, then the legs are extended vertically. There should be no break in rhythm after the eyes are focused on the basket. The arms and the body follow-through are pointed directly toward the basket.
6. The ball should be released with a slight backspin, which will make it easier to catch on the rebound and may cause it to go into the basket from the board or back rim. A correctly delivered shot will make several revolutions before reaching the goal.
7. The ball must be tossed softly in harmony with the rhythm of the entire body.
8. The eyes should not follow the ball in flight, but should be fixed on the target. However, if a player can concentrate on the target until after the ball is released from the hands, the accuracy of the shot is not affected if the ball is followed visually in flight.
9. The shooter should be sure not to step toward the basket too soon. This can be prevented by keeping at least one foot firmly on the floor until the ball is released.
10. Producing the least amount of extraneous movement possible aids in the accuracy of the shot. A rhythmic, smooth movement assures that a soft, accurate shot is accomplished.

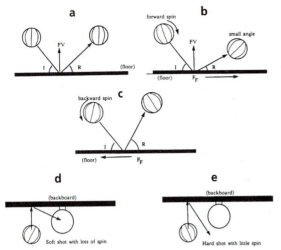

FIGURE 19.5 Angles of incidence and rebound of a basketball as measured from the rebounding surface. (*a*) Non-spinning ball, rebound angle (R) from floor or backboard will be slightly less than incidence angle (I) because elasticity coefficient is less than 1.0. (*b*) Forward-spinning ball against the floor (or inward-spinning ball against the backboard) will result in reduced angle of rebound because of friction of spin causing increased tangential speed (V_t). (*c*) Backward-spinning ball will result in an increased angle of rebound. (*d*) Low-velocity shots with high-velocity spins have a high percentage of rebounding into the basket. (*e*) High-velocity shots with low-velocity spins have a low percentage of rebounding into the basket. Complex spins, such as a backspin/sidespin combination, are more difficult to diagram. The ratio of the two spinning frequencies or the resultant direction of spin will need to be diligently measured.

Angle of Incidence. **Angle of incidence** and **angle of basket reflection** are the striking and rebounding angles of an object (ball) contacting a surface (backboard or floor). If the two objects come in contact with one another and if the impact is perpendicular, there is no friction because friction is parallel to the interacting surfaces. If the impact is not perpendicular to the floor, then the force of friction changes the rebound angle so that the parallel component of the rebound is reduced. If there is any spin on the ball, this modification is a bit more complicated.

Angle of Reflection. The angle of incidence is equal to the angle of reflection only when a ball is thrown against the backboard in a near-perpendicular line, such

as is sometimes done by a high-jumping player near the basket from a position in front of the basket. The ball will rebound directly forward, and gravity will bring it down onto the court. However, if the ball impacts the backboard at an angle (oblique angle of incidence), the angle of incidence will be different from the angle of reflection because the vertical velocity is affected by the coefficient of restitution and the horizontal velocity is affected by friction. (See Figure 19.5.)

Usually, the change in the angle of reflection makes it easier to rebound or tip in the rebounding ball. This is particularly true with the common high angle of reflection of a shot with a soft backward spin. Incidentally, a ball thrown from one side of the basket that misses the basket but strikes high on the backboard will rebound to the opposite side more than 50% of the time. Players know this and try to position themselves to catch the rebound.

MINI-LABORATORY LEARNING EXPERIENCE

1. Duplicate the situations depicted in Figure 19.5. Use lay-up or close-to-the-basket shots and try to predict the rebound of the ball. Experiment with different movements and types of spin, different placements on the backboard, and different types of backboards.
2. List other sports in which these principles are applicable. Name an activity in which precision in achieving correct angles of incidence and reflection determines success of the action.

Path of Trajectory. The **trajectory** of the basketball is predictable. It is the path of an object (ball or person) moving in space. For example, a ball thrown into the air will rapidly move upward until its velocity is zero. If an object lands at the same height that it has been released, the velocity at release and the velocity at (immediately prior to) landing will be identical. During shooting, the basketball follows a curved parabolic path.

■ The horizontal and vertical displacements are dependent on the angle and speed at takeoff.

In the case of a basketball launched toward the basket, the speed and angle of release determine the distance the ball will travel. A basketball player, desiring to shoot the ball at a higher angle than usual, may have a slower speed of release and a decrease in distance. However, a low angle of release means the ball is traveling too fast to ordinarily score a basket. A small player driving toward the basket and confronted by a taller player will change the angle of release to a higher one to avoid the shot being blocked. Such a player is close enough to the basket that distance is of no concern, angle of release and softness of shot being the more important factors.

Keep in mind that, given a constant velocity, as the angle of release is increased in degrees, the object will increase in displacement, up to a release angle of approximately 42–43°. In mathematical terms, a theoretical angle to use when throwing for a distance is approximately 43° from a player in a set position. With a constant speed, any release angle above or below that theoretical angle should result in diminished distance. In basketball, a ball released with controlled speed from a height of seven feet probably should be released at a 46–55° angle except when very near or above the basket, where a release angle up to nearly 90° can be used. This principle is true because maximum distance is not usually the object in shooting a basketball, and the landing target is three feet above the seven foot release height. Hudson found the proper angle of release in a free throw may be as high as 62°.

From a theoretical point of view only, the ball that is descending vertically into the basket has the best opportunity to go through the basket and to score a goal for a player. A slam dunk, where the ball is elevated directly above the basket, is the easiest position from which to score. It obviously favors the taller and/or the high-jumping player. The farther the distance the ball is launched away from the basket, the more "arch" (angle of release) is necessary for the best descent toward the basket.

Jumping

Jumping is the act of projecting the body upward by means of the force produced by the foot (feet), pushing against the floor and the floor pushing back. The amount of G is often three or four times greater than body weight. A person jumping either forward or backward in space will go up vertically but travel horizontally, too. The vertical impulse at floor takeoff contact determines the height of the jump (force × time). The angle of takeoff is also a factor in determining the horizontal distance from takeoff to landing. Most jump shooters try to jump as nearly vertical as possible.

The preliminary movements prior to jumping into the air involve the following:

1. The required takeoff speed
2. The angle of projection, which depends on the desired outcome
3. The force exerted against the floor and the amount of time the force is applied. Force × time equals impulse. The greater the impulse, the higher the jump. Most top jumpers exert a maximum force in a minimum time. What they lose in time, they gain in force production.

A player who cannot jump high makes it a point to correctly judge the rebound angle or path flight of the ball and to attempt to be inside the opponent under the basket area for a rebound. Low jumping height and slow feet still may be offset by quick hands and effective body position under the basket.

Takeoff Velocity. It is known that increased takeoff velocity results in a longer and/or higher jump. The basketball player may not wish to jump as high as possible because of the defensive player's height, location on the court, the position of all the other players, or the distance the ball is from the basket. The jumper, defensive or offensive, takes a reading of many situations and factors, and by virtue of many experiences, intuitively decides how to jump. A shooter may decide not to drive and jump because of a congestion of players. A fade-away shooter may want a displacement to the rear at takeoff in order to elude the defensive player, but this requires greater force in shooting the ball and an adjustment to maintain balance. A defensive player may wait and jump to try and steal the ball or not jump at all, but to steal the ball if the rebounder brings the ball down and in toward the body. Many rebounders spread their legs to block out opponents as they jump for the ball.

Airborne Action. While airborne, having one arm up and then moving the other forcefully downward causes the raised arm to move higher. This is termed "diagonal and spiral movement" of the trunk and elevated arm. As much as six inches can be added to arm-hand reach. Even if the off arm isn't forcefully moved downward, as much as three to four inches in height are gained by the use of a one-hand reach rather than the two-hand.

There are several types of jumps that a basketball player may use; however, our emphasis is on the vertical jump. From a standing position, the feet should be placed apart approximately equal to the width of hip sockets (10–12 inches). The angle at the knee should be approximately 115° for maximum lift. An explosive movement will increase the height of the jump.

The swing of the arms, first downward to add force to the floor push, and then upward for position to catch or bat the ball away is used. A shooter brings the ball downward by flexion of the arms and then elevates it to shoot. It has been shown (Williams 1983) that with the feet against the floor, the downward movement of the arms first adds force that later helps in the upward movement. The upward movement of the arms then raises the center of gravity of the player still higher within the body.

Vertical Height. The reports of vertical leaps of 44 to 48 inches from a standing position with feet parallel seem to be grossly exaggerated. A vertical jump is measured by the difference in the standing hand reach and height of the hand reach in the vertical jump without a "crowhop" or a run. The highest height recorded for an entire basketball conference was 29 inches. The mode was 25 inches.

A jump preceded by a run can cause the player to jump higher. A run, however, introduces other factors into the jump. The most notable is the conversion of horizontal velocity into vertical lift. The runner-jumper attains a certain velocity toward the basket in preparation for a shot. The run must be fast enough to attempt to outdistance the defense, yet the player must be under control. If the player is running too fast, it will be impossible to jump off the floor in an effective manner.

The tendency is for the jumper's center of gravity to move forward as the jumper shooter goes into the air. The jump should be as vertical as possible to gain height and to avoid jumping into defensive players. The center of gravity and the parabolic flight path must be controlled. The parabola or the path of the center of gravity must be a high elevated one, not a long low one. There is also a rotational component present in run-jump situations. This rotational aspect is overcome by moving the torso backward and attempting to jump as nearly vertical as possible. The jump shooter's takeoff and landing angles are similar, about 160°.

The layup usually involves a run and a jump toward the basket. This action is best accomplished more as a high jump than as a long jump. The takeoff angle is 165°. The jumper shooter travels horizontally in the air about one-and-a-half feet. The path of the center of gravity is a parabola.

In the driving layup the takeoff is by one foot with a minimum of reduction in momentum. The penultimate (next to last) stride should be longer and lower than the final stride to direct the jumper upward. The player going up for a layup must jump more up than out and shoot quickly if guarded.

The dunk shot is unique in that it is similar to a running high jump. The performer of this shot jumps vertically but, because of a run, has a parabolic path. Some jumpers can execute the shot from a standing position because of great standing height and/or outstanding jumping ability. The player throws the ball downward from a position above the rim. From this high position, it is an easy shot to execute.

Guarding

Defense is a team effort, as well as an individual effort. The most exacting so-called individual defense is that played in a player-to-player style. One player is accountable for one opponent. Zone defense can be individual to a degree, but is less precise, less demanding, and not as clearly delineated with respect to individual responsibility. It is not as easy in a zone-style defense to pinpoint accountability as it is in a player-to-player style. A delineated space is defended and different opponents enter this space. Since the mechanics of action in a player-to-player are more easily recognized and definable, this discussion is limited primarily to player-to-player defense, known as guarding. Even though the style of play can be a zone, press, a combination of player-to-player, or a helping type of player-to-player defense, all involve individual defensive maneuvers.

Cooper and Siedentop (1969, pp. 107–8) have listed the following principles of individual defense:

1. Playing good defense in a competitive situation is more (often) a matter of attitude, desire, and concentration than it is proper execution of skills. Perhaps this statement has some truth in it, yet the mastery of defensive skills is essential.
2. The main purpose of individual defense is to contain the player who has the ball and to prevent the player and the offensive team from scoring.
3. Individual defense can be aided by the use of a mechanically sound stance.
4. Variations in defensive stance used may depend on the immediate situation and the planned team strategy. It is possible to assume a defensive stance in which the offensive player is overplayed to one side, forcing certain responses from the offensive team.
5. The use of proper eye focus and concentration is essential to a good defensive player.
6. The manner in which the first defensive stride (step) is taken as the offensive player moves and the angle of pursuit used are fundamental to displaying good defensive play.
7. The footwork used by the defensive player should be continuously altered depending on the needs of the situation.

Movement skills used in defensive play are not difficult to execute, yet some players are slow in reacting to clues given by the offensive player. It may take such slow-reacting players several years to learn to play individual defense intuitively.

Change of Position. If a basketball player who has played inside positions (forward or center) is shifted to a guard position, the footwork and actions change, especially with respect to the defensive distance that must be traveled both forward and backward. It becomes more difficult to keep up with an opposing player who moves a much greater distance. There are some players who are quite capable defensively when they move forward or laterally but who have difficulty moving backward when trying to guard a cutting player. This problem is mainly due to the fact that they are unable to move their feet and shift their center of gravity quickly enough in the

rear direction to counteract the drive of the offensive player. Furthermore, when they are moving sideward or forward, they step in the desired direction with the center of gravity projected in that direction. To slide or step in a backward direction, unless the center of gravity is also shifted quickly backward, leaves them vulnerable to a drive toward them. They are, in a sense, polarized.

Stance. The stance of a defensive player out on the court is at best "liable to attack." It is a compromise between being balanced and stable and being unstable enough to move quickly in any direction. It becomes a guessing game between the defensive player and the offensive player. To limit the offensive possibilities, the defensive player may cause the offensive player to move in a path less desirable or make a move too soon.

If an opponent has dribbled, it is expected the player will pass, fake, or shoot. If the defensive player moves a hand close to the ball, the offensive player will be forced to turn and may make a mistake. Some offenses begin with defense, waiting until the offensive team makes a mistake. Defensive players take stances that do not hamper their possibility of movement. They are geared to take chances.

Cooper and Siedentop (1969, pp. 108–9) state, "The stance must be a stable one so that a slight reaction (counteraction) by the defensive player to a false (or fake) move by the offensive player will not throw the defensive player off balance. Increased stability (balance or equilibrium) is achieved by widening the base of support and lowering the center of gravity. Stability can be considered in direct proportion to the vertical and horizontal distance the center of gravity is from the base of support (feet). The feet (often in a stride position) are usually spread a distance just beyond the width of the shoulders (or even more, depending on the speed of the offensive player). The defensive player may assume a wide enough base in a stride position to stop a speedster. The legs are flexed to an angle at the knee between 90–120°."

Cooper and Seidentop continue:

If the defender increases the angle of flexion, thus lowering farther the center of gravity, the defender would gain additional stability but at the expense of mobility. Also, the increased low position makes the player unable to raise the center of gravity and the body, including the arms, fast enough to defend against a jumpshooter.

Other principles of guarding are:

1. The guarding position is similar to sitting in a chair. Weight is equally distributed between the feet.
2. Each type of guarding stance has its advantage. For example, a parallel foot stance is best to use in guarding lateral movements. The stride stance is best to use against a cutting player because the center of gravity is more toward the rear. The fencer's stance with the rear foot turned sideward gives the defensive player an opportunity for quick forward movement, since the player is able to push with greater force against the floor (action of the feet and reaction from floor), but is not too adaptable to use against lateral or backward movements. The stride position of the feet is the best all-around stance.
3. A defensive player should not leave the floor to block a shot until the offensive player is fully committed to jumping and shooting or passing. A player in the air cannot alter the flight pattern until returning to the floor. The defensive player is almost helpless while in the air. To leave the floor is usually a mistake unless done at the very last second. Some coaches don't permit their player to jump into the air to block a shot.
4. The defensive player focuses the eyes on the offensive player's belt-buckle area (which is approximately the center of gravity). This is especially true when the offensive player is a cutter or driver.
5. The arms of the defensive player are placed where best to counter a pass, shot, or dribble. This means that one hand might be held high to protect against a shot or high pass and one low to counter a dribble or low pass. Zone players should keep both arms extended overhead to help close open gaps in defense.

    In case of a non-cutter, both hands might be held high, and against a dribbler-cutter and passer both hands might be kept very low.

Each change in arm position changes the position of the center of gravity and has its advantages and disadvantages. The ability to move the hands through the full range of arm movement without unduly altering the position of the center of gravity is also essential to guarding mechanics.

6. It is possible for a defensive player to "close the gap" and be very close to the offensive player. This may be disconcerting, especially if the defensive player shifts so the favorite driving path is closed and only an alternative direction is available. For example, over-shifting of the upper body, but not the feet, may cause the offense to respond favorably for the defense, that is, move toward the sidelines. Thus, it is evident that defense should be considered in terms of the total body rather than just the position of the feet and arms. This is done by over-playing one way and leaving the alternative open for easy movement.

A defensive player has to be careful not to shift the feet, particularly in a forward direction, just as the offensive player starts a drive for the basket. He or she could not recover until the movement of the shifting of the foot (feet) is completed, and this would be too late to stop the drive. If a foot is raised into the air only a few centimeters off the floor in the so-called slide, the center of gravity of the defensive player is so far forward that, until the foot is firmly planted on the floor again, no movement can be made by the player to correct the mistake. Even a lean of the body in one direction (which is a shift of the center of gravity) in response to a fake may leave the opposite side open for a move by the offensive player.

The trunk is held essentially upright in a defensive stance. In this position, the defensive player is able to quickly lean the body (shift the center of gravity) in any desired direction. It is also possible to anticipate the direction the offensive player will move and be mentally moved before the actual movement takes place.

Movements of Defensive Players. In the past, there has been much discussion about the defensive player always using the slide step rather than a crossover step when moving on defense. This is true when the defensive player is moving laterally a short distance. However, if an offensive player cuts quickly for the basket, the only way the defensive player can hope to stay with the offensive player is with the use of a crossover step and to run the shorter distance to the basket. This is especially true if a "back-door" situation is taking place. In any situation that involves moving a large distance, the crossover step is faster than the slide step. However, when using the crossover step, recovery in the opposite direction is difficult because the center of gravity is projected quite far in the one direction. It may then be best to use the slide step in short quick counter-movements. The closer to the floor the step is made, the less the center of gravity is raised and the less likely it is that the offensive player will be able to drive by the defensive player.

The defensive player also has to be alert to offset a screen set by one of the offensive players. Teammates should notify the involved defensive player. This defensive player should be able to "feel" an offensive player coming up or across the floor to screen. Continually shifting the body to fight through a screen is necessary for a skilled defensive player.

Guarding a Player without the Ball.

Guarding a player without the ball means the defensive player may retreat to a certain distance from the defensive player out on the court. Nevertheless, the defensive player must know the location of the ball and, if possible, keep it in view at all times. This is done by constantly moving the body so the ball is seen peripherally. The defensive player focuses the eyes (or looks out of the corner of the eyes) on an object somewhat distant such as a spot on the floor. Since objects are seen more quickly with peripheral rather than with direct vision, this is an asset. The ball can be seen, yet the player being guarded can also be seen. If one is to sacrifice seeing one thing, however, it should be seeing the location of the ball, not the offensive player. Yet in the zone defense the location of the ball is usually the number-one priority.

The hand to use when attempting to knock the ball out of the hands of the offensive player is normally the lead hand, not the trail hand. To move the trail hand forward toward the ball causes the body to move a greater distance in one direction, so the defensive player may be out of position if the ball is missed. In most instances, a foul will be called. The movement of the hand should be up, not down, as it moves to knock the ball loose.

Playing Inside Players.

Guarding inside players is normally easier since the inside offensive players cover less distance. Many of the principles previously mentioned also apply. If the offensive player's back is to the basket, the defensive player guarding from behind should concentrate on a point on the body near the belt line (center of gravity). If the offensive player's belt line, from the rear, starts to move up when in possession of the ball, then it is possible the player is shooting. The defensive player must be prepared for this eventuality. It should be kept in mind that the offensive player cannot move without taking the belt line along.

Guarding a much taller inside player means the defensive player must slide from one side to the other in line with the ball to prevent the taller player from receiving a pass. Playing behind such a player can be difficult because of the height differential. Help from teammates may be necessary. Sometimes two or three players sink back toward the taller player to prevent the taller player from receiving the ball.

Team Handball*

Team handball features skills such as catching and throwing (to a degree) similar to those used in basketball, as well as some elements of soccer, with many notable execution exceptions. The game involves quick steps, crisp passes, rugged picks and physical contact. This section will concentrate on the offensive aspects of the game, which involve both jump and set shots.

Jump Shots

Jump shots usually occur on the move after taking three steps. Seldom does the performer move in a straight line when executing the three steps except when there is an unobstructed path down the court at the end of a fast break. Most movements during the three steps are made

---

*Contributed by Terence M. Freeman

in a zigzag fashion as the offensive performer tries to avoid defensive players and goes through the team defensive alignment.

■ A balanced position is essential—and difficult to achieve for shooting—since the horizontal momentum of approach is curvilinear.

Players seek alleys to the goal rather than shooting over the defensive player. However, shots are made from different offensive positions and the demands of each are different. The technique of shooting for a goal changes drastically, depending on position on the court, in contrast to basketball, in which similar techniques are used in many different situations.

For example, a shot at the goal from the backcourt must have greater velocity because of the distance from the goal. Circle runners and wings don't have to use as much power in their throws as do backcourt players.

Backcourt Jump Shot. The backcourt jump shot is executed with a wide range of motion of the throwing arm. (See Chapter 17 on throwing.) Players gain momentum by the leap since they not only leap up but forward slightly, with the center of gravity projected beyond the body.

At the instant of the execution of the second step the hips are rotated so the trunk (chest) is placed at a right angle to the direction of the throw. An erect position of the head is maintained at all times so a rotating motion about the body will not be introduced.

As the player leaps on the lead foot for the third step, the hips begin to move toward the rear. The trail foot is brought forward and the strong muscles, such as the latissimus dorsi and pectoralis major (chest muscles attached to the arm) are put on a stretch preparatory to accomplishing the throw. This is similar to the biomechanics of javelin throwing.

The ball is moved slightly behind the body and above the head. The shot occurs when the ball (not the head) is at the peak height. The hand is moved to flexion and then extension (often called the whip of the wrist), dictating line of aim. As the thrower reaches the peak height, the ball is often thrown downward at the goalie's feet, which brings into play the momentum of the jump and gravity in the downward throw. Good players shoot low because the goalie's feet can't move as rapidly as the hands in blocking the shot.

Wing Jump Shot. The wing jump shot is more acrobatic because the angle of the proposed shot is acute. To shoot around the body, arms, and feet of the goalie (who is usually positioned to prevent the direct shot to the near post), the wing player attempts to leap out into the goalie's protected six-meter circle. In reality, wing players hold the ball in the same manner as backcourt players when they shoot. However, there is a tendency for the hand holding the ball to move down. To overcome this tendency, the hand holding the ball should be moved to the rear and behind the head at the end of the backswing. Many experienced players are almost horizontal to the floor, inclining the body toward the throwing arm as the ball is released. (See Chapter 17 on baseball pitching.) There is medial rotation of the humerus and pronation of the forearm and hand during the throw. In such a throwing action most of the major muscles of the thorax, upper back, and upper and lower arm are activated. The thigh and lower leg muscles are also involved in the jump.

Circle Jump Shot. Circle runners work in very close quarters with defensive players crowding them on one or both sides. They often build momentum by twisting into small gaps in the defensive alignment; this twisting is not unlike what a shot-putter might do. But then the circle runner tries to get the shoulders at least square to the goal and perhaps even into a conventional throwing position. Squaring to the goal prior to the throwing action eliminates the full contribution of the chest muscles and limits the velocity of the throw essentially to that produced by the arms and wrist, which is not necessarily ineffective since the distance is short. Some circle runners seem to dive into the goalie's protected area to make their shots. Their bodies are almost prone to the ground when releasing the ball before hitting the floor.

■ Biomechanical principles of landing must be practiced and used by players executing jump shots.

Set Shots

Set shots exist in team handball. The shooter simply does not go airborne. Some set shots are opportunistic, straightforward throws through an open alley. Set shooters often create the alley by faking one vector and then twisting into another vector.

Set shots in team handball do not resemble the set shot in basketball. There is no sport widely played in America that prepares players for these types of shots except water polo. A great deal of time is spent in helping players unlearn mechanics that have become habitual to them in performing other sports. First-year players of both sexes often appear awkward as they try to bring all the movements into harmony.

Fleck et al. (1992) examined the relationships between ball velocity during set shots and jump shots and the isokinetic torque of selected upper body movements. Torque capabilities of horizontal adduction, shoulder flexion, and elbow extension were found to have a positive relationship to set shot peak ball velocity. Torque capabilities of the shoulder internal rotators, elbow extensors, and shoulder horizontal adductors showed the strongest positive relationships to jump shot peak velocity. The elbow flexors were not prime movers in the throwing of the jump shot. The relationship between torque capabilities of the elbow flexors and peak ball velocity may be related to the ability to decelerate the limb without injury after release of the ball.

Soccer*

Soccer is a team game in which the players strike a ball with the feet, head, or body in order to move the ball downfield or to a teammate. An exception is the goalie, who can use his hands within a confined area. The main skills involved are kicking (which is discussed in Chapter 18) and heading, as well as the chest trap and the throw-in. This section looks at the last three.

Heading

Heading skills can be divided into two categories: heading with the feet on the ground (see Figure 19.6) and jumping to head the ball. Each of these categories has many skill variations that permit the player to pass, shoot, or receive and control the ball. The following analysis will focus on heading technique in which the purpose is to impart maximum velocity to the ball from a standing position. Basically, this is an impact problem

in which the player attempts to maximize the preimpact velocity vector of the forehead relative to the preimpact momentum of the ball in order to redirect the ball.

Preparatory Phase. The legs should be spread in a comfortable forward-backward alignment with the knees slightly flexed. The body weight is on the balls of the feet. This is a relatively stable position in line with the path of the approaching ball and in line with the intended direction of projection. From this stance, players can adjust their body positioning. The arms are held out to the sides and in front of the body to assist with balance. Prior to contacting the ball, the body weight is shifted toward the back foot by pushing off the front foot and arching the trunk backwards. The arching movement stretches the anterior muscles of the trunk and hip and facilitates their subsequent contraction.

Activity Phase. The body weight is rapidly shifted forward toward the front foot by extension of the back leg and contraction of the previously stretched trunk and hip flexors. Additional forward velocity is attained by simultaneously flexing the neck and extending the forehead into the ball. On impact the neck muscles tighten to prevent the head and neck from recoiling. Just prior to contact, the arms are forcefully drawn back to enhance the forward momentum of the trunk and head.

Method of Contact. Contact with the ball should be made with the forehead. This generally flat region of the head permits ball control. The frontal bone of the skull, which encompasses the forehead, is also a relatively thick and strong bone. The eyes should be kept open and focused on the ball throughout the performance to ensure contact with the forehead. Contacting the ball with other regions of the head may be painful and injurious. The mouth should be kept open but held firmly in place. Some authors have suggested closing the mouth. However, the force of ball contact with the head establishes a shock wave that may injure the teeth if they are held together and vibrate against each other.

Soccer Chest Trap

In receiving a projected ball with the chest, the player attempts to reduce the ball's velocity by cushioning it with

---

* Contributed by Eugene W. Brown

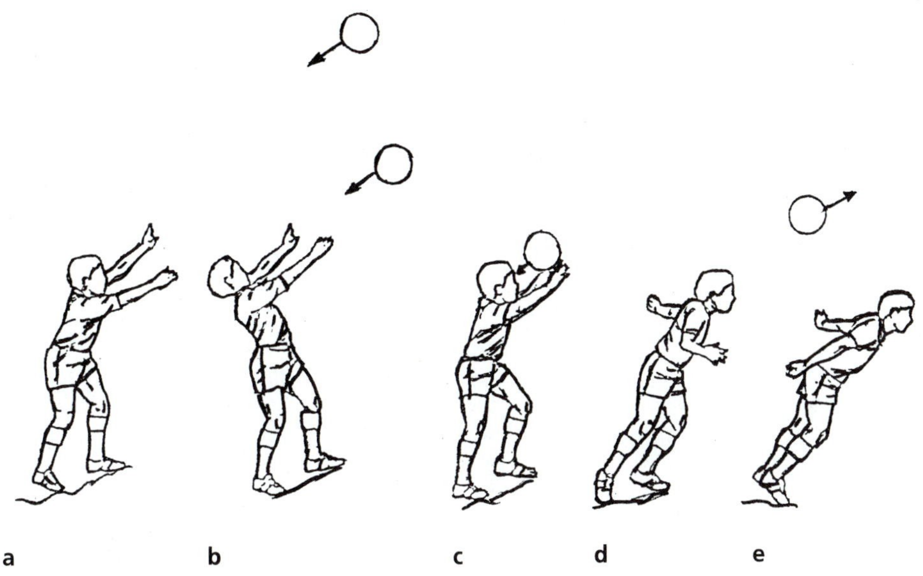

FIGURE 19.6 Soccer heading. (From Eugene W. Brown, *Youth Soccer,* Copyright © 1992 Wm. C. Brown Communications, Inc., Dubuque, IA. All rights reserved. Reprinted by permission of the publisher and the author.)

a   b   c   d   e

the chest and to redirect the ball to where it can be subsequently played. As the ball approaches, the player should assume a forward-backward straddle of the feet to increase the base of support and stability in the direction of the path of the ball (see Figure 19.7). If the feet are straddled to the sides of the body, impact of the ball may cause the player to fall backward. Initially, the body weight is mostly supported by the front foot. Just before and during impact the trunk is arched backward, shifting the body weight toward the back foot. If properly timed, this movement cushions the impact of the ball.

Ball contact should be made high on the chest, above the level of the nipples. At ball contact, elevation of the arms to the front and sides of the body will depress this region of the chest. This helps to absorb the impact of the ball and also forms a cup that aids the player in controlling the rebound of the ball. Orientation of the trunk in receiving the ball should be determined by the path of the ball. A ball with a shallow arc may be received with the trunk nearly perpendicular to the ground, while the trunk should be inclined backward when receiving a ball with a steep arc. After contact, the ball will rebound forward. The forward and backward straddle position of the

feet permits the player to push off the back foot and move forward for subsequent play. If the feet were straddling to the side, this would not be possible.

Soccer Throw-In

The rules governing the throw-in were designed to restrict this event to merely a means of putting the ball back into play after it has gone out of bounds over the touch line (side line), not to create a major advantage for the team taking the throw. The rules define the location (the point where the ball went out of bounds) and method (thrower facing the field of play, both feet in contact with the ground when the ball leaves the hands, two-handed throw with each hand applying approximately equal force to the ball, and one continuous movement in which the ball is taken from behind the head and released over the head for returning the ball to play). However, even with these restrictions, physically strong and skilled players are able to project the ball from the touch line to the front of the opponent's goal (distances of 35 meters or more), where their teammates can redirect the ball for a score.

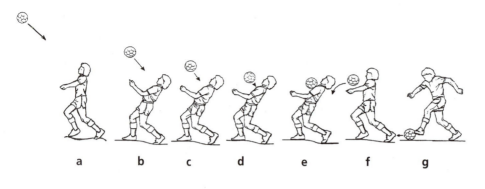

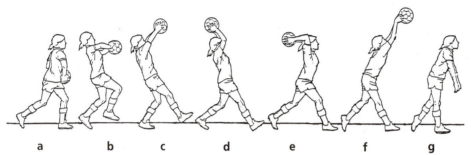

How can a soccer player achieve projectile distances of 35 meters or more with such a restricted throw-in? Aside from the physical strength required, long throws are accomplished through a specific sequential pattern of movement that temporally integrates linear and angular velocities of the body and its segments to achieve maximum linear velocity of the ball at release. Specifically, the thrower takes a controlled approach run (see Figure 19.8) toward the touch line and in the intended direction of the throw with the ball held in front of the body. The run is not a sprint because a sprint would necessitate a rapid performance of subsequent events and attenuate the range of segmental movements that contribute to maximum projectile velocity. The approach run is followed by a hop, step, and throw. The hop provides time for the elevation of the ball over and behind the head and hyperextension of the trunk. This stretches the anterior muscles of the trunk and potentially facilitates their contraction as a result of their elastic property and stretch reflex. The long step forward positions the center of gravity considerably behind the front foot. This provides an opportunity for the thrower to control the forward momentum of the body so that the line of gravity does not go beyond the forward edge of the base of support, resulting in a lifting of the back foot and a foul throw. The step and subsequent extension of the knee of the step leg block the forward movements of the pelvis simultaneously with the initiation of contraction of trunk flexor muscles. This causes a rapid increase in angular momentum of the trunk. The arms continue to swing backward momentarily until the muscles of the shoulder joint and shoulder girdle are placed on stretch. Then the shoulder extensor muscles quickly and forcefully contract simultaneously with a contraction of the spinal extensors. These contractions retard the forward rotation of the trunk and facilitate angular acceleration of the arms about the shoulder joints. Note that at this point (see Figure 19.8), the upper extremity's moment of inertia is reduced because the forearms are flexed. Subsequently, the angular velocity of the arms decreases and the angular velocity of the forearms increases.

The overall proximal-to-distal link-segment pattern is similar to a whip action, beginning with the trunk and ending with a maximum angular velocity of the forearms at release (see Figure 19.9). When throwing for maximum distance, soccer players do not project the ball

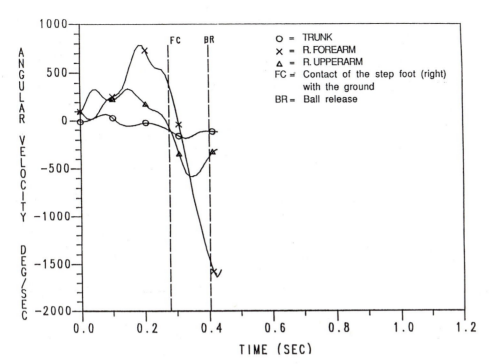

FIGURE 19.9 Segmental angular velocities in the soccer throw-in.

(From Brown, E. W., et al. 1987. Biomechanical comparison of the standard and handspring soccer throw-in. In *Biomechanics in sports III & IV*, eds. Terauds, J., Gowitzke, B. A., and Holt, L. E. p. 169. Del Mar, CA: Research Center for Sports.)

at 45°. This would give opponents additional time to intercept the throw-in intended for a teammate. Generally, the practical angle of projection is approximately 25°. This angle of projection is the result of a combination of the "ramp effect" movement of the center of gravity associated with a long step (drop in height of the center of gravity, as shown in Figure 19.8*d* and *e*) and sliding the back foot forward (rise in height of the center of gravity) and the release of the ball (see Figure 19.8*e–g*).

Field Hockey*

Field hockey is a striking game involving **linear** and **curvilinear** motion. Performance also includes changing direction while running and maneuvering and striking a field hockey ball with a flat, one-sided, curved shaft as shown in Figure 19.10. Men and women participate in

---

*Contributed by Lois Klatt.

the sport at all age levels throughout the world. American women have reached a high level, finishing third in the world at the 1984 Los Angeles Olympics.

In the linear running aspect of the game, performers must learn to use the same mechanics as do sprinters, with the exception that the performer runs under control, at about 80% maximum speed. This control is necessary because it enables the player to change direction, using maximum agility in response to movements of other players and the ball.

Curvilinear motion is incorporated as the ball carrier maneuvers the ball in the dribbling action. The curved running feature, which occurs frequently, involves moving the body's center of gravity laterally toward the inside portion of the curve and then accelerating after "setting" into the curve.

All these movements are made while the player is carrying or maneuvering a field hockey stick. The additional weight of the stick, combined with its length and

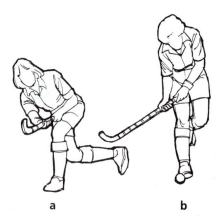

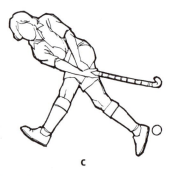

FIGURE 19.10 Note the differences in balance and positioning of the body parts in the execution of the following field hockey strokes: (a) the push pass; (b) the drive; (c) the drive on the run.

one-sided design (right-handed only), requires the player to have strength and considerable skill in manipulating the stick effectively.

The striking aspects are identical with those mentioned previously in other striking actions. The curved stick increases the length of the lever arm, allowing greater ball velocity than a straight stick.

Skills that must be mastered for effective and efficient play include achieving maximum ball velocity, being able to deliver the ball at a variety of angles, and being able to receive a ball coming in at a variety of

speeds. (See Chapter 1 on throwing and Chapter 14 on catching.) Patterns of movement include pushing and pulling as well as sequential joint action using the underarm and sidearm patterns.

During the 1984 Olympics in Los Angeles, Klatt (1984) studied all potential scoring opportunities of circle play: carry-in play; pass-in play; penalty corners; and penalty strokes. She used three-dimensional cinematography and computer simulation to determine temporal and kinematic characteristics.

Success in goal scoring off initial and follow-up shots was 6.5% for men and 7.0% for women. Significant results and biomechanical applications were categorized into technique, tactics, and game strategy as follows.

Techniques

1. Defensive players and goalkeepers, men and women, did not indicate a weak side, stick or non-stick side.
2. Offensive players demonstrated excellent speed but lacked maneuverability or change in direction.
3. On carry-in plays, offensive players averaged a 4.96 meters/sec velocity. Defensive players averaged 8.1 meters/sec at extreme angles, and movement was in all four planes.
4. Penalty corner data demonstrated greater accuracy on the pass-out and reception using a hit or drive-out compared to a push-out. Maximum shot/goal velocity was 31.6 meters/sec; an average time for the shot was 0.4 seconds.
5. The penalty stroke average velocity on the stroke was 21.1 meters/sec for men and 15.8 meters/sec for women. Execution of the flick stroke mechanically showed the men moving their center of gravity forward and into the stroke. Women executed the stroke moving back and away from the desired line of flight—possible reason for a lower velocity.

■ Environment and sport rules influence technique execution.

Tactics

1. Carry-in and pass-in plays on the offensive top left side of the circle showed defenders marking closely; on play developed down the right side, the defenders and goalkeepers interchanged responsibilities. Carry-into the circle (continuous ball control) resulted in "manufactured " fouls.

2. Second offensive players were available in support of the ball carrier on carry-in and pass-in play but were not used. Variables indicated that the ball carrier was pressured. Space and time appeared to be at a high premium.

3. Optimum scoring action on the penalty corner included the following:

   a. Designating a "corner team" of three players. The corner team must practice the drive or push-out so that the ball is received directly in front of the goal mouth.

   b. Holding the location of the reception consistent. Have the receiver move into the circle approximately one meter to reduce hit-out time and increase the angle open to the goal.

   c. Holding timing and direction of the shooter and shot on goal consistent; they must be practiced systematically.

   d. Positioning the defensive team so that no one crosses the visual path of the goalkeeper on the defensive rush.

   e. Having the goalkeeper move in direct line with the point of reception, moving out from the goal to decrease the opening to the goal mouth.

Game Strategy

Goals were scored on initial play into the circle (generally, a "fast break" situation); once play established itself in the circle, a dead ball situation usually occurred. Time means space—the strength and speed of today's players has "shrunk" the space inside the 16-yard striking circle. Rule makers in field hockey may need to consider increasing the size of the circle, goal cage, or both, for more success.

MINI-LABORATORY LEARNING EXPERIENCE

Use a stationary ball on the ground or batting tee and attempt to:

1. Contact the ball at the center of percussion. Include a variety of surfaces, e.g., floor, turf, and grass. Then contact the ball off center and observe the translatory motion that results.

2. Run carrying the hockey stick for 50 feet. Repeat without the stick. Repeat dribbling a field hockey ball. Run executing an air dribble. Time all runs and compare results.

3. Determine the distance a goalie can reach with the stick, with and without movement of the feet in relation to coverage of the entrance to the goal. Hint: draw a triangle with the apex at the center of the goal.

4. Try a flick (aerial) shot and a shot on the ground. Note the difference in the distance attained, especially in deep grass. Hint: friction may cause the difference.

5. Measure the dimensions of a field hockey stick and an ice hockey stick. Particularly note differences in length, blade portion, and curvature. Strike a hockey puck with the field hockey stick and strike a hockey ball with the ice hockey stick. Experiment with different sticks: goalkeeper sticks, floorhockey sticks, and weighted sticks. How do these sticks influence techniques, strategy, and general game play?

6. Discuss the effects or potential effects of the following on the game of field hockey.
   a. crowned synthetic turf playing field
   b. metal hockey sticks
   c. flat synthetic turf playing field
   d. changes in hockey stick weights: heavier, lighter, built up on back side of blade

Volleyball*

Volleyball is a striking activity and was transformed from an easy, recreational, fun game during the late 1950s and early 1960s to a complex, highly competitive game known as power volleyball. Top players developed high-level ability in striking, passing, jumping, and landing skills.

Some basic concepts involved in the game are as follows:

1. The various movements involved in the game must be understood since player positions are specialized, based on which movements the player can best execute.
2. Specificity of training must be recognized. A performer may be effective in one sport, but will need to perfect specific volleyball skills.
3. The better the feedback, the better the learning of motor skills.
4. Perhaps one of the most difficult skills in volleyball is spiking, since the performer must become airborne in an effort to exert maximum force on another airborne object, the ball. Often, otherwise perfected technique results in unsuccessful performance because of timing errors and inaccurate position relative to the ball.

The physical laws and principles involved in the various movements in striking, stopping an object, and passing, etc., apply in the game of volleyball. These will be discussed throughout this section. One of the most important concepts, the effect of impact on the ball or floor and these on the body, is determined by several factors:

1. The magnitude of the force can be reduced by prolonging the period of energy absorption.
2. The duration of the impact, if of high intensity, can be tolerated for only a brief period of time.
3. Spreading the forces over a large part of the body reduces the severity of the force.
4. A part of the body, such as the forearm, is best able to resist an impact if the focus of force is applied gently at first, and then gradually increased.

---

*Contributed by Mary Ridgway.

5. Striking a joint when it is at the extreme range of motion causes the joint to be moved beyond the normal range. Thus, not only the force of the blow, but the position of the body parts at the joint receiving the blow, determine the effect of the force.

Serving

All three basic patterns (underhand, overhand, and sidearm) of striking or projecting a ball can be used in executing the volleyball service. Although many players have been able to produce considerable spin using the underhand and sidearm services, the overhand service is the most effective type of service. The best type of service occurs when the ball travels with the fastest possible speed and flattest trajectory, forcing the receiver to respond in the shortest possible amount of time. Because of the law of gravitation—that is, all objects fall at the same rate—the overhand service will have the shortest air time and cause the receiver to make decisions and move more quickly than if either of the other two services are used. In addition, the lever systems and muscles used during the overhand service have the potential to create the greatest horizontal speed. Thus, the ball will be descending at a faster rate and a more horizontal angle, which is more difficult to receive than the sidearm and underhand services. For example, if the served ball is descending at a 30° angle, the arms of the receiver would need to be more vertical than horizontal. In terms of perception, this position is more difficult, and attenuation, by moving the arms in the same direction as the ball, is also more difficult.

To Increase Linear Velocity. In any style, it is important to hit with an optimally extended (not fully extended or locked) arm to increase linear velocity. It is also important to contact the ball in front of the body and to take a step or to shift the weight forward, thus transferring the momentum of the body to the ball at time of contact. By hitting approximately 6–12 inches in front of the body, the server can see the intended target area and the opponents' reception alignment.

Types of Serves. In volleyball, the most widely used types of serves are the over-floater, overhand topspin, roundhouse floater, and roundhouse topspin. The topspin serve is sometimes referred to as a drive or power serve. Accuracy as well as speed of travel are important considerations in serving. A taller player will have an advantage in serving because of increased linear velocity resulting from a longer system of levers. Additionally, the ball can be contacted at a decreased angle of projection, which increases the margin for error from an accuracy perspective and is advantageous in serving the ball to the specific target area. Another factor influencing a lower projection angle and a decreased time of flight is a fast arm swing. Beginning players often cannot generate the desired arm swing speed and, as a result, have to project the ball at a higher angle. Opponents, then, have more time to position themselves for the service reception. Since serving is a sequential striking skill, immature and ineffective patterns often appear as a push-like pattern with simultaneous segmental rotations occurring. In introducing overhand serving, it may be easier for the beginning server (sixth- or seventh-grader) to learn a roundhouse pattern since it is possible to achieve a longer lever action and produce more force on the ball with this pattern. It is a suitable choice of serve style, especially if the server is unable to develop the effective sequential pattern required in the traditional style of the overhead serve.

Float Serve. The float serve, equivalent to the knuckleball pitch in baseball, is an aerodynamic wonder and is often the serve style of preference because of the simplicity of the technique. It requires a lower projection angle and velocity than topspin serve styles because the ball is not dropping due to spin. Its unpredictable flight path can make it a difficult serve to receive and often requires the receiver to make last-minute positional adjustments because of a sudden deviation in flight path. Flight deviation may occur in a float serve as a result of the orientation of the seams and valve relative to the airflow. The nonsymmetrical surface of a volleyball gives rise to the turbulence and lower pressure zones that tend to shift around on the ball as it travels. Lift forces are produced at different areas, producing movements of the ball. Often players are instructed to position the air valve toward the opponent in order to induce greater movement on the ball. However, researchers have failed to validate this concept.

Since the ball is not perfectly symmetric with respect to weight, the type of flight obtained in a float serve will not maintain a parabolic curvature or a predictable modification because of spin, but will "wobble" or "float." The flight path depends on the ball's center of gravity, which may be to the right or left of the geometric center of the ball, or above or below it. A volleyball is relatively light in mass with a large, nonstreamlined profile and is usually out-of-round. In addition, it has patterned but irregular seams and an air valve. For the player to execute the float serve correctly, the ball must be struck through its center of mass so that rotation is not induced. The wrist should be kept extended (180°) at contact to minimize hitting the ball off center, in contrast to a topspin serve, in which hand flexion is important in producing an off-center hit.

Jump Serve. Another style of serving that is gaining popularity is the jump serve. This serve was initially used in the 1976 Montreal Olympic Games by several of the men's teams, and was common by the 1984 Olympic Games. Although this is a difficult serving style to master, the server can "spike" from the baseline at a higher velocity than is normally achieved in other patterns. It has a relatively short time of flight and often is hit with excessive topspin, which causes it to drop markedly during flight. A jump serve frequently results in an ace because the opponents do not make the necessary reception adjustments in time. Another factor that makes this service such an effective offensive weapon is that the server can actually be making ball contact from within the court, as long as the jump is initiated from behind the baseline. Two or three running steps may be taken to build up momentum for jump height. The coordinated action of trunk and shoulder rotation increases the range and speed of the sequential striking actions employed in serving.

Spiking

We will divide the spike into the following phases for analysis: approach; takeoff; body preparation during airborne phase; contact; follow-through; and landing.

Approach. For a regular high set, the spiker starts 8–12 feet from the net and takes a two- or three-step approach, which develops horizontal momentum. This horizontal momentum is converted to vertical momentum at takeoff to achieve jump height. In hitting from the side positions, the spiker should approach from outside the sideline in order to keep the ball in front of the hitting arm and to maximize the hitting area. Most hitters use a step-close or prejump approach and both are considered equally effective. On the plant step just prior to takeoff, the body is positioned at approximately 45° to the net when hitting strong side (left front) and middle (center front). This positions the hitting arm away from the ball, in addition to partially hiding the hitting arm from the opponent. The spiker can rotate through a large range of motion before contact, generating a high hitting velocity.

Takeoff. A forceful extension at the hips, knees, and ankles occurs as the spiker takes off from both feet. On quick sets, a one-foot takeoff is often used since jumping height is not as crucial. Quickness in getting to the set is a priority in hitting a front or back one-set. The one-foot takeoff enables the hitter to pivot and position behind the ball more effectively when running the various fast play patterns. A vigorous upward arm swing evokes additional force for takeoff propulsion. Estimations of arm swing contributions have been as much as 15% of the height of the jump. Spiking requires coordinating the jump and armswing in order to contact the moving ball in front of the body with an optimally extended contact arm.

Body Preparation During Airborne Phase. Once airborne, the spiker executes counter-rotation patterns on the backswing (forearm flexed, upper arm outwardly rotated, and hand hyperextended), which reduces the moment of inertia and increases the speed of rotation away from the ball prior to contact. The trunk is hyperextended, the hips and shoulders are rotated, and the striking arm is cocked, which increases the distance over which velocity is developed. The non-striking arm is extended upward. (See Figure 19.11.)

Contact. At contact, the body rotates and the left arm and shoulder drop quickly as the right arm moves toward the ball, with the elbow leading the motion. The striking shoulder elevates (left shoulder drops so right shoulder can get higher) to maximize a high ball-contact point. The trunk pikes (flexes), increasing momentum of the body. The more sequential the action of the trunk, upper arm, forearm, and hand, the more force produced.

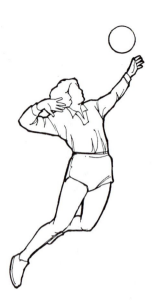

FIGURE 19.11 Position of the body and upper arm for a successful spike in volleyball.

The ball should be contacted in front of the body and with the arm optimally extended to maximize hitting velocity and to achieve the appropriate hitting angle. The distance through which the hand is accelerated is increased by inward rotation of the upper arm, forearm pronation, and hand flexion. "Snapping the wrist" (hand flexion) results in topspin being imparted to the ball as the hand wraps around the ball at contact producing an above-center eccentric force. Topspin results in a low pressure zone developing on the bottom of the ball, which causes the ball to drop more rapidly in flight and increase the chances of it staying in the court without compromising ball velocity.

Follow-Through. The follow-through of the spiking arm should be performed in a way that prevents violating the playing rules (e.g., hitting the net), losing linear velocity at contact by decelerating prior to contact, and preventing injury caused by the abrupt stopping of a fast-moving hitting arm that requires high-stopping forces.

Landing. Landing should be on both feet to increase the area over which landing forces act. Flexion occurs in the hips, knees, and ankles, which increases the time and distance over which force is absorbed.

Investigating spiking technique of elite and recreational female volleyball players, Ridgway and Hamilton (1991) reached several important conclusions:

For an effective spike, jump spikers should

1. develop a large horizontal velocity in the approach.
2. convert this velocity to a large vertical velocity at time of takeoff.
3. develop maximum tension during loading (the legs must withstand or minimize flexion of the knee during the setup phase).
4. not begin extension during the setup phase.

Furthermore, they indicated that the better spikers delayed premature extension during the loading phases, kept increasing their horizontal velocity throughout their approach, and generated higher angular velocities at the knee at time of takeoff. All of these factors result in higher jumps and a longer time of flight, which allow the spiker more latitude in adjusting to the set and successfully spiking the ball.

Volleyball Injuries and Prevention

Load. Load is recognized as a critical factor in the occurrence of pain and injury in volleyball. While most moves in volleyball occur without the ball, the highest loading occurs during landing movements associated with high intensity jumps at the net that are involved with spiking and blocking. A player may jump and land as many as 100 times per hour of play, and many of these landings occur on one foot. Many volleyball injuries occur in the lower extremity and back, usually as a result of landing on another player's foot. A sprained ankle can result from the unstable position of the ankle that occurs when the body is airborne. The relaxed foot tends to supinate, which is a most unstable position, and landing with the foot in this position makes it vulnerable to injury.

Impact Forces. Stacoff, Kaelin, and Stuessi (1986) report that impact forces in landing range from 1000 to 2000 N under the forefoot and from 1000 to 6500 N under the heel. The elastic limit of the cartilage is reached at approximately 5000 N. This limit was exceeded in almost 10% of the jumps they analyzed in their study. Clearly, shoes, surface, conditioning, and landing techniques should be scrutinized carefully. In volleyball competition as recently as 10–15 years ago, players preferred a thin-soled shoe that provided little cushioning and force absorption. Modern shoes can reduce landing forces by up to 30%. If a player, however, has weak ankles, the increased leverage provided by a thicker sole may cause the ankle to be more susceptible to sprains. If a player is suffering from jumper's knee, the extra cushioning provided by a thicker sole will minimize landing forces and is recommended. Athletes with ankle problems should train the peroneal muscles, wear thin-soled shoes, and use external devices such as high-topped shoes, ankle braces, and taping. Athletes with knee problems should wear thick-soled shoes, develop the calf muscles, and work on improved landing technique.

Preventing Injuries. In preventing injuries associated with floor skills such as diving and rolling, several factors should be considered. Split chins resulting from "bottoming out" (i.e., all body parts hitting the floor at the same time) in the dive can often be prevented through proper flexibility exercises in the neck and spine. In fact, certain players should not be taught to dive unless they have enough upper body strength and flexibility in the neck and spine to allow them to safely position the head off the floor when impact occurs.

Other factors often overlooked are the floor surface on which the dive is being executed and the jersey material and type and placement of the number on the player's jersey. Many of the synthetic surfaces impede the sliding of the player's body across the surface, which results in high forces being concentrated in certain areas of the player's body, namely, the chin, neck, and chest. If a player is wearing a jersey with a plastic number or logo that further increases the level of friction, the sliding action of the player during the floor move may be slowed, which decreases force absorption in the dive and increases stopping forces. More than one diver has had his or her chin stitched up as a result of sudden stopping action caused by a shirt number or rough textured, or even a dirty, sticky, floor. Additionally, proper technique must be emphasized in teaching floor skills. The worst scenario may involve a broken neck if the diver is unskilled and the dive is initiated from too high a position and too large an angle to the floor, negating proper dissipation of landing forces.

A major goal of the volleyball player is the replication of performance—the ability to continue successful execution of skills throughout the practice or competition. As fatigue occurs various performance variables are affected, which may result in pain, injury, or decrease in performance.

Jumping and Jump-Training in Volleyball

In the sport of volleyball, jumping depends not only on correct technique and leg strength but also on the ability to correctly load the muscles during the set-up phase. This phase begins when one foot hits the floor at the end of the approach and terminates when the legs reach maximum flexion. During negative work involved in the set-up phase, a certain quantity of elastic energy can be stored in the elastic elements in series found in the tendons and muscles. The energy stored during this eccentrically controlled work phase may be reused during the following concentric phase to improve jumping performance. A rapid lengthening of a muscle just prior to contraction results in a stronger contraction. This phenomenon is believed to be a result of the stretching of muscle spindles involving a myotatic reflex, which results in increased frequency of motor unit discharge, stimulation of other receptors, and an increased number of activated motor units. Other factors influencing the set-up phase include the velocity of the stretch and the time between the eccentric and concentric phases.

Depth Jump. For more than two decades, volleyball players have experimented with depth jumping (drop jumps or rebound jumps) as part of their jump training regime. Different drop heights are used, ranging from .3 m, which is recommended for first-year depth jumpers, to 1.10 m, which has been reported for training of elite athletes. Most researchers support the fact that depth jumping increases jump height, but fail to support that depth jumping is superior to other types of jump training. Bosco et al. (1981) were able to demonstrate that after 18 months of special plyometric training, eight volleyball players on the Finnish national team increased the elastic potential and stretch load tolerance of leg extensor muscles. Jensen and Russell (1986) report that depth jumping may be useful for teaching the regulation of muscle stiffness. They characterize optimum jump performance by high stretch velocities and short transitions between eccentric and concentric phases.

Based on research on the 1984 U.S. men's Olympic volleyball team, Colvin et al. (1984) suggest that optimum jumping technique is characterized by a forceful arm swing, a decisive blocking action with the arms (designed to transfer momentum developed in the arm swing to the body), and simultaneous extension at the hips, knees, and ankles during the extension phases. The less-skilled jumpers tended to extend at the knees and hips earlier than did the more-skilled jumpers. Time of support during the jump ranged from .26 sec to .38 sec.

MINI-LABORATORY LEARNING EXPERIENCE

1. Test jumping ability in a gymnasium volleyball situation.
2. Test jumping ability in a beach volleyball situation.
3. Compare and estimate magnitude of influence of environment and mechanics.
4. Observe locomotion during beach volleyball and gymnasium volleyball. Discuss friction, ground reaction forces, deformation, and other forces affecting movement.

Setting

Frequently, the setter in volleyball is compared to the quarterback in football—the "brains" of the outfit. Accuracy, speed of delivery, and deception are all necessary ingredients of good setting. Setting technique involves a push-like pattern, requiring simultaneous segmental rotations. As in other pushing patterns, the involved segments are aligned behind the object to be projected to allow for a flattening of the arc of the ball flight and greater accuracy. Finger action during the absorption phase involves stretching of the flexor muscles as a result of ball impact. This recoil action aids in ball projection.

In a study by Ridgway and Wilkerson (1986) of front setting and back setting, the investigators found that over 50% of the setters did not exhibit simultaneous extension of the legs and arms. The arms had begun movement toward the ball prior to leg extension. In high levels of quick, fast-paced play, frequently the setter has little opportunity to position in such a way that allows the use of the legs. As a result, the setter has an arm-dominated pattern. Quick sets such as the one-set or two-set are characterized by a greater ball absorption phase in the setter's hands and a slower projection velocity. The time of ball contact in the hands ranges from .054 sec for a low set to .072 sec for a high outside front set to .086 sec for a high back set. The volleyball official has a difficult task in judging the legality of a set because of two obvious factors: (1) the ball actually does come to rest in the setter's hands as it changes direction of motion during the absorption and propulsion phases; and (2) the setting technique, whether it be a high set or a quick set, often occurs in less than .01 sec. An official must not be too quick to make a judgment regarding an illegal hit because the setter appears to be poorly positioned for executing the set. Judging how long the ball rests in the hands is beyond the scope of this text.

Forearm Pass. Passing may well be the least glamorous of all volleyball techniques. Every offensive play, however, begins with a pass. Some of the variables influencing forearm passing success are the varying ball speeds, angles, and unpredictable flight paths associated with float serves and block deflections. In order to meet one of the goals of today's game, that of isolating hitters against only one blocker, passing must be quick, accurate, and consistent. The position of the setter should be such that there is a choice of several quick play-sets rather than a single choice through a double block.

Contour and size of contact area influence both the consistency of execution of the skill and the likelihood of injury to the body. "The greater the surface area, the less force per square centimeter" is a principle that can be applied to this skill. Injury is not likely to occur to hands; however, forearms do become bruised because the ball impacts against the flesh surrounding the radius and ulna. If there is insufficient adipose tissue or muscle, the deformation caused by the impact will force the small blood vessels against these bones, causing hematoma. Players often wear long-sleeved shirts to protect their forearms from bruises.

Receiving a Spike or Service in Volleyball

Served balls and spiked balls usually are received by means of an underhand hit termed a "forearm pass." In these situations, the volleyball has greater speeds, and, therefore, more kinetic energy and momentum, than in any other situation occurring in the volleyball game. Thus, the volleyball player uses the forearms as rebounding surfaces, rather than using the hands with the active flexion of the fingers (overhand passing technique). The speed and angle of the incoming spike and serve and the distance the ball must be passed determine whether the receiver will attenuate (absorb) the force or will apply force to the ball.

The first goal of the passer receiving a spiked or served ball is to establish a stable base of support. This base is best taken with the feet shoulder-distance apart with one foot slightly ahead of the other with the weight on the balls and insides of the feet. When it is not possible to play the ball off the midline of the body, a step with a pivot to the side is used to position the arms toward the path of the ball. Since spiked balls have a primarily downward flight, there is no need to widen the base of support in the anteroposterior direction to any great extent. Even in the case of served balls, the trajectory is apt to be 30–60° with the horizontal. Thus, the horizontal momentum is less than one-half that of a well-hit volleyball spike traveling 120 kmph (74 mph).

The type of contact and the surfaces of contact determine the amount of rebound velocity of the ball. Any forward motion of the arms will apply a force to the ball and impart additional velocity to it. If the arms are stationary at contact, the amount of tension and the amount of fleshy tissue determine the amount of attenuation of the force of the ball. For example, a ball dropped from a height of approximately seven meters will rebound almost two meters after impact on a wooden floor. The ball will rebound one meter (half that distance) if the impact is made on a maximally tensed, bony, tendinous surface such as the forearm. If, however, little effort is made to tense the arms, the rebound will be greatly reduced, to as little as, or less than 20 cm. If the shoulders are pulled back and the hips thrust forward, greater force absorption occurs in response to hard-hit balls. Thus, it is important both to develop kinesthetic awareness of the amount of tension in the arms, including the shoulder stabilization tension, and to be able to estimate the speed and angle of the incoming ball.

The flatness of the contact area is paramount for consistency in directing the ball. Theoretically, the anterior surface of the wrist and heel of the hand are best because of their flatness and large surface area. There is, however, the problem of stabilizing the two hands so that the forearms act as one unit. It is not normally recommended that the hands or the heels of the hands be used for contact on the forearm pass. The contact should be above the wrist and below the elbow, on the fleshy portion of the forearm, although some passers do clasp the hands together and use the radial surfaces of the forearms as the contact site.

Players position the rebounding surfaces for the desired angle of rebound primarily by means of shoulder flexion. The angle of the arms with respect to the trajectory of the ball determines, in part, the angle of rebound. For example, if the ball enters at a 90° angle to the arms, it will rebound at a nearly 90° angle. Angles of rebound and incidence are often dissimilar in volleyball, since balls have spin and are impacted with moving arms. This statement is based on Newton's third law and the coefficients of friction and elasticity. As the ball rebounds, the speed can be vectorally added to show the influence of spin, elasticity, and friction. Knowing the incoming speed and angle of the ball, we can predict the speed and angle of the rebound. Frequently, teams running fast offenses want low-trajectory passes to shorten the time it takes to run an offensive play. This decreases the time the defense has to set up against the attack. To accomplish this fast, low-arc pass, the passer has the arms pointing toward the floor and the back held straight. Projection angles of 30–50° are not uncommon, but, since the time of flight has been reduced, low passes require greater setter mobility.

Ridgway and Hamilton (1987) profiled low-skilled and high-skilled passers. The low-skilled passers were junior high and junior varsity players and their passing patterns were characterized by over-swinging at the shoulders; short ball contact time, which decreased force absorption of the ball; contacting the ball too close to the thumbs and wrists, thus decreasing force absorption, and passing too high (71° vs. 63°), which apparently resulted

from an erect head and upright trunk posture. Due to gravitational acceleration, high passes have a greater descent velocity, which makes it difficult for the setter to set. The setter must focus too high above the court, which interferes with the peripheral vision used in locating the hitters and opponents. High passes also have a longer flight time, which gives the opponents more time to set up their defense.

Blocking

Balls are blocked to prevent the opposing team from making a successful hit over the net; to reduce the force on a spiked ball; to force the opposing attacker to hit the ball toward the defense; or to take away the favorite shots of the opposing hitter. There may be one, two, or sometimes three blockers at the net. One blocker's action is described here.

The blocker is positioned close to the net so that the plane of the net may be penetrated in blocking the ball. In preparing for the jump to block the hit, the blocker places the feet approximately hip-width with legs flexed. The arms are first moved to bring force against the feet and then moved upward to aid in summation of the forces in the upward vertical jump to increase the height of the reach of the arms.

The arms of the blocker are elevated vertically and then the hands are flexed and moved forward above and across the net. The blocker's hands reach across the net to prevent the ball from coming down on the blocker's side. This arm movement takes away a larger portion of the hitting area of the court than if the hands are just above the net (see Figure 19.12).

The blocker jumps after the hitter jumps in order to time the block and to keep the ball from rebounding from the hands and going out-of-bounds. The blocker actually delays the jump for the block until the hitter is near the apex of the jump.

Since new ways of placing the hands during a block may arise, the main concept is to maximize hand area so a block can be successful. The wrists and hands should be firm at ball contact so injury to the finger joints does not occur.

Comparing the block jump and a counter-movement training jump performed by elite college and recreational female volleyball players, Ridgway (1990) found several differences between performance and training jump technique.

Major differences between the selected *training jump* (TJ) and *block jump* (BJ) included:

1. Use of arms in BJ is restricted. There is limited shoulder flexion in the BJ with exaggerated abduction moves employing different muscle groups than what would be used in the TJ, which uses large ranges of shoulder extension/flexion and a minimum of abduction.
2. Arms are decelerating at takeoff in TJs and are reaching maximum velocity at takeoff in BJs.
3. Head and trunk positioning varies greatly between the TJ and BJ, with more extension and less flexion used in the BJ.
4. Shorter landing times, smaller ranges of motion in the lower extremities, and greater landing forces may be occurring with the BJ as the player descends close to the net attempting to maintain balance.

Differences between *elite* and *recreational* players included:

1. Elite players use the arms differently in the BJ than do recreational players. As the legs flex prior to extension, the upper arms execute an arm pump by bringing the arms close to the body, then vigorous abduction occurs with takeoff.
2. Several of the recreational blockers took a hop or shuffle step forward before initiating the BJ.
3. Elite players, through the mechanics and motor integration of their jumping technique, reach a higher vertical velocity of their body mass center of gravity at takeoff, which results in a higher jump and a greater time of flight.
4. A greater time of flight may allow the player more options as to blocking technique, e.g., skilled jumpers usually pike during the block and have better arm penetration over the net. (See Figure 19.12.)

Training jumps and performance jumps share certain common technique characteristics, but there are also numerous critical differences. The coach and athlete should exercise caution in using generic vertical jumps

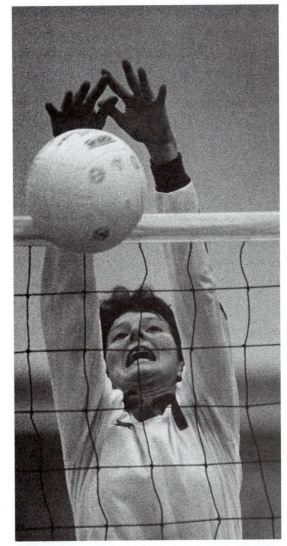

FIGURE 19.12 Blocking requires not only precise timing, but the appropriate positioning of the hands. This player has extended the upper body to its maximum after a forceful jump. The hands then reach forward toward the net fully extended to contact as much of the ball as possible.

as the nucleus of a jump training program. In designing an effective jump training program for success in both spiking and blocking, they should emphasize simulating performance requirements and rule restrictions imposed on the vertical jump under performance conditions.

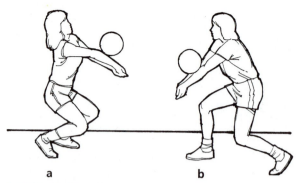

a   b

FIGURE 19.13 Examples of two volleyball players prepared to receive and pass the volleyball using a forearm bump type pass. Describe the differences and problems with the low-skilled technique (*a*) compared to that of the higher-skilled passer (*b*).

MINI-LABORATORY LEARNING EXPERIENCE

Study the low-skilled and high-skilled execution of a forearm pass. Discuss observable differences in technique and how these differences influence passing performance (Figure 19.13).

References

LEGENDS

BB   Basketball

VB   Volleyball

FH   Field hockey

HB   Handball

S   Soccer

BB   Allsen, P. E., and Ruffner, W. 1969. Relationship between the type of pass and the loss of the ball in basketball. *Athletic Journal* 49, September:105–7.

BB   Bergandip, T. A., Shryock, M. G., and Titust T. G. 1990. The basketball concentration survey: Preliminary development and validation. *Sport psychologists* 4(2): 119–29.

VB   Bosco, C., Komi, P., Pulli, M., Pettera, C., and Montonev, H. 1981. Considerations of the training of the elastic potential of the human skeletal muscle. *Volleyball*, 2:22–30.

BB   Brancazio, P. J. 1984. *Sports science physical laws and optimum performances*. New York: Simon and Schuster.

S   Brown, E. W., and Williamson, G. 1991. *Youth soccer: Complete handbook*. Dubuque, IA: Brown & Benchmark.

VB   Coleman, J. E., and Liskewych, F. N. 1974. *Pictoral analysis of power volleyball*. Hollywood CA: Creative Sports Books.

VB   Colvin, W., Beal, D., and Zier, D. 1984. A kinetic analysis of the vertical jump with arm swing. Paper presented at the 2nd International Symposium of Biomechanics in Sports, Colorado Springs, CO.

BB   Cooper, J., and Siedentop, D. 1969. *The theory and science of basketball*. Philadelphia: Lea and Febiger.

BB   Cousy, B., and Powers, F. 1970. *Basketball concepts and techniques*. Boston: Allyn and Bacon.

HB   Fleck, Steven J., et al. 1992. The relationships among ball velocity during set and jump shots and isokinetic torque of selected upper body improvements in team handball. *Journal of Applied Science Sports* 6(2).

BB   Hess, C. 1980. Analysis of the jump shot. *Athletic Journal,* November 1(3):30–58.

BB   Husdon, J. 1986. Shooting techniques for small players. *Athletic Journal* 66(3):40–45.

VB   Jensen, J., and Russell, P. 1986. Depth jumping and the volleyball spike. In *Biomechanics in sports III & IV*, eds. J. Terauds, B. Gowitzke, and L. Holt. Del Mar, CA: Academic Publishers.

BB   Kendalls, G., et al. 1990. The effects of an imagery rehearsal, relaxation and self-talk package on basketball game performance. *Journal of Sport and Exercise Psychology* 12(2):157–66.

FH   Klatt, L. A. 1977. Kinematic and temporal characteristics of a successful penalty corner in women's field hockey. Ph.D. dissertation, Indiana University.

FH   Klatt, L. A. 1984. A special study of male and female field hockey at the 1984 Olympics. Unpublished manuscript.

BB   Lehmann, G. 1981. *Basketball is my game: Lessons by Lehmann*. NJ: Riverside.

BB   Macauley, E. 1970. Anatomy of the jump shot. *Scholastic Coach,* December 8:11.

BB   Martin, T. 1981. Movement analysis applied to the basketball jump shot. *The Physical Educator* 3(38): 127–33.

VB   Ridgway, M. 1990. Comparison of the vertical jump utilized in the volleyball block with the standing vertical jump with arm swing. In *Biomechanics in sports VI*. Del Mar, CA: Academic Publishers.

VB   Ridgway, M., and Hamilton, N. 1987. The kinematics of forearm passing in low-skilled and high-skilled volleyball players. In *Biomechanics in sports V*. Del Mar, CA: Academic Publishers.

VB Ridgway, M., and Hamilton, N. 1991. Spiking technique of elite and recreational female volleyball players. In *Biomechanics in sports VII*. Del Mar, CA: Academic Publishers.

VB Ridgway, M., and Wilkerson, J. 1986. A kinetic analysis of the front set and back set in volleyball. In *Biomechanics in sports III & IV,* eds. J. Terauds, B. Gowitzke, and L. Holt. Del Mar, CA: Academic Publishers.

VB Sardinha, L., and Zebast, C. 1986. The effect of perceived fatigue on volleyball spike skill performance. In *Biomechanics in sports III & IV,* eds. J. Terauds, B. Gowitzke, and L. Holt. Del Mar, CA: Academic Publishers.

VB Stacoff, A., Kaelin, X., and Stuessi, E. 1986. Foot-movement, load and injury in volleyball. In *Biomechanics in sports III & IV,* eds. J. Terauds, B. Gowitzke, and L. Holt. Del Mar, CA: Academic Publishers.

HB *Team Handball USA Magazine,* January, 1990, March, 1991. Published by the US Handball Federation, Colorado Springs, CO.

BB Williams, W. 1983. The relationships of selected natural traits to statistical game performances. Ph.D. dissertation, Indiana University.

BB Wooden, J. R. 1980. *Practical modern basketball,* 2nd ed. New York: Wiley.

20 Biomechanics of Combatives

Two combatants face each other in close proximity, each attempting to outwit and defeat the other by means of striking, shoving, or throwing actions. Force vectors, timing, summation of forces, leverage, and center-of-gravity concepts are involved.

The smoke rises like solid grey beams in the hot light. All attention is focused on the two men in the small canvas square below, their bodies slick with sweat, faces distorted with mouthpieces, hands taped and gloved into shapeless weapons. What protection do they have from the blows of the opponent? Will conditioning and fast reflexes save them? How much force can a punch produce? How will the opponent minimize these forces?

What part will friction play? Who designed the shoes the way they are and why? Could they be better? What about the surface of the ring and the interface between the shoe-foot-ring surface? What are the ideal frictional values and what are the real ones?

In total silence, the two figures play each other up and down the narrow copper strip. Opponents, yet moving as partners, as though dancing an adagio in white. Each looks for a concentration break, one movement a little too large, and three feet of steel move forward at dazzling speed to find the open target with the tiny point. How fast is the attack? What is the time span between the decision to act and the act itself? Is speed more important than deception? The defense, how fast is it? Is it reflexive? How much force do fencers impart to the target? What is the line of force? Does it vary? Do skilled fencers produce and use forces differently than less-skilled fencers?

Answering Questions with Biomechanical Principles

The questions never stop. Each answer provides a small piece of information, which gives the next curious person a starting place. We know so little; we need to know so much more. Some of what we "know" may not even be true. We can be statistically positive, but we can never be sure. We must always remember to doubt. But the doubt must be informed; otherwise, it lapses into opinion.

How can we support the statements we make? Since the combatives can all be broken down into the basic movements of kicking, striking, pushing, and pulling, we can apply certain principles of mechanics to the questions we wish to answer. What are these principles? Certainly, the Newtonian principles of $F = ma$, impulse-momentum, work-kinetic energy, and potential energy apply. In defenses such as blocks and parries, the principles of stability and force absorption can be guides in answering questions. In each sport the action is that of two persons in close proximity to each other. Time, or timing of the actions, is very important. The techniques must be done skillfully, but will be of no value if performed a few milliseconds too early or too late. Analyzing combatives requires that the actions of both performers be analyzed in context with each other, as well as the determinants of success in the execution of each movement.

Karate*

The movements in karate are highly complex and often are represented in terms of descriptive models designed to depict particular points, phases, or events within a dynamic movement sequence. Concepts are often taught in the form of dichotomies. Nakayama (1977) alludes to three dichotomies that explain movement concepts of karate kata (formal exercise training). These may be extrapolated to all forms and aspects of karate: *Kata, Kihon* (basic technique training), *Kumite* (partner training), and sport karate competition.

Proper Use of Various Elements

Expansion and Contraction of the Body. The expansion and contraction of the body refers to the effective use of space and distance as a mode for accomplishing movement goals. The use of the body's full range of motion is necessary to cover distance to advance or retreat from an opponent, execute techniques at the optimal range, and provide an area in which force may be developed.

Use of Tension and Relaxation. Quality movement also requires graded interaction of tension and relaxation of musculature to provide for the expansion and contraction of the body and segments. Segment stability, coordinated agonistic and antagonistic tensions, and synergistic functioning are important to karate.

Use of Speed and Power. In karate, often only a fast movement is needed and, at other times, considerable power is required. The use of speed and power is dictated by the purpose of the technique.

*Contributed by Paul Smith.

Essential Movement Elements. Karate movement requires the integration of several basic factors to generate mechanical and aesthetic standards of quality. Elements of each of the following concepts are necessary in varying degrees for all movement.

Form. Form pertains to the outward, or visible, shape of a body (performer), which is molded by discipline and training. This may involve the whole body or segmental parts. Proper positioning for action is paramount. A certain level of aesthetic quality is associated with karate form and movement. Positioning of the body or its segments helps provide for the strength and/or stability of terminal body positions in preparation for the intermediate, transitional phases of a movement.

Balance or Equilibrium. Balance, or **equilibrium,** is necessary for the purposeful body positions and movements of karate.

Timing. Timing is a term used to denote synchrony or coordination. Internal timing is the coordination of muscular contractions to produce smooth, rhythmic movement. It is this quality that allows forces of individual segments to be summed up in such a way that the velocity of the fist, for example, is much faster than the speed contributed from arm extension alone. Body segments are coordinated so that the positive velocity of the center of gravity, hip rotation velocity, shoulder protraction velocity, and the linear velocity of the fist due to forearm extension are accelerated when the preceding segment in the chain is at its peak velocity to produce this effect. (See Figure 20.1.)

External timing simply refers to the coordination of movement of one system, such as a person, with another to meet a certain purpose. For example, correct timing is said to have taken place when a person counterattacks at an adversary's weakest position in a technique.

Rhythm. Rhythm is the regularity of beat, accent, rise, fall, or period of an event. In karate sparring, one partner may be noting the breathing rhythm of the opponent. This allows the first person to time the attack to impact when the second person is at the weakest point in the cycle—just as the opponent is finishing exhalation.

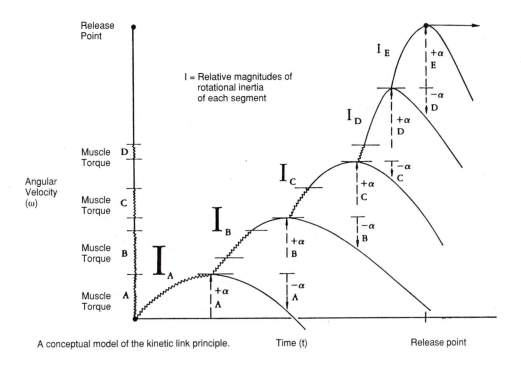

Release Point

I = Relative magnitudes of rotational inertia of each segment

Angular Velocity (ω)

Muscle Torque D
Muscle Torque C
Muscle Torque B
Muscle Torque A

I_A
I_B
I_C
I_D
I_E

$+\alpha$ A
$-\alpha$ A
$+\alpha$ B
$-\alpha$ B
$+\alpha$ C
$-\alpha$ C
$+\alpha$ D
$-\alpha$ D
$+\alpha$ E

A conceptual model of the kinetic link principle.

Time (t)

Release point

FIGURE 20.1 Conceptual model of summation of forces based on the kinetic-link principle of the human body. When each body segment begins its movement at the optimum time, the greatest velocity can be achieved at the final and distal body segment.

The establishment of a rhythmic movement greatly facilitates internal timing for a higher quality movement and allows the exploitation of the myotatic reflex to increase force generated by the body. Also known as the stretch reflex, the myotatic response prevents segments from moving beyond their range of motion by contracting antagonistic musculature when a segment is displaced rapidly. Rhythmicity and effective internal timing tend to maximize this effect. In snap kicking, for example, when the shank is smartly flexed prior to extension, the rapid stretching of the quadriceps muscle generates a violent contraction that serves to add considerable force to the kick. When the opposite or "draw hand" is quickly retracted in punching at the start of a punch, this effect takes place across the chest and serves to enhance the speed of the punching arm.

Speed. Speed is the rate at which a point changes position. As a scalar quantity, only the magnitude is specified and the object can be moving in any direction. The corresponding vector quantity, velocity, is probably a more appropriate term to use in karate since the magnitude and direction of the rate of change in position must be specified. As an example, the foot may be moving at 10 meters per second. But if it is moving in the wrong direction to accomplish a particular purpose, this speed is of little value. Though not technically correct, the term speed is often used interchangeably with velocity when the direction of movement is understood. In human movement, control of the velocity of the body and its segments is essential for techniques of high quality.

Power. **Power** is the time rate at which energy is converted into work. If a weight or force is moved a particular distance, work is being done. If that work is done quickly, in a short period of time, then a large amount of power is exerted. In karate impacts, it is often desirable to attack or counterattack with a great deal of power.

This entails not only striking the opponent with a quickly moving fist, but with a large amount of quickly moving weight connected to the fist. For certain types of impact, it is more desirable to maximize the velocity of the fist at impact—such as with a strike to a nerve center located close to the surface of the body or in the face. In other cases, such as when the nerve center is deeper within the body or greater penetration is desired, as with the trunk or ribs, more mass is needed to thrust the fist further into the target area. In these latter cases it may be beneficial to sacrifice some velocity in order to get more mass into the punch.

Focus. Focus in oriental martial arts refers to the concentration of energy. In karate the term *kime* can be translated to mean the concentration of energy at a particular point. *Kime* involves connecting the segments at impact to the body weapon, which is moving at its peak velocity. In striking or angular movements, body connection is accomplished by the body's natural mechanism to prevent joint damage, the stretch reflex. This braking system of the body starts the contraction of antagonistic musculature at approximately 70–80% completion of the full range of motion. By timing impact to occur within this range with a full-speed movement like a snap kick, the mass of body is connected to the leg segments by antagonistic muscle contractions taking place while the foot is moving at peak velocity. In this manner more energy and momentum are transmitted to the target.

With thrusting movements, considerable reaction force may be expected, particularly if deep penetration is desired or the impacted object has sufficient integrity. In this case it is important to prepare the body for the impact by stabilizing the joints firmly into their natural positions. By attempting to achieve a full range of motion and impacting the target at between 70% and 80% of full extension, the fist in a punch would be at maximum velocity. The effort of tensing agonistic and antagonistic musculature immediately at impact allows the body weight to be committed to the target with maximum velocity. It also helps to stabilize the joints to accept strong reaction forces generated by the target back to the fist. The fist is, in effect, thrust through the surface into the target. It is important to understand that focus is a very complex phenomenon and requires considerable practice to be executed in a natural, reflexive manner.

The Role of the Trunk in Karate

Vitally important to karate movements is the use of the most massive segment of the body, the trunk. Because the body center of gravity is located in the lower abdominal area of the trunk, movement is initiated with this segment. Three methods are used for this purpose: hip vibration, positive hip rotation, and reverse rotation.

Hip vibration is the sharp tensing of the lower abdominal area to stabilize the central body, to prevent its rotation. The person experiences a "vibration" feeling. The trunk becomes a firm base from which the limbs can push, throw, thrust, or snap. Correct stances provide firm support and motive forces for the trunk.

Positive hip rotation occurs when the pelvis rotates in the direction of the target. This contributes to the angular movement of the punching or kicking side of the body, during such skills as the reverse punch and jabbing punch.

Reverse rotation of the trunk takes place when the hip is rotated away from the target to be impacted. Used with many striking and blocking techniques, this action capitalizes on the force couple present about the shoulder joint.

Movement Patterns

Two general movement patterns are used to generate forces in karate skills: throw-like patterns and push-like patterns. Actually, a push-throw continuum exists, with movement tending to act as a function of the mass-velocity interrelationships of the objects or, in the case of karate, the body weapon and the target to be impacted, as well as the intended effect of the impact.

Throw-like Patterns. These are characterized by an angular application of force to the target. Examples of throw-like patterns are the "snapping" or "striking" techniques such as the backfist strike, knifehand strike, and front snapping kick. With this type of pattern, segmental movement takes place in a sequential manner from the more-massive to the less-massive segments. Retraction of the weapon follows a reverse order sequence. Forces are summed from segment to segment by the transfer of momentum to each succeeding link. This type of pattern is classified as an open-end system because the distal end of the chain is free to move during the execution, or force-generating, phase.

Throw-like, or "striking," patterns generate higher velocities at the hand or foot than push-like or "thrusting" movements, though less mass is involved in the strike at impact. With throw-like techniques, the force is delivered in an angular fashion and is particularly effective when more of a shock effect is desired. The relative mass relationship between the fist or foot impactor and the target is of great importance. In a perfectly elastic collision where both masses are the same, all the momentum will be transferred to the target with the impactor stopping and the target object moving away from the impactor at the same velocity the impactor was traveling. When the impactor has less mass, it will tend to rebound and the target will be displaced at a rate slower than the impactor was traveling. If the target has less mass, the impactor will still move in its previous direction, and the target will tend to bounce away faster than the impactor was moving.

Push-like Patterns. These patterns in karate, such as the side thrust kick and the straight punch, are located toward the push-like end of the continuum. Because penetration of more massive targets, or a crush, rather than a shock effect is desired, relatively more mass must be applied to the target, even with the loss of some velocity. In this case the segments tend to move in a more simultaneous fashion, and force is applied in more of a linear, rather than an angular, pathway. More of the body's weight is behind the impacting weapon. Because succeeding segments in the chain do not begin accelerating at the maximum velocity point of the preceding segment, the weapon does not reach the level of speed generated with the throw-like movement pattern. However, due to the more linear alignment of the body and weapon, more mass is directly involved at impact. Comparable levels of momentum may, therefore, be expected. But the lower peak force is applied for a longer period of time, assuming equal target inertia.

Maximizing Kinetic Energy and Momentum of Karate Skills

The training of striking and thrusting skills should be oriented toward the increase of velocity of the weapon in order to maximize both the momentum and kinetic energy of the system. Recall that:

$$KE = (\tfrac{1}{2})mv^2$$
$$\text{and}$$
$$M = mv$$

Because kinetic energy *(KE)* is the product of one-half the mass *(m)* and the square of the velocity *(v)* of the impacting system, and momentum *(M)* is the product of the mass *(m)* times the velocity *(v)* of the system, velocity can be considered a more critical element in the ability of the punch or kick to do damage to the target. An increase in the amount of mass involved in the impact, but not in the velocity achieved, appears to be a function of the skill level of karate punchers. The more-skillful punchers are better able to coordinate more mass into their movements.

Linear impact velocities for thrusting punches and kicks have been reported to range from about 7 m/s to 12 m/s. Tangential impact velocities for angular techniques reported from various studies have been about 2–4 m/s faster. One researcher reported a tangential impact velocity of 19 m/s for a roundhouse kick, an angular movement (Walker 1980).

Safety Equipment and Injury Probability

The nature of collisions, the probability of injury, and the impact attenuation effects of safety equipment are currently topics of study at several laboratories. Key variables of interest are impact velocity, effective mass during impact, resultant acceleration of tissues and segments, chest and head compression, force, and the momentum-impulse relationship. The probability of injury at different body locations, such as the head or thorax, varies according to the nature of the impact event and is a field of study in itself. The ability to inflict serious or critical injury, or even death, is well within the range of any expertly delivered karate technique. Therefore, the use of safety equipment and the control of contact are vital issues for sport karate competition.

Biomechanics of Combatives **431**

ID: 832WORH

832WORH

Date: 8-NOV-1991
Time: 12:02:52

FIGURE 20.2 Impact recordings of roundhouse (RH) and straight kick (SK) when wearing a chest protector.

Sternal (UP) Acc – SAE 180   Min = –41.824 @ 32. ms   Max = 44.397 @ 25. ms

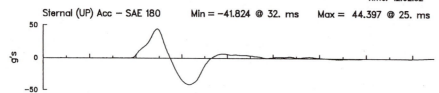

Sternal (LO) Acc – SAE 180   Min = –43.260 @ 30. ms   Max = 61.134 @ 24. ms

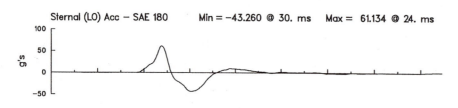

Spinal Acc – SAE 180   Min = –18.194 @ 29. ms   Max = 3.942 @ 38. ms

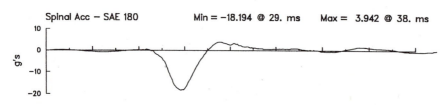

Deflection – SAE 60   Min = –14.397 @ 32. ms   Max = 0.019 @ 8. ms

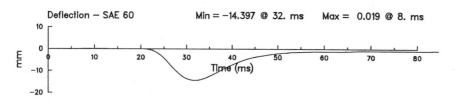

VC – SAE 60   Min = –0.066 @ 35. ms   Max = 0.105 @ 28. ms

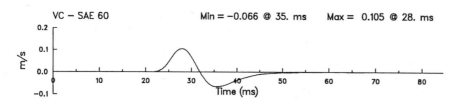

odim = 180. mm   karate2

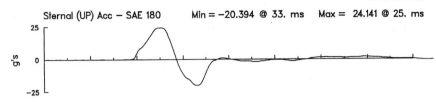

Sternal (UP) Acc — SAE 180   Min = −20.394 @ 33. ms   Max = 24.141 @ 25. ms

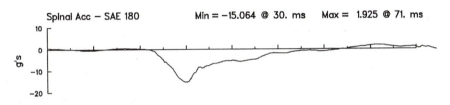

Sternal (LO) Acc — SAE 180   Min = −19.025 @ 29. ms   Max = 38.160 @ 25. ms

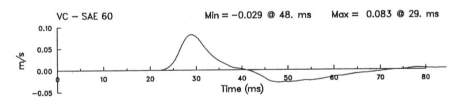

Spinal Acc — SAE 180   Min = −15.064 @ 30. ms   Max = 1.925 @ 71. ms

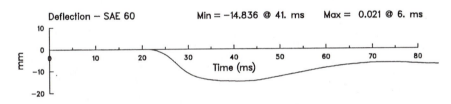

Deflection — SAE 60   Min = −14.836 @ 41. ms   Max = 0.021 @ 6. ms

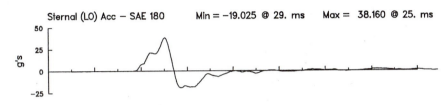

VC — SAE 60   Min = −0.029 @ 48. ms   Max = 0.083 @ 29. ms

odim = 180. mm   karate2

Biomechanics of Combatives   **433**

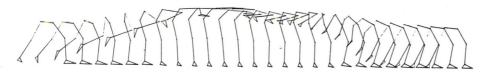

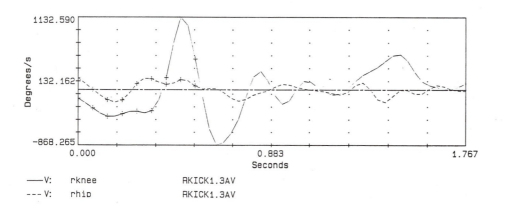

FIGURE 20.3 Angular displacement-time recordings of a karate kick.

Researchers have generally shown that safety equipment can reduce the probability of injury by absorbing impact forces or spreading the force over greater area, distance, or time. For example, it has been demonstrated (McLatchie 1981) that the use of a chest protector can make a difference in the nature of injuries that would occur from linear and angular punches and kicks of international-class karate athletes of third through seventh degree black belt levels. (See Figures 20.2 and 20.3.) Viscous Criteria (VC) index values were found to be below the point that would cause a medically severe injury (VC = 1) when using the chest protector. Without the chest protector, impact levels generated by these techniques were above the level that would cause severe injury. Characteristic shapes of acceleration and deflection waveforms tend to remain relatively unchanged for linear and angular technique types.

Punching Gloves and Karate. Punching gloves were originally devised to benefit the puncher rather than the person being hit. Most of us think of the glove as providing a safety margin for the person being impacted. This may be false because gloves provide support for the puncher's wrist and padding for the knuckles. Consequently, the natural limiting effect of pain from hitting something is lessened, allowing the karate participant or boxer to punch harder. The result can be counterproductive for the person being hit because greater momentum transferred to the head or thorax can cause higher accelerations of body tissues. Long-term serious injuries are more closely related to internal head and body tissue accelerations than injury from the forces that occur at the surface of the face or chest. Many injury effects are cumulative, and, from a safety standpoint, competition would be much less dangerous if contact between competitors was limited to low impact or no-contact situations, as with the classical forms of karate.

Whether different types of punching gloves could attenuate forces from karate blows below concussion levels for head impacts has not been fully demonstrated. The type of padding used in gloves and the nature of thumb stabilization are of major importance. Older style gloves with hair padding tend to "bottom out" with repeated impacts. Composite padding arrangements of materials with varying force-absorption characteristics tend to have better force-absorption response capabilities that cover the ranges of force generated by boxing and karate athletes. Thumbless glove designs or gloves in which the thumb is sewn to the fist are now required by most sanctioning organizations.

Boxing

Boxing has been practiced both as a sport and for self-defense since prehistoric times. Although professional boxing has waxed and waned in popularity, amateur boxing still enjoys a high number of participants. While the boxer can be among the fittest of athletes, some object to boxing on moral grounds. Since the object of boxing is to incapacitate the opponent, boxing can, by its very nature, cause injury. Boxers have much in common with karatekas in that they must impart and withstand forces and must move with precision and speed. The boxer, however, imparts a large amount of momentum to the entire mass of the opponent, while the karateka focuses power on one small body area.

Additionally, boxing involves the extraneous movements of bobbing, weaving, and ducking, either to avoid punches or set up the opponent. The boxer must carry the center of gravity higher than either the judo or karate participant, because boxing is more mobile than either of these sports. Additionally, the boxer does not always deliver power in a straight line, but often moves the hands in a circular type of motion to the target, as, for example, when delivering a roundhouse punch.

For the boxer, the problems of generating and absorbing force are of prime importance. From a position less stable than that of the judo or karate performer, the boxer must generate force and absorb it, not once but many times over. How does the boxer deal with these problems?

First, the boxer develops a great deal of musculature; the larger the muscle, the more strength available that can be used to generate power or to absorb the force of repeated blows. The boxer is also able to take advantage of the principle of the summation of forces. The amateur boxer especially counts on repeated impacts to "wear the opponent down." Here lies a basic problem with boxing: Although it actually ranks only tenth or eleventh in number of serious injuries, repeated impacts cause trauma that may not become apparent for a number of years.

■ **External collisions can cause unseen internal trauma.**

When a boxer sustains a blow to the head, the head is accelerated backwards. The brain, which is suspended in a cerebrospinal fluid inside the skull, moves the same way. The two main areas of the brain, gray and white matter, are accelerated, too, but at different rates. This difference in rate leads to shearing forces between the gray and white matter. Some nerve cells can be damaged and others can die, never to be replaced. Additionally, in the collision of the brain with the skull, both the front and back of the brain can be damaged. The common manifestation of this type of injury is the individual who appears to be in a stupor or drunk. Loss of memory as well as loss of functional ability may occur.

A primary concern is that the boxer could suffer a ruptured blood vessel in the brain. The bleeding from this rupture could lead to pressure on the brain, which could ultimately cause death. Such intracranial bleeding is thought by some authorities to be due to prolonged battering. Because of this possibility, amateur bouts are usually restricted in length to three rounds. Professional boxers, however, are often required to fight fifteen rounds (McLatchie 1981).

When studying boxing, questions always arise as to the amount of force that can be generated by a punch, the amount of force necessary to cause body damage, and the force-absorption characteristics of the boxing gloves and headgear. The Wayne State Tolerance Curve (WSTC) has established that forces sufficient to cause head accelerations of 80 G (784 N) of approximately 8 msec are of knockout proportions. A force of about 1100 N is required to break a mandible.

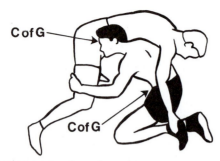

FIGURE 20.4 One form of wrestling takedown pattern. Visualize the relationships of the positions of the centers of gravity and line of gravity of the two wrestlers with respect to a takedown action.

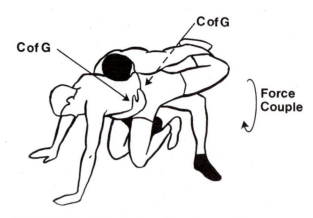

FIGURE 20.5 In the down position, the wrestler on top can compensate for lack of strength by using leverage.

Force Absorption of Boxing Impacts

Not only gloves but headgear, groin guards, chest guards, and instructor hand-held target pads have been developed for the absorption of forces during boxing and karate. Chapter 14 has additional information about collisions, punches, kicks, and other impacts between people.

Studies were conducted (Smith and Hamill 1985) on subjects punching a bag with no gloves, with karate gloves, and with boxing gloves. The boxing gloves imparted more momentum to the bag than did the bare fist, and the karate gloves imparted momentum similar to the bare-fisted condition. Peak forces transmitted to the target were also higher with the boxing gloves than with the karate gloves. For this reason, the boxing gloves tends to cause more damage to hard tissue, such as bone and cartilage. Additionally, boxing gloves lose much of their force-absorption characteristics after the first few impacts. Boxing gloves tested by Therrien (1981) lost as much as 50% of their force-absorption capability after only a few impacts. This is quite a serious liability, considering that a boxer may use one set of gloves for a number of fights. There were also large variations in force absorption characteristics between right and left boxing gloves of the same pair.

Finally, researchers suggest that neither boxing nor karate gloves offer much protection after the first few blows. Even low-skilled punchers could deliver blows of concussive force while wearing either type of glove.

Wrestling

Wrestling is a sport in which one performer attempts to throw and pin an opponent to the mat. The opponent resists and may in turn attempt to reverse the process. It involves each trying to maintain a state of equilibrium, that is, being stable. Stability is influenced by the height of the center of gravity in the starting stand-up position; all things being equal, the more stable the wrestler is, the better able he or she is to resist the opponent.

On the take-down, aggressive wrestlers attempt to attack below an opponent's center of gravity. They try to lift the opponent off their feet and throw him or her to the mat. (See Figure 20.4.)

Arm and leg strength are important to counter and counteract the moves, but leverage is also important. (For a review of lever concepts, see Chapter 4.) For example, in the down position (see Figure 20.5) the wrestler on top makes use of leverage; that is, the lever arms of the legs and arms of the opponent are kept in the least favorable position so strength can be offset.

In the stand-up starting defensive and attacking position, arms are held in front of the position with the forearms flexed and the hands pronated for greater strength. The CG of the wrestler must be low to resist the attacking wrestler. The position of the shoulders extends beyond the lead leg. The vulnerability to attack is enhanced since the arms are easier to grasp and the line of gravity is outside the body. The legs are flexed for greatest resistance.

The chin is held high so vision is not obstructed in the stand-up position. The wrestler should focus on the opponent's center of gravity, which is located at the belt line. In this concentrated focus, feints and fakes of the upper and lower body by the opponent become less effective.

Other wrestling techniques include using the body's momentum to advantage by letting a wrestler push or practically throw another wrestler. The pushed or thrown wrestler does not resist, but goes in the direction the opponent desires, then uses the momentum to escape. Also, moving rapidly from one position to another without pausing often confuses an opponent.

Weight reduction is common in wrestling, in order to meet a certain weight classification. The more weight lost, within limits, the more advantage the wrestler has. The high muscle, low fat ratio is best for executing more force. Also, being at the highest weight in the weight category is another advantage. However, excessive weight loss to gain biomechanical advantage may result in physical problems, particularly if wrestling meets are scheduled on successive days.

Many of the principles and concepts in judo are applicable to wrestling. Although some of the movement actions are different, they involve some of the same principles of execution.

Fencing

Fencing is unique in many ways. It involves no ball, but does involve a long striking implement (foil, epee, or sabre). This implement is not swung, but used as an extension of the arm. A sport of body propulsion, it involves neither running, jumping, or kicking. Yet the body is propelled rapidly forward and backward during the course of the bout. Speed is very important, and the line of action should be direct to the target, as previously explained in the karate section.

■ The fencing stance must be balanced, free from stress to the knee and trunk, and ready for mobility and force production.

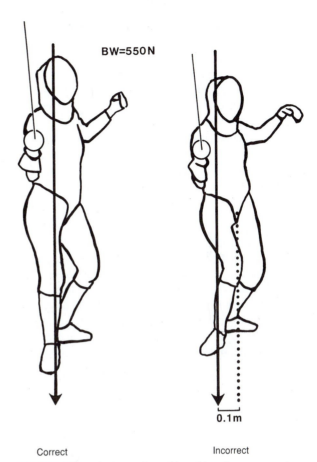

FIGURE 20.6 The en garde position of two fencers—one incorrect (greater stress on the knee) and one correct.

MINI-LABORATORY LEARNING EXPERIENCE

1. Measure the torque at the knee of the lead leg of the two en garde (basic stance position) positions of the two fencers in Figure 20.6.
2. Who is at risk? What tissues at the knee are at risk of injury? What type of tear would occur—compression, tension, etc.?
3. Measure the torque at the lumbar sacral spine of the two fencers.
4. Who is at risk? What tissues are involved in preventing injury?

Biomechanics of Combatives   **437**

The basic stance in fencing has little similarity to other sports, except certain positions in the martial arts. In the basic stance, the feet are at right angles to each other, with the lead foot facing the opponent.

This stance provides both lateral and sagittal stability. The width of the feet is such that the center of gravity may be lowered for stability, and increased flexion at the knees is possible in order to execute a forceful lunge. In addition, the knees should be above the feet to reduce the moments of force and stress at the knee joints. The feet should also be spread a distance that provides optimum mobility.

The Lunge

The method of delivering the attack in fencing, and in some cases the attack itself, is termed the lunge. The force produced in the lunge is obtained through extension of the rear leg and movement of the lead leg and rear arm. The more directly horizontal this force can be directed, the faster and more effective the lunge. Note in Figure 20.7 the differences in peak forces of the rear leg during the lunge of a skilled performer and that of an unskilled performer. The skilled performer developed 355 N of peak force and five times more impulse in the horizontal direction than did the unskilled fencer. The skilled fencer showed no vertical force greater than body weight. Observe the differences in the movement kinematics (stick figures) and speculate why the forces were so different. What did the unskilled fencer fail to do with the rear leg? What differences can you deduce about the vertical forces of the two fencers?

Research on horizontal work and power in the lunge was carried out on fencers of university varsity caliber (Klinger and Adrian 1987). The amount of work done and power produced were calculated. Power ranged from 1988 watts to 2105 watts, and work done ranged from 1196 joules to 1256 joules. These values can be interpreted as equivalent to lifting approximately 1000 newtons a distance of one meter in one-half second.

Electromyographic and electrogoniometric data on both correctly and incorrectly performed lunging are depicted in Figure 20.8. Note the differences in muscle action potentials with respect to position of the knee. Such data not only can assist a fencer in determining performance faults but can also be used to determine which muscles are vulnerable when the performance is incorrect. High speed photography can be used to observe changes in muscle shape and position, indirect evidence of muscle function.

Further analyses of elite performers in the lunge were carried out on three male members of the 1984 U.S. Olympic team (Klinger and Adrian 1985). The duration of their lunges, from start to finish, ranged from 250 to 600 milliseconds, and were fastest when they responded to conditions that simulated actual bouts. The velocity of the fencers varied from a low of 1.2 meters per second to 4 meters per second, with the greatest velocity again being recorded in the bout simulation condition.

Acceleration in the attack is important since varying speeds are difficult for the opponent to judge and defend against. To determine acceleration, the researchers investigated hip translation. In elite performers, acceleration did occur in the lunge, but it occurred in different phases of the lunge with each performer. These individual differences may be due to anatomical factors, age, weapon fenced, or other variables.

Blade Work

There is almost no research on blade work, that is, the intricate actions fencers make to defend and to deceive their opponent in order to hit the valid target. The velocities of different arm extensions to initiate the attack, however, have been investigated to determine the optimum arm position for initiating an attack. For example, if the arm is flexed in the en garde position (see Figure 20.9), it will develop moderate horizontal speed and strike the target in a fairly quick time. If the arm is flexed further, a greater velocity can be developed, but

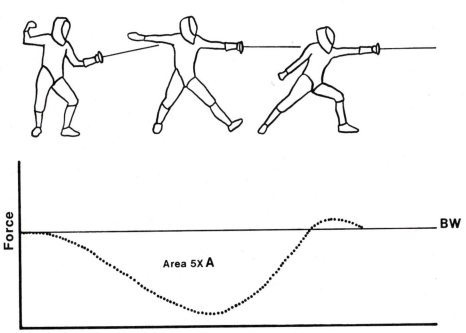

FIGURE 20.7 Horizontal force-time patterns for unskilled fencing lunge (a) and skilled fencing lunge (b). The horizontal impulse for b is five times that of fencer a (Area = 5 × a).

a

Area 5X **A**

b

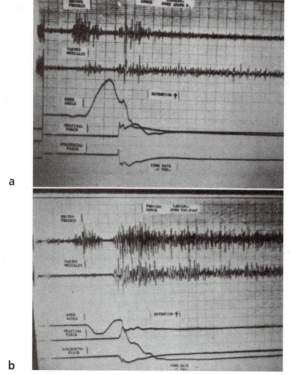

a

b

FIGURE 20.8 Comparison of electromyographic and electrogoniometric recordings as a function of the position of the knee during landing after two fencing lunges. (a) Knee is above base of support (foot) at end of lunge and muscular activity is low in the rectus femoris and vastus lateralis muscles. (b) Knee is outside base of support at end of lunge and muscular activity is high in both muscles. **Why is this so?**

the time will be longer to reach the target. Conversely, if the move is begun with the arm in a more extended position, the velocity is low, but the time is short. An optimum position appears to be nearly extended in the epee and semiflexed in the foil and sabre.

Judo*

Judo is a sport of high force and impact. While judo is comprised of pins, chokes, and elbow locks, it is most commonly recognized by its throws. The basic principle

*Contributed by Michael Purcell.

of off-balancing opponents and using their weight against them is well known, although not as commonly achieved. In biomechanical terms, the opponent's center of gravity must be moved outside the base of support, and sufficient torque applied to complete the throw.

Balance

Traditionally, off-balance in judo is created in eight directions: forward, backward, right, left, and to the four corners (diagonals). Force-application patterns used to produce an off-balance include push, pull, push followed by release, pull followed by release, push-pull (force couple), pull-push (force couple), and combinations of all of the above. Combinations of the push-pull and pull-push force couple actions typically produce rotation of the opponent's body about its longitudinal axis.

There are two basic postures in judo: "natural" (*shizentai*) and "defensive" (*jigotai*). In the natural posture, the body is kept upright, with feet slightly greater than hip-width apart and the legs slightly flexed. When shifting to a defensive posture, judo players (*judoka*) lower their center of gravity by exaggerating the flexion at the knees, and spreading their base of support. The resulting position is similar to the fencer's stance, but in judo, the torso is kept facing the opponent and the weight remains centered.

As *judoka* face each other, they grasp each other's uniform (*judogi*), typically by the lapel and sleeve. The material is held most strongly with the third and fourth fingers (like holding an ice cream cone). This grip permits a great range of motion. Grasping the lapel controls the midline of the opponent's body, while the sleeve grip allows a moment of force to be applied to the torso.

Since a *judoka* must always be prepared to meet an attack, locomotion is performed by short, sliding steps, with flexion at the knees to lower the center of gravity. The feet should never be crossed, or even brought close together.

Preparation for a throw consists of an interplay between opponents in which they search for the timing and position needed to create an off-balance. For example, after a series of movements and push-pull combinations, one *judoka* may push forward. The other *judoka* will match and use this movement with a pull in the same direction, creating a strong off-balance.

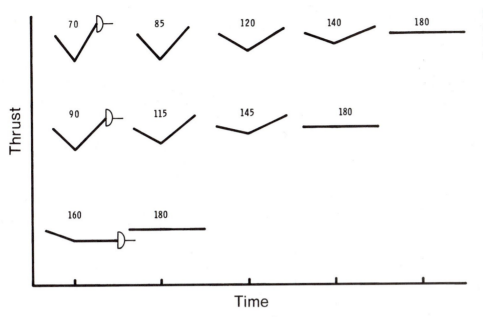

FIGURE 20.9 Relationship of displacement, velocity, and duration of execution of the arm extension in fencing.

Torque

Since judo throws are rotational, they rely on the development of torque. **Torque** is simply rotational force. To calculate torque, it is necessary to know two factors: (1) the force acting to cause rotation; and (2) the lever arm (movement arm) between this force and the pivot point (fulcrum). The two factors are multiplied together to calculate torque. In judo especially, after the opponent is unbalanced, torques are primarily caused by the force of gravity.

Classifying Judo Techniques

Because there are so many diverse throws in judo, leading *judoka* and biomechanists have long looked for a way to classify judo throwing techniques (called *nage-waza*). Dr. Jigoro Kano, the founder of judo, established the Kodokan classification, which, with some modifications, is still used in judo practice halls (*dojo*) the world over. Dr. Kano further suggested that the judo throw can be subdivided into three parts: (1) preliminary unbalancing with the hands; (2) final unbalancing; and (3) the execution of the throwing movement. These movements are known in judo as *kazushi, tsukuri,* and *kake*.

MINI-LABORATORY LEARNING EXPERIENCE

Study Figure 20.10.

1. Identify the force acting to cause rotation.
2. Identify the pivot point and estimate the length of the moment arm.

Looking for a way to classify judo movements biomechanically, Sacripanti (1987) suggests that all the throws in judo can be divided into two categories. The first category includes all techniques in which the thrower (*tori*) employs a force couple. This class contains, for example, leg sweeps. The second category includes techniques in which *tori* primarily uses principles of leverage. This encompasses all throws that occur as the result of turning the receiver's (*uke*) body around a pivot point, like *tai-otoshi* (body drop). This method of classification enables researchers to use two sets of easily understood physical principles to analyze the majority of judo throws. To illustrate the usefulness of this system, a judo throw, *seoi-nage* (shoulder throw, Figure 20.11) will be analyzed.

Biomechanics of Combatives **441**

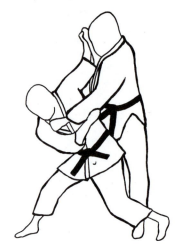

FIGURE 20.10 The tai-otoshi.

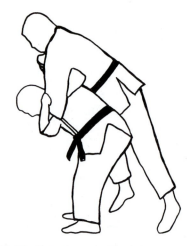

FIGURE 20.11 Note the use of both linear and rotary movements to position the center of gravity of the uke in a favorable position to execute the seoi-nage throw.

Basic Principles Applied to *Seoi-nage*

Refer to Figure 20.11 as you read the description of proper execution of *seoi-nage*. After a high forward pull, *tori* drops low and rotates in front of *uke*. By the time contact is made, *uke* is well off-balanced, and *tori* need only continue the rotation forward to execute the throw. The following principles are important to this throw:

1. Maintain a low center of gravity.
2. Take short preparatory steps to maintain equilibrium.
3. Move continuously and in a circular manner.
4. Unbalance the opponent.
5. Draw the opponent to you, rather than moving back into the opponent.
6. Throw in the direction of *uke's* movement, bringing *uke's* body over you in a curved path, keeping your feet and hips underneath the flight of the throw.

As *uke's* weight is moved forward outside the base of support, just the gravitational pull on the opponent's body could cause a fall. As previously explained, torque is the product of force multiplied by the lever arm. In this case, the force is *uke's* weight and the lever arm is the amount of unbalancing. The greater the lever arm, the greater the off-balance.

As *tori* turns and brings the unbalanced *uke* over the hip (*tori's* fulcrum), a second torque is applied, which causes *uke* to roll over *tori's* hip. It should be pointed out, however, that in a well-executed throw, *tori's* primary concerns are getting below *uke's* center of gravity and applying a strong forward pull to lengthen the lever arm. Most of the force of the throw is supplied by gravity.

Breaking the Fall (*Ukemi*)

Since all throws involve a landing, the basic concepts described in Chapter 14 are applicable. The hand slap is, however, unique to judo. Although the slap does not absorb a great deal of force, it is a useful aid in timing and placing the rest of the body, especially the trunk. The goal of the landing is to absorb the force of the fall over the greatest possible body area and for the longest amount of time. In flat falls, it is essential to land on relaxed muscle masses. In rolling falls, the body is curved to produce a low resistance to rolling.

Sports Medicine Problems

Judoka are typically handed, that is they perform most of their *nage-waza* to one side. As a result, *judoka* may become asymmetrically developed. Scoliosis due to the shortening of muscles on one side of the spinal column may result. Another common sports medicine problem is also seen in *judoka*. *Seoi-nage* elbow is similar to pitcher's elbow and tennis elbow. It is caused by allowing the trailing elbow to lead the hand and shoulder in the execution of a forward throw.

References

Adams, S., Adrian, M., and Baylise, M., ed. 1987. *Catastrophic injuries in sports avoidance strategies.* Indianapolis: Benchmark Press.

Adrian, M., and Klinger, A. 1977. A biomechanical analysis of the fencing lunge. *Swordmaster,* July.

Basmajian, J. V. 1957. New views of muscular tone and relaxation. *Can. Med. Assoc. J.* 77:293.

Basmajian, J. V. 1984. *Muscles alive: Their functions as revealed by electromyography,* 2nd ed. Baltimore: Williams & Wilkins.

Klinger, A., and Adrian, M. 1985. Effect of pre-lunge conditions on performance of elite male fencers. In *Proceedings of ISBS biomechanics in sports II,* ed. Terauds and Barham. Del Mar, CA: Academic Publishers.

Klinger, A., and Adrian, M. 1987. Power output as a function of fencing technique. *International series on biomechanics,* vol. 6B. Champaign, IL: Human Kinetics Publishing Co.

Klinger, A. K. 1977. Teaching mechanical principles through self-defense. In *Proceedings, kinesiology: A national conference on teaching,* ed. C. Dillman and R. Sears. Urbana: University of Illinois.

Kodokan. 1968. *Kodokan judo.* Tokyo: Kodansha.

McLatchie, G. R. 1981. Injuries in combat sports. In *Sports fitness and sports injury,* ed. T. Reilly. London: Faber & Fisher.

Nakayama, M. 1977. *Best karate: Comprehensive.* Tokyo: Kodansha.

Sacripanti, A. 1987. Biomedical classification of judo throwing technique. Unpublished paper presented at International Society of Biomechanics in Sports Symposium, July.

Schroeder, C., and Wallace, B. 1982. *Karate: Basic concepts and skills.* Reading, MA: Addison Wesley.

Smith, P., and Hamill, J. 1985. Karate and boxing glove impact as functions of velocity. In *Proceedings of the ISBS Biomechanics in Sports II,* ed. Terauds and Barham. Del Mar, CA: Academic Publishers.

Therrien, R. 1981. Energy absorption and force transmission characteristics of boxing gloves. Trois Rivieres. Quebec, Canada.

Walker, J. 1980. The amateur scientist: In judo and aidido application of the physics of forces makes the weak equal to the strong. *Scientific American* 243:150–61.

Walker, J. Karate strikes. *American Journal of Physics* 43(10).

Westbrook and Ratti 1980. *Aikido and the dynamic sphere: An illustrated introduction.* Rutland, VA: Charles and Tuttle Co.

PART

V

Sports Movements in Air, Ice, Snow, and Water Environments

21 Biomechanics of Aquatic Activities*

The discussions in this chapter focus on the most important aspects of moving through the water: (1) characteristics of water; (2) floating; (3) resistive drag; (4) propulsive forces; (5) using sculling motions effectively; (6) stroke rates and stroke lengths; (7) starts and turns; and (8) special training devices for improving swimming speed.

Characteristics Of Water

Three characteristics of water are pressure, density, and flow. Knowledge of water pressure and density is important to the understanding of how water supports the body during aquatic activities. Knowledge of water flow is necessary to understanding the resistive and propulsive forces that occur during aquatic activities. Discussions of these topics follow.

Water Pressure

In this case, pressure is defined as the amount of force water exerts against an object immersed in it, divided by the surface area of that object. When divers descend in the water, the pressure on their bodies increases because

of the weight of the water above them. This increase in pressure is felt when it compresses the volume of air in the middle ear and sinus cavities. Divers equalize or compensate for this increase in pressure by "popping" their ears.

Water Density

Water **density** describes the weight of water. Water is weighed in a container, and its weight density is expressed in terms of a given volume such as newtons per liter (NII). The weight density of fresh water is 9.9 NII and the weight density of salt water is about 10.2 NII. Salt water has greater density than an equal amount of fresh water because the dissolved salt gives it more mass. Density remains constant at various depths.

Water Flow

Water flow can be described as either laminar or turbulent. Water molecules tend to flow in smooth, unbroken streams. This smooth flow has been termed **laminar** because the streams of water molecules are packed one on top of the other like laminated sheets of plywood. Laminar flow has the least resistance associated with its movement because all of the water molecules travel in the same direction at a uniform rate of speed.

The laminar flow of water molecules can become **turbulent** when they encounter some solid object that suddenly interrupts their movement. This sudden interruption of their forward motion can occur when

* Contributed by Cheryl Maglischo and Ernie Maglischo.

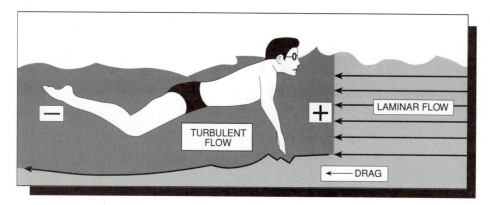

FIGURE 21.1 Turbulence caused by a swimmer's body moving into laminar streams. The straight lines represent the laminar streams. Turbulence is depicted by the swirling lines. The swirling water increases the pressure in front of swimmers relative to the pressure behind their bodies where the flow is more laminar. This pressure differential between front and rear will slow the swimmer's forward velocity.

laminar streams encounter swimmers' poorly stream-lined bodies. The impact causes the water molecules to become turbulent as they rebound wildly in all directions as they are diverted around the swimmer.

■ Water molecules that have become turbulent intrude on other laminar streams and collide with the molecules in those streams, causing them to rebound in random directions as well. These randomly moving molecules, in turn, intrude on still more laminar streams in an ever-widening pattern of turbulence.

Turbulent flow is illustrated in Figure 21.1. When swimmers' bodies pass through water, the turbulence they create will continue downstream until laminar flow has been reestablished. This is because the holes they opened do not fill in immediately. This failure of water to fill in immediately behind leaves an area to the rear of swimmers where only a small number of water molecules are swirling wildly. Thus, the pressure of water in this area is relatively lower than the pressure in front and will remain so until the turbulence has dissipated and it has been completely filled in by the streams of molecules above and below the swimmer's body. The swirling molecules called **eddy currents** are also illustrated in Figure 21.1.

A procedure called **dragging** is common in swimming. During training and competition, swimmers will follow closely behind teammates or competitors, stroking in the area of eddy currents they produce. In these cases, the swimmer in front performs some of the work of propelling the swimmer behind. This happens

because the pressure immediately in front of the trailing swimmer is higher than the pressure in the "pocket" behind the leading swimmer; this imbalance creates a suction effect that pulls the trailing swimmer forward.

■ Swimmers use dragging techniques the same way cyclists and runners do.

Floating

A body cannot be supported by water; it will sink either wholly or partially until the weight of the displaced water equals the weight of the body. Two concepts important to the understanding of floating are **buoyancy** and *specific gravity*.

Buoyancy

The first person to recognize this concept was Archimedes (287-212 B.C.), who said "a body immersed in a fluid is buoyed up by a force equal to the weight of the displaced fluid." This concept, understandably, has become known as **Archimedes' principle.** The upward force, which counterbalances the weight (force) of the body, is called *buoyant force*.

Specific Gravity

The term *specific gravity* is used to describe the ratio of a swimmer's body weight to the weight of the volume of water he or she displaces. A person's specific gravity is 1.0 when the weight of the maximum volume of

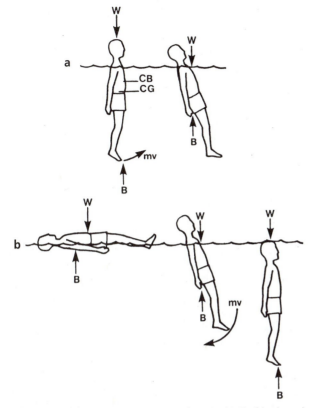

FIGURE 21.2 Relationship of center of gravity (CG) of body and center of buoyancy (CB) of body and floating ability. (*a*) Buoyancy force (B) and weight force (W) create momentum (mv) to rotate the body to floating position, which is the position of vertical alignment of the two centers. (*b*) When the body that does not float horizontally begins in the horizontal position, the momentum rotates the body into the water. The body tends to pass through the balancing (floating) point because of the momentum. This causes the body to submerge and assume a floating position with the complete body under water.

water displaced is equal to the weight of the person's body. Swimmers who displace a volume of water that weighs less than their weight have specific gravity greater than 1.0 and will not be able to float at the surface. A specific gravity less than 1.0 occurs when a swimmer displaces a volume of water that weighs more than body weight. Such persons are buoyant and will float easily at the surface.

■ The specific gravity of a human body is determined by its physical makeup. If the swimmer's body contains a large portion of fat, it will have a lower specific gravity because fat has more volume for its weight than muscle tissue. Conversely, a well-muscled swimmer will exhibit a higher specific gravity because muscle tissue is heavier than fat.

A swimmer's floating position depends not only on the specific gravity, but also on the relationship of the center of gravity to the center of buoyancy. The *center of buoyancy* refers to a point that represents the center of the body's volume. A swimmer will float in a position in which the center of gravity and the center of buoyancy coincide or are in vertical alignment. If the swimmer assumes a horizontal position, and the center of buoyancy and the center of gravity are not in alignment, the legs will sink until the correct position is reached. This is illustrated in Figure 21.2.

The center of gravity is lower than the center of buoyancy in an adult. Therefore, buoyancy can be increased by moving the center of gravity toward the head. This can be done by raising the arms overhead in line with the trunk or by flexing the lower legs.

Swimmers can also improve their ability to float by increasing their body's volume. They can take a large breath of air, which will increase the size of the chest area, displacing more water and increasing volume while having little effect on body density.

In synchronized swimming, including stunts, the performer who floats horizontally is more efficient than the one who floats diagonally because the more horizontal floater needs few if any sculling movements to maintain the floating position. An action such as a ballet leg, in which the leg is held perpendicular to and completely above the water, requires a force only equal to the weight of the leg. This stunt is more difficult for a person who does not float horizontally because muscular effort is needed to maintain the body position at the surface of the water and additional force is required to support the leg out of the water. Likewise, all the slow, propulsive strokes displaying exaggerated arm movements above the water require more effort by swimmers with poor buoyancy.

Resistive Drag

The forces opposing motion that swimmers encounter are known as *resistive drag*. Researchers have used both passive and active measuring techniques to determine resistive drag. There is considerable controversy as to the similarities between active and passive drag.

Passive Drag

Recent estimates of **passive drag** have been produced by measuring the force necessary to tow a swimmer through the water at a constant speed with the body in a prone position. It varies approximately with the square of the velocity of the body, ranging from about 30 N (at 1 m/s) to about 120 N (at 2 m/s) (Hay 1987).

Active Drag

Active drag is measured during actual swimming. Di Prampero and coworkers (1974) measured swimmers' oxygen consumptions during free swimming as a measure of active drag. They reported that it was 1.1 to 3.1 times the corresponding passive drag. Clarys (1979), towing swimmers attached by a belt to a vertical column that recorded the horizontal forces exerted against it when the swimmer did a front crawl stroke, reported that active drag values were at least 1.5 to 2 times the passive drag at equal velocities. Hollander and coworkers (1986, 1987), however, reported active drag values that were similar to or lower than values for passive drag.

Types of Resistive Drag Encountered by Swimmers

The resistive drag that swimmers encounter as they travel down the pool can be placed in three categories: profile drag, wave drag, and frictional drag.

Profile Drag

Profile drag is caused by the form or orientation of a swimmer's body to the water. It is a function of the space swimmers occupy, the shapes their bodies assume in the water, and their velocity.

The space swimmers occupy in the water has a significant effect on profile drag. This is because the swimmers interrupt a greater number of molecular streams when they occupy more space. The space they occupy has both vertical and lateral components. The vertical component is determined by the deepest point reached by a body part and the lateral component by the space swimmers occupy from side to side. Vertical size can be reduced by remaining as horizontal as possible (except when up and down movements add relatively more propulsive force). The effect of the vertical component on resistive drag is illustrated in Figure 21. 3. The effect of the lateral component is shown in Figure 21.4.

Where shape is concerned, tapered objects encounter less resistance than objects with square corners. This effect is illustrated in Figure 21.5. Both objects have the same surface area, but *a* is tapered at both ends while *b* is rectangular in shape. Object *a* encounters less resistive drag because its tapered front end allows the direction of the water molecules it encounters to change gradually as it passes through them. In addition, the tapered rear end allows the water molecules to fill in behind the object almost immediately. Therefore the small area of eddy currents behind the object quickly disappears after it passes through.

On the other hand, the square front end of object *b* pushes forward against several streams of water molecules at once causing them to rebound wildly. This sets up a pattern of turbulence that greatly increases the pressure of the water in front. The square rear end of object *b* does not allow the water molecules to fill in quickly after it passes through. This leaves a large low pressure area of eddy currents for a considerable distance behind the object. The combination of greater pressure in front and less pressure behind increases the pressure differential between front and rear, producing a greater retarding effect on the object. In spite of these observations, Clarys (1979) did not report a high relationship between body shape and drag measured during actual swimming.

Although heredity determines body shapes, swimmers can reduce profile drag by controlling the orientation of their bodies to the water. They should position their bodies so that all contours taper back gradually. They should also remain as horizontal as possible to the

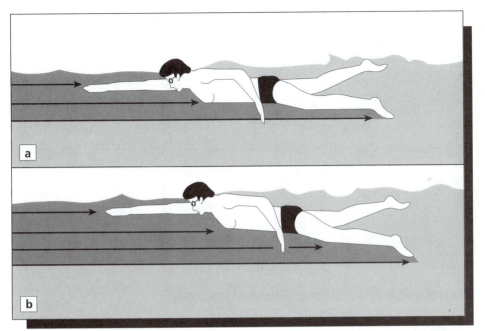

FIGURE 21.3 The effect of the space swimmers occupy in the water in the vertical component of resistive drag. Swimmers a and b are exactly the same size but their bodies are oriented differently to the water. Swimmer a, whose body is horizontal and streamlined, moves through a much smaller column of water than does swimmer b, whose body is angled downward.

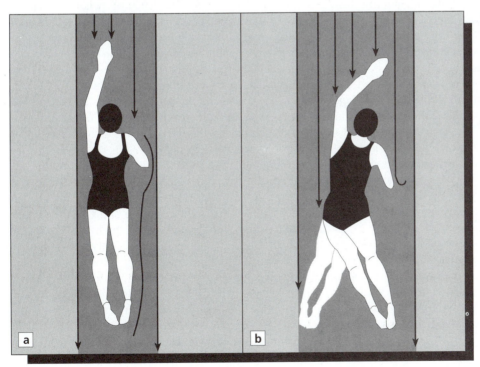

FIGURE 21.4 The effect of the space swimmers occupy in the water on the horizontal component of resistive drag. Swimmer a occupies less space because her body does not swing from side to side. Swimmer b is using faulty stroke mechanics that cause her body to swing from side to side so that she occupies more space in the water. She will encounter more resistive drag as she swims.

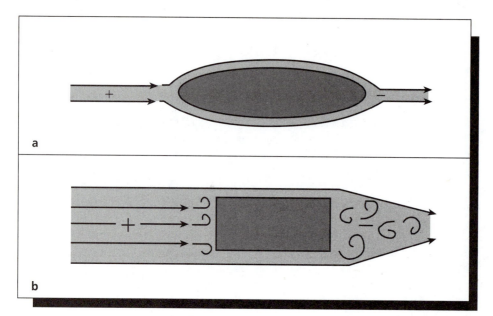

FIGURE 21.5 The effect of the shape of objects on resistive drag. Object *a* has a tapered shape that reduces resistive drag. Object *b*, which is rectangular, increases resistive drag.

surface. This is particularly true in the freestyle, sidestroke, and the backstrokes. When swimming these strokes, persons should keep their heads and trunks nearly horizontal while kicking deep enough to propel their bodies forward, but not so deep that they increase their vertical area unnecessarily.

Early researchers found when swimmers were towed through the water in flat and side positions the flat position created less profile drag (Counsilman 1955). This caused many swimmers to mistakenly keep their bodies as flat as possible while swimming the front and back crawl strokes. However, all top swimmers roll their bodies to some extent. Rolling from side to side allows them to apply more propulsive force with their arms and reduces reactive side to side body movements as their limbs travel up and down.

The butterfly and breaststroke present special cases where horizontal alignment is concerned. The effective production of propulsive forces requires a certain amount of body undulation in both strokes. While this undulation increases the frontal surface area presented to the water, the trade-off for increased propulsive force is probably a beneficial one.

The breaststroke is unique because of an ongoing controversy over the efficiency of swimming flat versus a style with somewhat more undulation. Traditionally, researchers have believed that undulating swimmers create more resistive drag than those who remain horizontal. This is probably not true. Swimmers who raise their heads and trunks somewhat above the water surface can maintain a more streamlined shape with their legs during their recovery and will not decelerate as much during this phase of the stroke. The breaststroke swimmer *a* in Figure 12.6 is recovering his legs in an undulating style. Swimmer *b* is using the flat-style. Both swimmers take up approximately the same space in the water. However, by lowering his hips and raising his trunk, swimmer *a* can bring his feet forward underwater without pulling his thighs underneath his body. On the other hand, the flat-style swimmer (*b*) must push his thighs forward under his hips in order to keep his hips at the surface and his feet underwater as he brings them forward. Pushing the thighs forward into a position that is nearly perpendicular to his hips will increase resistive drag much more than will the method used by swimmer *a*.

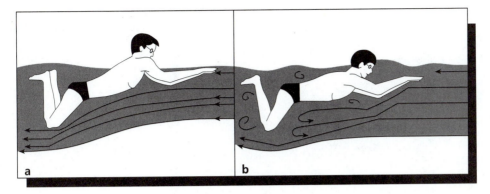

FIGURE 21.6 Two styles of leg recovery in the breaststroke. Swimmer *a* lowers his hips and raises his trunk while he recovers his legs. Swimmer *b* encounters more resistive drag by trying to stay horizontal because he must push his thighs forward against the water as he brings his feet up.

The third factor that influences profile drag is *swimming velocity*. This effect is so potent that doubling forward velocity will quadruple resistive drag.

Wave Drag

Some pools have more waves than others because of inadequate lane lines or poor construction. Waves of this origin are beyond the control of competitors. The bow waves that swimmers produce are also beyond their control because they are dependent on the swimmer's velocity. As swimming velocity increases, the "wall of water" rising in front of swimmers becomes larger. It then "presses back" against their bodies and slows their forward velocity.

■ Wave drag is caused by turbulence at the surface of the water.

Skilled swimmers can control the waves they produce when they push their arms forward against the water. When they drag their arms across the surface or smash them into the water, they push waves of turbulent water in front of them that finally swell and push back against them. The retarding force is even greater if their limbs are underwater because more water will be pushed forward. It has been shown that highly skilled swimmers produce less wave drag than recreational swimmers moving at the same speed (Takamoto, Ohmichi, and Miyashita 1985).

■ Wave resistance drag increases proportional to the cube of the swimmer's velocity: $V \times 2 = WD \times 8$.

Frictional Drag

Frictional drag is caused by the friction between the swimmer's skin and the water molecules that come in contact with it. As swimmers move forward, friction between their skin and the water causes some of the molecules to be carried along with them. The streams of water molecules affected by frictional forces are called the **boundary layer.** Molecules in the boundary layer collide with other molecules immediately in front of them and rebound off in random directions causing turbulence. The boundary layer is said to separate, or "break away," when this turbulence becomes great enough. Figure 21.7 shows the actual movement of fluid past an immersed sphere.

The principal factors that influence the amount of frictional drag exerted on objects are the surface area of the object, the velocity of the object, and the roughness of its surface. Swimmers have no control over surface area, and velocity can only be controlled to the extent that early portions of a race are paced. Therefore, surface smoothness is the source of frictional drag that is amenable to reduction. Since smooth surfaces cause less friction than rough surfaces, some experts have suggested that the almost universal practice of shaving their body hair before important competition improves the performance of swimmers by reducing their frictional drag. Not everyone agrees that these improvements are due to reductions in frictional drag, however. Some believe that shaving down has become "big meet" ritual that accompanies, but does

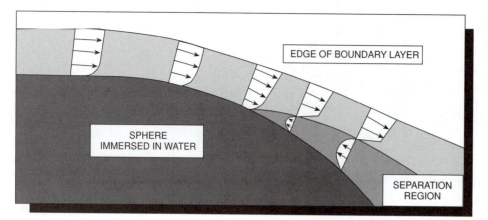

FIGURE 21.7 The effect of frictional drag on the boundary layer. The area of turbulence at the right side of the illustration is where the boundary layer has separated.

not cause, improved performances. Another popular explanation is that shaving down increases kinesthetic sensitivity, which results in improved stroke mechanics.

Clarys (1979) believes that frictional drag is negligible where humans are concerned. He believes they are so poorly streamlined compared to aquatic mammals that wave and form drag cause the boundary layer to separate almost immediately when water starts around their bodies.

Sharp et al. (1988) and Sharp and Costill (1989) have presented findings that suggest that frictional drag may have a potent retarding effect. They had a group of swimmers compete identically paced submaximal swims before and after shaving the hair from their bodies. Blood lactate samples were drawn to measure the effort of the paced swims, and the researchers also calculated stroke lengths.

When shaved, the swimmers completed their paced swims with significantly lower blood lactate values and greater stroke lengths. Following the paced swims, average blood lactate values for the group were 8.48 mmols/l before shaving and 6.74 mmols/l after shaving. Average stroke length increased from 2.07 meters per stroke cycle before shaving to 2.31 meters per stroke cycle afterward. This increase in the average distance traveled during each stroke cycle was presumed due to reduced frictional drag; however, it could also have been the result of improved stroke mechanics.

Sharp and Costill (1989) used a similar protocol in a second study to resolve the question of whether improved performances were due to reduced frictional drag or improved kinesthetic sensitivity. They included a tethered swim test before and after shaving down in which the swimmers' energy costs were assessed by measuring oxygen consumption during several incremental stages of work. They reasoned that the effect of frictional drag would be negligible because the swimmers were not moving through the water during the tethered swims.

The swimmers did not reduce their energy cost for the tethered swimming tests after shaving. This would seem to rule out better kinesthetic feel for the water as a reason for their improvements on the paced swims since the oxygen cost of the tethered swims would have decreased if they were swimming more efficiently after shaving. Thus, a reduction of frictional drag seemed the logical cause for the swimmers' reduced efforts on the paced swims after shaving down.

As part of this study, Sharp and Costill (1989) also measured the rate of deceleration following a push-off, before and after shaving down. They used a device called a velocity meter for this purpose because it could accurately measure small changes in velocity while swimmers were moving through the water. The swimmers pushed off the wall and glided until their velocities fell from greater than 2 m/s to less than 1 m/s. The rate of decline was significantly more rapid before shaving. The authors believed that the swimmers did not slow down as quickly after shaving because frictional drag was lower.

Swimsuit manufacturers also believe that reducing frictional drag can improve performance; they are in competition to produce suits made of the smoothest and thinnest materials that do not absorb water. The "fit" of swimsuits also influences frictional drag. They are designed to fit smoothly over the skin with no gaps or wrinkles that "catch" water. Furthermore, suits are designed to reduce body contours where water might be trapped and become turbulent. Finally, some swimmers cover their bodies with oil and other substances to reduce friction. However, no lubricant has yet been proved to reduce frictional drag.

Propulsive Forces

The physical laws that govern swimming propulsion remain a mystery, although several theories have been advanced over the years. Early attempts to describe the propulsive movements of competitive swimmers were based on the premise that swimmers used their arms like oars. Swimmers were taught to keep their arms straight during the propulsive phase of the stroke and to move their hands and arms in a semicircular pattern that resembled the sweep of a paddle wheel. This theory proved incorrect when underwater motion pictures showed that swimmers were flexing and extending their limbs as they pushed them against the water.

Drag Theory

Counsilman (1968) and Silvia (1970), in two separate publications, proposed that these limb motions were used to apply Newton's third law of motion to swimming propulsion. They reasoned that athletes alternately flexed and extended their arms during the underwater portions of various swimming strokes so they could use their hands like paddles to push water straight back over a longer distance. This became known as the drag theory of propulsion.

Although this theory was widely accepted, Counsilman was not satisfied that he had discovered the true nature of swimming propulsion. In 1971, he and Brown reported the results of a landmark study that revolutionized the teaching of stroke mechanics (Brown and Counsilman 1971). They filmed swimmers wearing lights on their hands while swimming in a darkened pool. The

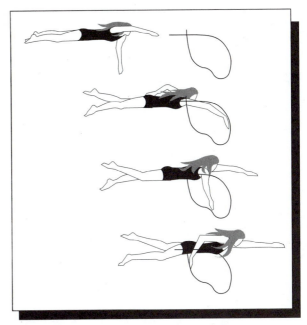

FIGURE 21.8 A front crawl stroke pattern drawn relative to a fixed point in the pool.
(Adapted with permission from Schleihauf, R. 1978. *Swimming propulsion: a hydrodynamic analysis*. In R. Ousley (Ed.), 1977 *ASCA World Clinic Yearbook*. Ft. Lauderdale, FL. p. 85.)

stroboscopic effect of the light flashes that appeared on the developed film showed the patterns of the swimmers' hands and feet relative to the water. Before this, the movements of swimmers' arms had always been described relative to their moving bodies.

Brown and Counsilman showed that the propulsive movements of swimmers' hands and arms were made in primarily lateral and vertical directions, with only minimal backward motion. They seemed to scull their hands in and out and up and down much more so than they pushed them backward. A typical freestyle stroke pattern, viewed from the side, is shown in the series of illustrations in Figure 21.8.

Lift Theory

Several other researchers have provided evidence that substantiates the fact that swimmers are using sculling motions for propulsion (Barthels 1979; Barthels and Adrian 1975; Van Tilborgh, Stijnen, and Persyn 1987).

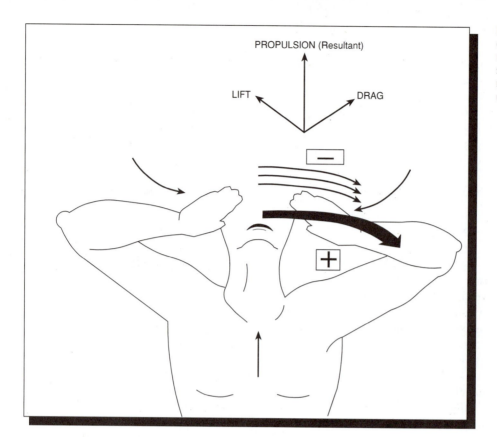

PROPULSION (Resultant)

LIFT   DRAG

FIGURE 21.9 The application of Bernoulli's theorem to swimming propulsion. A butterfly swimmer is shown from underneath as his hands sweep in under his body.

This became known as the **lift theory of propulsion** and Bernoulli's theorem was used to explain the manner in which the lift forces were produced. Daniel Bernoulli, a Swiss scientist, was the first person to identify the inverse relationship between the velocity of fluid flow and pressure. **Bernoulli's theorem** proposes that the pressure of fluid flow over a foil will be reduced when its speed is increased. Brown and Counsilman (1971) suggested that swimmers shaped their hands like foils to produce lift as they sculled them through the water. An example of swimming propulsion according to Bernoulli's theorem is shown in Figure 21.9.

The swimmer's hands are sweeping in so the relative direction of water flow will be out from the thumb— toward the sides of the little fingers. According to

Bernoulli's theorem, the water flowing over the longer upper surface of the swimmer's hand will accelerate so that it reaches the little finger side at the same time as the water flowing underneath. Consequently, the pressure of the water is lower above the hand than underneath the hand, where the flow is slower and the molecules packed together more tightly. The pressure differential between the palm and knuckle sides of the hand, indicated by the + and − signs in Figure 21.9, is thought to produce a lift force that acts in the direction shown by the lift vector in Figure 21.9. This force, in combination with the drag force, acting opposite the direction the hand is moving (shown by the drag vector), is believed to produce a resultant force that accelerates the swimmer's body forward.

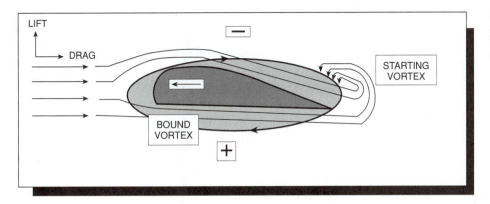

FIGURE 21.10 The formation of a bound vortex around a foil and its effect on producing lift forces and subsequent propulsion.

Vortice Theory

Recently, Colwin (1985a, 1985b, 1984) proposed a theory of lift propulsion based on the formation and shedding of vortices. Vortices are swirling, rotating movements, in this case, of water. Colwin studied movements of the water and their effect on propulsion and proposed that efficient swimmers use two types of propulsion, foil and fling-ring. He believes that foil propulsion takes place in the first half of the underwater armstroke, and the fling-ring mechanism takes place in the second half.

Foil Propulsion.   Foil propulsion is a result of the lift forces produced by a bound vortex, which is a mass of rotating fluid that circulates around a foil. The manner in which a bound vortex is thought to be formed is illustrated by the flow of water around a foil in Figure 21.10.

Notice that the water begins circulating up and back when it reaches the trailing edge (little finger side) of the swimmer's hand-foil after passing underneath his palm because, according to Bernoulli's theorem, the pressure of water is lower above the hand. Thus, the water tends to flow toward the region of lower pressure until it meets the water flowing over the top of the swimmer's hand. Because its pressure is less, that water begins to curl up and flow in the opposite direction. This reversal of direction of flow creates a so-called starting vortex, which, in turn, produces a counter-vortex of equal strength that circulates around the swimmer's hand. The counter-vortex becomes the bound vortex, which reacts with the fluid flowing past the hand to further lower the pressure

on the upper surface while increasing it on the underside. This is because the rotating fluid in the bound vortex is traveling in the same direction as the adjacent fluid over the knuckle side. Therefore, it causes that fluid to travel faster and reduces its pressure. The vortex is moving in a direction opposite that of the fluid under the palm. This slows the rate of water flow and increases pressure underneath the palm. Accordingly, the pressure-differential between the knuckle (–) and palm (+) sides of the hand will be augmented and the magnitude of the lift force increased.

Fling-Ring Propulsion.   The creation of a bound vortex is dependent on conditions of steady circulating fluid flow, which are impossible in certain phases of the competitive strokes such as the downbeats of the butterfly and flutter kicks and the final propulsive phases of the butterfly, front crawl, and back crawl armstrokes. Rapid changes of direction cause the boundary layer of fluid to break away during these phases, producing a condition of nonsteady flow where lift propulsion is no longer effective. The fling-ring mechanism comes into play in these cases. It is illustrated during the downbeat of the dolphin kick by the butterfly swimmer in Figure 21.11.

The swimmer maintains a bound vortex around his feet during the downkick. However, the fluid in that vortex is rapidly shed backward when the downward velocity of the feet becomes zero at its completion of the kick. The backward movement of water, in turn, creates a counter-force that propels the swimmer forward.

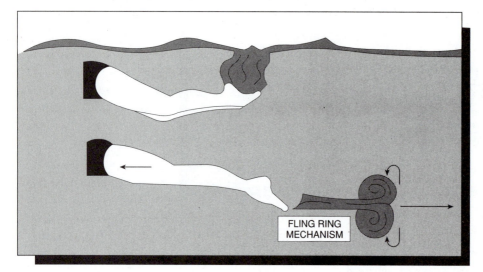

FIGURE 21.11 An example of the fling-ring mechanism of swimming propulsion. A butterfly swimmer is shown accelerating water backward while completing the downbeat of the dolphin kick.

(Adapted with permission, from Colwin, C. 1984. *Fluid dynamics: Vortex circulation in swimming propulsion.* In T. E. Welsh (Ed.), 1983 ASCA *World Clinic Yearbook.* Ft. Lauderdale, FL.)

Sculling Theory

Although both the lift and vortex theories are plausible, it is still possible that Newton's third law of motion may be the principal physical law that swimmers apply when propelling themselves through the water. In the past, the principal reason for rejecting Newton's law of action-reaction was the discovery that swimmers used diagonal sculling motion rather than backward pushes to propel themselves forward. This caused researchers to search for another explanation. Newton's action-reaction law may have been interpreted too narrowly. It was believed that swimmers had to push their arms and legs back like paddles in order to push water back and it was not considered that they could also move water back with sculling motions.

The illustration in Figure 21.12 shows how swimmers can displace water backward with sculling motions during mid-stroke in the front crawl stroke. Notice that the swimmer's hand is angled (pitched) in so that the thumb side is slightly higher than the little finger side. This angle causes water to be displaced backward by the palm as the hand passes through the water from thumb to little finger sides. The backward force imparted to the

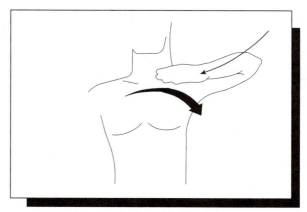

FIGURE 21.12 A method for displacing water back with diagonal stroking motions. An underneath view of a freestyle swimmer is shown as he sweeps his hand in under his body as indicated by the upper arrow behind it. The relative flow of water takes place in the opposite direction; that is, the water is traveling out as indicated by the lower arrow.

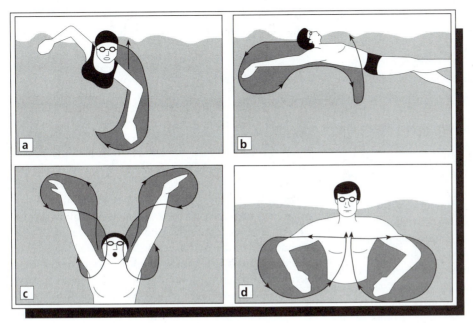

FIGURE 21.13 Patterns for the four competitive armstrokes drawn relative to the water. Shown are (a) a front view of the front crawl; (b) a side view of the back crawl; (c) an underneath view of the butterfly; and (d) front view of the breaststroke.

water produces, in accordance with Newton's third law of motion, a counter-force of equal magnitude that should propel the swimmer's body forward. This backward displacement of water also increases pressure under the swimmer's palm that, in turn, will increase the lift effect. That effect may be secondary to the effect of the backward displacement of water, however.

At present, Bernoulli's theorem is the most accepted explanation for swimming propulsion. However, it may not play as great a role as an explanation based on Newtonian physics. While Bernoulli's theorem is probably operating, any acceleration of fluid flow over the knuckles probably plays a minor role in propulsion compared to the displacement of water backward that is caused by the angle of attack of a limb. You can demonstrate this for yourself by sticking your hand out of the window when riding in a car. You will find that the angle of attack plays a larger role in producing lift than does the shape of the hand. Your hand will be pushed up immediately if you angle it down from front to back. You will feel little effect, however, if the hand remains perfectly flat, at a 0° angle of attack, no matter how much you may curve it. Consequently, Bernoulli's theorem may be a needlessly complex method of describing the production

of lift and propulsive forces (Koehler 1987; Sprigings and Koehler 1990). On the other hand, the concept of using sculling motions to displace water back is much easier to comprehend and probably more accurately describes the most important propulsive mechanisms.

Using Sculling Motions Effectively

There are three very important aspects of limb movements that determine the effectiveness of the diagonal stroking motions of swimmers: limb direction, angle of attack, and velocity.

Limb Direction

The best way to visualize the direction of the propelling movements swimmers make with their arms and legs is through the examination of stroke patterns. These patterns can be expressed either relative to the water or relative to a swimmer's body. Patterns drawn relative to the water provide the most accurate representation of propulsion. Front, side, and underneath patterns for the four competitive strokes are shown in Figure 21.13. They were drawn relative to the water from films of world-class athletes swimming at competition speeds. Their hand movements are three-dimensional, moving up and down, forward and backward, and inward and outward from the midline of the body (Counsilman 1977; Barthels 1979; E. Maglischo 1982; E. Maglischo 1984). There are several aspects of these patterns that deserve mention.

Notice that in all four competitive strokes the swimmers' hands travel in predominantly lateral and vertical directions. While some backward motion is needed to ensure that optimum amounts of water are displaced backward, it should be kept to a minimum. Reischle (1979) reported that the best swimmers exhibited the least backward hand movements in their strokes.

Swimmers make two or more major changes in the direction their hands are moving during the underwater portions of each competitive stroke. These changes are probably made in order to find undisturbed water that can be displaced back once previously encountered water has been accelerated to the rear (Counsilman 1977; E. Maglischo 1982). Counsilman (1977) stated, "Greater efficiency in water is achieved by pushing a large amount of water a short distance rather than by pushing a small amount of water a great distance."

All of the stroke patterns are elliptical. This is because swimmers use less muscular effort to change directions when they stroke in curvilinear paths. According to Newton's first law of motion, an object moving in one direction has inertia and must be reduced to zero velocity before its direction can be changed. A great deal of force is required to "brake" the inertia of a limb that is moving in one direction and to accelerate it in a new direction and the required effort is greatest when the change of direction is sudden and sharp.

■ Curvilinear stroking paths allow swimmers to change the directions of their limbs gradually and with less effort.

Curvilinear stroke patterns are also superior to linear patterns for maintenance of body alignment. With linear stroking motions the sudden braking effect on a limb moving in one direction creates a force of equal magnitude in the opposite direction. That force is transferred to swimmers' suspended bodies, forcing them out of alignment. Any loss of alignment increases drag and reduces forward velocity.

Angle of Attack

The **angle of attack** is the angle formed by the inclination of the hand and arm (or leg and foot) and the path of motion of the hand. Angles of attack for the hands of a breaststroke swimmer are shown from underneath and side views in Figure 21.14.

The hands, when angled in this manner, can be likened to hydrofoils. The movements of foils through fluids are identified by their leading and trailing edges. In the side-view example shown in Figure 21.14, the thumb side of the swimmer's hands is called the leading edge because it is the first part to encounter undisturbed streams of water as it sweeps down. The little finger side is the trailing edge because it is the last part of the hand-foil to have contact with that water. The leading edge can be the fingertips, wrist, thumb side or little finger side at various times during the underwater armstrokes of swimming strokes.

The angle of attack has great significance to the production of propulsive forces. Propulsion will be diminished if the angle of attack is too great or too small (Barthels 1979; Hay 1987; E. Maglischo 1982; Schleihauf 1978), substantiated by information gained from studying foils suspended in wind tunnels and water channels. How propulsion increases and decreases with changing angles of attack is illustrated in Figure 21.15. Hands are shown from an underneath view as though they were sweeping in under the swimmer's body at mid-stroke.

The amount of propulsion is minimal when the angle of attack is zero because swimmers' hands pass through the water without displacing it backward to any great extent. Consequently, there is only a small counter-force to propel them forward. This is illustrated by the small pressure differential between the palm and knuckle sides of the swimmer's hand. The small sizes of the + and − signs are indications that the magnitudes of these forces are not great.

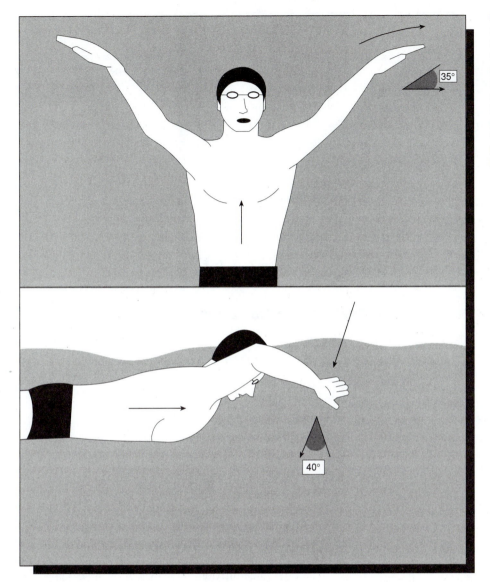

FIGURE 21.14 Underneath and side views of a breaststroke swimmer showing how the angle of attack of the hands is measured at the catch. These directions are indicated by the solid black arrows above his hands. His hands are inclined or pitched out and down. His palms are facing out to the side and they are inclined down slightly from thumb to little finger sides.

Propulsive force is increased when the angle of attack approaches 40°. This is because a considerable amount of backward force is imparted to the water as it passes under the swimmer's palm from the leading (thumb side) to trailing (little finger side) edges. This produces a counter-force of equal magnitude that propels the swimmer forward. The angle of attack shown here is probably very close to the ideal that swimmers should use when sweeping their hands under their bodies.

The palm presents a surface that is too flat when the angle of attack approaches 70°. Consequently, the water cannot change directions gradually. The effect is not unlike throwing a bucket of water against a wall. Some of the molecules "squirt" wildly away from the hand in random directions, while a good portion of the those remaining water molecules have their motion reversed. Forward propulsion is reduced because only a small amount of water is displaced backward.

Biomechanics of Aquatic Activities **461**

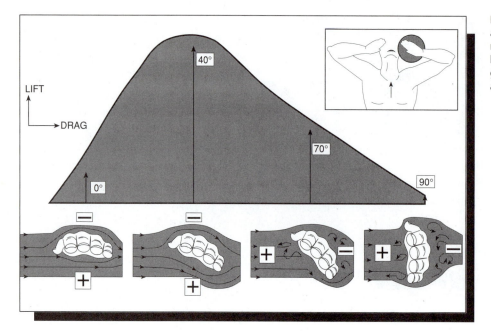

FIGURE 21.15 The effect of angle of attack on water movement during swimming. The hands are sweeping in with angles of attack of 0°, 40°, 70°, and 90°.

This loss of propulsion is even greater when the palm is perpendicular to the sideward direction in which it is moving. In this case, the hand acts like a paddle. There is no leading or trailing edge, only the large flat surface of the palm pushing sideward. The counter-force simply pushes the swimmer to the side in the opposite direction. A perpendicular angle of attack is only effective for propulsion when a swimmer's hands are traveling backward.

Researchers support these observations on angle of attack. For example, Schleihauf (1979) studied the effects of different angles of attack on lift by suspending plaster models of a human hand in a water channel. The water was forced past the hands at flow velocities similar to the hand speeds measured during competitive swims. He demonstrated a coefficient of lift curve for the hands that was similar to the one shown in Figure 21.15. His most significant findings were:

1. The coefficient of lift increased steadily up to an angle of attack of 40° and then decreased as the angle approached 90°. Angles of attack between 20° and 50° had very high coefficients of lift.
2. The coefficient of drag increased steadily as the angle of attack increased toward 90°.

3. Having the fingers together, or no more than ⅛ in. (.32 cm) apart was superior to finger spreads of ¼ in. (.64 cm) and ½ in. (1.27 cm) for producing lift.
4. Separating the thumb from the hand by a small amount produced more lift than a wide thumb spread.

Wood (1979) used a wind tunnel and plaster models of swimmers' hands and forearms to perform a series of studies similar to those conducted by Schleihauf. His findings were generally the same concerning the effects of different angles of attack on the coefficient of lift and drag. One interesting aspect of Wood's research is that he used three different directions of air flow across the hand. The most effective angle of attack was between 55° and 60° when the air was flowing across the hand from thumb to little finger side. The largest coefficients of lift occurred between angles of 15° and 35° when the flow was directed from little finger to thumb side. In the final series of experiments, the air was forced across the hand from fingertips to wrist. In this case, the optimum angle of attack was between 50° and 55°.

Remmonds and Bartlett (1981) also used a wind tunnel to study the effects of angles of attack on plaster models of swimmers' hands. They calculated the maximum lift force at an angle of attack of 50° with the fingers together and the thumb slightly separated from the hand.

Measuring angles of attack during actual swimming is a complicated and laborious procedure fraught with difficulty. Nevertheless, it has been attempted by several researchers over the years (Hinrichs 1986; Luedtke 1986; C. Maglischo et al. 1986; Schleihauf et al. 1983, 1984, 1988; Thayer et al. 1986). Schleihauf (1978) indicated that swimmers use angles of attack as slight as 15° and as great as 73° during various phases of the four competitive strokes. The swimmers in the study ranged in ability from good to world-class.

A team of researchers attempted to ascertain the best angles of attack for producing propulsive force in the front crawl stroke (C. Maglischo et al. 1986). Subjects were four male and four female distance freestylers who were members of the 1984 U.S. Olympic swimming team. The following observations were reported:

1. Angles of attack between 33° and 37° were most effective during the inward sweep under their bodies. Their hands and forearms moved across the water with the thumb side as the leading edge and the little finger side as the trailing edge. Swimmers who used angles of attack between 50° and 60° were not as effective during this phase.

2. Angles of attack between 30° and 46° were also most productive when the swimmers swept their hands out and up toward the surface in the final third of their underwater armstrokes. Angles between 50° and 70° were less productive during this sweep. Their arms moved through the water with their elbows as the leading edge and their fingertips as the trailing edge during this stroke phase.

Limb Velocity

Counsilman and Wasilak (1982) were the first to investigate the relationship between limb velocity and swimming speeds. They made us aware that the best swimmers accelerated their hands from the beginning to the end of their underwater armstrokes. These researchers reported maximum hand velocities in the range of 5.4 to 6.4 m/s (18.0 to 21.0 ft/s).

Later research by Schleihauf (1984) and Maglischo et al. (1987) showed that this concept was accurate but oversimplified. The swimmers did not accelerate their hands smoothly from start to finish. Rather, hand speed was accelerated in pulses, decreasing and then increasing with each major change of direction. The fastest velocities usually occurred during the final propulsive portion of an underwater armstroke.

Schleihauf (1974) presented the hand-velocity patterns of Mark Spitz, as shown in Figure 21.16. The hand-velocity patterns are depicted in relationship to still water and not the body. The hand velocity pattern in Figure 21.16 is typical of patterns used in the remaining three competitive strokes. In all cases, swimmers accelerate and decelerate their hands in pulses each time they change direction during the stroke. As you would expect, swimmers accelerate their hands more in sprints than in longer races. Also, females generally do not attain the same maximum velocities as males (C. Maglischo et al. 1986).

Stroke Rates and Stroke Lengths

The total time swimmers take to complete a race depends on their average swimming velocity. Swimming velocity is determined by multiplying a swimmer's stroke rate by stroke length. Stroke rates are usually expressed according to the number of stroke cycles swimmers take each minute (strokes/min), while stroke length is calculated as the number of meters the swimmer's body moves forward during each stroke cycle. The relationship between stroke rate and stroke length is negative because stroke length tends to decrease as stroke rate increases or vice versa. Nevertheless, the best swimmers generally cover more distance with each stroke cycle at competition stroke rates (Craig et al. 1985; Letzelter and Freitag 1983).

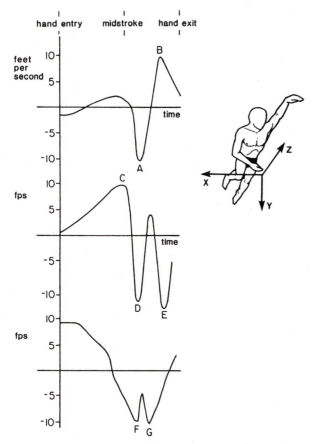

FIGURE 21.16 Hand velocity curves of Mark Spitz during crawl swimming. (*a*) Medial and lateral velocities; (*b*) upward and downward velocities; (*c*) forward and backward velocities. The ranges in all cases are ± 10 feet per second. **Visualize the direction and velocities at the points labeled A through G.**
(Modified from Schleihauf, R. 1974. A biomechanical analysis of freestyle. *Swimming Technique*, 11, p. 93.)

Males, on the average, have longer strokes than females. The stroke rates for males and females, however, are nearly the same for a particular race distance. In one study the stroke length for male competitors was, on the average, 18 cm (7 in.) greater than for females, while stroke rates were similar (Letzelter and Freitag 1983).

Hay et al. (1983) found that improvements in velocity during a season were due to increasing stroke length without decreasing stroke rates. Kreighbaum and

Barthels (1985) suggested that the reasons for these changes in stroke length might include the improvement of propulsive lift force through slight changes in hand path and hand angle of attack, along with a decrease in body drag caused by changing the swimmer's head and body position.

Faster swimmers not only cover more distance with each stroke early in races, they lose less distance per stroke when they become fatigued late in the race (Weiss et al. 1988). While the stroke length tends to become shorter for all swimmers when fatigued, the most successful swimmers shorten their strokes least.

Swim Starts and Turns

Start times account for approximately 25% of the total time spent swimming 25-yard races, 10% of the time in 50-yard races, and 5% of the time for 100-yard races. In addition, freestyle swimmers spend between 20% and 38% of their time turning in short course races that range from 50 yards to 1650 yards respectively. Breast-strokers, in short-course 200-yard races, spend 39% of their time turning and completing their underwater arm-stroke (Thayer and Hay 1984; Craig et al. 1988).

On the average, improving the start can reduce race times by at least 0.10 second. Improving turns can decrease race times at least 0.20 second per pool length. The act of turning involves the rapid somersaulting of the body and the rapid pushoff by the legs. The flexion of the legs to a near-45° angle gives the strongest angle for forceful and rapid movement.

Over the years, swimmers have used many starting styles. Initially, swimmers took a starting position with arms extended back. However, they soon found they could get their bodies moving toward the water faster by starting with their arms forward and then swinging them back. This technique made use of the action-reaction principle. The straight backswing start was later replaced by a circular backswing that provided more momentum during the takeoff from the starting platform.

The circular backswing has now been replaced by a faster method, the grab start. This start, introduced by Hanauer in the late 1960s, has rapidly gained in popularity

(Hanauer 1967). In this method, swimmers grip the front edge of the block. When the starting signal sounds, they pull their bodies forward with their arms.

Circular Backswing Start and Grab Start

Many researchers have verified that the grab start is faster than other methods (Winters 1968; Jorgenson 1971; Rotter and Nelson 1972; Michaels 1973; Bowers and Cavanaugh 1975; Cavanaugh et al. 1975; Thorsen 1975; Van Slooten 1975). This is because swimmers can get their bodies moving toward the water faster by pulling against the starting platform. Although they decelerate more quickly once they enter the water, the ability to get their bodies in motion quickly with a grab start outweighs any loss of momentum that occurs after entry. For example, Thorsen (1975) found that horizontal and vertical velocities were greater with the circular backswing start, yet the grab start was faster by 0.10 seconds to the point of entry. Bowers and Cavanaugh (1975) reported that swimmers left the block 0.17 sec. faster on the average when they used the grab start, compared to the circular backswing method. That measure accounted for practically all of the difference in time between the two starts at a point 10 yards down the pool.

Most of the studies comparing the grab and circular backswing starts have involved front crawl and butterfly swimmers. There is some doubt that it is the best starting style for breaststroke races because the deep entry and long underwater glide breaststrokers use allows more time for deceleration. Some coaches and swimmers have reasoned that it might be advisable to sacrifice a quick departure from the starting platform and use a circular armswing to gain more momentum during the glide.

Beritzhoff (1974) tested this theory by comparing the starting speeds of breaststroke swimmers using the grab start and the circular backswing start. The grab start was faster. Breaststroke swimmers reached a point 12.5 yards from the starting end of the pool on the average 0.150 seconds faster when they used a grab start. This advantage was noted despite the fact that, prior to taking part in the study, all but one of the subjects preferred the circular backswing start in competition.

Pike (Scoop) Dive

Another important change in starting technique is the adoption of the pike or scoop dive. In this starting style, swimmers travel through the air in a high arc, after piking (bending) at the waist, so they can enter the water at a very steep angle with minimal turbulence. Prior to the advent of this style, swimmers were advised to dive almost straight out and to enter the water at a very slight angle. The differences between the two dives are illustrated in Figure 21.17.

The major advantages of the pike dive is that swimmers encounter less drag at the point of entry. Consequently, they travel faster during the underwater glide.

However, a word of caution is in order regarding the pike dive. It has proven to be very dangerous when used in shallow pools. Several accidents have been reported where swimmers hit their faces and heads on the pool bottom. Some of these swimmers suffered serious neck injuries that left them paralyzed. Since the depth that swimmers reach with the pike dive varies from 3 to 5 feet (1.0-1.7 meters) (Counsilman et al. 1988), this dive should not be attempted in pools that are less than 6 feet deep.

Track Start

Another recent adaptation of the grab start is the track start, which has been used by several swimmers on the international level. The major difference between this and the traditional grab start occurs in the preparatory position on the starting platform. The swimmer in the drawings of Figure 21.18 performs the track start.

Two major advantages of the track start may be:

1. Swimmers can get into the water faster because the center of gravity travels almost straight forward beyond the starting platform until it begins falling toward the water. With the pike dive, the center of gravity travels up a greater distance after leaving the block and then down into the water. This increases the time it takes for swimmers to reach the entry position.
2. Swimmers' legs can deliver a greater forward thrust with two impulses rather than one. Swimmers get their bodies moving with their rear leg and then accelerate it forward even more with the front leg.

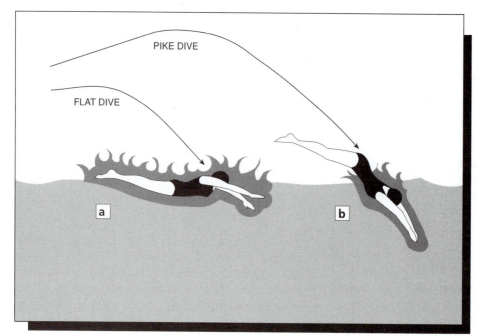

FIGURE 21.17 A comparison of the pike and flat dives. Swimmer *a* is shown entering the water after a flat dive. Swimmer *b* is using a pike dive. Swimmer *a* will hit the water in several places at once, causing her body to decelerate quite rapidly during the glide. Swimmer *b*'s entire body should enter the water at nearly the same point, causing her body to slip underwater with less turbulence, which, in turn, will allow her to glide much faster.

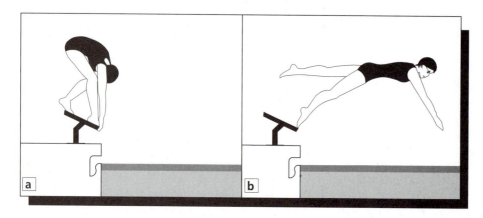

FIGURE 21.18 The track start in swimming. The swimmer has one foot back. For the traditional grab start, both feet are over the front edge of the starting block.

Three studies have compared the track start to other styles. In one, there was no difference in speed to 5, 10 and 12.5 yards between the flat grab start and the track start (Counsilman et al. 1988). In another, swimmers left the block significantly faster with the track start, but there was no difference in time between it and the regular grab start to a distance of 5 meters (approximately 16 feet) (Ayalon et al. 1975). In a third, the track start was significantly slower than the grab style for a distance of 5.5 meters (approximately 18 feet) (Zatsiorsky et al. 1979). Apparently, swimmers who use the track start seem to "get off the block" faster, enter the water at a somewhat "flatter" angle and lose time during the glide. Swimmers who use the conventional starting position (both feet at the edge of the block) are slower leaving the block but enter the water at an angle that permits a faster glide.

Hay et al. (1983) and Zatsiorsky and his associates (1979) reported that the gliding speed after entry accounts for most of the difference in starting times. Zatsiorsky and coworkers reported a significant relationship of 0.94 between starting speed and gliding speed. By comparison, the correlation between starting speed and speed off the block was 0.60. Although research is contradictory, the conventional grab start may be the potentially faster method because it permits a faster glide after entry.

One aspect in which the track start is clearly superior, however, is in preventing false starts. Swimmers have a more stable position on the platform and are not as likely to lose their balance if they pull early.

Special Training Devices for Improving Swimming Speed

Swimmers and coaches have used many practices to increase the work required of the athletes. Tethered swimming, swimming in a water treadmill, or swimming with hand paddles, drag suits, or other resistance devices have all been tried. Since force characteristics change in these situations compared with free swimming, one may assume that the mechanical characteristics of the stroke itself may change. For example, when a swimmer is tethered, the water is churned up and the same water is engaged with each stroke, causing turbulence. This turbulence causes the water particles to move in a haphazard fashion, increasing the resistance but varying it in unknown amount from one stroke to the next. Thus, the application of force by the swimmer will not be the same for each stroke.

Sprint-Assisted and Sprint-Resisted Training

E. Maglischo and Maglischo (1985) studied the use of surgical tubing as a means of sprint-assisted and sprint-resisted training. One end of the tubing was attached to an end wall and the other to a waist belt. In sprint-resisted training the swimmer would don the belt and swim away from the wall. This resulted in increased resistance as the tubing was stretched. In sprint-assisted training, the swimmer would first stretch the tubing and then swim back with the snap-back of the tubing allowing him to swim faster than he could during free swimming. Definite changes in free swimming stroke mechanics were reported in both sprint-assisted and sprint-resisted trials. Those changes appeared to improve mechanics with the sprint-assisted training. Changes in mechanics that occurred during the sprint-resisted training were considered detrimental. Stroke length and stroke rate both tended to increase during sprint-assisted training, while both decreased during sprint-resisted training.

Other Resistance Devices

Nelson (1976) attached a resistance training device to the waist of women being towed in the prone position. The average resistance recorded by strain gages during towing with the device was 90% greater than without the device. One group of swimmers trained with the device, and one group trained without it. The following conclusions were drawn:

1. The resistance while a swimmer is wearing the device will vary among subjects because of the size of the sagittal-thorax area, which is the primary cause of turbulent flow into and around the device.
2. Wearing the device will drop the lower half of the body, causing a change in the body orientation. This movement could prevent the swimmer from practicing the specific movements of stroking needed to train effectively.
3. The evidence suggests that swimmers who continue to use the device believe that it is beneficial in spite of perceived problems with specificity training.

Hand Paddles

Swimmers have used **hand paddles** to increase the area of the hand. This in turn increases the volume of water displaced backward while slowing the stroke rate. Hand paddles have been proposed as a stroke-teaching aid and as a form of resistance training for the muscles of the shoulders and trunk. Stoner and Luedtke (1979) reported that varsity swimmers who use hand paddles do not seem to make major alterations in either front or back crawl stroke patterns, although the amount of time spent in pulling is increased. Experts recommend that paddles be selected carefully so that they are similar in shape to the hand. Bollens and Clarys (1986) reported that the best shape was a rectangle with the finger-tip end rounded and bent slightly out of plane.

Flume Training

A **flume** is a swimming treadmill housed in a large tank in which the water moves in a circular manner and the swimmer swims in accordance with the speed of the water. The flume supplies a controllable laminar flow. It is like an environmental chamber in which water depth can be simulated with air and water temperature control. The swimmer in action can be biomechanically analyzed three-dimensionally through the use of two underwater cameras. The force applied by the swimmer can also be determined. Strengthening of body parts should be introduced in the training program and computer technology and video analysis are a part of the process. It is easy to understand that such an apparatus would be valuable in rehabilitation of disabled people and those recovering from injury.

MINI-LABORATORY LEARNING EXPERIENCE

1. Perform several underwater pushoffs and glides. Use the same leg extension force but vary the position of your arms from wide apart to close together and the position of your head from high to low. Discuss the differences in the amount of water resistance encountered.
2. Swim the length of the pool and record your time and stroke rate. Calculate your body velocity and the average distance covered per stroke.
3. Hold your hand out of a moving car's window. Vary the position of the fingers and the hand's angle of attack. Discuss the differences in the lift forces encountered.

References

Ayalon, A., Van Gheluwe, B., and Kanitz, M. 1975. A comparison of four styles of racing starts in swimming. In *Swimming II,* ed. L. LeWillie, and J. Clarys. Baltimore, MD: University Park Press.

Barthels, K. 1979. The mechanism for body propulsion in swimming. In *Swimming III: Proceedings of the third international symposium on the biomechanics of swimming,* ed. J. Terauds, and E. Bedingfield. Baltimore, MD: University Park Press.

Barthels, K., and Adrian, M. J. 1975. Three dimensional spatial hand patterns of skilled butterfly swimmers. In *Swimming II,* ed. L. LeWillie, and J. Clarys. Baltimore, MD: University Park Press.

Beritzoff, S. T. 1974. The relative effectiveness of two breaststroke starting techniques among selected intercollegiate swimmers. Master's thesis, California State University, Chico.

Bollens, E., and Clarys, J. P. 1986. Front crawl training with hand paddles: A telemetric EMG investigation. In *Biomechanics, the 1984 scientific congress proceedings,* ed. M. Adrian, and H. Deutsch. Eugene, OR: University of Oregon Microform Publications.

Bowers, J. E., and Cavanaugh, P. R. 1975. A biomechanical comparison of the grab and conventional sprint starts in competitive swimming. In *Swimming II,* ed. L. LeWillie, and J. Clarys. Baltimore, MD: University Park Press.

Brown, R. M., and Counsilman, J. E. 1971. The role of lift in propelling swimmers. In *Biomechanics,* ed. J. Cooper. Chicago: Athletic Institute.

Cavanaugh P. R., Palmgren, J. V., and Kerr, B. A. 1975. A device to measure forces at the hand during the grab start in swimming. In *Swimming II,* ed. L. LeWillie, and J. Clarys. Baltimore, MD: University Park Press.

Clarys, J. P. 1979. Human morphology and hydrodynamics. In *Swimming III: Proceedings of the third international symposium on the biomechanics of swimming,* ed. J. Terauds, and E. Bedingfield. Baltimore, MD: University Park Press.

Colwin, C. 1984. Fluid dynamics: Vortex circulation in swimming propulsion. *ASCA world clinic yearbook,* ed. T. Welsh. Fort Lauderdale, FL: American Swimming Coaches Association.

Colwin, C. 1985a. Essential fluid dynamics of swimming propulsion. *ASCA Newsletter,* July/Aug.

Colwin, C. 1985b. Practical application of flow analysis as a coaching tool. *ASCA Newsletter,* Sept/Oct.

Counsilman, J. E. 1955. Forces in swimming two types of crawl stroke. *Res. Q.* 26:127–39.

Counsilman, J. E. 1968. *The science of swimming.* Englewood Cliffs, NJ: Prentice-Hall.

Counsilman, J. E. 1977. *Competitive swimming manual for coaches and swimmers.* Bloomington, IN: Counsilman Co., Inc.

Counsilman, J. E., Counsilman, B. E., Normura, T., and Endo, M. 1988. Three types of grab starts for competitive swimming. In *Swimming science V,* ed. B. Ungerechts, K. Wilke, and K. Reischle. Champaign, IL: Human Kinetics.

Counsilman, J. E., and Wasilak, J. 1982. The importance of hand speed and hand acceleration. In *ASCA world clinic yearbook,* ed. R. Ousley. Fort Lauderdale, FL: American Swimming Coaches Association.

Craig, A. B., Jr., Boomer, W. L., and Skehan, P. L. 1988. Patterns of velocity in competitive breaststroke swimming. In *Swimming science V,* ed. B. Ungerechts, K. Wilke, and K. Reischle. Champaign, IL: Human Kinetics.

Craig, A. B., Jr., Skehan, P. L., Pawelczyk, J. A., and Boomer, W. L. 1985. Velocity stroke rate and distance per stroke during elite swimming competition. *Medicine and Science in Sports and Exercise* 17(6):625–34.

Di Prampero, P. E., PaPendergast, D. R., Wilson, D. W., and Rennie, D. W. 1974. Energetics of swimming in man. *Journal of Applied Physiology* 37:1–5.

Hanauer, E. 1967. The grab start. *Swimming World* 8:5, 42.

Hay, J. G. 1987. Biomechanics of swimming. *Swimming Technique* 24(4):18–21.

Hay, J. G., Guimaraes, A. C. S., and Grimstan, S. K. 1983. A quantative look at swimming biomechanics. *Swimming Technique* 20(2):11–17.

Hinrichs, R. 1986. Biomechanics of butterfly. In *ASCA world clinic yearbook,* ed. T. Johnston, J. Woolger, and D. Scheider. Fort Lauderdale, FL: American Swimming Coaches Association.

Hollander, A. P., de Groot, G., and Van Ingen Schenau, G. J. 1987. Active drag in female swimmers. In *Biomechanics X–B,* ed. B. Jousson. Champaign, IL: Human Kinetics.

Hollander, A. P., et al. 1986. Measurement of active drag during crawl armstroke swimming. *Journal of Sports Science* 4:21–30.

Jorgenson, L. W. 1971. A cinematographical and descriptive comparison of three selected freestyle racing starts in competitive swimming. Ph.D. dissertation, Louisiana State University.

Koehler, J. A. 1987. Bernoulli, and on how aircraft fly. Unpublished manuscript, University of Saskatchewan.

Kreighbaum, E., and Barthels, K. 1985. *Biomechanics: A qualitative approach for studying human movement.* New York: Macmillan.

Letzelter, H., and Freitag, W. 1983. Stroke length and stroke frequency variations in men's and women's 100 m freestyle swimming. In *Biomechanics and medicine in swimming,* ed. A. Hollander, P. Huijing, and G. de Groot. Champaign IL. Human Kinetics.

Luedtke, D. 1986. Backstroke biomechanics. In *ASCA world clinic yearbook,* ed. T. Johnston, J. Woolger, and D. Scheider. Fort Lauderdale, FL: American Swimming Coaches Association.

Maglischo, C. W., Maglischo, E. W., Luedtke, D., Schleihauf, R. E., Higgins, J., Hinrichs, R., and Thayer, A. 1986. A biomechanical analysis of the 1984 U. S. Olympic swimming team: The distance freestylers. *J. Swimming Res.* 2(3):12–16.

Maglischo, C. W., Maglischo, E. W., Luedtke, D., Schleihauf, R. E., Higgins, J., Hinrichs, R., and Thayer, A. 1987a. The swimmer: A study of propulsion and drag. *SOMA (Engineering for the human body)* 2(2):40–44.

Maglischo, E. W. 1982. *Swimming faster.* Palo Alto, CA: Mayfield Publishing.

Maglischo, E. W. 1984. A 3-dimensional cinematographical analysis of competitive swimming strokes. In *1983 ASCA world clinic yearbook.* Fort Lauderdale, FL: American Swimming Coaches Association.

Maglischo, E. W. 1986. Sprint freestyle biomechanics. *ASCA world clinic yearbook,* ed. T. Johnston, J. Woolger, and D. Scheider. Fort Lauderdale, FL: American Swimming Coaches Association.

Maglischo, E., and Maglischo, C. 1985. The effects of sprint assisted and sprint resistive training on stroke mechanics. *Journal of Swimming Research 1.*

Michaels, R. A. 1973. A time distance comparison of the conventional and the grab start. *Swimming Technique* 10:16–17.

Nelson, L. J. 1976. Drag and performance analysis of a resistance device in swimming. Master's thesis, Washington State University.

Reischle, K. 1979. A kinematic investigation of movement patterns in swimming with photo-optical methods. In *Swimming III: Proceedings of the third international symposium on the biomechanics of swimming*, ed. J. Terauds, and E. Bedingfield. Baltimore, MD: University Park Press.

Remmonds, P., and Bartlett, R. M. 1981. Effects of finger separation. *Swimming Technique* 18(1):28–30.

Rotter, B. J., and Nelson, R. C. 1972. The grab start is faster. *Swimming Technique* 18(1):28–30.

Schleihauf, R. E. 1974. A biomechanical analysis of freestyle. *Swimming Technique* 11:89–96.

Schleihauf, R. E. 1978. Swimming propulsion: A hydrodynamic analysis. In *1977 ASCA world clinic yearbook*, ed. R. Ousley. Fort Lauderdale, FL: American Swimming Coaches Association.

Schleihauf, R. E. 1979. A hydrodynamic analysis of swimming propulsion. In *Swimming III: Proceedings of the third international symposium on the biomechanics of swimming*, ed. J. Terauds, and E. Bedingfield. Baltimore, MD: University Park Press.

Schleihauf, R. E. 1984. Biomechanics of swimming propulsion. In *1983 ASCA world clinic yearbook*. Fort Lauderdale, FL: American Swimming Coaches Association.

Schleihauf, R. E., Gray, L., and DeRose, J. 1983. Three-dimensional analysis of hand propulsion in the sprint front crawl stroke. In *Biomechanics and medicine in swimming*, ed. A. Hollander, P. Huijing, and G. de Groot. Champaign, IL: Human Kinetics.

Schleihauf, R. E., Higgins, J., Hinrichs, R., Luedtke, D., Maglischo, C., Maglischo, E., and Thayer, A. 1984. Biomechanics of swimming propulsion. In *ASCA world clinic yearbook*, ed. T. Welsh. Fort Lauderdale, FL: American Swimming Coaches Association.

Schleihauf, R. E., Higgins, J., Hinrichs, P., Luedtke, D., Maglischo, C., Maglischo, E., and Thayer, A. 1988. Propulsive techniques: Front crawl stroke, butterfly, backstroke and breaststroke. In *Swimming science V*, ed. C. Morehouse. Champaign, IL. Human Kinetics.

Sharp, R. L., and Costill, D. L. 1989. Influence of body hair removal on physiological responses during breaststroke swimming. *Med. Sci. Sports and Exerc.* 21(5):576–80.

Sharp, R. L., Hackney, A. C., Cain S. M., and Ness, R. J. 1988. The effect of shaving down on the physiologic cost of freestyle swimming. *J. Swimming Res.* 4(1):9–13.

Silvia, C. E. 1970. *Manual and lesson plans for basic swimming, water stunts, lifesaving, springboard diving, skin and scuba diving*. Published by the author.

Sprigings, E. J., and Koehler, J. A. 1990. The choice between Bernoulli's or Newton's model in predicting dynamic lift. *Int. J. Sport Biomechanics* 6(3):235–45.

Stoner, L. J., and Luedtke, D. L. 1979. Variations in the front crawl and back crawl armstrokes of varsity swimmers using hand paddles. In *Swimming III: Proceedings of the third international symposium on the biomechanics of swimming*, ed. J. Terauds, and E. Bedingfield. Baltimore, MD: University Park Press.

Takamoto, M., Ohmichi, H., and Miyashita, M. 1985. Wave height in relation to swimming velocity and proficiency in front crawl stroke. In *Biomechanics IX-B*, ed. D. Winter, R. Norman, R. Wells, K. Hayes, and A. Patla. Champaign, IL: Human Kinetics.

Thayer, A., Schleihauf, R. E., Higgins, R. E., Hinrichs, J. R., Luedtke, D. L., Maglischo, C. W., and Maglischo, E. W. 1986. A hydrodynamic analysis of breaststroke swimmers. In *Starting, stroking & turning*, ed. J. G. Hay. Iowa City, IA: Biomechanics Laboratory, Dept. of Exercise Science, University of Iowa.

Thayer, A. L., and Hay, J. G. 1984. Motivating start and turn improvement. *Swimming Technique* 20(4):17–20.

Thorsen, E. A. 1975. Comparison of the conventional and grab start in swimming. *Tidskrift Før Legenspuelset* 39:130–38.

Van Slooten, P. H. 1973. An analysis of two forward swim starts using cinematography. *Swimming Technique* 10:85–88.

Van Tilborgh, L. V., Stijnen, V. V., and Persyn, U. J. 1987. Using velocity fluctuations for estimating resistance and propulsion forces in breaststroke swimming. In *Biomechanics IX-B*, ed. D. Winter, R. Norman, R. Wells, K. Hayes, and A. Patla. Champaign, IL: Human Kinetics.

Weiss, M., Reischle, K., Bouws, N., Simon, G., and Weicker, H. 1988. Relationship of blood lactate accumulation to stroke rate and distance per stroke in top female swimmers. In *Swimming science V: International series on sports sciences*, vol. 18. Champaign, IL: Human Kinetics.

Winters, C. N. 1968. A comparison of the grab start in competitive swimming. Master's thesis, Southeast Missouri State College.

Wood, T. C. 1979. A fluid dynamics analysis of the propulsive potential of the hand and forearm in swimming. In *Swimming III: Proceedings of the third international symposium on the biomechanics of swimming*, ed. J. Terauds, and E. Bedingfield. Baltimore, MD: University Park Press.

Zatsiorsky, V. M., Bulgakova, and Chaplinsky, N. M. 1979. Biomechanical analysis of starting techniques. In *Swimming III: Proceedings of the third international symposium on the biomechanics of swimming*, ed. J. Terauds, and E. Bedingfield. Baltimore, MD: University Park Press.

22 Biomechanics of Rolling and Sliding Activities

Gliding, sliding, and rolling devices must be controlled for successful performance in sports such as skiing, skating, and cycling. Both the equipment and the environment of ice, land, sun, snow, or water are important considerations in the biomechanics analysis of these sports.

The multitude of new rolling and sliding activities introduced during the past two decades are numerous. In-line skating, sandboarding, snowboarding, boardsurfing, skateboarding, and many types of dance and acrobatic competitions in both traditional and new sports have been created. The activities sometimes require jumping, twisting and turning around obstacles, moving to music, and traveling at high speeds. For example, skateboarders skate up a vertical wall and add an acrobatic stunt before skating down. The same activity can be done on bicycles. In-line skaters can travel more than 117 kmph (70 mph) in the tuck position and speed skiers go almost 232 kmph (140 mph). Indeed, on a testing area in Chile, one speed skier was clocked at slightly over 333 kilometers per hour (200 mph) at the finish!

What new devices will we see in the future? How many new types of competition will become Olympic-approved sports in this group of activities in which people have an interfacing device between their shoes and the ground or water?

Definitions

For ease in biomechanical analysis, those forms of locomotion that use some type of device to produce gliding motion can be placed into one of the following two categories: rolling or sliding. Examples of locomotion with *sliding* devices (boards and blades) include downhill skiing, cross-country skiing, other forms of snow skiing, water skiing, board surfing, snowboarding, bobsled, toboggan, luge, and ice skating of all types.

Examples of locomotion in which rolling devices are used are of two types: devices that roll as a result of a gliding of the body and devices that roll as a result of pedaling action of the person. Examples of locomotion in which the body glides on roller devices include roller skating, in-line skating, and skateboarding. Examples of rolling devices that use pedaling actions are unicycles, bicycles, tricycles, wheelchairs, and other human-powered machines.

Commonalities of Gliding Activities

1. A pedal/step/stroke produces momentum (gliding of the body) proportional to the produced impulse (sum of $Ft = mv$). The greater the force-time product, the longer the glide and the fewer strokes necessary to traverse a predetermined distance.

2. Maximizing the stroke-frequency is dependent on optimum timing of the next stroke prior to losses in speed. This is similar to loss of momentum in gliding action during swimming.

3. Since the base of support may be narrower (e.g., skates) or longer (e.g., skis), equilibrium may be more difficult to maintain or regulate. This is especially true during changes in direction.

4. When executing turns, the greater the arc, that is, the longer the radius of the turn, the greater the tangential velocity. This creates problems when executing a wide turn on a steep downslope.

5. In order to change direction, stop, or start, there must be a change in friction and reaction forces.

6. Waxing is required to change the surface friction and will facilitate maneuvers on water and snow. Snow does not pack under a properly waxed ski, but turns to water and maintains a more laminar flow across the ski bottoms.

7. With every change in body position (or body parts), there is a change in the center of gravity and gravitational line. The active forces between the ground and the gliding device change.

8. The body position influences the form and surface area drag, thus increasing or decreasing the velocity of the person. Body position also influences the magnitude of any required propulsive forces.

9. Expected and unexpected changes in the coefficients of friction occur between the gliding devices and the gliding surfaces. For example, the changing of compact snow to slush may cause greater friction, stopping the momentum of the ski and catapulting the skier in a forward rotational movement. Likewise, pedaling a bicycle too fast may cause tires to spin due to decreased friction on wet pavement, losing forward momentum.

10. Since tactile and kinesthetic sensations may not be recognized as readily when using gliding devices, precise fit between foot and device is imperative.

Skating*

Skating is considered to be a form of stepping; however, its mechanics differ in several ways from those of walking. In ice skating, the differences are caused by two aspects of the situation: (1) the base of support is much smaller (the width of the skate blade compared to that of the shoe or foot); and (2) the supporting surface offers little resistance to a horizontal push (ice compared to ground or floor). In roller skating, the base is wider, but the lack of friction between rollers and the supporting surface is comparable to that in ice skating. The major adjustment to this low coefficient of friction for the skater is to always keep the center of gravity over the supporting foot. The center of gravity cannot be allowed to fall ahead, since backward rotational movement and slippage of the foot will result, and balance is likely to be lost.

The muscles involved in skating are the leg extensor muscles, the abdominal muscles, and the arm/shoulder flexor muscles. The leg extensor muscles used in skating are the gastrocnemius and soleus muscles acting at the ankle joint, the quadriceps femoris muscles group at the knee joint, and the gluteus maximus and upper hamstring muscles acting at the hip joint (for pushing the leg back). The hip joint flexor muscles (the rectus femoris, the pectineus, and the iliopsoas) are used to lift the leg and place the foot on the ice for the forward glide. A strong midsection (the abdominals and the erector spinae) is needed in order to keep the body in the desirable position (either erect or flexed trunk) and to be able to transfer the force of the arms and legs in order to propel the body forward. A person can skate faster when the legs and trunk are flexed. To facilitate shoulder action and full range of motion of the arms, the following upper body muscles are used: the anterior deltoid, the pectoralis major and minor, the serratus anterior, and the trapezius.

Speed skaters use certain techniques to reduce drag. Examples are having the upper body flexed almost parallel to the ice to reduce the frontal area, keeping one

*Contributed by Sharol Laczkowski.

arm tucked behind the back to reduce the drag, and swinging the other arm to maintain balance. They also wear tight-fitting clothes to keep their body surface smooth.

Skating Research

In recent studies using a large subject sample, investigators secured film data with panning or fixed cameras. These cameras were on curves and straightaways, viewing from the sagittal and frontal positions. Approximately 19 kinematic variables, such as air friction, ice friction, and mechanical work per stroke/kg/body mass were measured. Models to predict power were developed. One such model was used to predict power as a function of trunk position, knee angle, body weight, body length, and speed of COG.

> Some basic skating principles are:
>
> 1. Speed is the ultimate result of a balance between minimal friction losses and maximal power production. Skating position is extremely important with respect to frictional losses and potential for power production. For example, plantar flexion of the foot causes increased friction as the blade pricks into ice.
>
> 2. Pushoff mechanics are very important on curves and straightaways to create effective mechanical work per stroke. Also important are the extension velocities at the hip and knee joints and the preextension knee angle.
>
> 3. Stroke frequency is used primarily to control speed. On the curves of oval courses, the stroke frequency is constrained by speed, work per stroke and radius of the curve.

De Boer and Nilsen (1989 a,b) analyzed kinematically gliding and pushoff techniques used in the 1988 Winter Olympics 1500 and 5000m races. In studies of more than 100 competitors, the only significant finding was that higher work per stroke is correlated with longer glide and more horizontal pushoff. They also found stroke frequency, consistent within one lap, to be the

major regulator of speed. They described the mechanics of speed skating the curves in a match model showing sideward pushoff characteristics of the propulsion and the cyclic nature of the motion.

In 500m races, the start is 80% of the variation of the total performance. During the first 4 seconds of these races, the skaters used a running-like technique until a speed of approximately 4 m/sec was attained. Then their technique changed to gliding actions. Females attained 8 m/sec and males attained 10 m/sec at the end of 4 seconds. Both male and female skaters can continue to accelerate and reach speeds of 11-15 m/sec. The effectiveness of the pushoff is more important than the high power-output values.

Speed Skating

Speed skating has the following phases: gliding (flight in running start), pushoff phase, and repositioning phase. Pushoff power of skaters has been measured as 2688 watts (average) for males and 1848 watts (average) for females on bike ergometers. Even when normalized to body weight, males produce more pushoff power. The start is very similar to that of the track sprinting start.

Marino (1983) investigated the factors that determine high acceleration rates obtained in the ice skating start. Although the regression equation for the relationship between technique variables and acceleration showed a multiple correlation of only 0.78, the following factors were identified as forming the ideal skating start pattern: high stride rate, significant forward lean, low takeoff angle, and placement of the recovery foot directly under the body at the end of the single-support phase.

Power Skating

Power skating is used in ice hockey and speed skating. Power skating requires mastering the use of the inside and outside edges of the skate blade and obtaining maximum leg power with minimum work and extraneous motion. Force applied correctly in a short period of time translates into power, which, in turn, is an important component of speed. The power-skating stride segments are divided into the areas of the wind-up, the release, the follow-through, and the return.

The wind-up is the preparation phase of the stride and prepares the skater to push by digging the blade edge into the ice and pressing the body weight down over the blade edge (coiling). The thrusting leg will provide great power if the edge is digging into the ice at an optimum angle (approximately 45°) ankle roll and if the leg is strongly flexed to approximately 45° at the knee. The feet are positioned in a V formation—toes apart, heels together. For an explosive start, both heels are lifted from the ice so only the front one-third of the inside edges of the blades are touching the ice and the upper body is angled forward with the legs flexed. The skater actually tries to fall forward while maintaining the body position. For explosiveness, there is no glide phase. Using the blade edges correctly in the windup prepares for rapid acceleration.

Release.   The release phase is the actual leg thrust in which power is applied. The thrusting leg must drive against the blade edge and must reach to full extension. The legs push (uncoil) quickly to reach maximum speed. The thrusting leg pushes on a side and back diagonal. The toe of the thrusting leg points outward (not down) at the finish of the push and very close to the ice surface. The support leg is flexed. Driving hard with the thrusting leg and reaching with the knees achieves power and distance with each stride.

■ The main power of the skating thrust is provided by the thigh muscles.

The return is a critical determinant of effectiveness of both the forward stride and the explosive start. The outstretched leg must return quickly, staying close to the ice surface and keeping the toes and knee pointed outward. Keeping the foot close to the ice surface helps keep the center of gravity low so speed will not decrease, and progress can be made in a straight line, which is more effective for speed. Keeping a strong "knee bend," the gliding foot will momentarily meet the returning foot in a V position as it sets down on the ice to become the gliding foot. Every push must start with the feet centered under the body.

■ Rapid leg turnover is essential to an explosive start.

Placement of the Foot.   In a study by Marino (1983) on acceleration in skating, it was found to be more im-

portant to place the foot directly underneath rather than in front of the body to aid in the next propulsive phase. This rapid striding pattern generates velocity. Getting a full extension at the knee during the pushoff results in the ability to cover a greater distance in less time. Also, rapid strides, rather than long strides, facilitate quickness in skating starts. The glide phase of the skating stride denotes a deceleration in the horizontal direction; therefore, for a quick start, very little gliding is used. To optimize the magnitude and the direction of propulsion, a low angle of forward body lean, approximately 42°, is desirable.

In speed ice skating, one of two foot positions is commonly used as the skater is waiting at the starting line for the starting signal. In one, the skates are placed shoulder-width apart one ahead of the other and both at an approximate angle of 40° with the starting line. In the other position, the front skate is pointed forward at 90° to the starting line, and the rear skate approaches a parallel position with the starting line. Skaters who use the second position believe that it saves a fraction of a second in the start, since the foot need not be lifted and turned to take the first step.

At the starting signal, the center of gravity is lowered by increasing flexion at the knee and hip. The weight is shifted to the rear foot so that the forward one can be lifted slightly for the first step. With this step, there is extension at the rear knee and hip. For a brief time, the center of gravity falls ahead of the supporting foot; this is possible because the angle of the skate resists the backward push of gravity and the extension continues until the rear limb is straight and inclined approximately 45° from the horizontal. After a short step, the front foot has in the meantime been placed on the ice and angled, as was the rear foot. The rear foot now steps. This type of stepping continues for three or four strides, each stride increasing in length over the previous one. During the beginning strides, the arms move as they do in running, in opposition to the lower-limb movements.

After the starting strides, the weight is carried over the front foot so that when the rear foot pushes, it does not affect equilibrium. As the push from the ice is applied to the body, a low center of gravity is advantageous. After the push, as the supporting foot glides, the rear foot is brought forward. As it passes the gliding foot, it takes the weight of the body by placing the foot in a forward direction and close to the other foot.

The Skating Stride. Ice skating is biphasic, with each stride consisting of alternate periods of single support and double support. In speed skating, the period of single support is the glide phase and propulsion occurs during the double-support phase. Because of the resistive forces of drag and friction, the body tends to accelerate when a propulsive force is applied and decelerate during the glide phase. A study by Marino and Weese (1979) revealed that the iceskating stride consists of two functional phases: (a) glide during the single support; and (b) propulsion during single and double support, beginning halfway through the single-support phase and lasting through the end of the double-support phase. In the technique of the skating stride, a long single-support time is related to relatively slow skating time and with a low rate of acceleration. A high stride rate was commensurate with fast skating time and a high rate of acceleration.

The mechanics of the skating action change somewhat with respect to the length of the race. Filmstrips prepared in 1962 by H. Freisinger, the 1964 U.S. Olympic team coach, showed that in the 500m race, the trunk is slightly above the horizontal. In longer races it is horizontal. Additionally, in the short-distance race, alternating flexion and extension of the spine is seen. At the end of the push, one limb is well back of the gliding foot, and the trunk is fully extended. At this instance trunk and limb balance each other over the supporting limb like two ends of a teeterboard.

■ The form (shape) of the body influences the magnitude of drag in a similar fashion to that of bicycling. The surface area encountering the air creates resistance that the skater must overcome with muscle force.

Stopping

There are many different techniques for stopping in skating. All of the different stopping positions consist of leaning the body backward and digging (sliding) the blades into the ice, causing an increase in friction.

Figure Skating

Basic figure skating involves the use of medial, lateral, inside, and outside edges of the skates. The inside edge is always toward the center of the curve and may be the medial or lateral edge, depending upon the situation. Skating in a curved path involves one medial and lateral edge, while fixing the skates in one position requires both medial edges or a flat blade (no edging).

The serrated toe of the skate is used to create friction and, thus, a change in direction and/or reduction in speed. Detailed exploration of edging and changes in friction are discussed in the skiing section.

Spinning, Turning, and Twisting in Figure Skating. The moment of inertia is the smallest about the horizontal axis and can be increased by extending the arms or legs or by flexing at the waist. A skater spins faster if the arms and legs are close and tight to the body. Positions of the arms and legs (e.g., planting the foot out to the side to provide an effective pushoff for turning, and swinging the arms horizontally in the direction of the turn/twist) provide torques needed to initiate spins. Raising the arms overhead increases the rate of spin. Unfolding the arms or a leg to the side while spinning brings about a deceleration.

ng and In-line Skating*

research does not exist on roller skating skills
cally, the information on ice skating and skiing can
e as a basic foundation for the analysis and improve-
ent of skating skills. In-line skating is presented here.

In-Line Skating. Because **in-line skating** is a relatively
new sport, little biomechanical research has been conducted on it. We can assume that it is similar to ice skating and snow skiing. The levels of performance vary in
purpose from recreational activity to cross-training for
other sports, such as cross-country skiing, ice hockey,
speed skating, surfing, skate skiing, and speed racing.
The activity imitates ice skating on dry land. In-line
skating is normally a form of low-impact aerobic exercise, which helps build strong leg, abdominal, and back
muscles. The footwear consists of ice skating boots or
plastic boots that grip the ankle to provide stability.

A skater can go much faster with the wheels in a row
(in-line skates) than with wheels side-by-side (roller
skates) and the skating technique is easier, smoother,
lighter, and quicker to learn. Three to five polyurethane
wheels are used, the most popular being four wheels to
provide an almost frictionless ride. On one or both
skates there is an attached brake on the heel designed to
give control. Bearings on the wheels can be interchanged to give more or less resistance as desired.

The four-wheeled in-line skates and the five-wheeled
racing skates (are detachable, having varying lengths
and heights) are made of strong, lightweight space-age
materials. For racing frames, the material is composed
of titanium and carbon graphite. The shorter rails are for
sprinting, climbing, and cornering. The longer rails are
for high-speed runs, long straight courses, and down-
high runs. Rails positioned more medial to the others are
for long glides. The back of each boot is placed above or
slightly forward of the rear-most axle.

Speed limits. In most city parks there is a limit of 15
mph set on in-line skating. Without speed limits, the
performer may reach 50 mph (80 kmph) from a standing

---

*Contributed by Sharol Laczkowski.

position. John Svensson attained a speed of 72 mph (116
kmph) in a tuck position on the six-mile run down
Steven Pass in the state of Washington.

Striding. The performer starts with one foot turned
outward and the other foot pointed straight ahead. The
arms are extended out in front of the body and held low
for better balance. The weight is centered on the balls of
the feet with the lower legs flexed, shins held against the
boot tongues. The body is crouched forward a little for
better control. The skater pushes out to the side with the
sideways skate and places the weight on the forward
foot. He or she brings the feet close together and then
pushes out with the other foot, transferring the weight
onto the forward foot pointed straight ahead. The push
outward is made more forceful and higher with the sideways foot. The weight is kept on the support foot as the
glide is performed.

Turning. The weight is placed over the inside edge of
the turning foot. (If turning left, this is the right foot.)
The lower leg is flexed to increase force on the edge and
increase the speed of the turn. Knees should face the direction of the turn. To slow down for a turn, skaters use
the brakes on the heel of the inside foot. The motions are
similar to those of ski turns and skate skiing.

Uphill Striding. Short strides are taken to keep the
weight over the balls of the foot, but the lean forward
should be only to a small degree.

Downhill Striding. The upper body (shoulders) is kept
square with the hill. The waist is flexed with the weight
over the total foot. The arms are extended out in front of
the body for balance, placing the center of gravity in the
abdominal region. Balance control in-line skating consists of transferring weight from one leg to the other and
keeping the weight on the inside edge. Going faster (taking quicker strides) means keeping the weight on the
balls of the feet, flexing 90° at the knees, and having a
slight forward lean.

Braking. Brakes on most in-line skates are on the right
skate heel. (Beginner skates come with brakes on both
skates.) To use the brakes properly, the right foot (brake

foot) is placed slightly in front of the left. The waist is flexed and tilted, with the right foot up and exerting pressure on the right heel. The lower legs should be flexed and the arms extended in front and away from the body for better balance. The more pressure exerted, the more the momentum is decreased. It is difficult to come to a complete stop gracefully wearing in-line skates, unlike on ice skates.

Protective equipment is advised when in-line skating. Helmets, knee and elbow pads, and wrist guards are available.

Skiing

Snow skiing includes many types: cross-country, downhill, slalom, jumping, and freestyle. The analysis of freestyle activities requires the understanding of dancer airborne flight and moguls; there are gliding, turning, and aerial techniques to study.

The latest invention is known as upskiing, a new adventure sport that combines a parachute-type sail with skiing. The sail has a vent to control the force of the wind acting on the chute. People have skied up mountains at speeds of 35 mph (57 kmph). They have raced across frozen lakes at 60 mph (97 kmph), and "jumped" 100 ft (30m) horizontally and 30 ft (9m) upward. But in this chapter we will concentrate on the basics of ski-snow interfacing and the slope and terrain of the hill. We will describe some applications of jumping, but you'll have to use your own ingenuity to analyze upskiing.

Effect of Steepness of Slope on Movement

What is the optimum slope angle for executing skiing techniques? Is one slope best for all ski levels? Once again, a free body diagram in which all the forces are identified is useful in understanding the movement situation. Before motion begins, there are two major forces acting: body weight (gravity) and friction. Additionally there are two forces that react to body weight and friction (termed reaction forces). These forces with respect to zero slope (level ground) are depicted in Figure 22.1. Notice that there is no propulsive force because gravity acts at right angles to the ground. Therefore, the skier would have to exert an additional force—for example, pole plant and push—to initiate movement. Friction is

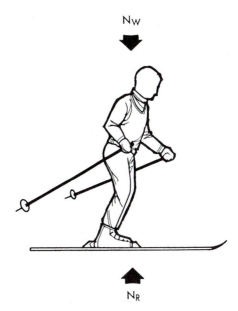

FIGURE 22.1 Contourogram of natural gliding posture of skier. Free body diagram of forces applied when slope is level and skier is stationary. (NW, Normal force of light; NR, normal reaction force.)

equal to the coefficient of friction times the normal force. The normal force in this case of zero slope is equal to body weight.

Alterations in force occur with the introduction of an incline or slope (Figure 22.2). As the slope increases, the normal force is now that component of the body weight that is perpendicular to the slope. Since the normal force decreases, the force of friction also decreases. Movement is therefore facilitated and occurs with less resistance or opposition than on a level surface. In addition, there is a component of body weight acting parallel to the slope. This component is termed the propulsive force because it causes the skier to be accelerated down the slope. This propulsive force increases in direct proportion to the increase in the slope. A skier, then, will have an acceleration in direct relationship to the slope of the hill.

■ The analysis of skiing involves resolving one force vector into pertinent components, in this case with respect to the slope of the hill.

The optimum slope for skiing varies with the individual and the techniques to be performed. There must be propulsive force to cause motion, but this force must not

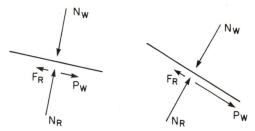

FIGURE 22.2 Free body diagram representing magnitude and types of forces acting on a skier under two different inclinations of the ski slope. (NW, normal force; FR, friction force; PW, propulsive force, NR, reaction force.) Some portion of the body weight vector (not shown) constitutes the normal force and the other portion is in the propulsive force. **Calculate these portions knowing that the slopes are 10° and 20°, respectively.**

be so great that the body accelerates so rapidly that the skier panics or does not have time to react and execute desired techniques. A slope that is too gentle is less dangerous, although equally difficult in terms of performance, than a slope that is too steep.

Concomitantly, one cannot disregard the type of snow and the surface of the skis. The interaction of these two materials produces a coefficient of friction that affects movement on a slope. An excellent treatise on this subject has been published as a result of the Winter Olympics in Sapporo, Japan and the organizers' concern for optimizing snow conditions for that event (Society of Ski Sciences 1972). The advent of indoor areas, artificial snow machines, and other advanced technology could result in ideal conditions for enhancing performance of both the beginning and the competitive skier.

Too often, the environment is ignored by the analyst of animal and human movement. Snow skiing, waterskiing, and surfboarding are excellent examples of activities in which the environment plays a dominant role in the success of the performer. Throughout this book, we have tried to show the importance of the environment in mechanical and anatomic considerations. Truly, the best performer is in harmony with the environment.

Balance

People are more stable on skis over packed snow than on shoes having the same type of surface as skis because the base of support of skis is three to six times longer than that of shoes. This greater stability on skis is primarily in the anteroposterior direction, which is an asset when a skier is sliding down a steep slope. Keeping the skis apart, about hip-width, provides greater lateral stability than placing the skis together. This wide position, called wide tracking, places the hips directly above the knees and the knees directly above the feet. This position ensures that there will be equal weight on both skis and that the line of gravity of the skier will be midway between the skis when the skier is going down the fall line (line of the slope that is the most direct). The weight of the body is distributed on the whole of both feet, the skis are flat, and the body is in a "natural position." This position places the center of gravity of the body lower than does the erect standing posture, thus increasing body stability. The term *natural position* means that the body segments are slightly flexed and able to respond easily to bumps and other changes in the terrain or the changes in the snow. This semiflexed position of the legs allows both further flexion and extension. The body faces squarely in the direction of travel, and it is in a state of differential relaxation: only a minimal number of essential muscles are contracting, and these muscles are contracting minimally.

Turning on skis, walking on level ground, stepping around, and climbing the slope all necessitate transference of the line of gravity from between the skis to a position over one ski. The shift of bodyweight should involve as little modification as possible in the trunk, arm, or leg positions, since the shift is a lateral shift of the total body. Fundamental to being able to achieve skill in skiing is the ability to change the body weight line (line of gravity) from one ski to the other, and from one ski to both skis. This ability, known as *dynamic balance,* can be achieved by placing the skier in situations that require combinations of single and double balance conditions. Skiers can practice achieving dynamic balance in such situations as stepping out (walking) at the end of a straight run (descent down the fall line), deliberately lifting one ski and then the other while in a straight run, and executing two steps to the side and back again during a straight run.

Steering

Steering refers to turning or changing direction of the slide of the skis. Since a turn requires greater movement of the tail of the ski than of the ski tip, the sliding action

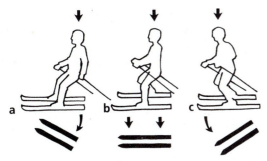

FIGURE 22.3 Effect of shift of body weight on flat skies set across the ski slope. (*a*) Backward shift causes ski tails to slide down slope faster than tips, producing a clockwise rotation; (*b*) balanced position causes skis to slide down slope in a parallel position; (*c*) forward shift causes ski tips to slide down slope faster than tails, producing a counterclockwise rotation. The change in friction is the primary factor explaining these movements.

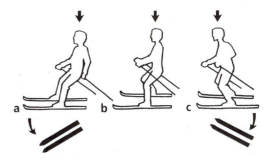

FIGURE 22.4 Effect of shift of body weight on edged skis set across the ski slope. (*a*) Backward shift causes ski tips to slide faster; (*b*) balanced position prevents sliding; (*c*) forward shift causes ski tails to slide faster. The change in reaction force is the primary factor explaining these movements or lack of movement.

of a turn is also called skidding. Short skis, or the graduated ski-length method (GLM), will provide greater success in learning the technique of skidding than will long skis. The reason is that longer skis have a greater radius and greater arc of turn for the same angle of turn. There also is more time to commit errors, and greater centrifugal force is developed when long skis are used than when short skis are used.

Regardless of what length ski is used, the wedge, or V position, is recommended to facilitate turning. This position presets each ski at an angle to the fall line, creating a turning angle. Shifting the weight from the center of the V to one ski will cause the skier to execute a turn in the direction of the ski's tip. Skiers can execute a series of turns by alternately shifting body weight from a position above one ski to above the other ski. The speed and magnitude of the turn depend on the slope, snow, duration of single ski support, and edging, that is, tilting the ski so that one edge penetrates the snow while the other edge is elevated.

Edging and Moments of Force

When skis are in the traverse position (across the slope), they tend to slide down the fall line if they are flat. The cause is the effect of gravity, which translates the skis as a unit. The speed of the slide is directly related to the steepness of the slope and inversely related to the amount of friction between the ski and the snow.

The friction is affected by such factors as the type and temperature of the snow and the type of wax used. In addition, the direction and speed of the slide can be regulated by the position of the line of gravity of the skier with respect to the ski length and to the amount of edging of the skis. If the skis are flat and the body weight is shifted forward, this places the line of gravity forward in relation to the balance point of the skis and creates a **moment of force,** causing the tips to rotate downward. By the same reasoning, if the skis are flat and the skier leans backward, the tails will rotate downward. In both instances, the results are caused by the creation of a moment of force. An analogy could be made to loading one end of a teeterboard with more weight than the other end. The weighted end rotates downward and the lighter end goes upward. (See Figure 22.3.)

The introduction of ski edging, however, creates a reactive force that can be greater than the moment of force produced by body weight. Edging the skis while leaning backward increases the friction on the tails, which prevents their rotation and causes the tips of the skis to rotate upward. Forward lean, with ski edging causes the tails to rotate downward. (See Figure 22.4.) It is evident that the skilled skier has learned to create the precise moment of force required for a turn by regulating the amount of edging and shifting the line of gravity in the anteroposterior plane of the body.

Biomechanics of Rolling and Sliding Activities   **479**

Methods of Initiating Turns

The three major methods for initiating a turn, that is, shifting the weight and rotating the skis are rotation of body parts, use of the external environment, and unweighting. We look at the anatomical, mechanical, and environmental considerations for each. There usually is more than one biomechanically correct way of performing a skill. There probably is, however, one *optimum* way for a given set of constraints, environment included.

Rotation of Body Parts. Almost any body part can be used to initiate a turn. Rotations at the shoulder, spinal column, hip, knee, and ankle are executed in a direction counter to the turn and then in the direction of the desired turn. These actions are similar to the preparation, coiling, or backswing of many throwing movements. Each rotation can be forceful enough and in the correct direction to cause turning. Knee steering (rotation at the knee) has two advantages over all the other rotations. First, the knee is at an equal distance between the center of gravity of the body and the ski. Thus, the rotation at the knee is easy to control and does not displace the line of gravity excessively. Second, the knee is an important joint in the balance phases of walking; the use of the knee for locomotion is familiar.

Rotation of Heel or Foot. Likewise, rotation of the feet (heel thrust or foot steering) is an effective means of producing a turn because the feet are used in walking. Although closer to the ski than the knee, the foot has the disadvantage of being far from the center of gravity of the body. In addition, the range of motion at the ankle is limited, as is the force. Some people have difficulty in performing the heel thrust technique. The heel thrust, however, is useful in deep powder snow and advanced turns and usually is combined with the method of unweighting.

Arm and Trunk Rotation. Arm and trunk rotations, initiated by movements at the shoulder, hip, and spinal column, cause the skis to turn if the action is forceful enough. This necessity for force, acceleration, and large motions is a source of "overturning" and loss of control. Why is loss of control apt to be more prevalent with this method than the others? When the trunk is moved, approximately half the body weight is moved. Usually the line of gravity is displaced a greater distance than necessary, thus causing the turn to be greater than 90° and inhibiting the second turn or causing a straight run backwards.

Use of External Environment. A bump, or mogul, may be used to effectively initiate a turn. The ski tips or the area under the feet can be used as a pivot point as the terrain elevates tips, tails, or both from the snow. Change in body lean or the use of knee steering or heel thrusts can produce the pivot. Release of the edges of the skis may be the only action necessary to have an effective turn on a mogul.

The use of one or both poles may also produce a turn. The friction between the ski and the snow may be decreased by transferring some of the body weight to the pole, or it may be eliminated altogether by transferring all of the body weight to two poles. The initial pole plant is nearly vertical but downhill from the position of the feet, so that the most effective reaction forces can be attained.

Unweighting. There are two types of unweighting: **up-unweighting** and **down-unweighting**. Each has its use, although many beginning skiers find up-unweighting to be a more familiar or natural movement. In both cases the principle underlying the method is that the acceleration of the body mass can create a force that reduces the normal force, thus decreasing the reaction of the skis with the snow and decreasing the resistance to turning:

$$F = ma + BW$$

If the acceleration is fast enough, the person can completely unweight, that is, have zero force between the snow and skis. This can occur without the skier becoming airborne. Acceleration of body mass is an outcome of rapid flexion or extension at the knee. The hips, trunk, and arms maintain their position of the line of gravity. The unweighting method makes it possible to turn with the skis in the wide-tracking (parallel) position.

$$F = Bw - ma = 0$$

The up-unweighting technique consists of an acceleration of the body due to leg extension. There is an initial overweighting followed by an unweighting as the legs reach the extended position (Figure 22.5).

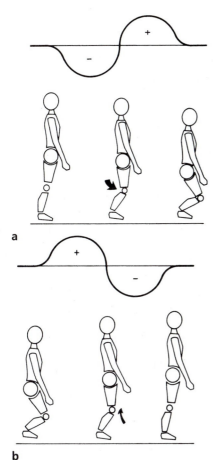

a

b

FIGURE 22.5 Effect of fast flexion movements (down-unweighting in skiing) and fast extension movements (up-unweighting in skiing) on ground reaction forces. These force-time histories were obtained from a force platform recording system. The horizontal line is the body weight line, also termed the body weight reference, and extends as a time continuum. The + depicts the positive impulse produced by the duration and magnitudes of forces greater than body weight. The – depicts the negative impulse produced by forces less than body weight. (*a*) Negative and positive impulses occurred in that order during flexion at the ankle, knee, and hip. (*b*) Positive and negative impulses occurred in that order during extension at the ankle, knee, and hip. Since *a* represents down-unweighting and *b* represents up-unweighting it is readily apparent that the down-unweighting style of skiing in turn must be initiated earlier than the up-unweighting style.

The turn must be executed in the latter part of the upward movement of the body, when the friction is least. This fact, and the fact that, in general, upward movements are thought to be lifting, or unweighting, movements, probably are the reasons why beginners more easily learn to turn with this method than with the down-unweighting method.

The down-unweighting technique (Figure 22.5) creates an unweighting in the initial part of the movement. The turn must be executed in the early part of the downward movement. If the turn is attempted later, as in up-unweighting, the reaction force is greater than body weight, and friction has increased proportionately, causing great difficulty and possibly preventing turning. Timing, or fast reaction time, is the key factor to success with this technique. Since the down-unweighting technique uses gravity and has the potential for attaining greater acceleration than is possible with up-unweighting, down-unweighting can be a more effective and efficient turning technique.

General Concepts. Turns may be executed from the wedge, stem (one ski in partial wedge position), and parallel positions. Wedges and stems provide a slowing-down capability useful on steep slopes or difficult terrain. Edging, whether in parallel position or not, reduces the skier's speed.

■ The method of turn is dependent on the steepness of the slope, the type of snow, the radius of turn desired, the speed of turn, and the skill of the skier.

Human beings tend to be asymmetric, that is, they perform a turn more successfully in one direction than in the other. Leg dominance with respect to balance usually determines the preferred turning direction. Turns are easier to perform when the skier is going fast and is close to the fall line. However, the acceleration rate and ultimate speed the skier's leg muscles and mind can tolerate determine the skier's need to check speed by stemming, edging, or deviating from the fall line. The larger the radius of rotation of the turn, the greater the speed and centrifugal force created and, therefore, the more difficult it will be for the skier to remain in control of the turn. The major danger is that the skier will be unable to turn from the fall line to complete the turn. The reason is that centrifugal forces cause the skier to "fly off at a tangent," that is, to continue in the tangential velocity at the midpoint of the turn, which is the fall line position. Beginning skiers should not attempt large-radius turns on steep slopes because they will not be able to adjust their speed appropriately and soon enough.

Speed Skiing

Downhill racing with gates (giant slalom) taxes the strength of the skiers as they try to go as fast as possible, turning at prescribed distances marked by poles (gates). A speed of 80 mph (133 kmph) is common as the skier assumes a bullet-like tuck with 18 pounds of drag resistance. On the turns it is common to have 220 times body weight on the turning leg.

The muscles must be strong and fast as they produce 1400 watts of power. Minimal movements of the shoulders occur as the skis turn a large curve. The free body diagram of a skier executing a slalom turn is shown in Figure 22.6.

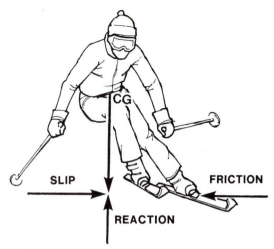

FIGURE 22.6 A downhill skier on a giant slalom course. Note the force vectors superimposed as a free body diagram of the kinetics to be considered at this instant in time.

MINI-LABORATORY LEARNING EXPERIENCE

Using the information in Figure 22.3 determine the propulsive force and speed of the skiers on the two slopes.

1. Assume body weights are 650 N each (143 lbs).
2. Determine the propulsive forces.
3. Assume the coefficient of friction to be 0.12 for each slope.
4. Determine the net propulsive forces.
5. Assume that the force acts for 0.1 sec and calculate the velocities for each condition.

Speed skiing requires a symmetrical tuck to reduce the drag as much as possible and prevent any deviation from the path. At 110 mph, (177 kmph) the skier planes a fraction of an inch above the snow. Speed skiers almost always plane.

Ski design is of absolute importance to attain these fast speeds. The stiffness, camber, and width of skis and edges must be customized for the skiers' body weight and the type of skiing. (Design is equally important for decreasing the turning radius for the giant slalom and slalom courses.)

MINI-LABORATORY LEARNING EXPERIENCE

Ski Jumping. The three most important determinants of success in ski jumping are: (1) the takeoff conditions, that is, velocity and position of skier and skis; (2) the aerodynamic characteristics of the jumper/ski system as it is oriented throughout the flight; and (3) muscle effort to create the velocity at takeoff and muscle effort to position the body during flight.

Based upon this information, complete the following experiments:

1. Find newspaper clippings of airborne jumpers and estimate the frontal area of drag.
2. Describe the best configuration for airborne jumpers.
3. Conduct some tests of leg explosive power and determine which members of the class would have the ability to produce the most forceful thrust at takeoff.
4. Calculate the vertical velocity of the experiments in step 3.
5. If the horizontal speed were 24 m/sec in ski jumping, how much farther would a jumper travel if the vertical velocity in #3 were vectorally added to the horizontal speed?

Surfboarding

Balance, or attaining a position or a series of positions of equilibrium on the surfboard, is the first skill in acquiring surfboarding expertise. Practice in still water and in a towing situation before beginning small-wave surfboarding will allow the person to realize similarities between the principles of equilibrium specified for walking, running, standing, and other land locomotion patterns and those used in surfboarding.

Low Center of Gravity

A low center of gravity produces greater equilibrium. A change in vertical position of the center of gravity is made without horizontal displacement when the surfer moves from the kneeling position to the standing position. The line of gravity remains near the midpoint of the base of support to provide the greatest distance for adjustments. Surfers position the feet slightly more than hip-width apart to provide control of the front and rear of the board without excess movement of the feet. The feet are set in a forward and backward stride position to provide control of the hydroplaning of the board. Surfers achieve lateral stability by a lateral spread of the feet approximately hip-width apart. When riding the crest of a wave that elevates the surfer and the board, the surfer lowers the center of gravity by assuming a semi-squatting position.

Depending on the weight of the surfer and the length, width, weight, and design of the board, the riding position of the surfer will vary. This position, however, is closer to the rear of the board than to the front of the board. Standing here, the surfer is able to keep the "nose" of the board above water, which produces a hydroplaning effect comparable to that of the skis in powder snow. Any displacement of the tips of the skis or nose of the surfboard below the surface level causes the snow or water to act as additional drag. It will stop or decrease the motion of the tips, while the body and rest of the skis or board continue to move and are rotated upward. This action plunges the ski tips or board nose deeper and causes the person to fall or capsize.

MINI-LABORATORY LEARNING EXPERIENCE

Place a short stick in water. Place a large bolt or nut on the stick at varying distances from one end. Note the results.

To keep the correct degree of hydroplaning, walking on the board is necessary as the velocity and height of the wave diminish. The board must be positioned to ride the wave and the leading edge (nose or side) must be prevented from plunging under water. Once the surfboard is positioned correctly, the surfer glides just as on snow skis. A turn is executed according to the basic principles of motion in a curved path.

The rear foot is placed at a right angle to the line of the board, while the leading foot remains in the direction of the board. This stance resembles the fencing stance. To execute a turn, the surfer counter-rotates toward the rear of the surfboard and then, using hip, knee, and foot steering as described in the section on snowskiing, rotates in the direction of the tip of the board. Once set, the surfer adjusts balance with body lean and rotation while maintaining contact with both feet, especially the ball of the rear foot.

Basic biomechanical principles may be even more important to the surfer than to athletes on land, since the former must shift bodyweight in response to a moving environment that is also the base of support. The water and waves are a constantly changing medium that would be difficult to understand without formulating some general principles about motion and forces. The waves are not repetitive; each is different in height, direction, and place of occurrence. The surfer must "read" the waves and adjust the position of the surfboard by shifting the line of gravity right, left, forward, or backward, depending on the crest and direction of the wave with respect to the surfboard. In addition, the environment represents a four-surface frictional environment. The coefficient of friction between the feet and the surfboard and the coefficient of friction between the surfboard and the water may be two very different values. This difference, as well as the newness of the skill, often causes beginning surfers to experience muscle aches and cramps resulting from excessive tension in the muscles of the lower extremities, especially the feet.

■ Snow boarding is a new sport: a combination of surfboarding and skiing.

Skateboarding

Surfboarding and skateboarding have several similarities, but there are also several major differences. The balancing techniques and shifting of weight front, back, right, and left are similar. When a performer is executing a turn, both activities require the same type of body position, the C-shape. This position also is commonly used in snow skiing and waterskiing. The skateboarder, however, uses the hands to pull up or down or turn the board to perform acrobatic stunts. Another major difference between surfboarding and skateboarding are the greater speeds achieved by skateboarders and the static environment of the ground used for skateboarding. Speeds of 62 mph (100 kmph) have been recorded for skateboarding competitors. Such speeds allow a person to skate around the inside of a cylinder, becoming upside-down during the mid-point of the loop. At such speeds the potential for serious injury exists if the person loses control and falls. Elbow and knee pads, wrist and hand protection, and helmets are some of the devices necessary to the safety of skateboard competitors. Should the body weight shift quickly to one or two wheels, causing a proportionately greater friction on these wheels than on the other wheels, turns can occur. If the friction is too great, these wheels will be prevented from rotating and will "lock," causing the person to be catapulted from the skateboard at the velocity achieved before the wheels stopped. This is another instance in which the safety of the performer depends not only on performance but also on equipment.

Bobsled*

The sport of bobsled is the only sliding event in which the athletes travel downhill in a seated position. Two- and four-person teams ride in a sled on a banked track that is usually close to one mile in length. The sled can weigh anywhere from 300 to 500 pounds (not counting the weight of the athletes) and can reach speeds in excess of 90 mph (145 kmph). In some of the sharper turns on the course, the athletes may experience forces up to five times that of their body weight. The average amount of time required by a bobsled team to complete a one-mile run is one minute, which means that the average speed of the slide is 60 mph (97 kmph).

The bobsled is made of steel with a fiberglass cowling to provide an aerodynamic form. It is articulated in the middle so that the rear of the sled can rotate slightly on the long axis relative to the front of the sled. There are four blades beneath the sled; the front blades pivot slightly, providing the driver with the ability to steer the sled. The rear blades are fixed. Steering is accomplished by pulling on one of two handles connected to either side of the front "axle" by means of an aircraft cable. Braking is accomplished by means of a simple mechanism mounted on the rear of the sled. The designated sledder (brakeman) pulls up on the handle of a lever, which has a row of triangular teeth on the opposite end. The teeth simply bite into the ice to slow the sled.

The brakeman pushes the sled via push-bars that protrude from the rear of the sled. These bars are part of the steel framework and do not change position during the run. The driver (and passengers in the four-person event) push on a single bar that protrudes from the side of the sled and then retracts into the cowling once the driver is in the sled. Retracting this bar insures that no objects protrude from the sled and that the aerodynamic properties are optimized.

The sledders are able to push the sled on ice because of a unique type of shoe they wear. The front half of the sole of this shoe looks very similar to the nylon portion of a velcro surface. There are hundreds of long thin spikes that enable the sledders to run on ice almost as well as on concrete. The remainder of the uniform consists of a skin-tight suit, which may have several layers of padding underneath. In addition, the sledders wear a helmet very similar to a motorcycle helmet.

In order to ensure fair competition between sledders, each sled is required to have its blades below a specified temperature (dependent on outdoor temperature) at the time of the start. Warm blades provide an unfair advantage because of a decrease in blade/ice friction, and their detection results in the elimination of that sled from competition. This prohibition also applies to all other sliding events.

---

*Contributed by James Richards.

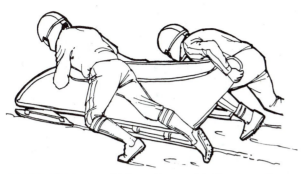

FIGURE 22.7 A world-class driver and brakeman perform a start in the 2-man bobsled event. The brakeman is behind the sled and the driver is on the side. **Measure the angles of each leg thrust in support of one aspect of their skill in starting.** Note the aerodynamically designed bobsled and headgear. (Courtesy of James Richards.)

The event starts when the athletes push the sled through a starting gate. In the two-person event (Figure 22.7), the brakeman pushes the sled from behind while the driver pushes from the side. In the four-person event, the driver is joined on the sides by two passengers. As in other sliding events such as luge, the start in bobsled is one of the major determinants of performance and must be perfectly executed. Because of the large mass of the sled, bobsled athletes must be large, strong, and fast. In addition, they need to coordinate their efforts with other team members.

The athletes push the sled until they approach their maximum sprinting speed. At this point, they board the sled and assume a low-profile position. The driver then has the responsibility of guiding the sled down the track, keeping it off the walls and as low as possible in the turns. The event ends when the sled crosses the finish gate. The sledders are in tremendous danger if the driver loses control of the sled and it overturns. When this happens, the sledders may end up rolling around a narrow channel of ice with a 500-pound sled at speeds greater than 60 mph. Broken bones and severe lacerations (from the ice) are common in crashes.

Current Research

Current research in the sport of bobsled is focused on three primary areas: sled design, start technique, and course simulation. Engineers and biomechanists are trying to surpass old competition records by applying the latest technologies to this event.

Sled Design Research. Effects of improvement in sled design consist of reducing the longitudinal friction of the blades, increasing the steering capabilities, improving safety, and reducing the wind resistance of the sled and riders. Researchers are performing extensive wind-tunnel tests in order to accomplish the latter goal. Design changes are being made to the cowl (the covering over the front of the sled), the push bars, and the blade housings in order to minimize wind friction.

Technique Research. Scientists are using instrumented sleds to measure and optimize forces exerted on the sled by the athletes during the starts. As with most other sports, success in the starts has been found to be heavily dependent on technique and on the coordination efforts between team members. Although the start represents a very simple mechanical problem (producing a maximum acceleration on a constant mass), the large mass of the sled and the fact that the performance is on ice dictates that the forces exerted during the start have to be precisely directed and controlled. (See Figure 22.8.)

Simulation Research. Another group of researchers have been working on the development of a mathematical model of the bobsled's performance. They have developed a three-dimensional model of several competition tracks, complete with turns. Using this model in conjunction with known properties of the sled, including parameters such as drag and lift coefficients, blade friction, and mass, researchers have been able to calculate performance histories of the sled, including both force and motion data, and to determine the amount of time required by the sled to complete selected turns. They are also trying to incorporate the steering actions of the driver into this model.

This is a rather extensive process, which, in theory, has wonderful implications for both bobsled and luge. The model allows researchers to calculate the optimum turn path for the sled. And, since virtually any track can be modelled, they can accurately and objectively determine strategies for the fastest performance times well in advance of the competition. Knowing this in advance would allow the athletes to eliminate the trial and error phase of establishing a race strategy and enable them to concentrate on practicing a single-run path. The model also moves researchers a step closer toward the development

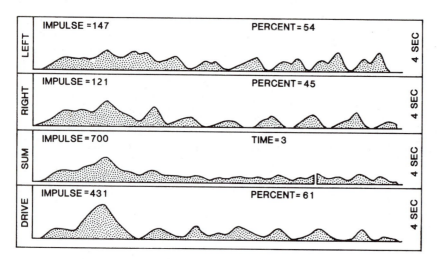

FIGURE 22.8 A graph of the forces produced on the starting bars by the brakeman (left and right upper graphs), the driver (bottom graph), and the sum of both (graph above the driver's graph). The percent value in the driver's graph represents 61% of the team impulse; whereas it is more typical among world-class teams that the brakeman exerts that amount. The symmetry of the right and left force production of the brakeman can be evaluated.

(Courtesy of James Richards.)

of a truly interactive simulator in which athletes can repeatedly race on one or more tracks, providing an enormous supplement to limited practice opportunities.

Luge*

The sport of luge involves a sledder maneuvering down a channel of ice containing extremely sharp turns and high arching banks. The event consists of both one- and two-person teams for men and single-sledder events for women. Sledders travel through a frozen maze while lying feet first on their backs on top of a 50-pound sled, which may reach speeds of greater than 60 mph (97 kmph) at various points throughout the run. The object of the sport is simple: travel the entire track, from top to bottom, in as short a time as possible.

Several factors are involved in accomplishing this objective. First, the sledder must have an effective start. This provides the sledder with a high initial velocity on the track which, when all other factors are accounted for, results in a fast finish time. Second, the sledder must minimize wind resistance while riding the sled by adopting and maintaining an efficient sliding position. Third, the sledder must have a "clean" run; that is, no part of the body should touch the ice at any time. In addition,

the sledder must stay low in the turns, as this has the effect of shortening the track. A sledder who stays low in the turns has a shorter distance to ride than a sledder who takes the turns high. Heavy persons obtain greater maximum velocity if frontal drag is reduced. Finally, the sledder must have equipment that is technologically competitive with the competition's. The sled should have an efficient aerodynamic design and offer minimum resistance to the ice surface. In addition, it must also have very controllable and predictable steering qualities. The uniform the sledder wears must provide some degree of protection, while at the same time offering a minimum amount of wind resistance to the rider. This is currently a skin-tight glossy Lycra suit with booties and a low-profile helmet with a visor.

The sled itself consists of a semi-rigid framework that encompasses two steel blades and a fiberglass pod on which the sledder lies. The overall structure resembles a high-tech version of an old recreational sled, except that it is much heavier and aerodynamically designed. The blades mounted on the sled are slightly convex, so that only a few inches of the blade are in contact with the ice at any time. This design allows the sledder to steer the sled by bending the frame. For example, if the sledder pushes down on the sled simultaneously with the right shoulder and left leg, the sled will steer to the right. Pressing with the left shoulder and right leg steers the sled to the left.

*Contributed by James Richards.

Equipment

The equipment components of luge must be optimized in order for the sledder to achieve competitive results. Equipment components can be categorized as aerodynamic properties of the sled or frictional properties of the sled. In addition, the steering properties of the sled, governed by the flexibility of the frame and the design of the blades, must fit the style of the sledder in order to ensure a clean run and a fast time on the track.

The human element in luge is the additional obvious factor that accounts for a sledder's success or failure. The sledder must perform three primary tasks: (1) produce a maximum starting velocity; (2) accurately steer the sled down the track; and (3) maintain an efficient aerodynamic profile throughout the entire run down the track. Of these three tasks, the generation of a maximum starting velocity may be the most difficult for many sledders to perform.

The luge start is performed with the sledder in a seated position on the sled, facing the run and positioned between a set of starting bars. The starting bars are large handles attached to the track that allow the sledder to overcome inertia by pulling and then pushing out of the starting gate. The race does not start when the sledder leaves the starting bars but rather several meters later; the sledder is already moving when the timing of the race begins. The object is to enter the first timing photocell with as high a speed as possible and to maintain a maximum speed throughout the course. The speed reached at the start plays a major role in determining how fast the sledder can complete the rest of the run.

Based on research on the luge start, the start consists of two separate phases, a pull phase and a push phase. (See Figure 22.9.) The pull phase is the power phase and accounts for approximately 75% of the impulse (and thus velocity) generated at the start. The push phase, as well as the transition into the push phase (from the pull), accounts for the remaining 25% of the starting impulse. In addition, researchers indicate that the start, despite its simplistic appearance, is extremely technique-dependent. Carefully designed technique changes employed by several members of the United States national luge team accounted for as much as a 20% increase in starting velocity during the 1986–87 season.

Additional research in the sport of luge centers around the design of the sled and the clothing worn by

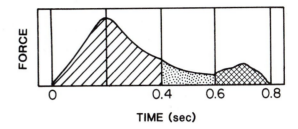

ORIGIN OF IMPULSE (traditional start)

☑ PULL PHASE

▦ TRANSITION PHASE

▨ PUSH PHASE

FIGURE 22.9 A typical force pattern created by a luger on the starting bars. Note that the pull phase has the greatest impulse and is the primary determinant of success of the start. (Courtesy of James Richards.)

the sledder. Wind-tunnel research tests the aerodynamic qualities of various types of fabric and different sled designs, as well as of varying styles of helmets and face shields.

Bicycle Racing*

In recent years, improvements in bicycling world record times have mainly occurred due to improvements in aerodynamic efficiency of the bicycle frame and wheels. Significant changes in both the bicycle and riding attire of competitive cyclists at the 1984 Olympic games included aerodynamic helmets, skin-tight clothing (body suits), and solid (disc) wheels.

Since then, we have witnessed such technological innovations as the three-bladed tri-spoke, and five-bladed front and rear composite material wheels; aerodynamic handlebars (aero bars), borrowed from the sport of triathlon; lightweight pedals that allow a degree of lateral as well as anteroposterior movement of the cleat attachment; extremely lightweight, stiff composite bicycle

---

*Contributed by Douglas Briggs.

I. Using a bicycle, skis, skateboard, skates, toboggan, or other gliding device in an appropriate environment, perform the following:

   A. Glide in a straight line and experiment with various body positions. Describe the balanced position of the body that appears to be best. State why.

   B. Assume different amounts of lateral lean of the body when gliding in a curved path at three designated speeds: slow, moderate, and fast.

   C. Estimate the amount of lean possible for each of the speeds, and discuss the basic principles involved in determining lean.

II. Take a small toy car or truck and attach a weight to the front.

   A. Push the weighted car down an incline.

   B. Describe the path of the car.

III. Repeat step II, changing the weight from the front to

   A. the rear

   B. the right

   C. the left

   Describe what happens to the path of the car for each situation and explain why.

IV. Apply the information in this chapter to the following sports:

   A. Cross-country skiing

     1. differences with respect to walking

     2. differences with respect to slope

   B. Ski jumping

     1. determine the velocity at takeoff

     2. compare differences in drag with respect to different body configurations

---

frames constructed from materials used to build modern jet fighters; and significant improvements in shock-absorbing suspension systems for mountain bike racing.

In 1984, Italy's Francesco Moser started a technical revolution when he used a 72 cm (28.33 inch) diameter front disc wheel and a 1 meter (39.37 inch) diameter rear disc wheel to set the current world one-hour record of 51.151 kmh (31.67 mph) on the Stuttgart indoor wooden banked velodrome. In 1992, Chris Boardman of England set world and Olympic records using a uniquely crafted single front fork, termed the "uniblade."

In an attempt to improve world records in cycling, experts in many fields are cooperating. These include engineering (drag reduction); biomechanics (predictive modeling and simulation of the rider-bicycle system, and study of the techniques for optimization of force application at the pedal-cleat interface); physiology (effectiveness of different training programs); nutrition (specific dietary requirements of endurance athletes); sports psychology (mental preparation for training and competition); physical therapy, orthopedics, and applied kinesiology (specialists in preventive and corrective measures); and coaching.

Forces that Propel or Retard Forward Motion of the Cyclist

The magnitude of mechanical power output (W) that a cyclist must generate at the pedals to maintain a given speed can be predicted by developing a power equation. (See Figure 22.10.) Using a free body diagram, the internal muscular forces required at the pedal at a given leg speed (rpm), designated FP or force of propulsion, must exceed the combined effect of those forces acting on movement of the rider-bicycle system (termed frictional, retardational, or external forces). Thus, the internal force(s) minus the external forces equal the ma of the system. This is termed the power balance-equation. We can use this to calculate the effects of rolling friction (wheel resistance to motion) and aerodynamic drag (profile or form drag). We can also calculate the mechanical power output (W) required to achieve a given speed using different combinations of wheel type and size (diameter), type of bicycle tubing (round or elliptical), crank arm length, and bicycle fit to the cyclist. Because the propulsive power and average trip speed a cyclist can generate for any given distance are closely correlated, improvements in bicycle design and pedaling technique are important to optimize the "power balance."

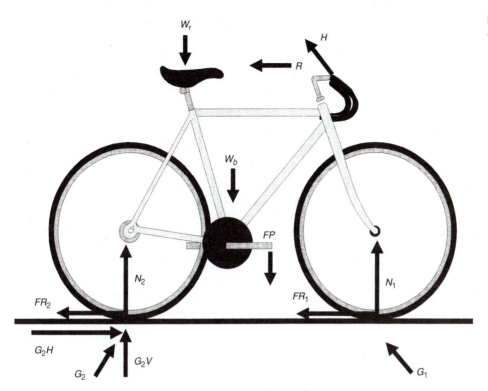

FIGURE 22.10 External forces acting on a bicycle.

The horizontal force component at the rear wheel ($G2H$) is the only force that powers both wheels forward riding on a flat surface in still air. It is a ground reaction force that opposes the propulsive force (FP) generated by the cyclist at the pedals. For horizontal motion to occur, $G2H$ must exceed the sum of external or resistive forces.

Forces of Retardation

Among the retarding elements in bicycling is the air resistance (R), which is due to the friction between the air and the moving bicycle (which includes the cyclist). Also, other factors such as drag (cd = coefficient of drag), surface area, relative velocity (V), air density (V^2), wind effect, and the speed attained by the cyclist are retarding ingredients.

Frictional resistance varies with surface roughness of clothing, skin, hair, and bicycle components. The result is that differential velocities of boundary air layers in contact with the system create turbulent eddies, and, therefore, differential pressures called *dynamic pressure*. Dynamic pressure (resistance) multiplied by surface area of the system equals drag force (lbs.) and is formulated in Bernouilli's principle, which expresses the inverse relationship between relative velocity and relative pressure in a fluid flow. Therefore, those areas or regions of the rider-bicycle system about which fluid flow is high, experience low(er) pressure(s) because the streamlining effect is enhanced. The reverse also applies.

■ Drag force increases as the square of the velocity, contributing 90% of the force retarding a cyclist outdoors at racing speeds exceeding 32.2 kmh (20 mph).

Rolling Friction. Rolling friction (wheels) equals coefficient of resistance of rolling (crr) and maximum force between tires and ground surface, that is, $N = (N_1 + N_2)$. crr is inversely proportional to wheel diameter as well as tire type, tire pressure (psi), tire width (mm), and nature of the ground surface in contact with the wheels.

The rolling resistance, or coefficient of rolling resistance (crr), is almost directly proportional to the weight placed on the tire. A bicycle tire resists being put into motion until a force initiated at the pedals is transmitted

Biomechanics of Rolling and Sliding Activities **489**

to it. The coefficient of rolling resistance is a measure or expression of the relationship that exists between drag force (lb) at zero velocity and weight (lb) placed on the bicycle tires, where:

$$crr = \frac{\text{drag force at zero velocity (lb)}}{\text{weight placed on the tire (lb)}}$$

Integrating the rolling friction and air resistance concepts with power concepts, we can estimate the effective mechanical power of a cyclist riding a slope. Another way of expressing the conditions faced by a cyclist follows.

$$P_{\text{cyclist}} = \tfrac{1}{2}\, p\, A\, P\, cd\, (v + \triangle v)^2 - crr.\, N\, v + (g \cdot \sin\theta\, v)$$

where, above the terms: perp. surf. area, drag coeff., air velocity, normal force between tires, gravity effect of slope; below the terms: ½ air density, air press., speed rel., coeff. rolling resistance, speed rel.

Simplified, this equation becomes:

$$P_{\text{cyclist}} = 0.19\, (v) + 4\, v$$

Di Prampero et al. predicted force(s) opposing motion of a bicycle from calculations of rolling resistance and aerodynamic drag in a similar way.

According to di Prampero et al., an expression of mechanical power or P, measured in watts, (where $P = Fv$) for a cyclist riding on a flat surface can be obtained by multiplying the retardation forces by the groundspeeds.

Reducing Drag

Much of the emphasis in bicycling research has been placed on technological innovation allowed within rules formulated by the international governing body for cycling (Union Cycliste Internationale) and the International Triathlon Federation (I.T.F.). Wind tunnel experiments continue to focus on improving the design of frames, wheels, and components in an effort to reduce *structural drag*, which accounts for 30% of the total wind resistance, and *frontal surface area* and the frontal drag component of the cyclist seated on the bicycle, which accounts for 70% of the total wind resistance.

Kyle and Burke (1984) conducted numerous wind-tunnel experiments using both the bare bicycle and bicycle with rider. They maintain that there are only two ways to decrease the wind resistance of bicycle components:

1. reduce the frontal surface area exposed to the air by lowering the body position on the bicycle.
2. streamlining (contouring) the bicycle components; smoothing the surface of the components to reduce air turbulence.

Narrowed Elbows, Flat Back, Work

A series of wind-tunnel tests using different aerodynamically designed bicycles, with combinations of aerodynamic bar widths (wide, regular, and narrow), heights, and reaches, were conducted on Greg LeMond at a wind tunnel speed of 48.3 kmph (30 mph). LeMond posted some extremely low drag figures, suggesting he has an aerodynamic advantage over most professional cyclists. The researchers felt LeMond has the potential to exceed Moser's existing one-hour world record of 52 kmph.

Significant findings of this experiment were:

1. On every bicycle and in every different reach-height position, LeMond recorded an extremely low drag force of 5.7–6.4 lb.
2. The key to LeMond's low drag factor was the extremely flat-backed position he was able to assume "along" the bicycle (see Figure 22.11).
3. The flat-backed position works for three reasons:
   a. Smaller frontal area reduces the amount of air that needs to be pushed out of the way; that is, turbulent flow is reduced.
   b. A more pointed rear end reduces turbulence behind the rider, and fairings on the side of the saddle, as evidenced in the 1991 Tour de France, direct the airflow behind the rider rather than allowing it to spiral behind the back.
   c. Concave backs tend to increase drag because they create "scoops" for the air.

Having a low drag figure translates into either a lot more speed on the road, or a lot less energy expended to maintain a given speed. Narrow elbows (forearms

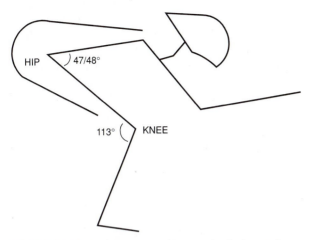

FIGURE 22.11 Body position and joint angles for lowest drag.

touching along their entire length), provide a fast profile because the upper arms block the wind. Analysts maintain that LeMond is successful because he combines high oxygen-use capability (percent VO^2 max.) and high mechanical power output (W), with very low aerodynamic drag measurements. He is able to maintain a low, flat position on the bicycle that is both aerodynamic and comfortable for him.

Significantly, the researchers did not measure and compare mechanical power output for the various bicycle-elbow width-reach combinations used by LeMond in the wind tunnel experiments.

Drafting and Wind Resistance

Drafting is the act of riding closely behind another cyclist in order to take advantage of an artificially created tailwind. It is used in women's 50km time-trial, the men's 100km time-trial, the men's 400m team pursuit, and the men's point race. If the drafter has the front wheel within 0.2 m (8 in.) of the rear wheel of the lead rider, wind drag can be reduced 44%. At a 2 m gap, wind drag is reduced 27%.

Although the effect of spacing between cyclists in a pace line decreases wind resistance for the drafting riders by about 40%, their overall drag and required mechanical output are only effectively lowered by about 30%, since rolling friction does not change. The Russians were the first to use bicycles with a 27 inch-diameter rear wheel and a small 24 inch-diameter front wheel for the men's 100km time trial in an attempt to get closer to each other during the race. The United States later tried both 24- and 26-inch wheels. Kyle and Burke (1984) maintain that the problem is not making a practical bicycle with small wheels, but finding small tires with a rolling resistance sufficiently low that they do not cause the advantage obtained by drafting to be negated. Paula Newby-Fraser, the leading female triathlete in the world, used an elliptical tube frame set, two 24-inch aero wheels, and aero bars for the 112-mile bicycle segment when she set an unofficial world's best for a woman in the 1989 Ironman competition in Hawaii.

Other Factors Influencing Speed

Tailwinds, Crosswinds, and Headwinds. Pure tailwinds or headwinds speed up or slow down the rider slightly more than half of the wind speed (di Prampero et al. 1979; Kyle and Burke 1984). A rider capable of averaging 32.2 kmph (20 mph) will average 41.86 kmph (28 mph) with a 15.1 kmph (10 mph) assisting tailwind. A 18.1 kmph (10 mph) headwind will reduce the average speed of the same rider to about 22.54 kmph (14 mph). Crosswinds increase drag, as shown by wind-tunnel measurements taken to assess the effect of yaw angle and speed.

Weight of the Bicycle and Rider. Van Ingen-Schenau (1988) explains that although initially the world of cycling concentrated on reducing the weight of the bicycle and streamlining the frame, other factors such as body posture and clothing influence speed to a much greater extent. He estimates that by using a 6 kg (13.2 lb) bicycle, a cyclist can travel approximately 45% faster than on a bicycle weighing 9 kg (19.8 lbs). (Note: In this section, the kilogram is used as a force unit equivalent to 2.2 lb, not as a mass unit. This equivalency is common in the literature of cycling.) He emphasizes that the weight of the rider is more significant than that of the bicycle because the same weight difference (3 kg/6.6 lb) equals a speed differential of 0.6%, taking air friction into account. Both figures are for cycling on a flat road, with weight assuming much greater significance when cycling uphill. A typical racing cyclist producing 350W at 42 kmph (26.25 mph) can decrease air friction by using a skin suit, resulting in a 1–1.5% increase in speed.

Altitude. As elevation increases, air density and wind resistance decrease. Bicycle speeds in Mexico City, where air density is 20% lower than at sea level, are 3–5% higher than at sea level. Bicycling records at altitude would improve significantly were it not for the counter-effect of reduced oxygen availability acting to reduce the rider's aerobic power level.

Rolling Resistance

Friction and Balance. The coefficient of friction between two tires, the supporting surface, and the weight of the bicycle determine how easily the bicycle can be accelerated. Low friction and lightweight bicycles are the goals for racing. Depending on prevailing windspeed and direction and skill of the cyclist, the lateral stability of the bicycle may become a problem. If the cyclist has difficulty in balancing a bicycle, a wider-track tire may be required. The rolling resistance or resistance at zero velocity of bicycle tires is nearly constant at normal bicycling speeds. Rolling drag becomes less important than wind drag as speed increases. Typically, rolling drag of bicycle tires varies from less than 0.5 lb. for fine tubular tires to over 2 lb. for balloon tires with knob treads.

Today's racing tires are either tubular ("sew-ups"), in which the tube is sewn into the tire, eliminating the need for rim flanges, and glued to the rim before use, or "clinchers" that use a rim flange with a separate tire and tube.

Typically, drag force is measured in a wind tunnel. Once we know the coefficient of rolling resistance of the tire type, tire width (mm), weight (grams), and maximum inflatable pressure (psi), we can calculate the total resistance force or drag for any type of tire, in lbs. where:

$$\text{drag (lb) of a tire type} = crr \text{ tire type} \times \text{weight placed on the tire (lb)}$$

Reducing Rolling Resistance. Although information detailing the effect of different road surfaces on rolling resistance is scarce, the rolling resistance of bicycle tires can be decreased in several ways (Kyle and Burke 1984). Smoother, harder road surfaces, large (r) diameter wheels, higher tire pressures, smoother surfaced thinner profile, and suitable choices of wall and tread materials have all been used by competitive cyclists in an attempt to reduce rolling resistance. Recent experimentation includes development of a 12 mm-thick solid rubber tire for use in the men's 100km time trial; use of helium-filled racing tires to significantly reduce weight; and routine use on the velodrome of tires inflated as high as 225 psi. Small diameter wheels are superior to large diameter wheels for several reasons: they are lighter and accelerate faster; they are stronger and can be built narrower with fewer flat-bladed spokes; they have less wind resistance; they permit closer drafting; and because of their size, can accommodate a lighter weight bicycle frame. The only disadvantage is their invariably higher rolling resistance compared with larger wheels over irregular surfaces. This occurs due to the greater deformation of the narrow tire.

Cyclists who compete in velodrome events spend many hours improving their bike-handling skills. They seek to improve their ability to steer their lightweight, aerodynamic "funny" bicycles around a banked track, in an attempt to minimize rolling resistance contributed by inadequate steering. In particular, the rider is responding to the opposing forces on the combined cyclist-bicycle center of mass; centripetal force inward-pulling or center-seeking, or radial force, versus the centrifugal force outward-pulling, or tangential force.

Selecting a Bicycle

Competitive cyclists usually have bicycle frames built for them depending on the type of race or event they participate in, including velodrome, road stages, timed trials, ultraendurance (RAAM-Race Across America), criteriums, biathlons, short and long triathlons, mountain biking, cyclocross, or touring. Computerized instructional videotape systems, like the one put out by the New England Bicycling Academy (the "Fit Kit"), are available at local bike shops. These tapes help adequately fit individuals to event-specific frames and components.

Sometimes, however, the most aerodynamically efficient position on a bicycle is not always the most comfortable one. Within the rules governing bicycle design for competition, bicycle design engineers, biomechanists, and physiologists work to achieve a compromise between aerodynamics and comfort. Bicycle frames are now being built specifically for women as well as for men, due to anatomical differences in effective lever arm lengths. Simple adjustments in saddle and handlebar positioning alone alter distribution of the body weight along the bicycle, and affect the ability of the cyclist to apply force to and through the pedals.

Saddle Height and Bicycle Posture

A qualitative measure of saddle height is 107–109% of the symphysis pubis height from the floor. It has been suggested that the saddle height of 109% is conducive to greater power output, and therefore useful for sprint racing. The height of 107% is preferred for minimum energy expenditure and for long-distance races. Analysis of actual performance speeds, energy required (fatigue level), and comfort, as well as trial and error, make it possible to determine the optimal saddle height for an individual. The handlebars are placed in a position to enable the body to lean forward, reducing the hip angle in flexion, which allows optimal use of the powerful gluteus maximus muscle during cycling. Briggs and Rink (1985) have shown that there is greater electrical activity in the extensors when the cyclist is in the low crouching position (termed the "racing position"), as opposed to the upright trunk position.

Ability of the cyclist to exert greater force in the racing position has also been substantiated by research in which strain gauges were used to measure forces exerted on the pedals. The upright body position may be the preferred trunk posture for older persons with kyphosis or those who wish to isometrically contract the abdominal muscles while cycling, thus improving strength in the affected muscles. This position may also be preferred by those who have excessive tension in shoulder, neck, or upper back because of habitual work or sport postures. Conversely, the person with low-back pain may prefer the flexed-trunk position to relieve stress in the lumbar spine. Body postures with respect to the vertical, greatly influence the value of $AP \times Cd$ (perpendicular surface area exposed to the prevailing wind × the drag coefficient of the system). Because the trunk makes the largest contribution to $AP \times Cd$, a cyclist can lose as much as 1mph (almost 2.5%) of velocity for every 10° deviation of the trunk from optimal posture. Reducing the angle of inclination of the trunk from the typical angle of 30° from the horizontal reduces the magnitude of $AP \times Cd$ considerably.

MINI-LABORATORY LEARNING EXPERIENCE

Using eyesight and a goniometer, obtain and record the following data from subjects riding bicycles with the saddle height set at approximately 105% and at 80% of leg length. (TDC = top, BDC = bottom)

Measured angle at:	105%	80%
Knee TDC:		
BDC:		
Hip TDC:		
BDC:		
Ankle TDC:		
BDC:		

1. Estimate the action of the muscles crossing these joints in these two conditions. Why is the 80% height not as effective or mechanically as efficient as the 105% height?
2. If the following instrumentation is available, use it to gain further understanding of the effect of saddle height on performance.
   a. Electrogoniometry: measure changes in angles, angular velocities, and ROM.
   b. Electromyography: measure relative duration and relative magnitude of muscle tension.
   c. Videography and photography: measure changes in angles, angular velocities. ROM, sequencing, and total body contourograms.

Developing Maximal Mechanical Power Output in Cycling

Using known pedal forces, Yoshitaku and Walter (1989) developed a model (Figure 22.12) to predict mechanical power output. This model consists of five rigid bodies located in a single plane (pelvis, thigh, shank, crank, and seat tube), and four smooth pin joints (hip, knee, pedal shaft, and crank shaft). They assume maximal muscle power output in bicycling to be a function of rider position, disposition of body weight along the bicycle, pedalling rate, and muscle length. In turn, the design parameters that significantly affect the mechanical power output are crank arm length (mm), fore and aft adjustment of the cyclist on the seat, seatpost angle, seat height, handlebar position, and gear ratio.

Okajima (1983) developed the concept of "impedance matching;" which is the benefit obtained by selecting the optimal gears for terrain-dependent cycling, using his elliptically shaped chainwheel. He found that the best speed for the muscles varies. Sprinters spin at 160 rpm; pursuiters spin at 120 rpm; road racers vary the rate of spinning from 70–130 rpm, depending on the terrain, race distance, and tactics used at different stages during a race. To increase the mechanical power output cyclists increase their cadence (rpm) more than they increase the gear size. If the cyclist cannot spin using a higher gear ratio, the power will drop; ideal spinning speed seems to reflect the power required for a given event, bearing in mind that rapid leg speeds increase friction within the muscle, resulting in a loss of kinetic energy. Muscle contraction speed during pedaling is relatively slow, about one-third as fast as that of running at a similar level of effort; this implies that the opportunity for increasing power output is also limited. Okajima maintains that the traditional chainwheel, requiring a circular path of the foot, reduces the velocity of muscle contraction and requires the direction of the useful force on the pedal to be perpendicular to the crank. He maintains that these conditions are not easy or natural. So, although bicycling is effective for locomotion, it does not permit muscles to reach their true force-generating potential. From beginners to champions, improvement of the ratio between pedal force and crank torque is less than 10% at 60 rpm. Thus, up to a critical point, higher

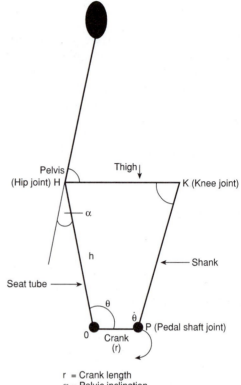

FIGURE 22.12 Maximum muscle power output in bicycling. (Adapted from Yoshitaku.)

leg speeds induce higher muscle contraction velocities. These velocities make it less difficult to spin the pedals and improve the mechanical efficiency of the cyclist, such that competitive cyclists tend to spin 50% faster than untrained cyclists. A cyclist should experiment with leg speed and gear ratio combinations to determine the optimum propulsive torque for each event.

Relationship Between Pedal Force (*FP*) and Rear Wheel Propulsive Force (*G2H*)

Forces applied to the pedals rotate the crank arms, creating a "turning effect," force moment, or torque. Torque generated at the pedals is transmitted via the chain wheel through the chain to the rear sprocket. This process causes the horizontal ground reaction component *G2H*

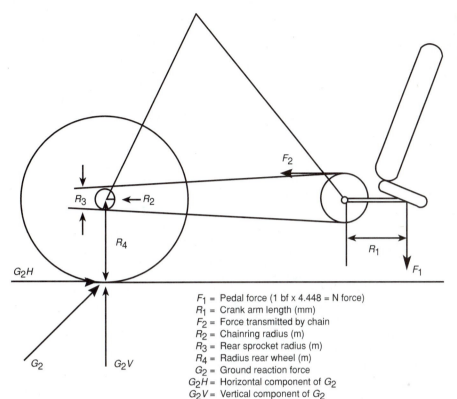

FIGURE 22.13 Forces and lever arm lengths required to calculate: A, force moments ($M_1 - M_4$) and B, rear wheel propulsive force (G_2H).

F_1 = Pedal force (1 bf x 4.448 = N force)
R_1 = Crank arm length (mm)
F_2 = Force transmitted by chain
R_2 = Chainring radius (m)
R_3 = Rear sprocket radius (m)
R_4 = Radius rear wheel (m)
G_2 = Ground reaction force
G_2H = Horizontal component of G_2
G_2V = Vertical component of G_2

to propel the rear wheel forward with minimal dissipation of force (3–5%) between the pedal and the rear wheel. (See Figure 22.13.)

■ The turning effect of applying a force at a perpendicular distance from the line of action of the force to the center or axis of rotation is called torque, or force moment. The effective force moments operating in a bicycle are (F) (Lever arm lengths).

Four force moments are generated between the applied pedal force ($F4$) and the ground reaction force at the rear wheel ($G2$), to propel the bicycle forward. Finding rear wheel ground reaction force ($G2H$) from pedal force (FP), assuming zero force dissipation between the pedal and the rear wheel, is calculated in this way:

$$F4 = F1 = (R1/R2)\ (R3/R4)$$

MINI-LABORATORY LEARNING EXPERIENCE

Example: Given: R_1 (crank arm length) = 170 mm
R_2 (chain ring radius) = 100 mm
R_3 (rear sprocket radius) = 22.5 mm
R_4 (rear wheel radius) = 350 mm

Find: F_4 the rear wheel reaction force

Solution: F_4 = $F1$. (170 mm/100 mm)
(22.5 mm/350 mm)
F_4 = $F1$. 0.109
F_4 = 0.109.$F1$.; that is, the ground reaction force is only 11% of the pedal force.

Biomechanics of Rolling and Sliding Activities   **495**

Handlebar Forces. Soden and Adeyefa (1979) measured pedal forces three times body weight, which they attributed to the cyclist pulling on the handlebars. Apparently, the pedal forces could not be accounted for by acceleration of the rider because during the pedal stroke, the body accelerated downwards, reducing the pedal forces. The vertical forces calculated in the hands were:

starting: 1.08 times body weight in one hand and

0.4 times body weight in the other

hill climbing: 0.36 and 2.7 times body weight

uniform velocity cycling: 0.11 and 0.17 times body weight

In all three situations, the unequal forces reported prevented overbalancing due to offset pedal loads. The authors concluded that the hands generate significant forces during cycling. Based on results of this study, strategic placement of strain gauges along the handlebars may provide further insight into disposition of body weight. But determination of the force distribution, or "pressure points," within the new triangular aerodynamic handlebars is not a simple task.

> Ideally, the cyclist who can generate maximum propulsive torque at the pedal-cleat interface per crank arm revolution, with minimum energy expenditure above and beyond resting oxygen consumption level, riding the most aerodynamically stable, stiff, lightweight bicycle should win.

Modeling Forces of the Leg. The functions of the human leg during cycling can be modeled as a three-link mechanical system of rigid levers (thigh, shank, and foot) rotating about axes. Since the bicycle imposes constraints on the leg, the movement is almost totally predetermined. By means of a computer, any saddle height, handlebar position, and anthropometric body configurations (e.g., thigh-shank-foot length) can be modeled and the pedaling action simulated.

The leg then is modeled to move in a circular path. The angle at each joint changes in order to effectively push the pedal with the foot. The vector for the pushing force would be tangential to the circle. Ranges of motion at the three joints would be approximately 42° at the hip, 73° at the knee, and 25° at the ankle for an average leg. Moments of force and forces acting at the joints including muscle forces, can be predicted at selected speeds and gear-ratios if the forces at the pedal are known. For example, the moment at the ankle is equal to the force at the pedal times the distance from the ankle times the angular acceleration of the foot (provided there is some) times the moment of inertia of the foot. This moment of force at the foot is countered by an equal and opposite moment created by the muscles.

A three-dimensional model is useful to determine frontal deviation of the leg and, therefore, predict stress to the foot or knee soft tissues, such as medial collateral ligaments. The three joints are now assumed to be pin-type, rather than the hinge-type of the two-dimensional model. Anatomical characteristics such as bowleggedness, knock-knees, forefoot and rear foot valgus and varus can be investigated using this model. Muscle forces are used to maintain straight leg alignment. Any deviation from this straight line places the force line outside the mid-joint position creating greater stress at these sites. Orthopedic bicycle pedals that allow for anatomical anomalies and correct foot alignment have been developed.

Pedal Forces. Pedals and crank arms instrumented with strain gauges, miniature one-, two-, or 3-dimensional force sensing devices have been used extensively over the years in an attempt to

1. quantify the magnitude and direction of forces produced during cycling.
2. describe an "efficient" pedaling action for both separate and combined-leg efforts in terms of force distribution per 360° of crank arm revolution.
3. describe the impulse of force or "pattern" of force distribution exhibited.
4. identify and measure the magnitude of unused force (*FU*) and effective force (*FE*), and if necessary, take steps to modify impulse by noting changes in force patterns that can occur with changes in variables such as frame size and geometry, seat height, seat

fore and aft position, seatpost angle, different front and rear wheel diameters, changes in cadence dictated by terrain-dependent gear-ratio selections, disposition of body mass "along" the bicycle (between-forearm spread with the forearm supported on pads attached to the handlebars, and so forth).

"Effective force" represents ". . . that component of the resultant pedal force which is responsible for generating ground reaction/propulsive force at the rear wheel (*F4* or *G2H*)." It is the applied force component that is always perpendicular to the crank arm and is used to calculate the force moments. *FE* can be either positive, when it is responsible for propelling the bicycle forward, or negative, when it acts to retard pedaling. *FU* is designated as "unused force" because it is the force that is directed along the long axis of the crank. As such, it cannot generate crank arm torque. Pedal force applications of *FE* and *FU* for elite cyclists for successive lb degree sectors are represented as a criterion diagram in Figure 22.14.

Faria and Cavanaugh (1978) found that more than 50% of the total propulsive impulse was applied between 60° and 120° past top-dead center, with a slight negative impulse noted between 120° and 165° past TDC. Briggs et al. (1989) found that for a given pedal rate (95–140 rpm), instantaneous crank arm force magnitudes increased between 30° and 150° past TDC with "matched" increases in gear size. But the pattern of force distribution, or impulse of the force over this sector, did not alter, suggesting that elite cyclists learn force patterns. Faria and Cavanaugh (1978) suggest that the criterion the cyclist should attempt to achieve is reduction of every bar on the criterion without affecting propulsion. Reduction of the size of the axes radiating outward from the diagram means that less propulsive force (*FP*) is wasted as the cyclist attempts to eliminate or reduce the negative force component during a recovery of each foot (BDC through TDC) without actually pulling up on the pedal-cleat interface. Such pattern analysis is valuable for analyzing left and right leg symmetry too, since most riders exhibit different force patterns in each leg.

Experimentation designed to measure between-leg imbalances in instantaneous torque magnitudes at precise points within each crank revolution and in impulse should be made for individuals. Imbalances may simply

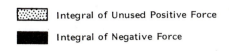

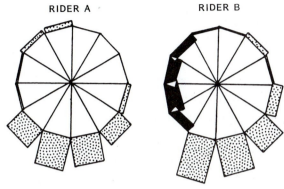

FIGURE 22.14 These pedal force patterns can be used to compare cyclists with respect to effectiveness of application, that is, the amount of effective negative force application and the amount of unused (ineffective) positive force application. **Which is the more effective rider? At which areas of the pedal cycle are the riders most effective?**

be due to factors such as differences in leg length and the need for minor separate adjustments of cleat position on the pedal. Should the leg lengths differ, the cyclist should experiment with very minor differences in crank arm length (mm) or elect to build up the pedal surface or shoe thickness on the side of the bicycle supporting the shorter leg.

Current research in pedaling technique aims to provide instantaneous, on-line visual, and/or audible feedback for impulse "smoothing," reduction of the negative, or counterpropulsive, force component, resulting in improved symmetry (R/L leg % power symmetry) for a given leg speed (cadence), and gear size.

Instrumentation: Quantification of Crank Arm Forces

A portable, battery-operated, real-time indoor-outdoor bicycle computer has been designed to measure two-dimensional crank arm bending moment and tangential force to learn more about the kinetics of cycling during competition and training. The system is equally effective indoors attached to a microcomputer or portable laptop, where immediate adjustment of impulse can be made using digital computer assisted systems. Indoors, real-time, on-screen moving stick figures (stickplots) are generated immediately in view of the cyclists as they attempt to reduce any net power asymmetry that might exist.

Optimization of Pedaling Mechanics

■ One thing clear at the elite level is that the significance of the average fades; each athlete must be examined as a case study (Faria and Cavanaugh 1978).

Little information exists regarding the magnitudes or manner in which mechanical power is produced, or the nature of force patterns produced by individual cyclists during outdoor competition and training. The latest in performance data-acquisition systems for cycling was designed by Irish. It measures and records 28 parameters real-time, beneficial for assessment of an individual's potential to optimize propulsive power output (W). Information stored and retrieved by the computer can be displayed on the handlebar LCD (liquid crystal display) and subsequently dumped into a laptop computer outdoors or a microcomputer indoors. The current 110 gram (4 ounce) combined weight LCD and sprocket indoor-outdoor computer, can display and store two-dimensional crank arm bending moments for a maximum of five hours. (See Figure 22.15.)

■ The portable computer provides instant feedback for optimization of pedaling technique and documentation of mechanical power output obtained using different leg speed (rpm)-gear size combinations during training and competition.

The computer displays and stores counterpropulsive forces (N) real-time, from which applied software calculates torque (m); power (1 nm/sec = 1/watt) for each leg separately and combined leg or net power per crank revolution, gear ratios used, a mechanical efficiency rating, heart rate, current trip speed (kmph/mph), elapsed time (h/min/s.), and elapsed distance.

Much of the published research conducted outdoors using portable on-bicycle computers has been conducted by Briggs and colleagues. Results of research conducted by Briggs, Fedel, and Foulke using the battery-operated computer outdoors with members of the United States cycling team and professional triathletes are as follows:

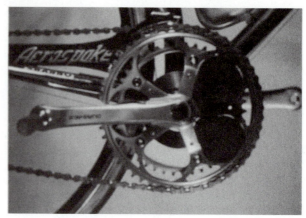

a

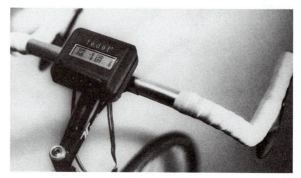

b

FIGURE 22.15 Portable sprocket-mounted indoor-outdoor bicycle computer and LCD.

1. Eleven of fifteen national-caliber cyclists reduced their negative torque by 10–18% without altering their posture on the bicycle when using 83–102 inch gear sizes at leg speeds of 90–110 rpm.

2. Ten of the subjects produced similar total work magnitudes during 50-minute outdoor time trials, but total negative work magnitudes varied considerably between subjects. They appeared to increase when the total average net power asymmetry for each individual was significant (15% bilateral/R-L leg differences).

3. The cumulative R/L% net power asymmetries of an American Tour de France competitor performing an 80-km (50-mile) time-trial outdoors confirmed what appeared to the naked eye to be a "smoother" pedaling action than the other riders tested. In direct contrast was the large negative force component of another Tour de France cyclist, producing an asymmetrical or "butterfly pattern." Two equally successful riders can produce force at the pedals in distinctly different ways.

4. A direct relationship existed for all subjects tested between increase in leg speed and increase in negative torque magnitude generated for gear sizes eliciting power outputs of 320-449 watts.

5. The most significant increases in average power output for the group (40 W increase) occurred with increases in leg speed from 104–109 rpm in the 53:17 to 56:14 gear-ratio range.

It appears that crank arm force distribution is learned and that cyclists tend to maintain identical individualistic patterns even when they increase their propulsive power output. If the assumption is made that the "smoothing" of impulse patterns is the key to improvement in pedaling

mechanics and reduction in performance times, more research is needed to determine that combination of biomechanical parameters that will achieve the desired goal.

The bicycle portable computer adequately highlighted individual cyclists' left and right leg contributions to total power output, as well as variations in velocity-dependent forces produced at different power outputs.

References

Legend: SK—skating

SKI—skiing

BS—bobsled

L—luge

CY—cycling

CY Bergmaiser, G., Hediger, F., and Marki, M. 1989. Force measurement in competitive cycling with mobile equipment. *XII Int. congress of biomechanics proceedings* Abstract 207. Los Angeles: U.C.L.A. Press.

SK de Boer, R., and Nilsen, K. 1989a. The gliding and push-off technique of male and female Olympic speed skaters. *IJSB* 5 (2):119–134.

SK de Boer, R., and Nilsen, K. 1989b. The gliding and push-off technique of male and female Olympic speed skaters. *IJSB* 5 (2):135–50.

SK Brancazio, P. 1984. *Sport science.* New York; Simon & Schuster.

CY Briggs, D. W., Fedel, F., and Foulke, J. 1985. Microstrain assessment of composite frame olympic bicycles. Unpublished Study. Dayton, OH: Huffy Corporation.

CY Briggs, D. W., Fedel, F. J., Wooley, C., and Foulke, J. 1988. Measurement of competitive cycling performance using an on-board computer. *XI Int. congress of biomechanics proceedings.* Amsterdam, Netherlands: Free University Press.

CY Briggs, D. W., Fedel, F. J., and Irish, L. 1989. Design validation and use of two indoor-outdoor sprocket-mounted portable cycling computers for evaluation and modification of pedaling technique. *XII Int. congress of biomechanics proceedings.* Los Angeles: U.C.L.A. Press.

CY Briggs, D. W. and Rink, L. 1985. Computerized metabolic assessment of elite cyclists using a VO2 max. with ventilatory threshold protocol. Unpublished study, United States Cycling Federation.

MINI-LABORATORY LEARNING EXPERIENCE

Converting Analog Values into Pounds Force

Given: Crank calibration for both cranks is 35 force units = 25 lb. Baseline for R crank = 51 force units; baseline for the L crank = 50 force units. Convert, R. TDC value for sample 1 (58 force units) into lb force.

Solution: 58 force units-R. crank arm baseline (51 force units × crank calibration factor (35 force units = 25 lb force)

Thus: $(58-51)/35(25)=7/35(25) = 5$ lb force (proof)

Note: When the force unit value is less than the baseline value (either crank), then the force will be negative or counterpropulsive. (Example: sample 2; L. leg; 112.5 degree position: $22-50/35(25) = -28/35(25) = -20$ lbs. force.

CY di Prampero, P., Cortilli, G., Mognoni, P., and Saibene, F. 1979. Equation of motion of a cyclist. *J. Appl. Physiol.* 47:201.

CY Faria, I., and Cavanaugh, P. 1978. *The physiology and biomechanics of cycling.* New York: John Wiley and Sons.

SK Feinman, Neil. 1990. Roll into shape. *Women's Sports and Fitness,* Sept:50.

SK Feinman, Neil 1991. Training tips—Get in-line. *Women's Sports and Fitness,* Sept:68.

SK Feinman, Neil 1992. Rolling thunder. *Men's Fitness,* Jan: 96.

L Hahn, M. R. 1980. A kinematic analysis of selected body segments during the start in luge. Masters thesis, University of Illinois.

SK Howe, J. 1987. *Skiing mechanics.* Laporte, CO: Poudre Press.

BS Hubbard, M., Kallay, M., and Rowhani, P. 1989. Three-dimensional bobsled turning dynamics. *International Journal of Sport Biomechanics* 5(2).

SK Iizuka, K., Kobayashi, T., and Miyashita, M. 1985. Ski robot for parallel turning: Comparison with skier's movement. In *Biomechanics IX-B,* Winter, ed. D. R. Norman, R. Wells, K. Hayes, and A. Patla. Champaign, IL: Human Kinetics.

CY Kyle, C., and Burke, E. 1984. Improving the racing bicycle. *Mechanical Engineering* 105 9: 34–45.

BS Leonardi, L. M., Dal Monte, A., Faina, M., and Rabazzi, E. 1982. Quantitative and qualitative measurement of the force exerted on a bobsled in the push-off phase. Vienna, Austria: *Proceedings, XXII world congress of sports medicine.*

SK Marino, G. W. 1983. Selected mechanical factors associated with acceleration in ice skating. *Research Quarterly for Exercise and Sport* 54(3).

SK Marino, G. W., and Weese, R. G. 1979. Systematic analysis of the ice skating stride. In *Science in skiing, skating & hockey,* ed. J. Terauds. Del Mar, CA: Academic Publishers.

SK Monahan, T. 1991. In-line skating: Does it improve fitness? *Physician and Sports Medicine Journal* 17(2): 89.

BS Morlock, M., and Zatsiorsky, V. 1989. Factors influencing performance in bobsledding. I: Influences of the bobsled crew and the environment. *International Journal of Sport Biomechanics* 5(2).

CY Okajima, Shinpei. 1983. Designing chainwheels to optimize the human engine. *Bike Tech.* 2(4): 1–8.

BS Paul, J. C. 1986. Progress in bobsled technology. *The Bobsledder* 3(1).

BS Richards, J., Tyler, J., Walter, J., Lapham, E., and Higgs, C. 1986. An analysis of forces involved in the 2-man bobsled start. *The Bobsledder* 3(1).

L Rogowski, P. and Wala. 1978. *The sport of luge.* Baltimore: University Park Press.

SKI Society of Ski Sciences. 1972. *Scientific study of skiing in Japan.* Tokyo: Hitachi, Ltd.

CY Soden, P., and Adeyefa, B. 1979. Forces applied to a bicycle during normal cycling. *J. Biomech.* 12:527.

CY Stein, P. D., Briggs, D. W., Kuznecov, A., Kono, T., and Schairer, J. 1992. Echocardiographic and ECG evaluation of left ventricular function and size in elite soviet cyclists. *Proc. VIIIth European Society of Biomechanics,* Rome.

SK Strauss, R. 1990. In-line skating: A new path to fitness and fun. *Physician and Sports Medicine Journal* 18(8): 36.

SKI Terauds, J., and Gros, H., ed. 1979. Science of skiing, skating, and hockey. Del Mar, CA: Academic Publishers.

CY Van Ingen-Schenau, G. J. 1988. Cycle power: A predictive model. Endeavor, New Series (1). Pergamon Press, Great Britain.

CY Yoshitaku, Y., and Herzog, W. 1989. Rider position, rate of pedaling, and definition of muscle length. *Proc. XII Int. congress of biomechanics.* Los Angeles: U.C.L.A. Press.

23

Biomechanics of Airborne and Arm-Supported Activities*

Rotating, twisting, falling, and moving through the air are uniquely different from land and water movements. These movements, as well as balancing on the hands, create unusual and inverse orientations in space.

The movements of gymnasts, acrobats, and divers not only differ from the majority of other sporting and physical activities by being primarily nonlocomotor, they are also usually performed in inverted positions and off the ground. Gymnasts and divers seem to defy the very biomechanical factors that govern bipedal motion. In reality, participation in these two sports, as well as in ski acrobatics and circus performances, requires strict adherence to many interacting mechanical factors. Adhering to these mechanical factors allows performers to somersault and twist in consecutive or simultaneous rotations while attempting to maintain execution details that are aesthetically pleasing to the judges! The apparent overcoming of gravity and other restrictive forces makes these sports not only difficult and at times dangerous, but also highly entertaining events for spectators.

Diving, acrobatic, and gymnastics elements can be initiated from force applications to resistances of various magnitudes. For example, diving boards are springy while towers are hard and unresponsive to applied force.

Still rings are actually very unstable while balance beams are solid (yet do give a little), although extremely narrow surfaces. While action forces are often applied by the feet to the surface or apparatus in question, elements are also initiated from the hands, knees, back, and hips. Actions begin from stationary positions, locomotion, or swinging actions.

The performance success of airborne and arm-supported performers depends most on the position of their body and the forces generated at takeoff, which determine the projectile characteristics of the athlete. Most important in this regard are the shape of the parabolic path of the center of mass and the time available for flight. These two factors are critical in achieving sufficient time for the completion of aerial rotations and preparation of body position for landing. Body position and applied forces (torques) are also important to ensuring sufficient angular impulse to generate the optimum angular momentum. Athletes must also consider conservation of angular momentum in free rotations and swinging activities.

Planar movements in either supported activities or aerial rotations are relatively easy to analyze. Activities that consist of movements in two or more planes (about two or more axes of rotation) are more difficult to analyze. We can study these complex activities by separating each rotary component and defining the basic mechanical principles and anatomical considerations involved in each component. We must also investigate the combinations, however, because while somersaulting and twisting are not difficult to understand on their own,

*Contributed by Dayna Daniels.

the relationships between these activities are critical for the success of both when performed in the same skill. Athletes who are apparently expert at somersaulting may find it difficult to combine this activity with twisting and vice versa.

Basic Principles Relating to Airborne and Swinging Activities

Some of the basic principles of rotary aerial elements and swinging activities are as follows:

1. Rotation can be produced only by the application of an eccentric force (torque); that is, the force must create a moment about the axis of rotation. For aerial rotations, the axis of rotation passes through the center of mass. For swinging activities, the axis of rotation is primarily through the grip of the hands on the bars, rings, or other surface. In either case, the action force must be applied some distance from the axis of rotation to create the moment.

$$\text{Moment } (M) = \text{Torque } (T) = \text{Force} \times \text{Distance}$$
$$\text{(perpendicular)}$$

2. The moment of force must be optimized. Performers must generate sufficient torque to provide an impulse that will produce sufficient angular momentum to complete the desired number of rotations in time to prepare for landing. The athlete must be prepared for the speed and duration of the rotating actions without becoming disoriented.

3. Sufficient vertical height must be produced to facilitate the aerial portion of the element. The time of flight can be determined using a number of equations.

   If we know the approximate time of flight, we can use the law of falling bodies to determine the minimum vertical height required to complete the skill:

$$S = \tfrac{1}{2}\,at^2$$

   where t is equal to the time needed in the airborne phase to complete the desired number of rotations.

   If a more sophisticated method of recording, such as film or video, has been used for skill

analysis purposes, we can determine the projectile qualities of the skill. In this case, we can predict the potential height the diver or gymnast can attain from the equation:

$$S_v = \frac{(V \sin O)^2}{2a}$$

   where $(V \sin O)$ is the vertical component of the takeoff velocity.

4. While the gymnast or diver is airborne and during swing elements, the principle of conservation of angular momentum can be applied. Performers can change their angular velocity by changing body position (moments of inertia) about appropriate axes of rotation.

5. The flight path of the center of mass is determined at takeoff or release and cannot be adjusted once the athlete is airborne. Changes in body position during flight occur through internal forces only; thus, the sum of all these forces is zero. The body position about the center of mass can change, causing both desirable and undesirable actions.

   Asymmetrical body movements about a single axis of rotation could cause nutation, or wobbling. If a performer desires to initiate a twist from a somersault, for example, this would be useful. But in other circumstances wobbling could be disastrous as the performer could be off balance at landing and either fall or be injured.

6. The time required for the successful execution of an element depends on a number of factors including the body position used and the desired number of rotations to be completed. If factors affecting the amount of time of flight are altered, the athlete might be forced to alter performance in order to avoid injury. If the angle of takeoff is too low, horizontal velocity will be enhanced, but time in the air will be diminished. The athlete will need to reduce the number of rotations to be completed or change the position of the body to reduce the moment of inertia about the axis of rotation to complete the somersault. Failure to conserve angular momentum or change body position could lead to unsafe landings and injury.

7. Movements of body parts, including hand position changes (such as grip changes on the uneven bars or

high bar), are most easily performed at times of zero angular velocity in swinging activities. These times occur when gravity, as a torque-producing force, is minimized at the end of the ascent phases of the swing.

8. Producing simultaneous rotations about two principle axes is a complex phenomenon.

MINI-LABORATORY LEARNING EXPERIENCE

A gymnast/diver is ready to learn a full-twisting backward somersault from the feet. Should the athlete emphasize initiating the somersault or the twist at takeoff?

Determine:

1. primary axis for each rotation
2. relative moments of inertia about each axis
3. relative angular impulse to generate angular momentum for each rotation
4. nutation factors when axis of momentum and the axis of rotation are no longer coincidental
5. differences in body position changes when somersaulting is emphasized over twisting
6. differences in body position changes when twisting is emphasized over somersaulting.

Trampolining, Tumbling, and Diving Skills

The purpose of the skill determines the desired trajectory of the center of mass in flight. Trampolining and diving require maximizing the height gained (vertical projection). As dives become more complex (include larger numbers of somersaults and twists), divers are often forced to restrict their attempts to higher and higher springboards or towers. This adds to the vertical component of the diver and increases the amount of time the diver has available.

There are four factors to consider when attempting to gain height from a trampoline (or other pushoff surface). First, trampolinists are restricted by the amount of "bounce" they can produce from the bed or surface of the trampoline. Some gymnasts have been known to bottom

TABLE 23.1 Comparison of first, second, and third bounce heights and resultant depression on the trampoline. Note that the trampoline appears to have reached its maximum depression on the second bounce.

	Height	Resulting Net Depression
First bounce	0.53 m (21 in.)	0.51 m (20 in.)
Second bounce	1.14 m (45 in.)	0.76 m (30 in.)
Third bounce	1.50 m (60 in.)	0.78 m (31 in.)

out the trampoline (jump so high that deformation of the surface at landing causes the bed of the trampoline to hit the floor before recoil) in an attempt to generate greater height for more complex skills. Thus, the mass of the trampolinist could be a restrictive factor in the development of height; a lighter gymnast might be unable to deform the surface of the trampoline enough to gain any greater heights. More massive jumpers need to use caution to avoid extreme deformation of the bed, which could lead to injury.

Trampolinists use repeated bounces to gain increases in bed depression and, therefore, higher jumps. Table 23.1 presents data from skilled performers that shows the measured changes in the height of the bounce and the resulting depression of the bed. Due to the fabric used for the bed surface and the springs, tension is nonlinear. Therefore, heights gained from bed depression cannot be predicted accurately.

Second, force production must be such that only vertical impulses are generated. To accomplish this, the center of mass should be directly over the feet whenever the jumper is in contact with the trampoline. The direction of the landing force, straight downward, maximizes the depression of the bed.

Third, to avoid absorbing any of the force at landing, thus reducing the force available to depress the surface, the jumper must keep all the joints in the lower extremity extended. The potential jarring of landing in such a position is avoided as the surface deforms.

Fourth, as the bed deforms, the jumper flexes all the joints in the lower extremity and lowers the arms. This provides additional downward force to depress the bed of the trampoline. As the surface recoils, the jumper extends all of the joints in the lower extremity and flexes the upper extremity at the shoulder to help attain greater upward force in the jump. It is important that all body position changes take place in such a way as to keep the center of mass over the base of support. "Travelling," or horizontal displacement, must be kept to a minimum in trampoline skills.

Projectile Direction

Because the trampolinist desires to minimize any horizontal deviation, body position as the bed recoils and the gymnast is projected airborne is critical. The vertical velocity of the center of mass of the jumper is equal to the vertical velocity of the bed. Additional upward force can be generated by the extension of the legs and flexion of the upper extremity prior to takeoff.

Although the desired parabolic path of the center of mass is as vertical as possible, the jumper must generate angular impulse for the creation of angular momentum for somersaulting on the bed. Body position at takeoff determines the direction of rotations.

Rotations and Twists in Flight

As somersaulting takes place in the sagittal plane about an axis of rotation with the greatest moment of inertia, it is important that the gymnast (or diver) place the body in a position to optimize the desired rotation—forward or backward. The amount of lean depends on the desired number of rotations during flight. Angle of lean of the takeoffs of an expert diver planning to execute forward and backward somersaults during flight are presented in Figure 23.1. For the forward rotation, the center of mass has been moved in front of the feet by hip and shoulder flexion. This body position, coupled with the extension thrust at takeoff, produces a counter-clockwise moment. For the backward rotation, knee flexion and hip extension (causing a backward lean) move the center of mass behind the toes. Rotation in a clockwise direction results. Once airborne, changes in body position act to conserve angular momentum, allowing the gymnast to increase or decrease angular velocity as needed to complete the element.

Symmetrical changes in body position about the principal axis of rotation result in speeding up or slowing down the angular velocity of a somersaulting gymnast. The moment of inertia of a gymnast about a transverse

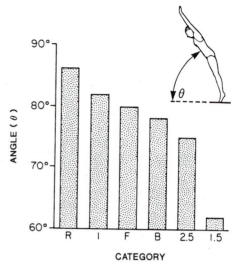

FIGURE 23.1 Relationship of body lean to type of dive. R, Reverse layout; I, inward layout; F, front layout; B, back layout; 2½ somersault back layout; 1½ somersault front pike. Although these precise values may not be true for all divers, the trend (ranking) should be the same. For example, the diver's height will influence angle of body lean prior to takeoff. **What other factors will influence body lean?**

axis in a tuck position is nearly 2.5 times less than the moment of inertia about the same axis with the body in a layout position. Thus, the speed of rotation in tuck is sufficiently greater than the speed of rotation in a layout somersault.

Asymmetrical body changes about the principal axis of rotation cause an unbalanced rotation, or nutation. Gymnasts must apply this concept carefully when initiating a twist from a somersault position.

Rotary Capabilities of the Human Body

The human body can rotate about three principal axes: vertical, frontal-horizontal, and sagittal horizontal. The rotations are termed:

1. pitch, demonstrated by forward or backward somersaulting rotations about the frontal axis
2. yaw, illustrated by sidewards rotations such as cartwheel-type elements about the sagittal axis
3. roll, or twisting rotations about the longitudinal axis.

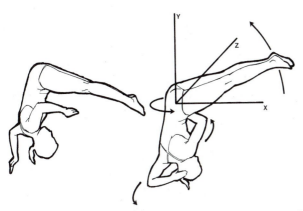

FIGURE 23.2 Mutation or rotation about nonprincipal axis of body.

In addition, the body may rotate about a nonprincipal, or diagonal axis, or about more than one axis in a single element (see Figure 23.2). It is possible for a gymnast who is rotating (somersaulting) about a horizontal axis to redistribute the body mass in such a way as to cause rotation (twist) about the vertical axis. This is accomplished through asymmetrical changes in body position, which cause the principal axis of rotation to deviate from the principal axis of momentum. This causes the body to wobble, or nutate, in a conical fashion about the axis of momentum; it also causes the body to rotate about more than one axis simultaneously.

Angular momentum is produced by an angular impulse generated when the gymnast is in contact with some surface, e.g., the floor or other apparatus. Rotations actually begin before the performer has left the ground. Twisting segments, which appear to begin later in the skill, well after the performer has become airborne, are actually generated by angular impulses about the vertical axis while still in contact with the ground. "Delay" in the twisting action can be attributed to keeping the moment of inertia about the vertical axis as large as possible, slowing the rotation. Forces used to initiate the twist are also less than the forces used to initiate the somersault. As a result the body rotates through a much greater range of rotation about the horizontal axis than the vertical axis in the same amount of time.

It is possible for the human body to be rotated without any angular impulse once the body has left the supporting surface. However, this takes place through a transfer of momentum from the local axis of momentum to a remote axis about which no angular momentum has been generated. The body cannot rotate more than a few degrees about an axis for which no moment has been generated.

Gymnastics and Rotations

In contemporary gymnastics, the most commonly used method of initiating the twisting action from the somersaulting action is referred to as a "tilt twist." The twist is achieved through an asymmetrical change in body position. Generally, one arm is lowered causing a reduction in the moment of inertia about the vertical axis and a subsequent tilting of the body. This asymmetrical action also reduces the moment of inertia about the original horizontal axis of rotation and increases angular velocity on that side of the body.

MINI-LABORATORY LEARNING EXPERIENCE

How does a gymnast decide which arm to drop to initiate a tilt twist from a somersaulting action?

1. If a gymnast is rotating backwards about a horizontal axis of rotation and wants to initiate a left twist about the vertical axis:
   a. Which arm should the gymnast drop?
   b. How does this action affect the moments of inertia about the horizontal and vertical axes?
   c. How will the principle of conservation of angular momentum enhance the twisting action?
2. Answer the three previous questions if the same gymnast desires to initiate a left twist about a vertical axis from a forward somersault.

To initiate a left twist from a backward somersaulting action, the gymnast would drop the left arm. This causes the body to tilt slightly to the left. Simultaneously, through conservation of angular momentum, the left side of the body speeds up in the direction of the original rotation. That result, coupled with the tilt, causes the gymnast to twist to the left while continuing to rotate backward.

Artistic gymnasts must concern themselves with a number of actions that affect performance. The biomechanical factors are not difficult to identify. However, the gymnast must also be concerned with the aesthetics of the performance and the potential for injury that accompanies activities that take place above the ground. The gymnast must pay attention to all three of these conditions at all times—this makes gymnastics (and gymnastics analysis) complicated.

A gymnast wishing to execute a back handspring, for example, can consider the desired flight path of the center of mass, the differences to takeoff position, forces and timing depending on whether the skill is to be performed in combination or independently, and the landing position for the same reasons. At the same time however, the gymnast knows that although bending the knees will conserve angular momentum and cause the rotation to be speeded up if the skill is short, it will also cause marks to be deducted in performance. If this back-handspring is being performed on the balance beam, the questions become more complex: *Do I break form and lose points? Do I try to maintain form, take the hard way out biomechanically, and risk injury?* Avoiding injury should always be of prime consideration. But in the heat of competition, gymnasts usually emphasize performance.

Determinants of Skilled Gymnastics Movements

George (1980) identified four basic principles that differentiate between skilled and unskilled performers in gymnastics and help to solve the problems indicated above.

1. **Amplitude.** This refers to the "bigness" of movements. The gymnast should strive to optimize internal and external amplitude. The gymnastics judge (and the biomechanical analyst) is trained to evaluate amplitude factors.

MINI-LABORATORY LEARNING EXPERIENCE

1. Spin a person standing in the anatomical position on a freely rotating platform. Next, repeat steps in the previous Mini-Laboratory Learning Experience, but vary the starting position from the anatomical position. Begin with the arms/legs abducted, etc. Note the differences in torque production required to initiate rotation of the body in various positions.

2. Hang suspended by your hands from a set of gymnastics still rings. Have a partner rotate you until the ropes above the rings are twisted a number of times. As the ropes begin to uncoil, abduct and adduct or flex and extend the legs at the hips. Note the changes in angular velocity as angular momentum is conserved. Vary the starting position by beginning with the legs abducted. Note the differences in torque production to initiate the rotation. Adduct and abduct the legs during rotation. Note changes in angular velocity as angular momentum is conserved.

External amplitude can be considered to be the range covered by the center of mass of the gymnast with respect to the apparatus (see Figure 23.3). Height off the ground in tumbling, lengths of vaults, and size of circling radii on the bars are indicators of external amplitude. External amplitude is dependent on the impulse (force × time) of the propulsive actions of the gymnast. Usually lesser-skilled gymnasts do not maximize their potential because of less power (force) and ineffective and reduced speed (time). These factors combine to limit momentum factors.

Internal amplitude indicates the relative range of motion of the gymnast's body segments in the performance of an element. The greater the segmental velocities and ranges of motion, the

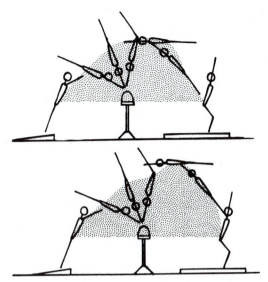

FIGURE 23.3 Comparison of amplitudes of two performances. Note how the stunt itself dictates amplitude. The amplitude pattern of each stunt can then be used as a criterion for success (both in technical execution and quality).
(Modified from George, G. 1980. *Biomechanics of women's gymnastics.* Englewood Cliffs, NJ: Prentice-Hall.)

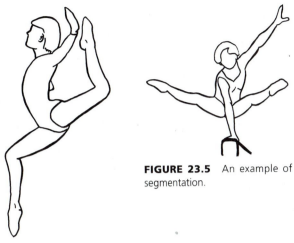

FIGURE 23.5 An example of segmentation.

FIGURE 23.4 An example of internal amplitude.

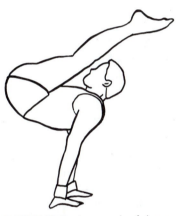

FIGURE 23.6 An example of closure.

greater the ability to perform complex elements and to complete elements in good form. An example of effective internal amplitude is shown in Figure 23.4.

2. **Segmentation.** The human body is made up of 14 segments. We have the ability to move many of these segments in different directions at the same time! Skill proficiency is inversely related to the number of segmental body parts used in the execution of a particular element. Another way to state this is that proficiency in skill performance is indicated by a reduction of extraneous or independent body segment actions. Symmetry of motion enhances this. Gymnastics elements, however, often require asymmetrical segmental movements. The gymnast must keep in mind that any action of any segment affects the location of the center of mass and the distribution of forces through the body and to the resistance surface. A skilled gymnast is able to use fewer body segments to complete even the most complex of skills (see Figure 23.5).

3. **Closure.** This factor relates closely to internal amplitude and is concerned with the absolute changes in body shape throughout a skill. The attainment of precise body shape is desirable for both aesthetic and mechanical reasons (see Figure 23.6).

4. **Peaking.** Peaking is concerned with the precise timing of body segment changes. The gymnast must be concerned with principles of impulse and conservation of momentum when executing body position changes. Peaking can be noted when a gymnast changes from a stretched to a pike position

Biomechanics of Airborne and Arm-Supported Activities   **507**

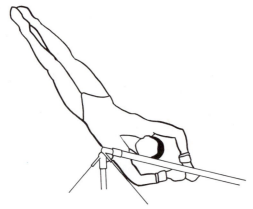

FIGURE 23.7 An example of peaking.

in a somersaulting action or when direction changes are initiated in swinging elements on the bars (see Figure 23.7).

Arm-Supported Skills

We will use gymnastics apparatus as examples for our analysis of arm-supported skills.

Mechanics of Arm-Supported Skills

In many gymnastics skills the body is supported by or suspended from the hands as it is rotated in a vertical or horizontal plane about the support. In some events, such as the uneven parallel bars, parallel bars, and rings, elements alternate between support and suspension. In other events, such as pommel horse and tumbling, elements are always in support above the hands.

Rotations in the vertical plane are affected by gravity in that this force is motive in the descent phases and resistive in the ascent phases of the skills. Maximizing the radius of rotation about the bar or rings on the down phase of a skill is accomplished by flexion at the shoulder and extension at all other joints. This allows for the maximization of gravity as a torque-producing force and for continued acceleration of the body through the bottom of the swing. On the upswing, the body position must be adjusted in order to conserve angular momentum to increase angular velocity, so that the effects of the resistive force of gravity can be minimized.

■ Rotations performed primarily in the horizontal plane get no motive impulse from gravity.

Skills must be performed quickly enough to maintain rotation, yet executed in such a way as to keep the center of mass over the very small base of support created by the hands. In skills where the base of support is a dynamic one, such as on the pommel horse, stability factors must be carefully considered.

Basic Underswing

The basic underswing, an oscillating motion of the body, is a preliminary movement used to prepare for the execution of more difficult and complex skills. The body is suspended below the base of support (the hands), which provides the axis of rotation. When the body is hanging below the bar, the force of gravity passes directly through the hands and, therefore, cannot provide any angular impulse to generate rotation. In order to begin rotation, either an external force must be applied to the gymnast (such as a coach spotting to begin the swing) or the gymnast must adjust body positions to displace the center of mass from below the axis of rotation. Flexion and extension at the hips and/or the elbows are common methods for beginning the underswing from a stationary hang. These actions shorten the radius of rotation and displace the center of mass. As the center of mass seeks to return to its most stable position, below the support, the swinging motion is enhanced by the shortened radius.

The most effective position for the body for the underswing and more advanced long swings is in a "hollow" position. To achieve this slightly curved position, the shoulder girdle is elevated and protracted as much as possible within the constraints of the apparatus. A backward pelvic tilt aids in curving the body from the neck to the feet. In this position, the center of mass is forward and may actually precede the body passing below the bar. This places the gymnast in a position below the bar as the unweighted bar begins to recoil from its deformed position. The recoil of the bar, generally inward and upward, acts as a motive force against the gymnast during the ascent phase of the skill.

Giant Swing

Increasing the external amplitude of the underswing eventually leads to the potential for a 360° rotation about the hands. This is known as a giant swing. (See Figure 23.8.) Although the giant swing is not an oscillating motion, full rotation of the underswing in both forward and backward directions is a critical lead-up to full circling movements on the uneven bars, parallel bars, high bar, and rings. The giant swing can be performed forward or backward and is frequently combined with turns. Many advanced elements, including reverse throws, somersaults, and dismounts, require precisely executed giant swings to provide the foundation for their performance.

The effect of gravity in the giant swing parallels that of the underswing, but is manifested in greater magnitudes at all points. The motive effect of gravity in the downswing should be maximized by extending the body to increase the radius of rotation. The acceleration of the body throughout the descent phase requires a strong grip, one that provides a secure link to the bar but does not increase friction to a point that tearing of the hands occurs. Centrifugal force increases throughout the descent phase of the swing, acting to both pull the gymnast away from the bar and to deform the rail. Properly timed body position changes to reduce the moment of inertia about the rail, coupled with the inward and upward recoil of the bar(s), aid the gymnast in overcoming the resistive force of gravity to complete full circling actions. Body position changes must be aesthetic as well as effective. Depression of the shoulder girdle or slight flexion at the hips (also known as "booting") just past the bottom of the swing are the best actions to meet both criteria.

Maintaining a secure grip on the apparatus is an important aspect of complete circling movements. As the gymnast reaches the top of the swing it is imperative that the hands be rotated quickly to establish a solid base of support on the top of the bar. This hand position allows the gymnast the possibility of pushing the body up to the final handstand position above the bar if there is insufficient angular momentum to complete the circle with swing. Being in a completely extended inverted position at the end of the circle maximizes the potential for developing sufficient angular velocity on the downswing of the next element to ensure a complete circle.

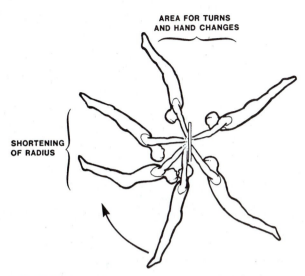

FIGURE 23.8 The back giant swing on the high bar has commonalities with giant swings on parallel and uneven parallel bars, the rings, and the front giant swing. Note the area of longest radius of rotation (body extension), the area of shortening of the radius, and the area in which hand changes and turning can occur.

MINI-LABORATORY LEARNING EXPERIENCE

1. Make a graph illustrating the changes in the factors of moments of inertia and angular velocity throughout a giant swing to conserve angular momentum.
2. A gymnast executing a giant swing on the rings attempts to abduct the rings to help complete the circle.
   a. What effect does abduction of the rings have on the execution of this skill?
   b. At what point in the giant swing should this abduction take place? Why?
3. Angular impulse is equal to torque × time. Explain how both factors of angular impulse change throughout the downswing of a giant circle. What can a gymnast do to maximize the potential for the development of the greatest amount of angular impulse?

Valliere (1973) reported the following kinetic findings on performers executing the backward giant swing on the still rings:

1. An increase in force was exerted during the descent phase.
2. A sudden increase of force coincided with the greatest shoulder joint velocity.
3. A drop in force coincided with the whiplike action of the legs, occurring at the bottom of the swing.
4. A sharp increase in force, moving to a maximum, coincided with the upward lift of the body in the ascent phase. (See Figure 23.9 for view of this special apparatus and the force-time curve.)

Elements on the Parallel Bars

The parallel bars provide for a unique set of elements, since skills can be performed from a cross-support position, with one hand on each rail and the body supported between the hands, or from a front-support position, with both hands on a single rail.

Due to the large pendulum and circling actions that can take place on the parallel bars and the relatively small base of support, the gymnast must be concerned with keeping the center of mass over the base. It is most important that the shoulders be kept in a straight line with the hands when in support or suspension, and that the forearms remain extended. For elements performed in the cross-support position, the body rotates through a greater range of motion about the shoulders than the shoulders rotate with respect to the hands. It is difficult for beginners to control a cross-support swing because the action about both the wrists and shoulders occurs simultaneously. Loss of balance, particularly if the shoulders move too far ahead of the hands on the prone portion of the swing or if there is too much hyperextension at the shoulders in the supine position, is a common execution fault in beginners.

In the swing from the support position on the parallel bars to a handstand, much of the skill depends on adjustments made to keep the body's center of gravity over (or near) the supporting hands. (See Figure 23.10.) Note that in the supine position the arms are tilted to the left and the legs are flexed; both adjustments move the body mass toward the vertical plane of the hands. In the prone position, flexion at the elbow occurs; this is a reversed muscle action that moves the upper arm and with it the upper portion of the trunk to the right to balance the lower limbs. In the final position, extension of the spine and backward rotation of the pelvis have moved the lower limbs close to the support to balance the head and shoulder girdle. As the arms moved to the right on the downswing, the effect of gravitational force increased by increasing the distance between the hands and the center of gravity. As the flexion occurs at the elbow on the first part of the upward swing, the moment arm was shortened to make better use of the momentum developed on the downward swing.

Elements on the Uneven Parallel Bars and the Horizontal (High) Bar

Contemporary work on the unevens is, to a great extent, indistinguishable from work on the high bar. The "asymmetric bars" were introduced into the Olympics in 1956 and have changed more than any other piece of apparatus. The original uneven bars were modifications of the parallel bars. Today, the apparatus look much more like the high bar. Elements originally performed were a combination of basic high bar moves and modifications of parallel bars elements. Routines included poses and even splits on the bars! Today, new equipment design and difficulty requirements require that women gymnasts be able to use their high bar in a manner quite similar to the way the men use theirs.

Performance rules stipulate that at least two elements must be performed on the low bar of the unevens. Often this requirement is kept to the minimum, with the majority of the routine looking primarily like a traditional high bar routine. Elements performed on the low bar are frequently modifications of high bar elements, including giant swings, Stalders, and twists.

Although the mechanics of swinging are the same for the unevens and the high bar, the application of successful movements is more complex on the unevens due to the presence of the low bar. Even the smallest of gymnasts often must execute more extreme changes in body position to avoid contacting the low bar during circling elements. Women gymnasts are also more limited in the directions they may face in executing circling elements.

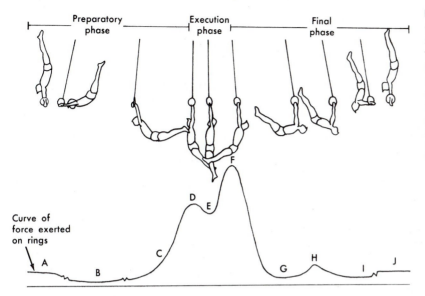

FIGURE 23.9 Kinetic and kinematic diagram of backward giant swing executed on still rings. Special strain gage transducers within the supporting cable structures of the rings were used to obtain the force-time curve. Selected points on the force-time curve were synchronized with corresponding body positions traced from movie film.
(From Valliere, A. 1973. Kinetic and kinematic analysis of the backward giant swing on the still rings in gymnastics. D.P.E. dissertation, Indiana University.)

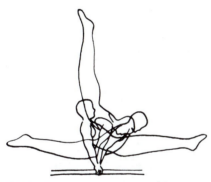

FIGURE 23.10 Swing from support position on parallel bars into a hand stand. Note the shift of the shoulders about the hands. The arms flex at the elbows when the body is in the prone position. This is an example of incorrect segmentation and judges would deduct a fraction of a point.

Because men on the high bar are not constrained by another bar, they can perform all elements forward or backward regardless of the way the gymnast faces. Women gymnasts are more constrained to face "out," or away from the low bar, when executing circling, release, or tangent dismount elements. It is most desirable to have the greatest radius of rotation possible on the downswing of circling movements such as a giant swing (see previous section on the giant swing). The woman gymnast is forced to flex at the hips on the downswing to avoid contact with the low bar. Facing "in" would solve this dilemma on the downswing, but the actions required by any gymnast to conserve angular momentum on the upswing would present a greater problem on the unevens.

Giant circles on the unevens are performed with less angular velocity. Therefore, momentum on the downswing requires greater execution technique on the ascent phase on the unevens than is required on the high bar. This also means that release elements and tangent dismounts are performed with less angular momentum as well. (See Figure 23.11.)

Representative elements of contemporary uneven bars and high bar routines come from the same three categories: circling elements with body position changes and/or twists, release elements, and tangent dismounts.

Circling Elements

These are elements in which the gymnast goes from an extended body position in the giant circle to piked or straddled positions during the circle, but extending back to the handstand at the end of the rotation. Stalders, Endos and "Toe on" actions fit this category. Partial circles with body position changes also precede a number of dismounts.

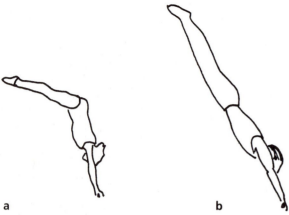

FIGURE 23.11 Differences in release positions of woman from uneven parallel bar (*a*) and man from high bar (*b*).

The Stalder is a common example of a giant circle with body position change executed within the circle. Beginning like a giant swing, the gymnast attempts to maximize the radius of rotation about the bar through flexion at the shoulder and extension of all other joints. As the gymnast circles the rail, the legs are straddled and maximally flexed at the hips. This position is maintained until the gymnast's center of mass passes the rail on the ascent phase of the circle; at which point the legs are extended at the hip to return the body to a handstand position on the top of the rail. (See Figure 23.12.)

The difficulty of this element and others similar to it are twofold. First, as the gymnast begins acceleration about the rail with a large moment of inertia, the angular impulse is high. As the gymnast begins the straddle-in action of the legs, the moment of inertia about the rail decreases. To conserve angular momentum, angular velocity increases. The increase in angular acceleration functions to increase the tangential forces tending to pull the gymnast away from the rail. This can be dangerous to a gymnast who might not be strong enough to maintain a solid grip on the rail. The most common problem is a further flexion of the legs and a closure of the torso to the arms.

Second, the straddle-in action of the legs functions as an internal angular impulse. The remote angular momentum of the rotating legs takes up some of the angular momentum about the principal axis of rotation in the conservation of angular momentum. This slows the rotation of the gymnast about the rail. As the gymnast extends from the straddle-in position back to the handstand position, the moment of inertia about the rail increases, reducing the angular velocity even more. A gymnast in a poor straddle-in position, or one who continues to flex throughout the skill, can actually take up enough remote angular momentum about the hips and shoulders to slow rotation about the rail to nearly a stop well before sufficient height in the upswing is reached to complete the circle.

The highly skilled gymnast uses the deformation and recoil of the rail throughout the execution of the skill. The high tangential acceleration possible in the downswing functions to deform the rail sideways, in the direction of the gymnast. As the gymnast reaches the bottom of the swing the rail is also deflected downward.

Standards established by the F.I.G. (International Gymnastics Federation) set the limits of rail deflection. For both rails of the uneven bars, a minimum deformation of 65 +/–10mm must be measured when a test load of 135 kg is suspended from the center of the 2400mm length bar. For the high bar, a minimum sag of 100 +/–10mm must be noted when a load of 220 kg is suspended from the center of the 2400mm rail. A gymnast suspended from any of these rails is likely to cause little deformation. However, a gymnast circling the rail with a large amount of angular momentum can significantly deflect the rail in the direction of the acting centrifugal force.

After the gymnast passes below the rail on the bottom of the swing, the unweighted rail begins to recoil, both inward and upward. Daniels (1981, 1982) noted a consistent increase in the angular momentum of 28 female gymnasts doing Stalders at the timing of the unweighting of the rail. The only explanation for the cause of this impulse was the recoil of the rail. (See Figure 23.13.)

■ Skilled gymnasts must learn to time the actions of body position changes in circling actions to maximize the deformation and recoil of the rail to aid in the completion of these skills.

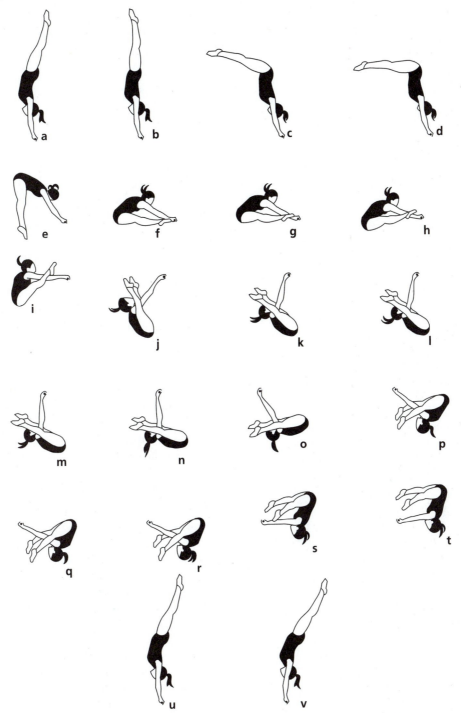

FIGURE 23.12 Sequences of contourograms of Stalder performance of woman executing a correct straddle position (initiated at f). (From Daniels, D. B. 1982. D.P.E. dissertation, University of Alberta.)

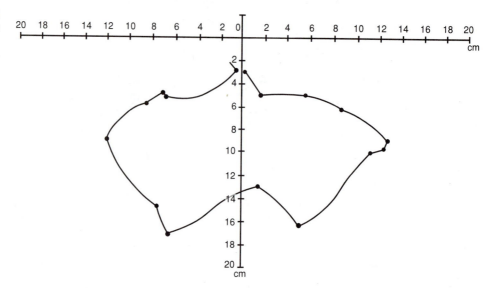

FIGURE 23.13 Plot of rail deflection Stalder performance on uneven parallel bars. (From Daniels, D. B. 1982. D.P.E. dissertation, University of Alberta.)

Release Moves

The most recent addition to difficulty elements on the unevens and high bar come from a family of elements called release moves. Although some of these elements have been used in competition for years, the new release moves are complex, spectacular, and often dangerous. Release moves are generally executed from a giant swing and involve a timed release of the bar so that the gymnast can either change body configuration with respect to the bar (such as a Tkatchev) or do a somersault with or without a twist (such as a Deltchev) in such a way as to the allow the gymnast to regrasp the rail and continue in the next element.

Top gymnasts are executing these release moves consecutively on both the unevens and the high bar. Many release moves performed on the high bar are initiated from one-arm giants—giant circles around the rail with a grip from only one hand.

The necessity of regrasping the rail following the release requires split second timing. If the rail is released too soon or too late, the gymnast, moving tangent to the arc of the giant swing might travel too far away from the rail to regrasp it or too high above the rail and risk coming down on top of it. The extreme risk taken by some gymnasts in the execution of release elements has caused rule changes. Thicker landing mats are now allowed under the high bar during competitive routines.

Also, coaches are allowed to be close to the apparatus to spot gymnasts. As long as the coach does not touch the gymnast there is no penalty. But the high risk of release elements necessitates the close proximity of a spotter to prevent any catastrophic injuries!

Obviously, release elements are among the most risky to be performed on any event. Coaches and gymnasts must have a solid foundation of the understanding of the mechanics of these elements to even begin to know how to develop the progressions for breaking them down.

Tangent Dismounts (Flyaway)

A variation on release elements are **tangent dismounts.** These are elements that use the tangent velocity of the release elements in such a way to carry the gymnast up and away from the rail far enough to execute a dismount and land on the mats without contacting the high bar or either rail of the unevens.

Tangent release dismounts can be fairly simple elements. (See Figure 23.14.) They can come from a full giant swing, but a gymnast with a good underswing can actually execute a successful flyaway. A single flyaway in tuck position begins as the gymnast swings below the rail. If there is sufficient angular velocity, the gymnast can maintain an extended body position until just before the instant of release. As the gymnast reaches sufficient height above the floor to complete a backward somersault

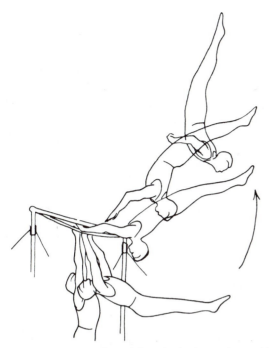

FIGURE 23.14 Flyaway (layout) from back giant swing on high bar. Head appears to extend too early, thus reducing maximum lift of body from the bar. The action of the arms after pushoff also is not appropriate to optimum performance since the arms remain slightly flexed.

Dismounts with numerous somersaults require that the tangent release from the bar be as vertical as possible to maximize the time in the air needed to complete the desired rotations and land safely. The tangent release must also be horizontal enough to guarantee that the gymnast will not contact the rail during the dismount.

MINI-LABORATORY LEARNING EXPERIENCE

A gymnast circling the rail to do a flyaway dismount is rotating about the rail with an angular velocity of 10 rads/second. If the CG of the gymnast is .8 m from the rail at the instant of release, what is the linear velocity of the gymnast at release?

If the CG of the gymnast is 4 m above the ground at release and the angle of release is 10° above a horizontal line drawn through the rail, how high will the gymnast go? How long will the gymnast stay in the air? How far from the apparatus must the coach place the landing mat to guarantee the gymnast will land on it?

---

and land well, slight flexion at the knees occurs, causing the gymnast to both speed up and begin to rotate about the center of mass. At this point, the gymnast releases the grip on the bar, continues the rotation about the center of mass, and completes the somersault by landing on the mats.

Tangent releases can also be much more complex, including numerous twisting, somersaulting actions to dismount from the apparatus. The more rotations and twists required in the flyaway dismount, the greater the speed needed in the lead-up giant swings. Particularly on high bar, gymnasts execute two or three progressively faster giant circles to gain enough angular velocity to maximize the linear velocity at the instant of release. The gymnast must conserve angular momentum on the ascent phase of each giant circle and maximize the radius of rotation on the descent phase to gain as much angular momentum as possible.

Elements on the Still Rings

Performance on the still rings is one of the most difficult events in men's gymnastics because the rings are not only *not* still, they are very unstable. The gymnast is required to be in support above or suspension below his hands, the base of support of the body. Yet the rings are suspended from their base of support, a freely moving joint, approximately 3 meters above the rings themselves. This configuration demands exactness in motion to prevent the rings from swinging—a serious fault—in competition and a potentially dangerous situation for the gymnast.

The two basic principles for successful performance on the rings are: (1) to shorten the moment arm (radius of swing, length of arms) for efficiency of energy use and balance; and (2) to use a continuity of motion between elements in the routine. Again, the principles are needed for efficiency, but also for success. The angular velocity and the final body position of the preceding movement have a direct effect on the success of the next successive element.

Biomechanics of Airborne and Arm-Supported Activities　**515**

Movements on the rings involve actions below the rings in suspension (usually elements seen at lower performance levels), actions that take the gymnast from suspension below the rings to support above the rings and circling movements, such as giant swings. Contemporary movements on the rings also involve twisting elements. As the rings are never released until the dismount, the twisting actions are developed from actions that actually twist and untwist the cables themselves throughout various elements.

Back Uprise to Handstand

This element illustrates skills that begin below the rings in suspension and end above the rings in support. The primary biomechanical principles applied for success in movements in this family are: (1) impulse directed as vertically as possible to minimize the possibility of generating undesirable movement in the rings; and (2) transfer of momentum through kip-like actions.

To execute the back uprise to handstand on the still rings (Figure 23.15), the gymnast executes an underswing from back to front. On the downswing (coming from either a hang at the mount or a previous movement in the routine), the gymnast extends at the hips and adducts the rings to maximize the moment about the hands through the bottom of the swing. Shortening the radius (the distance between the center of mass and the rings) on the upswing through hip flexion and ring abduction conserves angular momentum and allows the gymnast to increase the amplitude of the swing on the ascent phase.

The uprise is conducted by arching the back and in-locating the shoulders (Figure 23.15b). An in-locate is a rapid internal rotation of the humeral head in the glenoid fossa. This action helps to overcome the force of gravity and accelerate the gymnast upward. It also causes a rotation of the rings, which establishes the base of support for the gymnast when he or she reaches the cross-support position.

The body is moved forward, placing the center of rotation nearer to the support (hands), which is kept behind an extended line from the shoulders. Throughout this entire action, the center of mass is kept below the point of suspension to minimize ring displacement and cause swing. As the point of support moves over the

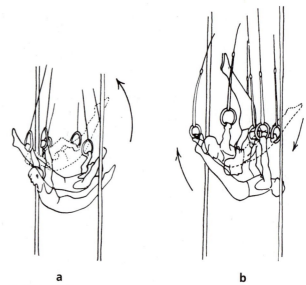

a   **b**

FIGURE 23.15 Movements on the still rings have high potential for injury to the shoulders, especially dislocations. Note the movements of the body about the shoulders in the back uprise to handstand (a) and the shoot to handstand (b).

point of suspension of the rings the center of mass is moved upward and inward at the same rate. The performer pulls the body upward through forceful scapular abduction and arm extension. At this point the legs are flexed forward. They swing down and back and the arms press to bring the body into a handstand support above the rings.

Since the rings should be as stationary as possible throughout the routine, the gymnast must execute each element in such a way as to minimize unnecessary forward and backward displacement of the rings and cables. Swing usually occurs when the gymnast fails to keep his center of mass under the point of support and along the suspension line of the cables. When unplanned swinging begins, it is difficult to stop, making all elements difficult, and possibly dangerous, to perform. Developing a certain amount of swing is inevitable in the course of a competitive routine. The accomplished gymnast learns to "kill" the swing, usually by controlling movements of the center of mass in the opposite direction of the movement of the rings.

Cross-hang Position on the Rings

The cross-hang, or Iron Cross, is a simple movement that requires extreme strength as the gymnast attempts to support himself by the rings with the arms almost fully abducted. The center of mass is below the base, but the arms are held horizontally making the point of rotation the shoulder girdle rather than the hands. To maintain the arm position the shoulder adductors must contract forcefully and maintain this isometric contraction for the duration of the hold—usually two seconds or longer. The elbows and wrists must be locked, but if the shoulder position is held, the muscular strength required to stabilize these joints is minimized. From the Iron Cross position, gymnasts can execute a number of variations. Upper trunk rotation to either the left or right is called an Olympic Cross. A gymnast may also flex the legs at the hips until they are parallel to the floor and hold the L-sit in conjunction with the Iron Cross. All of these elements require tremendous strength.

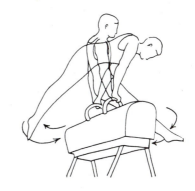

MINI-LABORATORY LEARNING EXPERIENCE

What advantage does the short-armed person have over the long-armed person performing on the rings? Refer to information in Chapter 4.

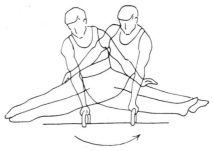

FIGURE 23.16 High double leg circles on side horse. **Is the circle symmetrical with respect to the different right and left circles?**

Pommel Horse Elements

The pommel horse is often considered to be the most difficult of the events in men's artistic gymnastics. Elements are composed from swinging and-or pendular actions, both of which are constrained due to the configuration of the apparatus itself. The circumpendular action of the legs and body about the frequently dynamic and small base of support requires tremendous upper body strength and balance.

The basic circumpendular element on the pommel horse is the double leg circle, the foundation movement for most other skills. (See Figure 23.16.) Takemoto and Hamaido (1961) liken this action to the spinning of a top. During the execution of the double leg circles, the center of mass must be kept over the point of support. As the body moves both forward and backward and side-to-side, the hands must release the pommels in well-timed sequence to allow the body to pass over the horse without being impeded by the arm.

The body rotates about the center of support by means of lateral trunk flexion, with the shoulders held more or less at the same elevation. The shoulders move side-to-side and front-to-back to help keep the center of mass over the support as amplitude of the circle increases. The higher the body and legs are held above the apparatus, the easier it is to complete the circle. However, this takes more strength and precise technique. No pause (or slowing down) may occur while the action takes place or the performer will fall from the apparatus or collide with it.

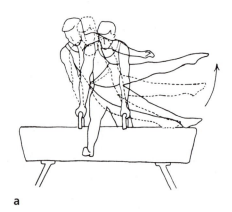

a

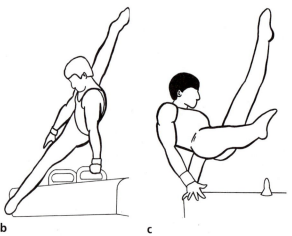

b   c

FIGURE 23.17 Scissors or leg cut actions with various support sites.

A more pendulum-like action, required in all competitive pommel horse routines, is the scissors or leg cut. (See Figure 23.17.) These actions generally are executed out of double leg circles. The gymnast must use proper timing and technique to move smoothly from a circular motion in a continuous direction to an oscillating pendulum action. The points of suspension of the pendulum are the shoulders—alternatively one, then both, then the other. The radius is shortened as the performer moves the center of mass nearer to the base of support on the upswing and is increased on the downswing to increase angular velocity. They accomplish this by flexing at the hip, accompanied by flexion and lateral rotation of the trunk. On the upswing, the top thigh is abducted. The resistant arm of the lever (distance from the point of support to the center of mass of the combined mass of the trunk and lower limbs) is also shortened on the upswing and lengthened on the downswing. As the upswing diminishes until velocity is zero (when the upward velocity and the downward pull of gravity nullify each other), the performer flexes the lower leg, flexes and laterally rotates the trunk, and executes the leg cross or scissor-like action. As the gymnast descends, the legs are split in a forward/backward stride over the horse through the downswing to the other side of the horse, where the actions are repeated.

Balance Beam

If the pommel horse is the most difficult of the men's events, balance beam is the most challenging of the women's. The gymnast is required to perform dance and acrobatic elements forward, backward, and sideways along a beam that is 1200 mm above the ground and only 100 mm wide on its top surface. In addition, the gymnast is also required to leave the beam through leaps, jumps, and tumbling elements and land solidly back on it without breaks in form or timing.

The most successful performers on the balance beam are likely those gymnasts with the highest levels of kinesthetic awareness and, possibly, intestinal fortitude! Posture at all times is a critical feature for work on the beam. The shoulders must remain over the hips in all upright work to keep the center of mass over the narrow side-to-side base of support. Because the gymnast is required to keep moving throughout the routine (only two choreographed stops are allowed without penalty), the base of support is a dynamic one and frequently changes from the feet to the hands to the back, knees, or torso. During the execution of most elements, the center of mass must move only in the direction of movement so that movement flows as progress is made back and forth on the beam (Wilkerson 1978).

Beginning and novice performers view the width of the beam as a requirement for precision of execution, but view the height of the beam fearfully. Analyses of movements on the balance beam should include direct or indirect measurement of muscular activity. Tension in extraneous muscles is a primary cause of unsuccessful or unskilled performances. If the actions can be performed on a line on the floor, why can't they be performed on the beam? This is a perfect example of the necessity of analyzing the affective aspects of performance within the biomechanical analyses of movements. Coaches might be encouraged to "raise the floor" rather than have gymnasts practice elements on lower-level balance beams. Piling landing mats up to the level of the beam increases the safety and feelings of confidence of the gymnasts, while allowing them to train at the competitive heights required.

MINI-LABORATORY LEARNING EXPERIENCE

One trick gymnasts can learn to help them to stay on the beam when balance is lost is taking advantage of various ways to take up remote angular momentum from the local angular momentum about the principal axis of rotation. When gymnasts lose their balance and begin to fall (rotate) forward over the feet, they can execute certain actions to take up angular momentum or increase stability.

What actions can gymnasts perform to stay on the beam (without grabbing the beam with the hands, which is a penalty) if they start to fall forward? Backward?

MINI-LABORATORY LEARNING EXPERIENCE

Observe, videotape, or record EMG from arm and trunk muscles, or otherwise record three skipping patterns with the following constraints:

1. skip forward on the floor
2. skip forward along a 4 in. wide plank
3. skip forward on a 4 in. × 4 in. × 6 ft board set on the floor
4. skip forward on the 4 in. × 4 in. × 6 ft board elevated from the floor

Record results in the form of a table or graph. Discuss results. Does the skip change? How? Estimate planes of movement, ROM, and sequencing of movement.

Vaulting

Vaulting is a complex event that demands that almost all of the requirements of a full routine be performed in one element. Vaulting contains locomotion, two springing actions—one from the feet on the board and one from the hand or hands on the horse, rotation about the transverse (frontal) axis frequently combined with rotation about the longitudinal (vertical) axis, and a controlled landing. The vault takes place over both horizontal and vertical displacement, which are related, to some extent, to the height of the gymnast as well as vaulting ability.

The success of most vaults, whether side horse for women (the horse is placed cross-wise to the run-up) or long horse for men (the long side of the horse is parallel to the direction of the run-up), depends on the ability to generate high linear velocity during the run-up and to lose as little forward momentum as possible through the generation of optimum vertical impulse on the board. The allowable run-up distance for both women and men vaulters is 25 m. This distance contains the space necessary for the hurdle onto the board and the board-to-horse distance. This distance does not allow for most gymnasts to attain maximum running speed prior to the hurdle onto the board. However, high running speeds require exact timing on the board to control both the horizontal velocity of the run-up and the vertical impulse of take-off. Average speeds of skilled vaulters immediately before contact with the vaulting board have been reported as between 6.09 and 7.9 m/sec. The difference between male and female junior elite vaulters in the United States was approximately .3048 m/sec (Sands and Cheetham 1986). The fast speeds of approach found in the performances of the men in the 1984 Olympics ranged from 7.6 m/s to 7.99 m/s. Investigations have been conducted of the changes in speed during the run-up. Theoretically, the speed increases until the hurdle is initiated. The following results, however, were obtained from the final four steps of elite juniors: increase in speed from the fourth-last step to the third-last step, lesser increase in speed from the third- to second-last step, and slight decrease in speed from the second-last to last step.

Little or no speed should be lost on the board during contact, because of the rebound capabilities of the board and the vaulter's ability to apply force during the contact phase. Kreighbaum reports complex deflection patterns of the board at contact and inconsistencies in deflection patterns with variation in contact points on the board. She reports that the smoothest deflection curves were obtained when foot contact on the board was midway between the front and back.

Less-skilled vaulters are not able to use high linear velocities by controlling the horizontal momentum well enough to use it to generate vertical impulse against the board. Therefore, they are likely to run more slowly or rapidly decelerate in the final steps before the hurdle. Studies of less-skilled vaulters indicate a loss of speed 1 or 2 m/sec during the final few steps leading to the hurdle.

The speed of the approach, coupled with the maintenance of the momentum on the board, is a major determinant of flight speed in the vault. The faster the approach speed, the greater the potential for horizontal displacement and vertical displacement throughout the action phase of the vault. Maximizing time in the air enhances the gymnast's ability to complete all necessary rotations and land with the body as erect and balanced as possible. The multiple correlation among the peak velocity of the run-up, number of steps in the approach, and score awarded was reported to be .953 for nine vaults by elite juniors (Daniels 1981). There is no doubt that gymnasts should attempt to maximize the length of the vault run-up and maintain speed or even accelerate into the board.

Dynamic control of the approach speed is the next determinant of skilled performance, since the takeoff determines the angle and speed of the preflight (airborne phase between the takeoff from the board and contact with the horse). In addition, the kinematics of the initial contact with the horse influence the flight characteristics of the postflight (airborne phase between the horse and landing). Placement of the board relative to the horse is an important factor in maximizing the qualities of the vault. This distance must be great enough to provide time for any preflight actions and allow space for the individual gymnast's body to extend and invert onto the horse. The type of vault and speed of the run-up also help determine the placement of the board.

The run-up also produces momentum, which has a direct effect on all phases of the vault. Dainis (1980) has shown that a decrease of 7% in the run-up speed results in a 13% decrease in postflight distance in a handspring

MINI-LABORATORY LEARNING EXPERIENCE

1. Set up a series of photocell timing devices and record the speed of run-up of vaulters at intervals of 1 meter. If photocells are not available, videotape the run-up and record the time to execute each step of the run-up. Plot the results on a graph using step numbers for the X axis and time for the Y axis. Assume equal length of steps. A digital time code on the videotape and single-frame advance capabilities on the playback unit are necessary. An alternate approach is to use an audiocassette recorder and record the sound of the steps. Estimate cadence or changes in time intervals. Qualitative assessment of positive and negative acceleration is probably all that is feasible in this case.

2. Observe and measure (during the performance or with a postperformance evaluation of a videotape) the distance of preflight and postflight. Compare these distances with respect to type of vault and score awarded for performance.

vault. In addition, he showed that a 7% decrease in vertical speed off the board resulted in a 25% decrease in postflight amplitude. Although the handspring is a vault rarely seen at higher levels of competition anymore, it is the foundation vault for almost all advanced vault families executed today. (See Figure 23.18.)

Vault families involve basic handspring actions with: longitudinal axis twist in preflight and/or postflight; somersaulting actions in preflight and/or postflight; and combinations of twists and somersaults in preflight and/or postflight. Yurchenko family vaults include all of the above rotations, but entry onto the horse is from a backward approach (a roundoff is executed onto the board rather than a hurdle, and an action resembling a back handspring rather than a front handspring is executed onto the horse), rather than a forward one.

Gymnasts attempting to execute these vaults require excellent kinesthetic awareness, primarily because the somersaulting/twisting actions in the postflight are initiated

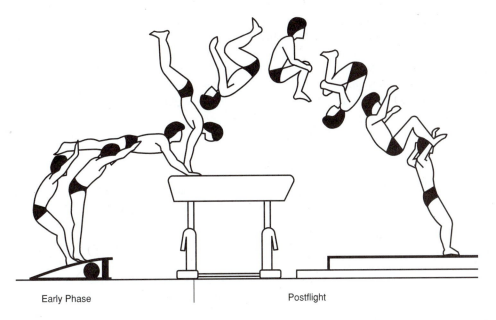

FIGURE 23.18 The handspring front one-and-a-half somersault vault.
(Reprinted by permission from Cheetham, P. J. 1982. The men's handspring front: One-and-a-half somersault vault: Relationship of early phase to postflight. In *Biomechanics in sports,* ed. J. Terauds. Del Mar, CA: Research Center for Sports.)

Early Phase   Postflight

from an inverted position on the hands from the horse. The ability to adjust body positions to conserve angular momentum is also a necessity:

Anthropometric Considerations for All Gymnastics Events

Internal amplitude factors directly affect not only the aesthetic, but also the biomechanical success of many gymnastics skills. Except for the floor area, balance beam, still rings, and high bar, all other pieces of artistic apparatus can be adjusted in certain ways to fit the various dimensions of the individual gymnast's body. It is important to use the proper amount of space to guarantee proper timing, force application, and direction of force production. A gymnast on the beam, for example, has practically no margin of error in sideways movement. If insufficient space is taken up along the length of the beam to accommodate the size of the gymnast, such as in the execution of a side aerial, then the gymnast will be forced to place her body in such a position to use sideways space to complete the skill. This will affect balance characteristics and certainly aesthetic ones.

Biomechanics and Safety

In the same way that body alignment is the key to biomechanically sound standing posture, it is also the key to gymnastics activities. The handstand and the long hand from the bars are considered the foundation for practicing straight body alignment. The arms, trunk, neck, and legs are in a straight line, and the shoulder girdle is depressed. A backward pelvic tilt is often seen in the hollow position when swinging.

Low back pain is a common complaint among gymnasts. Repeated and often excessive arching of the lumbar spine is a typical posture seen in numerous elements, particularly for women gymnasts. If such a posture occurs during dismounts from the apparatus or vault landings, trauma from impact forces is apt to cause chronic problems. Since gymnastics activities are replete with landings, and since point deductions are frequently taken for the force absorption actions of hip and knee flexion, special landing mats have been developed for each piece of apparatus.

More important than even mats is the necessity of teaching gymnasts (and all physically active people) how to land properly on the feet, hands, and back. Landing on the feet is the most common type of landing in gymnastics and other sporting activities. In gymnastics, landings can occur from forward, backward, and sideways momentum. They can come from common projectile-type motions of the body or from rotations. The two biomechanical factors that must be applied for all landings to control the movement and for safety reasons are: (1) absorb force over the largest possible surface area; and (2) absorb force over the longest amount of time possible. Both of these factors necessitate the use of joint flexion—a potential cause for deductions from a gymnast's

---

MINI-LABORATORY LEARNING EXPERIENCE

Work with a group of individuals so that each can observe a number of landings.

Execute two vertical jumps:

Land with the lower legs flexed on contact with the floor.

Land with a force absorption pattern of toes, ball of the foot, heels, knees.

What are the differences?

Jump from a variety of progressive heights—either forward or backward. Notice particularly your ankles and others'.

What differences can you note between landings in which the heels are kept in contact with the floor and landings where plantar flexion is allowed to take place?

Is there a difference in balance factors if the landing is from a forward or backward direction? Describe any differences and determine why they might be occurring.

What conclusions can you draw regarding the differences in landing forces in these two techniques?

If a force platform is available, repeat these activities. What differences in load are obtained?

---

score. Coaches of young gymnasts should forgo the quest for higher scores rather than risk permanent or chronic injury to their gymnasts.

The pattern of force absorption when landing on the feet should be toes, ball of the foot, heels, knees. The most common injury in foot landings is sprained ankles. Inversion sprains are a likely result of landing from a height and contacting the floor with the feet plantar-flexed and the lower legs flexed. It is important to instruct gymnasts to press their heels to the floor and keep them in contact with the floor before and throughout leg flexion.

Risk Analysis

What are the risks of trauma in the joints of the body in gymnastics and how would you estimate them? Follow this procedure.

Step 1. Hypothesize that the greater the landing forces, the greater the risk of injury. This is based on the stress-strain relationship, which, in review, can be stated as follows: As stress is increased, the strain increases. Thus, a body will deform positively with increased force applied to it until it fractures.

Step 2. Review literature to determine impact values and tools used to obtain these values. Too and Adrian (1987) found values of 5–6 BW (five to six times body weight) during landings from a vaulting box .85 m high. A change in the surface mat resulted in a difference of almost 20% BW with an increase in mat thickness. Mat 1 was 1 cm thick with a coefficient of restitution of .78 (as calculated from the rebound height of a dropped ball). The second mat was 5 cm thick with a coefficient of restitution of .58.

They also compared those gymnasts landing with a flat trunk (no increased curvature at the lumbar spine) and arched trunk. Mean vertical impact forces were 5.47 BW flat-trunk response and 6.62 BW arched-trunk response.

Step 3. Select subjects (people who follow standard test directions) to perform different types of landings. Measure the vertical ground reaction forces, using force platform or other force transducer. If neither is available, use an animal, truck, or other floor scale with a range of 0–1,000 lb. could be used. For relative estimation (ranking of different conditions), a sand landing pit could be used. Measure the depth of foot penetration for each condition and record and rank them. The deeper the penetration, the greater the impact force.

MINI-LABORATORY LEARNING EXPERIENCE

1. Execute a foot-to-foot forward roll while attempting to take up as little space as possible.

   Lie on the floor with your arms extended above your head. Have a partner mark the location of your hands and feet. Repeat the forward roll, beginning on the line where your feet were marked, and attempt to finish the roll where your hands were marked.

   What differences can you note in amount of force production, direction of resulting action, balance factors, and potential ease in executing a another element right out of the roll.

2. Using the lines drawn in step 1, attempt to execute the following skills:

   a. Handstand. Begin with the back foot on one line and attempt to place the hands on the second foot.

   b. Cartwheel. Begin with front foot on one line. Note where the first foot to touch the floor at the end of the cartwheel touches down.

   c. Back handspring. (Find someone who can do a standing back handspring.) Begin with both feet on one line. Note where feet touch down at end of the skill.

3. Discuss the results of the above experiments. What differences occur when less than the space between the lines is used to complete any movement?

Step 4. Observe, videotape, or film the kinematics of the subjects as they perform landings from different heights.

Step 5. Based on your data, derive one or more principles about impact force and body segment motion.

References

Bergemann, B. W., and Sorenson, H. C. 1979. Dynamic analysis of the kip on the high bar. In *Science in gymnastics,* ed. J. Terauds, and D. B. Daniels. Del Mar, CA: Academic Publishers.

Bovinet, S. L. 1979. The dynamics of the kip on the uneven parallel bars. In *Science in gymnastics,* ed. J. Terauds, and D. B. Daniels. Del Mar, CA: Academic Publishers.

Cheetham, P. J. 1982. The men's handspring front: One and a half somersault vault: Relationship of early phase to postflight. In *Biomechanics in sports,* ed. J. Terauds. Del Mar, CA: Research Center for Sports.

Cheetham, P. J. 1984. Horizontal bar giant swing center of gravity comparisons. In *Sports biomechanics,* ed. J. Terauds, K. Barttels, E. Kreighbaum, R. Mann, and J. Crakes. Del Mar, CA: Academic Publishers.

Dainis, H. 1980. Model and analysis of vaulting. International Gymnast 22(7):TS7–TS12.

Daniels, A. 1979. Cinematographic analysis of the handspring vault. *Res. Q.* 50:3.

Daniels, D. B. 1981. A Biomechanical analysis of the handstand to handstand stalder circle on the uneven parallel bars. Ph.D. dissertation, University of Alberta, Canada.

Daniels, D. B. 1982. Biomechanical analysis of the stalder on the uneven parallel bars. In *Biomechanics of sports,* ed. J. Terauds. Del Mar, CA: Research Center for Sports.

Daniels, D. B. 1987. Identification of critical features in gymnastics skills through biomechanical and statistical analysis. In *Diagnostic, treatment and analysis of gymnastics talent,* ed. T. B. Hoshizaki, J. H. Salmela, and B. Petiot. Montreal: Sport Psych. Editions.

Darda, B. 1986. Springboard diving. In *Encyclopedia of physical education,* ed. T. K. Cureton.

George, G. 1980. *Biomechanics of women's gymnastics.* Englewood Cliffs, NJ: Prentice-Hall.

Hay, J., Wilson, B., Dapena, J., and Woodworth, G. 1977. A computational technique to determine the angular momentum of a human body. *Journal of Biomechanics* 10:269–77.

Hennessy, J. T. 1992. And now comes trampoline! *ASTM Standardization News,* June 1992.

Kreighbaum, E., and Barthels, K. 1989. *Biomechanics.* Minneapolis: Burgess.

Landa, J. 1973. Shoulder muscle activity during selected skills on the uneven parallel bars. Ph.D. dissertation, Washington State University.

Montebell, G. M. 1992. Ice skating surfaces: The uncontrolled playing fields. *ASTM Standardization News,* June 1992.

Oglesby, B. 1969. An electromyographic study of the rectus abdominus muscle during selected gymnastic stunts. Ph.D. dissertation, Washington State University.

Osborne, G. 1979. A comparison: Two styles of straddle stalders. In *Science in gymnastics,* ed. J. Terauds, and D. B. Daniels. Del Mar, CA: Academic Publishers.

Miller, D. I., and Nissinen, M. A. 1985. Greg Louganis' springboard takeoff: II linear and angular momentum considerations. *IJSB* 1(4):288–307.

Miller, D. I., and Nissinen, M. A. 1987. Critical examination of ground reaction force in the running forward somersault. *IJSB* 3(3):189–206.

Prassas, S., and Terauds, J. 1987. Gaylord II: A qualitative assessment. In *Biomechanics in sports II & IV,* ed. J. Terauds, B. Gowitzke, and L. Holt. Del Mar, CA: Academic Publishers.

Rackham, G. 1975. *Diving complete.* London: Faber and Faber.

Reuschlein, P. 1962. An analysis of the forward somersault in the pike position. Unpublished paper, University of Wisconsin.

Sands, B., and Cheetham, P. 1986. Velocity of the vault run. *Technique* 6(3):10–14.

Stroup, F., and Bushnell, D. 1969. Rotation, translation, and trajectory in springboard diving. *Res. Q.* 40:812–17.

Swain, R. 1979. A comparison between coaching cues and the execution of that dive. Unpublished paper, Washington State University.

Takemoto, M., and Hamaido, S. 1961. Gymnastics illustrated. Tokyo: Ban-yu.

Too, D., and Adrian, M. 1987. Relationship of lumbar curvature and landing surface to ground reaction forces during gymnastic landing. In *Biomechanics in sports III & IV,* ed. J. Terauds, B. Gowitzke, and L. Holt. Del Mar, CA: Academic Publishers.

Valliere, A. 1973. Kinetic and kinematic analysis of the backward giant swing on the still rings in gymnastics. Ph.D. dissertation, Indiana University.

Wilkerson, J. 1978. Kinematic and kinetic analysis of backhand spring in gymnastics as performed on the balance beam. Ph.D. dissertation, Indiana University.

Yamashita N., Kumamota, M., and Okamoto, T. 1979. Electromyographic study of forward and backward giant swings on the horizontal bar. In *Science in gymnastics,* ed. J. Terauds, and D. B. Daniels. Del Mar, CA: Academic Publishers.

24 Visualizing the Future

Anything is possible. Today, sophisticated technology is too expensive and esoteric for everyday use. But in the future it will become available for practitioners and general society. We will use it to solve the problems of disuse, misuse, and abuse of our bodies, as well as problems of injury, asymmetry, physical dysfunction, and aging.

As a biomechanist, you have three projects to complete today. You begin work by speaking to your computer. You tell it to activate the Multidimensional Profiling Program. You feed in the split-screen videodisk of the performance of walking by a person afflicted with cerebral palsy (CP). Within minutes the computer has analyzed the video and drawn kinematically a 3-D animated regeneration of the walk. It then generates a kinematic profile.

You then ask the computer to access the Walking Database Network. It does so and instantly you have a comparison of your kinematic profile with the World Normative profile. Dysfunctional factors are identified and laboratories with CP databases are listed.

You videolink with E mail to Brazil, Germany, New Zealand, and China to see and talk with the researchers and discuss dysfunctional characteristics and procedures to improve the gait. One researcher suggests the use of an Enhancer Walker, the latest in supplemental devices. You ask the computer to link you with the AutoDesign Program. You input anthropometric and strength data and the software custom-designs an Enhancer Walker. You electronically mail the design to a fabricator who will send it to you within an hour.

Your second project involves supervising an exercise program for a group of fitness clients. Each client approaches a body scanner that measures and records physical dimension, range of motion, bone density, and lean body mass data. Before the client begins a strength exercise, the strength machine automatically adjusts to the client's physical parameters, conducts a strength evaluation, searchers for prior exercise results, and creates an optimum computer-controlled exercise program. The client exercises according to the computer program. All exercise results are stored in the computer and can be graphically portrayed for client profiles.

The last project of the day is a sports class. Each student is given a microprocessor to wear in a waist pouch. The student will activate the microprocessor with coded inputs for each practice activity, for example, batting, pitching, and running bases. The kinetic energy of the bat swing is recorded during batting practice, the velocity of the ball is measured during pitching, and the accelerations during five steps after batting and during two steps stealing a base are calculated. At the end of the class, the microprocessors are interfaced with a computer and data inputted into student databases. The computer can generate a profile of today, last week, six months ago, etc. In addition, it can produce comparison profiles.

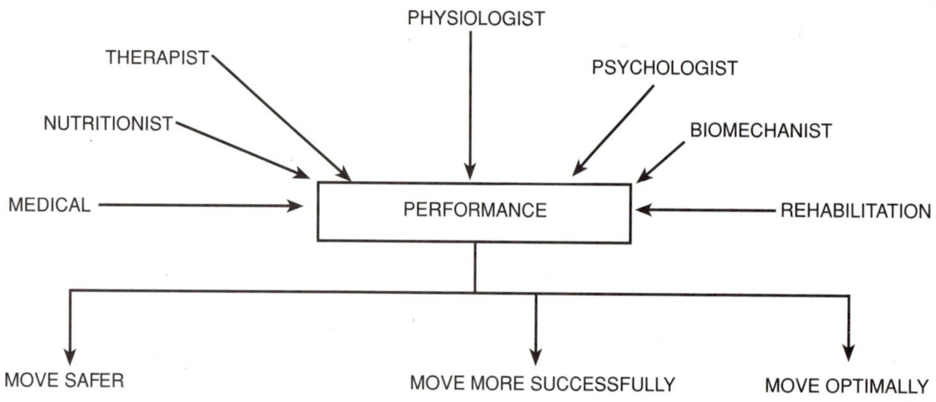

FIGURE 24.1 The movement science specialists involved in enhancing performances of athletes.

A Vision or Reality?

Do the above examples seem unreal or impossible? They shouldn't! All components exist now, but have seen only limited use and not on the grand scale depicted.

■ The scenarios exist now. The breadth of use is the only visualization into the future.

The advances in human movement analysis and the dissemination and interpretation of analysis to athletes, clients, students and others has been, and will continue to be, made possible because of the rapid advances in computer technology. A complete system for video image-grabbing, 3-D graphics, windows for comparing several performances at the same time, animation, and data storage cost less than five thousand dollars in 1992. Software is still expensive. But in the future it will be so easy to write that it will be available to the average coach, clinician, and teacher. Commercial interactive video software will also be inexpensive and on the hard disk drive at purchase. High-speed videography will be commonplace, and movements of all types of all persons will be inputted into computer data banks. Five or more cameras are now being used. There are software packages specifically for analyzing feet, gait, spine, orthopedics, and lifting. Interactive books and videos that work with software have been developed.

Teams of Movement Analysts

More and more advances are made because of team approaches to human movement analysis. Under the sports science umbrella are the United States Olympic Committee, the International Olympic Committee, and many other separate sports-governing bodies. A flow chart of the sports science umbrella is shown in Figure 24.1.

The same team effort is being used in rehabilitation, aging, motor development, and education and programming for the disabled. The study of movement may be narrow, as with biomechanics, but the application of knowledge gained must be broad and comprehensive to provide meaningful information. We have the potential to create, and are doing so in many cases, mountains of data. Unfortunately, we have a dearth of understanding. We fail to synthesize the data. One of the needs for the future is to determine how to get the data from the laboratory and research journals into the field with the practitioners. New, low-priced automatic analysis devices are being developed to make the sophisticated technology accessible to the practitioner, fitness participant, athlete, worker, and home user.

New Fitness Equipment

Three major types of fitness equipment will become readily available at fitness centers, schools, and homes: customized-fit machines, computer-controlled exercisers, and simulators. In addition, linking fitness equipment to databases and to competitive situations will provide the user with information about progress and relationship to performances of others.

Customized-fit Machines

These include sizing to the physical dimensions of the user and the limits of ranges of motion. Accommodating loading is the concept that enables the user to perform prescribed work at each instant of range of motion and speed. Separate limb activation will provide greater loadings for the stronger limb and lesser loadings for the weaker limb. Eccentric enhancement and other types of special techniques for unique loadings can provide further individualization of the exercise workload.

Computer-controlled Exercisers

These machines can be set to vary the load, speed, or other parameters based on the preselected limiting value of any of the following factors: heart rate, range of motion, speed, distance, power, interval between signals, work rate, or pressure.

Simulators

These machines are designed to duplicate the movements required in sport, work, home activities, and any other movement pattern. Complete biomechanical assessment of the "real movement" must be obtained in order to produce a true replica of the movement pattern. The simulators have on-board and on-line data-acquisition units so that all the kinematic and kinetic parameters can be recorded in real-time (for an example see Chapter 22, the bicycling section). Graphic portrayals and comparisons with previous performances are outputted from the computer. This computer serves as a data processor for statistical treatment of data, data-storage bank, data-retrieval system, data manipulator and display system for 3-D graphics, animation, and force-kinematic interfacing. (See Figure 24.2.)

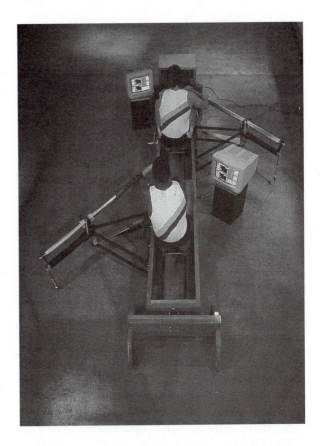

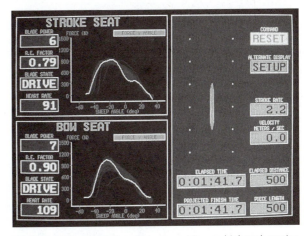

FIGURE 24.2 Simulation during exercising on high-tech rowing machines with feedback, adaptation, and graphics. (Courtesy of Simuletics.)

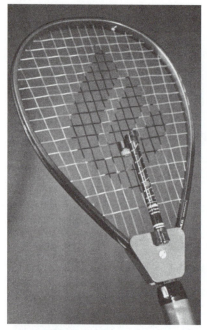 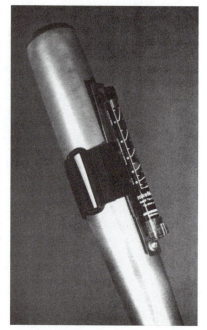 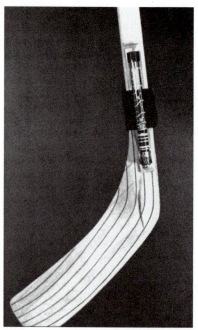

FIGURE 24.3 Strokemaxxer records speed of tennis racquet, bat, and hockey stick during play. An accelerometer is placed on the sports equipment.
(Courtesy of Golf Research Technology Corporation, Norcross, GA.)

Recording Movement Parameters in Sports

At last the technology has become available to monitor movement parameters of sports performances during teaching and training. Here are but a few of the devices currently available to the public at low cost.

1. In a karate class, the practice kicking pad has a force transducer that measures the kicking impact.
2. Sports players attach accelerometers to their sports equipment and are able to measure the swinging speed of each stroke (see Figure 24.3).
3. Forces are measured as the swimmer's hand and thigh are moved through the water (see Figure 24.4).
4. A microprocessor is used to measure the speed, direction, and impact angle of a golf club. It also measures the kinematics of the flight of the ball.
5. The impact forces are measured and recorded during boxing, kendo, and karate. These are summed and the winner of each round is determined by the frequency and magnitude of strikes to the opponent.

6. The table tennis player (or other racquet sports player) uses a Newgy table tennis robot to project balls with predetermined sequences of spins, speeds, and directions (see Figure 24.5). The Logic Handle, another table tennis robot, can actually be programmed to simulate the game strategies of the top players of the world.

Improving the Environment to Improve Athletic Performance

By studying exactly what is required of the athlete, we can make the equipment and environmental surfaces "match the person or the task." This creates optimum performance and, perhaps, a "super athlete." A few of the current and future inventions are

1. automatic shifting of bicycle gears in response to pedal pressure.
2. talking ropes for communication between linked mountain climbers.

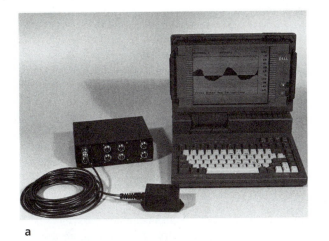

a

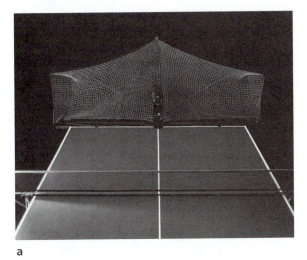

a

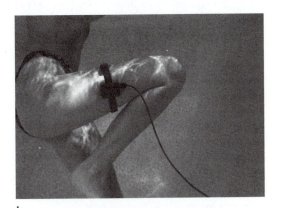

b

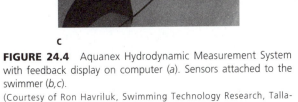

c

FIGURE 24.4 Aquanex Hydrodynamic Measurement System with feedback display on computer (*a*). Sensors attached to the swimmer (*b,c*).

(Courtesy of Ron Havriluk, Swimming Technology Research, Tallahassee, FL.)

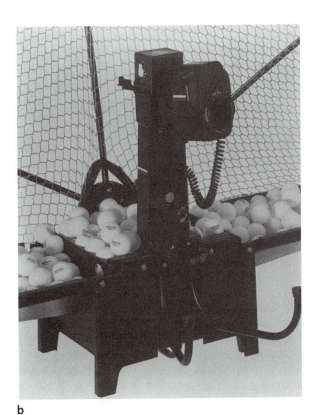

b

FIGURE 24.5 Newgy Table Tennis Robot. The table tennis balls are automatically projected to a player. Angle and speed of ball and time interval of "returns" can be prescribed.

(Courtesy of Newgy Industries, Inc.)

3. "sticky shoes" for rock climbing.
4. snap-on ski bases for the changing conditions of snow.
5. retracting arrow rests to eliminate interference with the flight of an arrow.
6. telemetered headphone input of the second-by-second status of an athlete's speed, range of motion, force production, heart rate, and lactate accumulation.
7. customized track surface/shoe energy tuning.
8. talking shoes for signalling excessive impact forces.
9. computerized simulators for rowing, bobsledding, cycling, canoeing, running, and skiing.

Expert Systems and Profiling

Highly productive and appealing expert system databases have been developed in the sports world. One of these is a biomechanical-physiological combination, developed exclusively in swimming, at the Evaluation Center for Swimmers in Belgium. Each swimmer is tested and a profile card is stored in the computer database. Each profile card consists of ranked anthropometric, flexibility, strength, and speed parameters (see Figure 24.6). Time-space, anthropometric, flexibility, strength, swim tests, and many other derived indices have been used to predict performance. In 1984, the Center organized the European Olympic Solidarity Program Seminar to teach coaches and researchers the procedure for developing and using their evaluative approach and database.

World consortiums have been founded for cooperative biomechanical analyses at International and Olympic competitions. The U.S. Olympic Committee Sports Science and Technology Committee are funding innovative projects that include the design of performance data-acquisition systems. Their projects include simulations of bobsled runs, modeling and simulations of paddles and oar blades for rowing and canoeing, and a real time data-collection system from a computer mounted on a boat. A profiling of locomotor performance during fencing competition has been developed through the United States Fencing Association. Fencers are video taped and their actions are encoded into a computer via a spreadsheet program. For example, an advance would be entered as #1. Distinct profiles for two fencers are seen in Figure 24.7.

■ We need a diagnostic database for every movement pattern.

Solving Movement Problems

Long-term problems of movement dysfunction and injury are now at the top of the list for solutions. Some of the important problems and actions that biomechanists can take to solve these problems are described in the following sections.

Assymetry

From birth, all human beings begin their assymetrical development. Body symmetry and harmony are disrupted in the search for specificity and success. For example:

1. We learn to write with one hand.
2. The majority of our sports are unilateral-type sports, that is, one side of the body is used differently than the other with forceful movements of one arm causing dysplastic development.
3. Our furniture, tools, and customs are geared to a right-handed world.
4. We habitually perform movements with the same side of the body "leading the movement."

■ Assymetry may begin with habits, but it is intensified and perpetuated as the body structure changes, reinforcing assymetrical movements.

Movement patterns are stronger and easier to do in one direction and one side of the body than the other. The center of gravity of the body moves toward one side, away from the midline of the body. This results in minor movement dysfunction. A major result of unilateral pattern perpetuation is scoliosis.

There is one ball sport, handball (not team handball that is played in the Olympics), that uses both hands in hitting the ball. This sport is played in a walled court similar to squash or racquetball courts, and the ball is hit with either hand. The resurgence of this sport would be one of the most important events in countering the unilateral development of the body.

Movement analysis of the right and left movement patterns of the body is needed. The body must be able to perform adequately with both limbs if we want to be

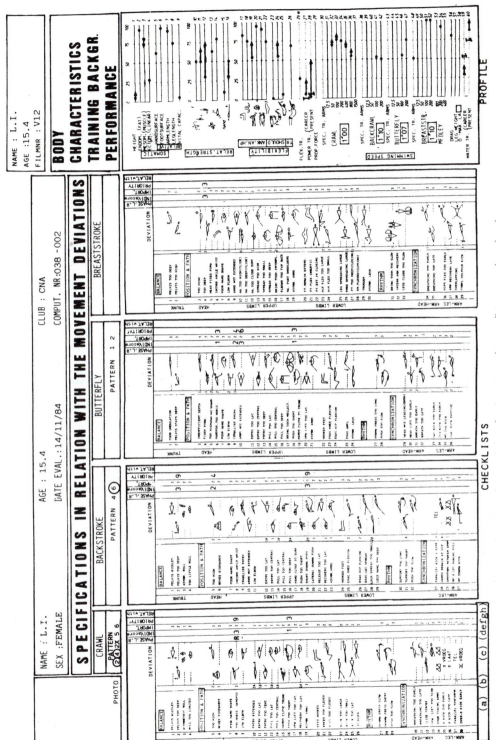

FIGURE 24.6 An example of profiling to determine characteristics of swimmers and to predict success in swimming. (Courtesy of Evaluation Center for Swimmers, Belgium.)

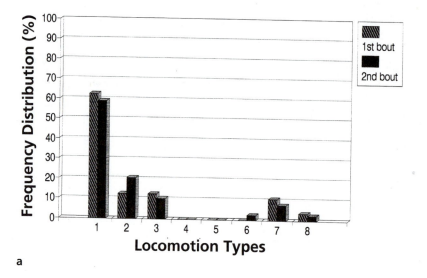

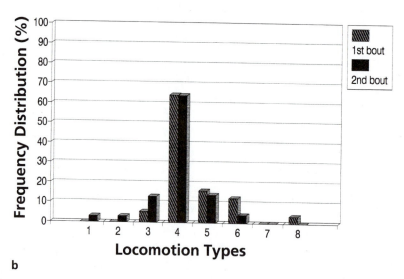

FIGURE 24.7 Two fencing profiles, unique to each fencer and consistent within each fencer. 1, advance, 2, retreat, 3, lunge, 4, fleche (all biomechanically correct), 5, advance, 6, retreat, 7, lunge, 8, fleche (all with foot and leg in misalignment and potentially unsafe).

"movement-fit." Loss of adaptability, especially inability to adapt after heart attacks, strokes, and other disruptions of dominant arm functioning, often results from assymetrical development. We have not begun to understand the ramifications of these changes. Does gross body movement assymetry affect eye use, hearing, general balance, and total body coordination? In the future we must find the answers.

The Epidemic of Injury

Injuries are the leading cause of death in sports and research is needed to help reduce the incidence of injuries. In the sports arena, injuries are a near-epidemic. In some sports, a large percentage of athletes have sustained moderate to severe injuries. Adequate identification of the forces during competition, practice and conditioning has not been made. The forces produced during a biomechanically correct movement pattern and an incorrect one (e.g., off-balance, improper sequencing of limb accelerations) are of different magnitudes and act at different body sites. Questions to ask include:

1. Do sports require greater force tolerances than the human body can achieve?
2. How does one assess individual performances?
3. Can a data bank of movement patterns include sufficient information to predict trauma?
4. Is it only a matter of scientifically determining the progression and intensity of training in order to prevent injury?

Two approaches are especially promising: the use of imaging techniques and the use of "real data." Imaging techniques are noninvasive and consist of information obtained from soft tissue not available in the past. Magnetic resonance imaging, including CAT scans, of joints can display positions, changes in position and, therefore, tensions and other stresses. One of the co-authors of this text has proposed a Dynamic Trauma Imaging Model to simulate the shoulder joint during baseball pitching as a way of analyzing potential injuries. The model would determine the reactive forces acting at the joint and relate these forces to stresses at the tissues created by different types of pitches and different speeds.

The video illustrator depicted in Figure 24.8 is not only a coach's tool to improve performance, but can be

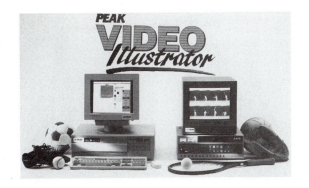

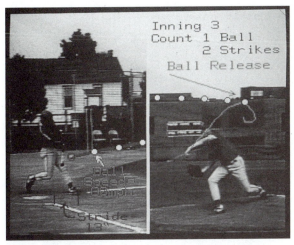

FIGURE 24.8 System for instant replay and manipulation of images.
(Reprinted with permission from Peak Performance Technologies, Inc., Englewood, CO.)

very important for identifying problems and risk of injury. This instant-replay system can be used to superimpose vectors, comments, and errors on the video image.

Sports for People with Physical Disabilities

While the existence of sports equipment, prostheses, and other devices that enhance the quality of life of people with physical disabilities is an extremely positive development, advances have unfortunately brought with them injuries and problematic new movement patterns. Training, conditioning, and rehabilitation are affected. We need to know more about the kinematic and kinetic characteristics of sports for the disabled. One recent area of research is the modeling of the arm during wheelchair propulsion

Visualizing the Future   **535**

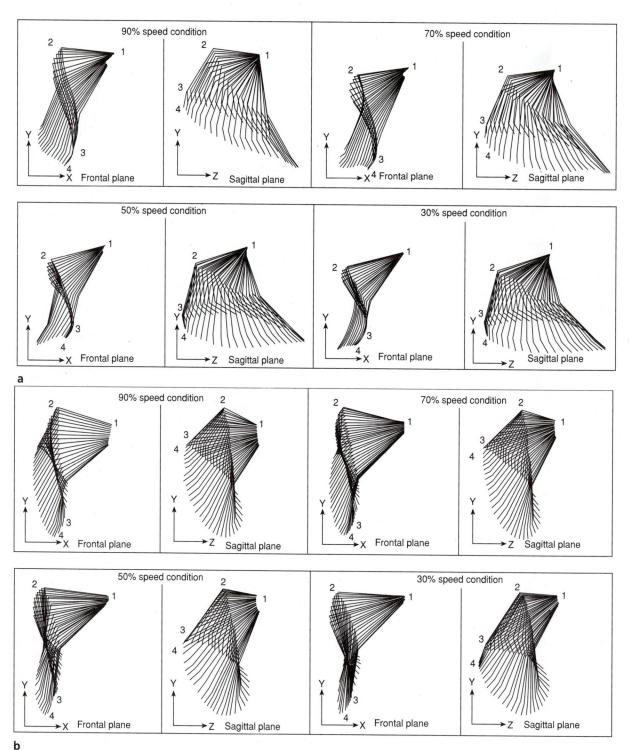

FIGURE 24.9 Mean cycle data of three-segment model (upper arm, forearm, and hand) of 10 wheelchair athletes during four speed conditions with respect to individual maximum speed. (a) Daily chair; (b) racing chair.

(Courtesy of Yong Tai Wang, Biomechanics Laboratory, Auburn University, AL.)

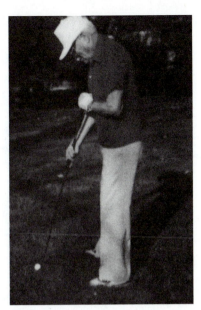

FIGURE 24.10 The posture of a golfer is more erect and less stressful to the spine when using a long-shafted putter.

TABLE 24.1 Changes in the human body due to weightlessness and living in space and suggested actions to alleviate or reduce these changes.

Change	Action
loss in body weight	exercise with this new body
upper trunk flexion	trunk extension exercises
flexion of lower legs	shank extension exercises
extension of thoracolumbar spine	spine strengthening
negative pressure in lower body	inversions-yoga, gymnastics
higher center of gravity	practice balance activities
bone mineral loss	strength exercises
bone strength loss	strength exercises
muscle strength loss	strength exercises
reduced work tolerances	training
disturbances in vestibular function	balance activities
disturbances in perceptual/ motor tasks	practice

under various loads and speeds. Wang studied the 3-D kinematics of the arm, related it to EMG of muscles, and postulated risk of injury to the shoulder complex. (See Figure 24.9.)

Physical Dysfunction and Aging

Maintenance of functional fitness of the older population is a goal of everyone in the health professions, including physical educators and biomechanists. More and more researchers are investigating movement capabilities and performances of older persons. Personalized profiles and criterion-based standards will be the emphasis in the future. Maintenance of movement skills that the individual older person needs and is interested in is important. Equipment is being modified for sports for older persons, which results in different movement patterns and postures. Note the difference in posture when using the long-shafted golf club depicted in Figure 24.10.

Space Living

Want to go to a space camp? The three-to-eight day experiences are based on NASA's astronaut-training program. People can experience cockpit simulators, space

station modules, weightlessness cabins, underwater astronaut trainers, and gravity chairs that mimic body weight on the moon. The complete space gravity environment can be simulated at these camps and academies. Biomechanists need to be familiar with potential changes in the human body and movement. A partial listing of these factors is given in Table 24.1.

Travel exercise kits for the space age are already on the market. Each year new devices are introduced. For example, in 1988, Quik-Fit introduced a set of sports-specific muscle strengthening and conditioning training kits. In 1991, a small portable stepping machine was introduced. Although all these devices can be used on earth, they have particular value in space environments.

New Perspectives

Scaling

Although researchers have used scaling techniques for decades, there appears to be a resurgence into identifying

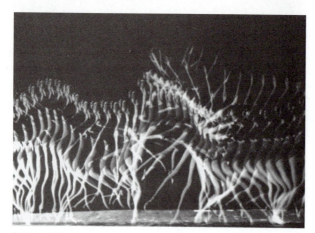

FIGURE 24.11 Form and motion merge to depict a nonnumerical quality of dynamics.

the most advantageous and informative approach to data interpretation. Greer (1992) and others have studied performances of children throwing balls of different sizes. They compared the anthropometry of the hand and the diameter of the balls with respect to ability to throw and to use one hand. Hudson (1988) has proposed some exciting ideas concerning scaling of running and swimming performances between men and women. When eliminated as a variable, anthropometry results in the reduction of differences in performance between the genders.

■ Chaos, nonlinear dynamics, and nonconservative concepts have become very popular in the physics world. Are they also valuable in the understanding of human movement? Time will tell.

Ecological Biomechanics

This is an energy approach to the analysis of goal-directed human behavior. Psychology and biology are fused to investigate the movements of people in known environments. The ecological biomechanist perceives space in multiple reference frames and considers movement as conservative or nonconservative.

Synergistic Biomechanics

Garrett (1986) coined this term in 1986 and produced computer graphics with artistry. Many observers viewed the images as more than mechanics, a combined art and science form. With newer techniques we now can

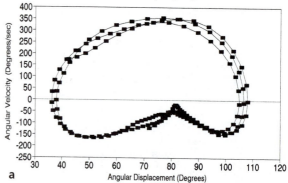

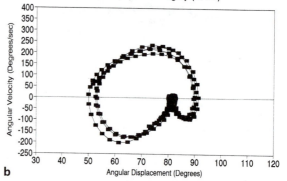

FIGURE 24.12 Angle velocity (phase portrait) diagrams of (a) normal subject walking at 90 steps per minute; (b) subject with cerebral palsy prior to surgery; and (c) autistic subject. Note the consistency of patterns for multiple steps and the deviation from normal for the subject with cerebral palsy.

(Courtesy of Eliane Mauerberg, Laboratory of Psychophysics of Action and Perception, UNESP, Brazil.)

538   The Future

visually reproduce exciting artistry of movement. The emergent entity is holistic, greater than its parts, and combines the metaphorical with the rational. An example is shown in Figure 24.11.

Dynamical Systems Theory

Such researchers as Clark, Truly, and Phillips (1990), Thelen (1989), and Kugler and Turvey (1987) are using this theory to understand motor development as well as general non-linear motion. Phase portraits are constructed to identify the attractors and invariants of a cyclic movement. Pattern recognition and other qualitative analyses form a prominent part of dynamical systems analysis. Its major contributions are new ways of perceiving the kinematics of movement and the kinetics, including energy. Phase portraits and angular velocity as a function of angular displacement are depicted in Figure 24.12.

■ Always look for new perspectives. Be innovative.

References

Clark, J. E., Truly, T. L., and Phillips, S. J. 1990. A dynamical systems approach to understanding the development of lower limb coordination in locomotion. In Sensory-motor organizations and development in infancy and early childhood, ed. H. Bloch, and B. I. Bertenthal. Klinver Academic Publishers, Netherlands.

Garrett, G. 1986. Synergistic biomechanics. In Biomechanics—The 1984 Olympic scientific congress proceedings, ed. M. Adrian, and H. Deutsch. Eugene, OR: Microform Publications.

Gillette Children's Hospital, St. Paul, MN. 1993. Normal walking, an interactive CD-ROM videotape and regular videotape.

Grabiner, M. D. 1993. Current issues in biomechanics. Champaign, IL: Human Kinetics Publishers.

Greer, T., et al. 1992. Commentary on movement and communication in human infancy. Jnl. Hum. Movement Sci. (Amsterdam):453–60.

Hudson, J. 1988. Scaling performances of men and women in selected sports. Report at AAHPERD convention.

International Journal of Sports Biomechanics (1985–present). Champaign, IL: Human Kinetics Publishers.

Journal of Orthopaedic and Sports Physical Therapy (1979–present). Baltimore, MD: American Physical Therapy Association.

Kugler, P. N., and Turvey, M. T. 1987. Information, natural law, and the self-assembly of rhythmic movement. Hillsdale, NJ: Lawrence Erlbaum Associates.

National Strength and Conditioning Association Journal (1980–present).

Soma, V. M. Engineering for the human body. 1988. Baltimore MD: Williams and Wilkins.

Thelen, E. 1989. Self-organization in developmental processes: Can systems approaches work? In Systems and development: The Minnesota symposia on child psychology, vol. 22. Hillsdale, NJ: Lawrence Erlbaum.

Thelen, E., and Ulrich, B. D. 1991. Hidden skills: A dynamic systems analysis of treadmill stepping during the first year. Monographs of the Society for Research in Child Development 56 (1) Serial No. 223.

Vaughn, C. L., Davis, B. L., and O'Connor, J. 1992. Gait analysis laboratory (An interactive book and software package). Champaign, IL: Human Kinetics Publishers.

Winter, D. 1987. Mechanical power in human movement: Generation, absorption and transfer. In Current research in sports biomechanics, ed. B. Van Gheluwe, and J. Atha. Med. Sport Sci. 25: 34–45.

Zhang, R. V. et al. 1987. A biomechanical study of supras pular nerve injuries in volleyball. In Biomechanics X-B, ed. B. Jousson. Champaign, IL: Human Kinetics Publishers.

A Metric-English Units

The International System of Units (Système International, or SI, is now the universal system of measurements. It is sometimes referred to as the metric system, since distance (meters) is one of the most common items measured. The basic units of measurement for the movement analyst are those measuring time, distance, force, and mass.

Table A.1 lists the standard SI unit and common multiples or fractions for each of the measures, together with equivalents from the English system of measurement.

Table A.2 shows some commonly used units derived from mathematical manipulation of the basic units or from a combination of time, force, distance, and mass units.

Conversions from English to SI appear in Table A.3.

TABLE A.1 SI units

SI Unit	English Equivalent
Linear distance	
Meter (m)	3.28 feet (ft)
Millimeter (mm), 0.001 m	0.0394 inches (in.)
Centimeter (cm), 0.01 m	0.3937 inches
Kilometers (km), 1000 m	0.621 miles
Angular distance	
Radian (rad)	57.296 degrees (°)
2π rad	360 degrees or 1 revolution
Time	
Minute (min)	Same
Second (sec), 1/60 min	Same
Hour (hr), 60 min	Same
Force	
Newton (N)	0.225 pounds (lb)
Kilonewton (kn)	225 pounds
Mass	
Kilogram (kg)*	0.0685 slugs*
Gram (gm), 0.001 kg	0.0000685 slugs

*Note that 1 kg is equal to 1 Nsec^2/m; 1 slug is equal to lb-sec^2/ft.

TABLE A.2 Derived units

SI Unit	English Equivalent
Velocity Meter per second (m/sec)	3.28 ft/sec or 0.447 mph

Acceleration
  Meter per second per
  second (m/sec^2)
	3.28 ft/sec^2 or
	0.447 miles/hr^2

Linear momentum (mV)
  Kilogram-meter per
  second (kgm/sec) (equal
  to newton-second)
	0.225 lb/sec

Impulse (Ft) Newton-second (Nsec)	0.225 lb/sec
Moment of force (torque) Newton-meter (Nm)	0.738 ft-lb

Work (energy)
  Joules (J) (equal to
  newton-meter)
	0.738 ft-lb

Power
  Watt (W) or newton-meter
  per second (Nm/sec)
	0.738 ft-lb/sec

Moment of inertia (I) Kilogram-meter^2 (kgm^2)	0.738 slug-ft^2

Angular momentum (I)
  Kilogram-meter^2 • radian
  per second (kgm^2 rad/sec)
	0.738 slug-ft^2 rad/sec

Pressure (Pa)
  Pasqual
  Kilopasqual
  Newton per centimeter^2
	0.689 lb/in^2

TABLE A.3 Conversions from English to SI.

To Convert From	To	Multiply By
inches	centimeters	2.54
feet	meters	0.305
yards	meters	0.91
miles	kilometers	1.61
pounds	newtons	4.45
slugs	kilograms	14.59
ft.lbs	joules	1.36

(same multiplier for torque, work, energy, and angular momentum)

B Trigonometry, Vectors, and Problems*

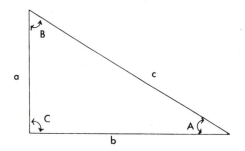

It is possible to solve many force and velocity problems by drawing vector diagrams. However, the degree of accuracy is dependent on the exactness of the drawing and measuring. In addition, this approach is time-consuming compared to the quicker, more accurate method using trigonometry. The word **trigonometry** literally means the *measurement of triangles*. Most problems in motion analysis involve the use of right triangles.

A right triangle is one containing an internal right angle (90°). The *sum of the three internal angles of a triangle always equals 180°*. Also, an *angle less than 90° is called an acute angle* and one *greater than 90° is an obtuse angle*. Two angles are said to be *complementary* if their sum equals 90°. Thus in a right triangle it is apparent that the two acute angles are complementary. (If the sum of two angles equals 180°, they are said to be *supplementary*.)

To understand the trigonometric functions, we must first be able to identify the parts of a right triangle. The following diagram of a right triangle will be used for the purpose of explanation.

The six component parts of the triangle consist of three angles and three sides. In the diagram, note that the longest of the three sides (c) is opposite the right angle (C). This longest side is called the hypotenuse. Since the hypotenuse is always opposite the right angle, it is very easy to identify. The other two sides are called the *legs* of the right triangle. A side may also be referred to as the *side opposite* a particular angle. In the diagram, the side opposite angle A is side a. The side opposite angle B is side b. *Adjacent side* is a term used to identify the side that, along with the hypotenuse, forms a given angle. Thus the side adjacent to angle A is side b. Likewise, the side adjacent to angle B is side a. It is important to understand that the hypotenuse never changes; which side is opposite or adjacent depends on which angle is being considered.

Of the six trigonometric functions, four are described here. These functions are based on the relationships between the angles and sides of the triangle.

The *sine* of an angle (pronounced "sign" and abbreviated *sin*) is defined as the ratio of the side opposite to the hypotenuse. Thus the sine of angle A is the length of side a divided by the length of side c, the hypotenuse ($\sin A = a/c$) and the sine of angle B is the length of side b divided by the length of side c ($\sin B = b/c$).

The second trigonometric function is the *cosine* (*cos*), defined as the ratio of the side adjacent to the hypotenuse. For angle A the cosine is b/c; for angle B it is a/c.

---

*Prepared by Jim Richards, Indiana University, 1979.

The *tangent* (*tan*) is defined as the ratio of the side opposite to the side adjacent. The tangent of angle A is a/b, and the tangent of angle B is b/a.

The *cotangent* (*cot*) is the ratio of the side adjacent to the side opposite. The cotangent of angle A is b/a; the cotangent of angle B is a/b.

These trigonometric functions have a specific, constant value for any given angle regardless of the size of the triangle. Since the values are constant, they can be compiled in tables such as Table B.1.

Since one angle in a right triangle is fixed, only five parts can vary (three sides and two angles). If either one angle and the length of one side or the lengths of two sides are known, we can calculate the remaining parts. The sides can be used to represent distance, magnitude of force, velocity, or other physical properties (vectors).

Example: Assume that the hypotenuse is 6 cm in length and angle A is 40°. Find (1) angle B, (2) side a, and (3) side b.

1. Angle B can be determined very readily since it is complementary to angle A, which is 40°:

$$90 - A = B$$
$$90 - 40 = B$$

2. To find side a, we must select the trigonometric function that involves side a (which is unknown) and side c, the hypotenuse (which is known). The sine of angle A equals side a (opposite) over side c.

$$\sin A = \frac{a}{c}$$

Since c is known to be 6 cm and $\sin A$ can be obtained from Table B.1, the only unknown is side a.

$$\sin 40 = \frac{a}{6 \text{ cm}}$$

$$.6428 = \frac{a}{6 \text{ cm}}$$

$$6 \times .6428 = a$$
$$a = 3.86 \text{ cm}$$

3. The same procedure is used to find side b.

The following problems are included as practice exercises. It may be helpful to make a sketch of each triangle to better understand the problem.

1. GIVEN: Hypotenuse = 10 cm; one angle = 30°
   FIND: Both legs (sides) of the triangle
2. GIVEN: One angle = 55°; side opposite = 4 m
   FIND: Hypotenuse and adjacent side
3. GIVEN: Hypotenuse = 4 in.; one side = 3 in.
   FIND: Both acute angles
4. GIVEN: One leg = 3 m; other leg = 5 m
   FIND: Both acute angles and hypotenuse
5. GIVEN: A ball projected at an angle of 25° with the horizontal; an initial resultant velocity of 10 m/sec (resultant equals hypotenuse)
   FIND: Vertical and horizontal components of the velocity
6. GIVEN: At takeoff, long jumper with a forward velocity of 32 ft/sec and a vertical velocity of 12 ft/sec
   FIND: Angle of takeoff and resultant velocity

Problems*

1. In the following triangle, label the sides (opposite, hypotenuse, and adjacent) with respect to angle a.

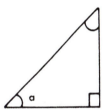

2. In the following triangle, complete the appropriate ratios.

$\sin a =$ _____

$\cos a =$ _____

$\tan a =$ _____

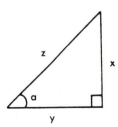

TABLE B.1 Trigonometric functions*

Degrees	Sines	Cosines	Tangents	Cotangents	Degrees
0	.0000	1.0000	.0000		90
1	.0175	.9998	.0175	57.290	89
2	.0349	.9994	.0349	28.636	88
3	.0523	.9986	.0524	19.081	87
4	.0698	.9976	.0699	14.301	86
5	.0872	.9962	.0875	11.430	85
6	.1045	.9945	.1051	9.5144	84
7	.1219	.9925	.1228	8.1443	83
8	.1392	.9903	.1405	7.1154	82
9	.1564	.9877	.1584	6.3138	81
10	.1736	.9848	.1763	5.6713	80
11	.1908	.9816	.1944	5.1446	79
12	.2079	.9781	.2126	4.7046	78
13	.2250	.9744	.2309	4.3315	77
14	.2419	.9703	.2493	4.0108	76
15	.2588	.9659	.2679	3.7321	75
16	.2756	.9613	.2867	3.4874	74
17	.2924	.9563	.3057	3.2709	73
18	.3090	.9511	.3249	3.0777	72
19	.3256	.9455	.3443	2.9042	71
20	.3420	.9397	.3640	2.7475	70
21	.3584	.9336	.3839	2.6051	69
22	.3746	.9272	.4040	2.4751	68
23	.3907	.9205	.4245	2.3559	67
24	.4067	.9135	.4452	2.2460	66
25	.4226	.9063	.4663	2.1445	65
26	.4384	.8988	.4877	2.0503	64
27	.4540	.8910	.5095	1.9626	63
28	.4695	.8829	.5317	1.8807	62
29	.4848	.8746	.5543	1.8040	61
30	.5000	.8660	.5774	1.7321	60
31	.5150	.8572	.6009	1.6643	59
32	.5299	.8480	.6249	1.6003	58
33	.5446	.8387	.6494	1.5399	57
34	.5592	.8290	.6745	1.4826	56
35	.5736	.8192	.7002	1.4281	55
36	.5878	.8090	.7265	1.3764	54
37	.6018	.7986	.7536	1.3270	53
38	.6157	.7880	.7813	1.2799	52
39	.6293	.7771	.8098	1.2349	51
40	.6428	.7660	.8391	1.1918	50
41	.6561	.7547	.8693	1.1504	49
42	.6691	.7431	.9004	1.1106	48
43	.6820	.7314	.9325	1.0724	47
44	.6947	.7193	.9657	1.0355	46
45	.7071	.7071	1.0000	1.0000	45
Degrees	**Cosines**	**Sines**	**Cotangents**	**Tangents**	**Degrees**

*For angles larger than 45°, be sure to use the headings that appear at the *bottom* of the columns.

3. Using Table B.1, find the following.

sin 30°   cos 30°   tan 40°
sin 60°   cos 60°   tan 60°

4. In the following triangle, find the value of angle *a*.

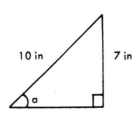

5. If angle *a* is 20° and side *A* is 10 inches long, find sides *B*, and *C* and angle *b*.

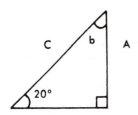

6. Find the two unknown sides and one unknown angle in the following triangle.

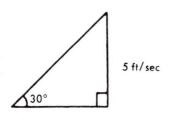

7. A woman walks 8 miles east, turns left, and walks 16 miles north. What is her resultant displacement?

8. The side of a mountain makes a 20° angle with the horizontal. If a man walks 1 mile up the mountain, how much has he increased his elevation?

9. A football is kicked with a resultant velocity of 12 m/sec at a 20° angle to the ground. What are the horizontal and vertical components of the velocity?

10. Without using trigonometric functions, determine the length of the hypotenuse (also called the resultant side) in the following triangle.

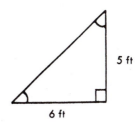

11. A man walks 36 km east and then 10.4 km north. What is his resultant displacement?

12. An automobile travels on a road 50° north of east. If the car goes 17 miles, what are the north and east components of the displacement?

13. The side of a mountain makes a 30° angle with the horizontal surface of the earth. If a man walks 2 miles up the mountain side, what is his vertical elevation above the horizontal surface?

14. Find the resultant of the four following vectors:
   a. 100 cm at 0°
   b. 80 cm at 40°
   c. 110 cm at 130°
   d. 160 cm at 210°

15. A runner changes speed from 20 ft/sec to 28 ft/sec in 4 seconds. What is the acceleration? The average velocity? The total distance traveled?

16. A stone is dropped from the top of a vertical cliff. It strikes at the foot of the cliff 3 seconds after it was dropped. How high is the cliff? With what velocity did it strike?

17. If the wheels of an automobile have a diameter of 60 cm, how far does the car move when the wheels in contact with the road turn through 9 radians?

18. If a plank 12 ft long of uniform cross-section and density and weighing 120 lb is placed so that 5 ft of it extends over the bank of a creek, how far out on the plank can a boy weighing 75 lb walk without tipping the plank? What is the minimum weight of stone that must be placed on the end on shore to permit the boy to walk to the end over the creek without tipping?

19. A player jumps into the air with both arms extended vertically overhead. Just before the maximum height is reached one arm is forcibly lowered so that the center of gravity is lowered 2 to 4 cm in the body. Do the fingertips of the other hand go higher or lower as a result? How much?

20. If a jumper jumps 2 ft high and takes off at an angle of 20° with the horizontal, how fast is he going forward after the takeoff?

21. If the shot is put at an angle of 42° with the horizontal and with a velocity of 10.8 m/sec in the direction of the put, what will be its upward velocity at the moment of release? What will be its forward velocity? What will be its time of flight from the point of release to the return to the same level at which it was released? How high will the shot go?

22. At the moment of takeoff, a broad jumper has a forward velocity of 9 m/sec. Her vertical velocity is 3 m/sec. What is the angle of her takeoff? How high does her center of gravity rise?

23. If the shot were projected horizontally at a speed of 40 ft/sec from a height of 32 ft, how soon would it hit the ground? How far from the starting point would it hit in horizontal distance?

APPENDIX

C Projectiles

Projection of an object or of oneself is the outcome—the product—of many actions. It is affected by gravity, velocity, and angle of projection. The effect of gravity on unsupported objects is the same regardless of the weight of the object (see Figure C.1). (Using SI measurements would mean a distance of 16.1 ft/3.28 = 4.9 m.)

The constant acceleration of gravitational force pulls the object downward a distance that equals in feet 16.1 t^2, in which t represents the time in seconds, during which gravity has been acting on the object. In 1 second an object would be pulled downward 16.1 ft (16.1 × 1^2); in 0.5 second the distance would be 4.025 ft (16.1 × 0.5^2). If the velocity and direction imparted by body levers are known, the path of flight can be determined. In Figure C.1 the horizontal line represents the projection of an object by means of force imparted by the body, a velocity of 80 ft/sec in a horizontal direction. Each dot represents an additional 8 ft in flight and also an additional 0.1 second of time. The effect of gravity at each time interval is represented by the vertical lines. The lower ends of the vertical lines mark the path of flight resulting from the two forces. The path of flight can be determined in like manner whenever the velocity and direction imparted by body force to an object are known.

With trigonometric relationships the measures of angles and velocities can be obtained in many ways; those which require the least calculation can be used. As one example, the angles of projection might have been determined before the velocities. When the angle is known,

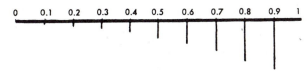

FIGURE C.1 Gravitational effect at each 0.1 second on object projected horizontally at 80 ft. 0.4 in. represents 8 ft.

another trigonometric value might be used to determine the length of the time to the high point and subtracting from the product, the 16.1 t^2 value for this time.

The processes described can be used to determine the position of the projectile at any time in its flight. When the projection has a downward component, the 16.1 t^2 value is added, instead of subtracted, in determining the height, and the resulting sum is subtracted from the starting height.

Knowledge of velocity, angle, and position at any time in flight can be applied to many situations and enable the instructor to set specific goals for development of skill in a given situation. One illustration is that of developing skill in a tennis serve. Most beginners are likely to direct the ball upward; yet a velocity of 80–90 ft/sec can be achieved by the average adult. Suppose that the height at which the ball is impacted is 8 ft and the ball has a velocity of 80 ft/sec. The net is approximately 40 ft from the impact, and the ball would reach it in 0.5 second. The 16.1 t^2 value for this time is 4.025 ft, so that, as the ball reaches the net, it would be 3.975 ft above the ground, thus clearing the net by 0.975 ft. The

547

ball would reach the ground when the 16.1 t^2 value was 8 ft; $8 = 16.1\ t^2$; $t^2 = 8/16.1 = 0.4969$; $t = 0.704$ second. The horizontal distance would be $80 \times 0.704 = 56.32$ ft, which is well within the service court.

Mortimer[1] has applied angle, velocity, and ball position in determining the projection most likely to make a basket from the free throw line when the starting point is 5 ft above the floor. She recommends a velocity of 24 ft/sec and an angle of 58°.

Optimal Projection Angle for Greatest Distance

A projection angle of 45° is often recommended as the optimum when the greatest possible distance is desired. This is true only when the vertical distance between the starting point and the end of the flight is zero. Bunn has shown this in discussing the projection of the shot put.

When the vertical distance between the start and the end of flight and the velocity of projection are known, the angle that results in the greatest distance is one in which the following applies:

$$\text{sine}^2 = \frac{\text{Velocity}^2}{2\ (\text{velocity}^2 - gh)}$$

In this formula, g is 32.2, and h is the vertical distance between the start and end of flight. If the start is higher than the end, h will be a minus quantity.

Bunn[2] gives a table of the distances that the shot put would reach if projected at angles from 37 through 44 degrees when released at a height of 7 ft at velocities from 20 to 50 ft/sec. If the shot were given a velocity of 30 ft/sec, the determination of the optimal angle would be as follows:

$$\text{sine}^2 = \frac{30^2}{2[30^2 - (32.2 \times -7)]}$$

In this case the end of the flight is below the starting point, and h has a minus value.

[1]Mortimer, E. 1951. Basketball shooting. *Res. Quarterly* 22:234.

[2]Bunn, J. 1955. *Scientific principles of coaching.* Englewood Cliffs, NJ: Prentice-Hall.

$$\text{sine}^2 = \frac{900}{2\ (900 + 225.4)}$$

$$\text{sine}^2 = \frac{900}{2250.8} = 0.39985$$

In this case the sine = 0.6323, which is the value for an angle of 39° 13′. For a 39° angle and for a 40° angle, Bunn's table gives a distance of 34.42 ft, the longest for the angles included in his table.

In jumping for distance, the center of gravity is higher at the beginning of flight than it is at landing. At the beginning of flight the body is extended, the arms are raised, and in an adult 6 ft tall, the height of the center of gravity can be estimated as 3 plus ft. If the landing is made with the thighs horizontal and some inclination of the legs, we can assume for this illustration that the center of gravity is 1.5 ft lower than it was at the beginning of flight. If the velocity of projection is 16 ft/sec, the optimal angle for greatest distance will be one in which the following applies:

$$\text{sine}^2 = \frac{16^2}{2\ [16^2 - (32.2 \times -1.5)]}$$

$$\text{sine}^2 = 0.4206$$

In this case, the sine = 0.645. This is the value of an angle of 40° 26′.

If the velocity is 12 ft/sec and the other measures remain the same, the optimal angle is 37° 43′. If the positions of the center of gravity are determined at the beginning and end of flight, as they can be from film, the value of h can be more accurately determined. The velocity of the center of gravity can also be determined from these film measures (Chapter 8). In calculating the angle of projection in better-than-average performers, we have found that this angle is less than 45°; this is another example of the body's making necessary adjustments without the person being aware that it is doing so.

Summary of Calculations and Other Comments

For ready reference the calculations discussed here and others that are related and useful are summarized here.

Range is the horizontal distance between the starting and landing point; time means the time in flight.

1. Horizontal velocity = Range ÷ Time.
2. In determining vertical velocity (V. vel.) consideration must be given to the vertical distance (VD) between the starting and the landing point. When VD is 0:

$$\text{V. vel.} = 16.1 \ t^2 \div \text{Time}$$

3. When the starting point is higher than the landing point:

$$\text{V. vel.} = (16.1 \ t^2 - VD) \div \text{Time}$$

Note that, if $16.1 \ t^2$ is less than VD, the minus quantity indicates that the projection is below the horizontal.

4. When the starting point is lower than the landing point:

$$\text{V. vel.} = (16.1 \ t^2 + VD) \div \text{Time}$$

5. For the projection velocity (Proj. vel.):
   a. When the horizontal velocity (Horiz. vel.) and vertical velocity components are known:

$$(\text{Proj. vel.})^2 = (\text{Horiz. vel.})^2 + (\text{V. vel.})^2$$

   b. When the angle of projection is known:

$$\text{Proj. vel.} = \text{V. vel.} \div \text{Sine}$$
$$\text{or}$$
$$\text{Proj. vel.} = \text{Horiz. vel.} \div \text{Cosine}$$

6. The angle of projection can be determined by use of trigonometric relationships. For the angle of projection:
   a. Tangent of the angle = V. vel. ÷ Horiz. vel.
   b. Sine of the angle = V. vel. ÷ Proj. vel.
   c. Cosine of the angle = Horiz. vel. ÷ Proj. vel.
7. The high point (h.p.) of the projection can be located by finding first the time to the high point.

$$\text{Time to high point} = \text{V. vel.} \div 32.2$$

8. The distance of the high point above the starting point = (V. vel. × Time to h.p.) − 16.1 (Time to h.p.)^2
9. The horizontal distance from the starting to the high point = Horiz. vel. × Time h.p.

The relationships used in finding the high point can be used to locate the projectile at any time and at any point in flight. For example, a tennis ball was projected from a height of 7 ft and 40 ft from the net at a velocity of 50 ft/sec and at an angle of 10° above the horizontal. Where was the ball when it reached the net? The horizontal and vertical velocity components must be known.

They can be found by rearranging the equations in 5b:

$$\text{V. vel.} = \text{Proj. vel.} \times \text{Sine}$$
$$\text{Horiz. vel.} = \text{Proj. vel.} \times \text{Cosine}$$

For an angle of 10° the sine is 0.173; the cosine is 0.984. In the described tennis situation the numerical values are as follows:

$$\text{V. vel.} = 50 \times 0.173, \text{ or } 8.65 \text{ ft/sec}$$
$$\text{Horiz. vel.} = 50 \times 0.984, \text{ or } 49.2 \text{ ft/sec}$$

Following is the time to the net:

$$40 \div 49.2, \text{ or } 0.81 \text{ second}$$

During this time the vertical velocity has moved the ball upward; gravitational force has moved it downward. The combined effect will be as follows:

$$(8.65 \times 0.81) - 16.1 \ (0.81)^2$$
$$7.00 - 10.573, \text{ or } 3.573 \text{ ft}$$

At the time the ball reaches the net, it will be 3.573 ft lower than the starting point, or 3.427 ft above the ground and 0.427 ft above the net, which is 3 ft in height.

The questions might also arise as to where the ball would be at a given time, such as 0.5 second after the flight began. From the starting point it would travel horizontally as follows:

$$49.2 \times 0.5, \text{ or } 24.6 \text{ ft}$$

Vertically it would travel as follows:

$$(8.65 \times 0.5) - 16.1 \ (0.5)^2$$
$$4.325 - 4.025, \text{ or } 0.3 \text{ ft}$$

In 0.5 second the ball would be 0.3 ft higher than, and 24.6 ft from, the starting point. The spinning ball in flight is affected by the amount and direction of force applied at takeoff and the type and amount of spin (see Figure C.2).

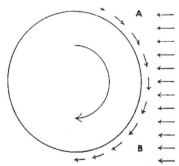

FIGURE C.2 Rapidly spinning ball in flight encounters more resistance at *a* than at *b* and in flight will curve toward *b*.

TABLE C.1 Gravity distance relationship: Given a specific free-fall time, a ball will fall a predetermined distance.*

Time	0.00	0.01	0.02	0.03	0.04	0.05	0.06	0.07	0.08	0.09
0.0	0.000	0.001	0.006	0.014	0.025	0.040	0.057	0.078	0.013	0.13
0.1	0.161	0.194	0.231	0.272	0.315	0.362	0.412	0.465	0.521	0.58
0.2	0.644	0.710	0.779	0.851	0.927	1.006	1.088	1.173	1.262	1.35
0.3	1.449	1.547	1.648	1.745	1.861	1.972	2.086	2.204	2.324	2.44
0.4	2.576	2.706	2.840	2.976	3.116	3.260	3.387	3.556	3.709	3.86
0.5	4.025	4.187	4.353	4.524	4.694	4.870	5.048	5.230	5.416	5.60
0.6	5.796	5.980	6.188	6.290	6.584	6.802	7.014	7.227	7.444	7.66
0.7	7.889	8.116	8.346	8.579	8.816	9.056	9.299	9.545	9.795	10.04
0.8	10.304	10.573	10.825	11.091	11.360	11.632	11.970	12.186	12.468	12.75
0.9	13.041	13.332	13.627	13.925	14.226	14.530	14.838	15.148	15.462	15.77
1.0	16.100	16.432	16.750	17.080	17.414	17.750	18.090	18.433	18.779	19.12
1.1	19.481	19.837	20.196	20.558	20.923	21.292	21.664	22.039	22.417	22.79
1.2	23.184	23.602	23.963	24.357	24.755	25.156	25.560	25.967	26.378	26.79
1.3	27.209	27.629	28.052	28.469	28.899	29.342	29.788	30.208	30.660	31.10
1.4	31.556	32.008	32.464	32.922	33.384	33.850	34.318	34.790	35.265	35.74
1.5	36.225	36.709	37.197	37.688	38.172	38.680	39.180	39.684	40.192	40.70
1.6	41.216	41.732	42.252	42.776	43.307	43.832	44.365	44.901	45.440	45.98
1.7	46.529	47.078	47.630	48.187	48.745	49.306	49.861	50.439	51.011	51.58
1.8	52.164	52.745	53.329	53.917	54.508	55.102	55.660	56.310	56.903	57.51
1.9	58.121	58.734	59.361	59.907	60.593	61.220	61.849	62.482	63.118	63.75
2.0	64.400	65.046	65.644	66.346	67.002	67.960	68.322	68.987	69.206	70.326
2.1	71.001	71.679	72.360	73.044	73.732	74.422	75.116	75.813	76.514	77.217
2.2	77.924	78.634	79.347	80.064	80.783	81.566	82.232	82.962	83.694	84.430
2.3	85.169	85.911	86.657	87.405	88.157	88.912	89.671	90.432	91.197	91.965
2.4	92.736	93.510	94.288	95.069	95.854	96.640	97.431	98.224	99.021	99.823
2.5	100.625	101.432	102.341	103.054	103.871	104.690	105.503	106.339	107.168	108.000
2.6	108.836	109.675	110.517	111.362	112.211	113.262	113.917	114.780	115.637	116.502
2.7	117.369	118.240	119.114	119.992	120.872	121.756	122.643	123.534	124.437	125.024
2.8	126.224	127.127	128.034	128.943	129.856	130.772	131.692	132.614	133.540	134.469
2.9	135.401	136.336	137.275	138.217	139.162	140.110	141.062	142.016	142.974	143.936
3.0	144.900	145.868	146.828	147.802	148.790	149.770	150.754	151.781	152.731	153.724
3.1	154.721	155.721	156.724	157.730	158.740	159.752	160.768	161.787	162.810	163.835
3.2	164.864	165.896	166.931	167.970	169.021	170.056	171.104	172.157	173.210	174.268
3.3	175.168	176.393	177.480	178.531	179.605	180.682	181.763	182.846	183.933	185.023
3.4	186.116	187.212	188.312	189.415	190.521	191.630	192.742	193.858	194.977	196.100
3.5	197.125	198.354	199.585	200.620	201.759	202.901	204.045	205.193	206.344	207.498
3.6	208.656	209.817	210.981	212.148	213.319	214.492	215.669	216.849	218.033	219.219
3.7	220.409	221.602	222.798	223.998	225.200	226.406	227.615	228.828	230.043	231.262
3.8	232.484	233.709	234.938	236.169	237.404	238.642	239.884	241.128	242.376	243.627
3.9	244.881	246.138	247.399	248.663	249.930	251.200	252.474	253.750	255.030	256.314
4.0	257.600									

*Distance in feet through which freely falling objects move in a given time, calculated as distance = $\frac{1}{2}gt^2$ (g = 32.2). Conversion to metric system: value in table, divided by 3.28.

D Maximum Moments of Force

TABLE D.1 Maximum moments of force (torques) acting at selected joints during various movement activities.

	Ankle		Knee		Hip		Shoulder		Elbow		Wrist	
	Flex.	Exten.	Flex.	Exten.	Flex.	Exten.	Flex.	Exten.	Flex.	Exten.	Flex.	Exten.
Badminton smash	270		39		44		22	17	6	7	2	2
Basketball, vertical jump	300	80	45	75	6	30	6					
Bicycling, 15 mph	3	3	3	40	22	14						
Fencer's lunge, front	275	185	81	130	75	25						
Fencer's lunge, rear	300	290	90	120		63						
Football block		300		240	30	125						
Football punt		300	16	90	75	35						
Golf drive, back arm	200		130				19	9	9	12	5	5
Hammer throw	500	500	300	240	150	200	100	45	90	90	50	90
Head spring					10		33	30	30	24	24	26
Rowing, 36/min	3		20		3		10	12	9	1	5	1
Swim start		59	11	87	56	26	11	13	5	5		
Tennis serve	150	300	5	95	49	70	27	24	16	14	5	6
Track start	400	400	240	230	60	115						

Measurement is in kgm of force; kg = 2.2 lbs.

E

Anthropometric Values

TABLE E.1 Comparison of 5th, 50th, and 95th percentile anthropometric values of different aged populations.

Variable	Age	Mean	Male 5	Male 50	Male 95	Mean	Female 5	Female 50	Female 95
Weight (kg)	1	9.5	7.8	9.4	11.1	8.9	6.4	8.8	10.6
	6	20.8	15.6	20.7	24.7	19.3	15.2	19.1	23.2
	13	40.7	28.1	39.8	53.4	48.0	35.7	45.9	59.7
	Adult	70.8	55.5	68.6	90.8	60.0	46.6	59.6	74.5
Height (cm)	1	73.5	68.6	72.4	79.8	72.4	67.5	72.7	76.3
	6	133.7	105.4	114.3	120.3	112.8	104.2	113.1	121.5
	13	149.5	137.9	148.3	160.3	155.1	144.0	154.7	164.4
	Adult	174.1	162.8	174.1	185.3	163.0	152.6	162.8	174.1
Sitting height (cm)	1	47.2	44.7	46.3	50.3	46.3	43.0	45.6	50.1
	6	62.4	56.8	62.8	65.8	61.3	56.9	61.2	65.0
	13	76.8	71.5	76.9	82.4	80.0	75.3	80.4	86.2
	Adult	89.3	83.5	89.3	95.4	85.1	79.0	85.2	90.8
Hand length (cm)	1	8.8	8.1	8.7	9.8	8.8	7.4	8.8	9.4
	6	12.6	11.4	12.6	13.6	12.4	11.3	12.3	13.5
	13	15.9	14.3	15.8	17.4	16.8	15.0	16.7	18.4
	Adult	19.0	17.4	19.0	20.6	17.4	16.1	17.4	19.0
Knee height (cm)	1	20.1	18.9	19.9	22.2	19.3	17.1	19.5	21.4
	6	34.1	30.7	34.0	36.8	34.0	30.4	33.8	37.4
	13	47.5	42.1	47.4	55.5	49.0	45.4	49.1	52.3
	Adult	55.1	50.2	55.1	60.2	51.0	46.9	50.9	55.5
Buttocks-foot (cm)	1	35.0	31.6	35.0	37.8	34.1	31.7	33.6	37.0
	6	62.5	57.1	62.7	67.1	63.0	50.9	62.4	69.0
	13	86.9	80.2	86.3	99.0	92.2	83.8	93.1	98.8
	Adult	N/A	N/A	N/A	N/A	N/A	N/A	N/A	N/A
Shoulder breadth (cm)	1	20.7	18.9	20.7	22.5	20.3	18.7	19.9	22.3
	6	27.8	25.2	27.5	30.6	27.3	24.6	27.1	29.8
	13	35.8	32.7	35.7	41.7	37.4	33.5	36.8	41.8
	Adult	45.1	41.2	45.0	49.4	42.1	38.4	42.0	45.7
Lower torso breadth (cm)	1	15.2	13.8	15.0	18.1	14.6	13.1	14.4	16.8
	6	19.6	17.3	19.5	21.9	19.8	17.7	19.7	22.0
	13	26.2	23.8	25.5	30.9	28.7	25.0	28.5	31.5
	Adult	N/A	N/A	N/A	N/A	N/A	N/A	N/A	N/A

GLOSSARY

Abduction: Movement away from the midline.

Acceleration: The rate of change in velocity.

Accelerometers: An instrument to record the acceleration of an object.

Accelerometry: The study of the aspects of acceleration.

Accumulative Trauma: Increased trauma.

Accuracy Throws: Throws aimed at a specific target.

Active Drag: Drag on a body that has moving parts (swimming).

Activity Phase: Involves motion.

Adaptative Devices: Devices altered so they can be used in specific situations.

Adduction: Movement toward the midline.

Adjusted Lean Body Weight: May be adjusted due to gender, age, and body build.

Adjusted Work: Workload adjusted to fit a person's body condition.

Aerobic Aerodynamic: The two words combined bring together the laws of motion in air situations and performing while breathing.

Afferent Motor Fiber: Carries messages toward the central nervous system.

Agonist: The muscle(s) that originate or cause movement.

Air Resistance: Resistance of the air to movement.

Airborne Activities: Activities that occur in the air.

Amplitude: The state of the swing of a body.

Analyses: The measurement of the actions of a body.

Angle of Attack: Angle between the longitudinal axis of a body and the direction of the fluid.

Angle of Incidence: Angle made by the path of the body with the surface at the point of impact.

Angle of Inclination: Deviation from a given direction from the vertical or horizontal.

Angle of Lean: Deviation of trunk from the vertical.

Angle of Reflexion: Angle made by an object and a target on rebound.

Angled Approach: A curved approach.

Angular Acceleration: Usually expressed in radians per second squared or degrees per second and is the change in angular velocity of an object (including a body) divided by the time over which the change occurs.

Angular Displacement: A change in position of an object moving in a circular path.

Angular Momentum: Momentum of an object moving in a circular motion.

Angular Motion: A motion that revolves around a central point or line.

Angular Velocity: Velocity of an object moving in a circular path.

Anomalies: Anything irregular or abnormal.

Antagonist: Muscle(s) that generate torque opposing the action of the agonist.

Anthropometry: The science and technique of human measurement.

Apex: The highest point in the trajectory of a projectile.

Archimedes' Principle: The buoyant force acting to support a body in a fluid is equal in magnitude to the weight of the fluid displaced by the body.

Arm-supported Activities: Activities such as gymnastics in which the arms support the body.

Artist: One who is skilled in any of the fine arts.

Asymmetric Lifting: Not symmetrical or not the correct way to lift an object.

Automatic Digitizing: Digitizing done by machine as contrasted by hand.

Autonomic Neurons: A plexus of neurons originating in the spinal column not subject to voluntary control.

Axis: A line around which a turning body revolves.

Axis of Rotation: An imaginary line about which all points in a rotating body describe circles.

Axons: A tubular process that arises from a neuron and transmits signals generated by the neuron.

Balance: A position where equilibrium is controlled.

Ballistic Movement: A movement or part of a movement in which the motion of the area involved is the result of its own momentum, not due to external force.

Basal Ganglia: Group of nuclei in cerebrum.

Base of Support: That area where a body and supportive surface are in contact.

Bending: Condition where a load applied to a structure causes it to bend about an axis. The result produces tension on one side of the longitudinal axis and compression on the other side.

Bending Moment: The moment found by the distance perpendicularly from the end of the bending-length to the point of the bending origin.

Bernoulli Theorem: Regions of relative high velocity fluid flow are associated with regions of relative high pressure. When these regions of low and high pressure are on opposite sides of the foil, a lift force is created perpendicular to the foil from the high-pressure zone to the low-pressure zone.

Biomechanics: A synthesis of biology and mechanics in the understanding of human movement.

Bipennate Muscle: Having two feather-like arrangements within the muscle.

Body Physique: Physical structure organization of body parts culminating in the appearance of the body.

Boundary Layer: The layer of fluid immediately next to a body.

Brain Stem: All of the brain except the cerebellum and cerebral cortex.

Braking Force: Force acting as a deterrent to speed or any motion.

Buoyancy: Tendency of a liquid to keep an object afloat.

Bursae: Sacs located around joints that secrete fluid to reduce friction.

Cardio-vascular Exercise: Exercise that involves the heart and all blood vessels.

Carpal Tunnel Syndrome: Cumulative pressure trauma to tendons, nerve, or artery at wrist cuff.

Center of Gravity: Imaginary point around which the mass and weight of a body has its total mass concentrated.

Center of Mass: Center of the total mass of a body.

Centrifugal Force: A counter-force to centripetal force.

Centripetal Force: A force directed toward the center of a rotating body equal to MV^2/r.

Cerebral Cortex: Thinking part of the brain.

Cerebrum: Upper anterior part of the brain above the pons and cerebellum.

Cinematography: Use of cameras to film motion.

Circumduction: Moving in a circle about a joint.

Clinical Diagnosis: Diagnosis by means of practical and experimental information.

Closed Kinetic Chain: *See* Chapter 11.

CNS: Central nervous system.

Coefficient of Elasticity: A number indicating the degree of magnitude when an object is compressed and regains its normal shape ratio of drop height to rebound height.

Coefficient of Friction: Ratio of the force required to slide one surface over another to the force that is acting perpendicular to the surfaces.

Coefficient of Restitution: Indicates the elasticity of an object.

Compression: Squeezing or pushing together.

Computer-aided Design and Modeling (CAD/CAM): Design created by computer programming with modeling techniques.

Computerized Optical Systems: A system involving computer and optics.

Concentric: The action involved in the shortening of muscle.

Concurrent: Involves meeting or intersecting in a point.

Conservation of Momentum: Maintaining relationship between velocity and mass.

Contourogram: Line drawings of body outlines.

Cosine: *See* table in Appendix B.

Couple: Involves a pair of equal, opposite forces acting on opposite sides of an axis of rotation to produce torque.

Curvilinear: Moving along a curved path.

Deformation: Change that occurs in original shape.

Density: Amount of mass per unit of volume.

Developmental Biomechanics: A study of change as a human develops toward maturity and beyond.

Diarthrodial Joints: Freely moving joints of the body.

Displacement: Changing position.

Down Unweighting: In skiing, the body of the skier moves downward on the skis to reduce force on ground.

Drag: Force on a body moving through a fluid.

Dynamics: That branch of physics that treats the motion of bodies and the effects of forces producing motion.

Eccentric: Action that takes place when muscle is lengthened.

Ecological Biomechanics: Study of relationship of an organism and its environment.

Ectomorph: Denoting a physical and personality type associated with leanness of the body.

Eddy Currents: A whirling or backward circling current of water.

Efferent Motor Fiber: Motor fiber receiving a message to move outward.

Effort Arm: That part of the lever system that indicates the distance of the effort from the axis.

Elasticity: The degree to which a structure, when deformed, returns to its original shape and size.

Elements of Gymnastics: Composed of all the actions involved with gymnastic action.

Endomorph: Denoting a physical and personality type associated with fatness of the body.

Epiphysis: The center of the bone that produces new bone until the entire bone closes completely.

Equilibrium: A state of balance among forces acting within or upon a body.

Excessive Force: Force exerted as more than should be used against an object.

Exercise: A set of systematic movements used to strengthen, train and develop people to perform more effectively.

Exercise Equalizing Equation: [Work performed = number of repetitions × (weight lifted + body segment lifted) + (displacement of weight) × adjusted lean body weight]

Falling: The act of moving downward caused by the pull of gravity.

Fatigue: A condition of lessened activity of an organism or any part caused by prolonged exertion.

Fixator: Muscle tending to fix the movement of a joint.

Flexibility: A qualitative term representing the range of motion at a joint in different directions.

Flexion: The bending of a joint so that the angle between the bones is decreased.

Flume Training: Performed in a swimming treadmill. It is done in a large tank in which the water moves in a circular fashion.

Follow-through Phase: Action that occurs after an object is released.

Force: The product of a body's mass and its acceleration.

Force-angle Curve: The curve showing force on one axis and the angle on the other axis.

General Motion: A term used when motion is involved in which rotation and translation occur at the same time.

Goniogram: Basic unit of mass (or weight) in the metric system. Gonio denotes a corner or angle.

Grade Running: Running uphill or downhill. This involves the inclination of the terrain.

Ground Reaction Forces: Forces generated against the ground, usually by the feet in running.

Hand Paddles: Paddles held by hands to increase swimming action.

High-velocity Throws: Throws in which the performer releases an object at high velocity.

Homonymous: An anatomical relation between sensory receptors and motoneurons that serve the same muscles.

Hyperextension: The maximum extension of an arm or leg beyond the plane of the body.

Imaging System: System used to find appropriate structures and materials by CAT scans with magnetic resonance equipment.

Impact: The forcible contact of a moving body with another object moving or at rest.

Impulse: The product of a force and the time that occurs during the action.

Inertia: That condition in which a body tends to remain at rest or in a state of constant velocity.

Inherent Motor Patterns: Inherent means to be inseparable and applies to qualities. So, motor patterns that are connected or similar are inherent; also means innate.

In-line Skating: A new form of skating using roller blades. It is similar to ice skating, but is done on land.

Instantaneous Velocity: Refers to velocity being attained immediately.

Involuntary Motor Patterns: Motor actions that are not controlled.

Isometric: Involved in strengthening muscles without movement of the joints.

Kineanthropometry: Focuses solely on the measurement of size, shape, proportion, composition, maturation and gross function as related to such things as growth, exercise, performance, and nutrition.

Kinematics: That branch of mechanics that deals with motion without reference to force or mass.

Kinesthesia: The perception or consciousness of one's own muscular movements.

Labyrinthine Reflex: The righting reflex that acts with others to maintain equilibrium.

Laminar Flow: A flow of fluid that is smooth and moves in parallel layers.

Landing Angle: The angle formed by an object with the surface when contacting it.

Lateral Rotation: Rotation to one side as opposed to medial.

Lever: A machine composed of a bar that can be caused to rotate about a center or axis.

Lever Arm or Moment Arm: The perpendicular distance from the point of application of a force to the center of motion in a relatively rigid structure.

Lift Force: The component of the fluid-resistance vector that acts perpendicularly to the direction of the fluid flow (for example, aiding a swimmer).

Ligament: A band or sheet of firm, compact, fibrous tissue closely binding bones together.

Linear: All parts of a body moving in the same direction and at the same time along a given path, either straight or curved.

Linear Velocity: Velocity of an object moving in a straight line.

Line of Gravity: Line of action or application of the force of gravity.

Line Segment Figures: Lines drawn to represent a body including head, trunk, and limbs (stick figures).

Locomotion: The act of moving from one place to another.

Magnetic Resonance Image: Image obtained by magnetic resonance procedure.

Magnus Effect: A spinning object in flight will deviate toward the direction of the spin.

Mass: The quotient of the weight of an object divided by the acceleration due to gravity.

Maximal Stimulus: Greatest stimulus that can be exerted.

Mechanical Advantage: This is the ratio of effort arm to the resistance arm. If the ratio is greater than one, the mechanical advantage is strength or force. Otherwise, speed and range of motion regarding movement are the advantage.

Mechanical Efficiency: Efficiency of a body or machine determined by mechanical means.

Mechanical Energy: Energy from a mechanical device.

Medial Rotation: Rotation around the middle.

Mesomorphy: Denoting a physical and personality type associated with physical prowess, such as an athlete possesses.

Meter: See international units of weights and measures in appendices.

Mobility: Ability to move with facility.

Modeling: A means of displaying action through a model.

Modulus of Elasticity (Young's): A ratio of stress to strain at any point in the elastic region of a load-deformation curve giving a value for stiffness.

Moment Arm: The perpendicular distance of a force from the line of application to the center of motion.

Moment of Force: Force that is determined by measuring the distance perpendicularly from the length of force arm to the point of application.

Momentum of Inertia: Involves rotating bodies and is increased with the mass and distance from the axis in rotation.

Motor Development: Development of the motor aspects of the individual.

Motor Map: The motor cortex. It is the topographic representation nerve center of the location of the muscle.

Motor Unit: Entire neuron and muscle fibers that it innervates.

Movement Time: Time that elapses after reaction to a signal has taken place.

Mover: Muscle that causes movement.

Multipennate: More than one arrangement of pennate-type fibers in a muscle.

Myotatic Reflex: Stretch reflex such as a knee jerk.

Neural Adaptation: Refers to possible changes occurring within the nervous system that allow production of strength and power.

Neuralizer: A muscle that aids in neuralizing action.

Neuromuscular Exercise: Exercises that involve the nervous and muscular systems.

Neuron: Each cell body in the nervous system with its fibers.

Occupational Biomechanics: Involves the study of the interaction of the worker and the industrial environment.

Optimization: To make the most of a situation or action.

Optimum Velocity: Velocity that is optimum for best performance.

Osteoporosis: A condition in which the bone loses material and becomes less strong.

Pacinian Corpuscle: Part of the receptors in the skin and tendinous insertion of the muscles of the joints.

Parabolic Flight: The curve path of an object in flight.

Parallelogram of Forces: Forces are shown in a four-sided plane figure whose opposite sides are parallel and equal.

Passive Drag: Resistance of water on body in singular position, e.g., gliding.

Patella Tendon Reflex: Reaction of the patella tendon to stimulus such as the tap of the knee.

Peaking: Nearing maximum.

Pendulum Swing: Swing of a body suspended from a fixed point and free to move to and fro.

Pennate Muscle: Fibers are arranged like a feather.

Peripheral Nervous System: Includes the cranial and spinal nerves and the peripheral portions of the autonomic nervous system.

Plyometrics: A form of training that uses the stretch reflex in improving, for example, jumping (known as depth jumping).

PNF: Proprioceptive neuromuscular facilitation.

Point Plot: Plotting points representing parts of the body such as knee joints.

Postural Sway: A body moving from side-to-side and front-to-back when standing upright.

Posture: Positions of a body in reference to its parts, a neuromechanical state that concerns the maintenance of equilibrium.

Potential Energy (PE): Stored energy.

Power: Production of work, which is calculated as work or movement accomplished divided by the time taken to complete the effort.

Proprioceptors: Nerve receptors located in the joints and tendons.

Propulsive Phase: That phase (often main) that is involved in the action.

Prostheses: Artificial parts attached to the body to enable action to take place.

Qualitative: Pertaining to quality as contrasted with quantitative; doesn't involve a numerical measure, only stated in general terms.

Quantitative: Involves use of numbers to evaluate something.

Race Walking: A form of walking that is close to running.

Raw EMG: Electromyogram that is not integrated or modified.

Reaction Time: Time elapsed before responding to a stimulus.

Receptors: Portions of the nervous system that receive messages.

Rectilinear: Involves movement along a straight line.

Rehabilitative Biomechanics: Study of movement pattern of injured and disabled persons.

Relaxation: The state of being relaxed.

Release Angle: Angle at the moment of release of an object.

Resultant: Single force that is the sum of a given set of forces with a common point of application.

Reversed Muscle Action: Muscle action that takes place in the direction that is not the common one.

Rolling Friction: Friction created as an object is moving across a surface.

ROM: Range of motion.

Rotator Cuff: Muscles (supraspinatus, subscapularis, teres minor, infraspinatus) that attach by tendon to the capsule of the glenohumeral joint.

Ruffini Endings: Nerve endings located in the joints that respond to pressure.

Running Economy: Running in a manner to conserve energy.

Sagittal Plane: Frontal, transverse, and sagittal planes are described in Chapter 2.

Sargent Jump: A vertical jump measured by the height reached by hand or center of gravity in the jump.

Scalar Quantity: Quantity that has magnitude but no direction.

Scale Method: The use of scales to find the equal distribution of body weight to determine the center of gravity.

Segmental Body Weight: The weight of each body part.

Segmental Method: A method of analysis in which the centers of segments of the body are used as points and a digitizing program is used to determine the path of the center of gravity.

Shear: Involves loading in which a load is applied parallel to structure, causing internal angular deformation.

Shunt Muscle: Possesses a larger stabilizing component than a moving component. The angle of pull is less than 45°.

Sine: A function of an angle in a right triangle expressible as the ratio of the side opposite the angle to the hypotenuse.

Somatotyping: Typing the human body according to certain physical and organic characteristics.

Spatial Angle: Angle in space.

Speed: Rate of motion without regard to direction.

Spin: The angular movement (rotation) of an object.

Spurt Muscle: This muscle has a larger moving component than a stabilizing component. Its angle of pull is greater than 45°.

Stability: State of being in stable equilibrium.

Static Posture: Posture of a human that is held as still as possible.

Statics: Branch of mechanics dealing with objects that are stationary, not subject to acceleration (in equilibrium).

Steeplechase: A race over a course of prescribed distance in which there are hurdles and water jumps or objects to be jumped during the run.

Steering: Having a body or object directed in the desired direction.

Step: One-half of a stride.

Straight Approach: Linear approach.

Strain: Change in dimension that occurs within structure in response to external loads.

Stress: Involves load per unit area that develops on a plane surface that results in deformation divided by the original length of surface.

Stretch Receptor: The muscle spindle is a type of stretch receptor, which when stretched, initiates and transmits nerve impulses to the spinal cord.

Stroboscope: An instrument for studying periodic motion by rendering the moving body visible only at certain points of its path.

Synapses: Connections that occur at each level of entry into the spinal cord and throughout the brain.

Synergist Muscle: A muscle working together with others.

Synergistic Biomechanics: Biomechanics concerned with artistry and holism of movement.

Synovial Fluid: Lubricating fluid, secreted by the synovial membrane of a joint.

Tangent Dismount: A dismount that follows a path of a line tangent to the curve of the dismount.

Tangential: Of, pertaining to, or moving in the direction of, a tangent.

Task Analysis: A planned analysis of a given task using certain criteria.

Tension: A condition in which equal or opposite loads are applied, causing the structure to lengthen and become narrow.

Three-dimensional Photography: Photography that shows three sides of an object or 3 planes of motion.

Torque: The rotary effect of a force quantified as the product of force and moment arm.

Torsion: Deformation of a body through twisting.

Total Body Center of Mass: Average of all the centers of mass of the various body parts.

Trajectory: A projectile's path in the air.

Translation: Indicates linear motion.

Transportation Devices: Devices constructed so that transportation from one place to another is made easier.

Trigonometry: Branch of mathematics that treats the relations of the sides and angles of triangles so that solutions to problems involving same can be made.

Triple Jump: A jumping event in which the jumper uses a hop, step, and jump, preceded by a run.

Turbulence: The irregular flow of a fluid caused by an outside object contacting it.

Up-unweighting: Occurs in skiing when the skier moves the body weight up vertically during the skiing action.

Valgus: A condition of outward deviation.

Varus: A condition of inward deviation.

Vector: A line representing a physical quantity that has magnitude and direction.

Velocity: A change in position in regard to time.

Vertical Jump: A jump upward measured by the height of center of gravity or hand reach.

Vibration: The act of oscillating.

Visual Artists: Artists who use tools, e.g., to sculpture, draw, or paint.

Walking: A mode of transportation in which at least one foot is in contact with the surface at all times.

Weight: The gravitational force the earth exerts on a body.

Work: A transference of energy from one body to another, resulting in motion or displacement. It is expressed as the product of the force and the amount of displacement.

INDEX